WA 1385332 5

D1757433

CHRONIC GRAFT VERSUS HOST DISEASE: INTERDISCIPLINARY MANAGEMENT

Chronic graft versus host disease (GVHD) is the most common complication of allogeneic bone marrow transplantation. Because of the protracted clinical course of chronic GVHD, transplant centers and hematology/oncology offices are inadequately equipped to manage these immuno-incompetent patients with a multisystem disorder. Practitioners need to be able to recognize and effectively manage chronic GVHD as a late effect of more than half of allogeneic transplantations. The text is oriented for the clinician, with chapters covering staging, organ site and system-specific manifestations, treatment options, and supportive care. Drs. Georgia B. Vogelsang and Steven Z. Pavletic have been pioneers in the recognition of the multiorgan complexity of this disease and have gathered the input of a variety of subspecialist physicians for this book. This book fills the gap in practical literature on chronic GVHD, providing a comprehensive, up-to-date, and clinically relevant resource for anyone who deals with cancer patients posttransplant.

Georgia B. Vogelsang, MD, is Professor of Oncology at the Johns Hopkins University School of Medicine, Baltimore, Maryland.

Steven Z. Pavletic, MD, is the head of the Graft versus Host and Autoimmunity Unit in the Experimental Transplantation and Immunology Branch of the National Cancer Institute, Bethesda, Maryland.

CHRONIC GRAFT VERSUS HOST DISEASE: INTERDISCIPLINARY MANAGEMENT

EDITED BY

GEORGIA B. VOGELSANG

Johns Hopkins University School of Medicine, Baltimore, Maryland

STEVEN Z. PAVLETIC

National Cancer Institute, Bethesda, Maryland

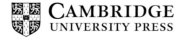

CAMBRIDGE UNIVERSITY PRESS
Cambridge, New York, Melbourne, Madrid, Cape Town, Singapore, São Paulo, Delhi

Cambridge University Press
32 Avenue of the Americas, New York, NY 10013-2473, USA

www.cambridge.org
Information on this title: www.cambridge.org/9780521884235

© Cambridge University Press 2009

This publication is in copyright. Subject to statutory exception
and to the provisions of relevant collective licensing agreements,
no reproduction of any part may take place without the written
permission of Cambridge University Press.

First published 2009

Printed in the United States of America

A catalog record for this publication is available from the British Library.

Library of Congress Cataloging in Publication data
Chronic graft versus host disease : interdisciplinary management / [edited by] Georgia B. Vogelsang,
Steven Z. Pavletic.
   p. ; cm.
Includes bibliographical references and index.
ISBN 978-0-521-88423-5 (hardback)
1. Graft versus host disease.   I. Vogelsang, Georgia B.   II. Pavletic, Steven.   III. Title.
[DNLM: 1. Graft vs Host Disease – therapy.   2. Chronic Disease – therapy.
3. Immunosuppression.   4. Immunosuppressive Agents. WD 300 C5565 2009]
RD123.5.C485   2009
617.9′54–dc22   2009007296

ISBN 978-0-521-88423-5 hardback

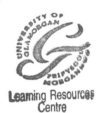

Learning Resources
Centre

13853325

Cambridge University Press has no responsibility for the persistence or
accuracy of URLs for external or third-party Internet Web sites referred to in
this publication and does not guarantee that any content on such Web sites is,
or will remain, accurate or appropriate. Information regarding prices, travel
timetables, and other factual information given in this work are correct at
the time of first printing, but Cambridge University Press does not guarantee
the accuracy of such information thereafter.

Every effort has been made in preparing this book to provide accurate and
up-to-date information that is in accord with accepted standards and
practice at the time of publication. Although case histories are drawn
from actual cases, every effort has been made to disguise the identities of
the individuals involved. Nevertheless, the authors, editors, and publishers
can make no warranties that the information contained herein is totally
free from error, not least because clinical standards are constantly
changing through research and regulation. The authors, editors, and
publishers therefore disclaim all liability for direct or consequential
damages resulting from the use of material contained in this book. Readers
are strongly advised to pay careful attention to information provided by
the manufacturer of any drugs or equipment that they plan to use.

CONTENTS

CONTRIBUTORS

GÖRGÜN AKPEK, MD, MHS Blood and Marrow Transplantation Program, Greenebaum Cancer Center, Department of Medicine, University of Maryland School of Medicine, Baltimore, Maryland

CLAUDIO ANASETTI, MD H. Lee Moffitt Comprehensive Cancer Center, Tampa, Florida

VIKI ANDERS, RN, MSN, CRNP Graft-Versus-Host Disease Clinic, The Sidney Kimmel Comprehensive Cancer Center at Johns Hopkins, Baltimore, Maryland

JOSEPH H. ANTIN, MD Department of Medicine, Dana-Farber Cancer Institute, Harvard Medical School, Cambridge, Massachusetts

SALLY ARAI, MD Department of Medicine, Division of Blood and Marrow Transplantation, Stanford Cancer Center, Stanford, California

MUKTA ARORA, MD Department of Medicine, Division of Hematology, Oncology, and Transplantation, University of Minnesota, Minneapolis, Minnesota

ANDREA BACIGALUPO, MD European Group for Bone Marrow Transplantation, Department of Hematology, Ospedale San Martino, Genova, Italy

KRISTIN BAIRD, MD Pediatric Oncology Branch, Center for Cancer Research, National Cancer Institute, National Institutes of Health, Bethesda, Maryland

JULIET N. BARKER, MD Memorial Sloan-Kettering Cancer Center, New York, New York

MICHAEL BOECKH, MD Fred Hutchinson Cancer Research Center, Department of Medicine, University of Washington, Seattle, Washington

JAVIER BOLAÑOS-MEADE, MD Department of Oncology, The Sidney Kimmel Comprehensive Cancer Center at Johns Hopkins, Division of Hematologic Malignancies, Baltimore, Maryland

PAUL A. CARPENTER, MD Fred Hutchinson Cancer Research Center, Seattle, Washington

KATHLEEN M. CASTRO, RN, MS, ACCN Clinical Center, National Institutes of Health, Bethesda, Maryland

LEIGHTON CHAN, MD Rehabilitation Medicine Department, Warren G Magnuson Clinical Research Center, National Institutes of Health, Bethesda, Maryland

NELSON J. CHAO, MD, MBA Departments of Medicine and Immunology, Duke University, Durham, North Carolina

JASON W. CHIEN, MD, MS Division of Pulmonary and Critical Care, University of Washington, Clinical Research Division, Fred Hutchinson Cancer Research Center, Seattle, Washington

YU-WAYE CHU, MD National Cancer Institute, National Institutes of Health, Bethesda, Maryland

DANIEL R. COURIEL, MD Stem Cell Transplantation and Cellular Therapy, M. D. Anderson Cancer Center, The University of Texas, Houston, Texas

EDWARD W. COWEN, MD, MHSc Dermatology Branch, Center for Cancer Research, National Cancer Institute, National Institutes of Health, Bethesda, Maryland

COREY CUTLER, MD, MPH, FRCPC Department of Medicine, Harvard Medical School, Dana-Farber Cancer Institute, Boston, Massachusetts

H. Joachim Deeg, MD Fred Hutchinson Cancer Research Center, Department of Medicine, University of Washington, Seattle, Washington

Anne Dickinson, MD NorthEast England StemCell Institute, Marrow Transplant Biology, University of Newcastle Medical School, Newcastle upon Tyne, United Kingdom

James P. Dunn, Jr., MD Division of Ocular Immunology, The Wilmer Ophthalmological Institute, Baltimore, Maryland

Jane M. Fall-Dickson, PhD, RN Symptom Management Branch, National Institute of Nursing Research, National Institutes of Health, Bethesda, Maryland

James L. M. Ferrara, MD Departments of Pediatrics and Internal Medicine, Blood and Marrow Transplant Program, University of Michigan, Ann Arbor, Michigan

Alexandra H. Filipovich, MD Department of Pediatrics, Division of Hematology/Oncology, Immunodeficiency and Histiocytosis Program, Diagnostic Immunology Laboratory, Cincinnati Children's Hospital Medical Center, Cincinnati, Ohio

Mary Evelyn D. Flowers, MD Clinical Research Division, Fred Hutchinson Cancer Research Center, Department of Medicine, University of Washington, Seattle, Washington

Juan Gea-Banacloche, MD Experimental Transplantation and Immunology Branch, National Cancer Institute, National Institutes of Health, Bethesda, Maryland

Lynn H. Gerber, MD Center for the Study of Chronic Illness and Disability, College of Health and Human Services, George Mason University, Fairfax, Virginia

Andrew L. Gilman, MD Department of Pediatrics, Pediatric Blood and Marrow Transplantation, University of North Carolina at Chapel Hill, Chapel Hill, North Carolina

Alois Gratwohl, MD Hematology Department, University Hospital, Basel, Switzerland

Hildegard T. Greinix, MD Medical University of Vienna, Vienna, Austria

Ronald Gress, MD National Cancer Institute, National Institutes of Health, Bethesda, Maryland

Ernst Holler, MD Department of Hematology/Oncology, University of Regensburg, Regensburg, Germany

Thomas Hughes, MD National Cancer Institute, National Institutes of Health, Bethesda, Maryland

Sharon R. Hymes, MD Department of Dermatology, M.D. Anderson Cancer Center, The University of Texas Medical School, Houston, Texas

Myra J. Jacobs, MA National Bone Marrow Transplant Link, Southfield, Michigan

David A. Jacobsohn, MD Department of Pediatrics, Northwestern University School of Medicine, Stem Cell Transplant Program, Children's Memorial Hospital, Chicago, Illinois

Madan Jagasia, MBBS, MS Department of Medicine, Division of Hematology-Oncology, Vanderbilt Ingram Cancer Center, Vanderbilt University Medical Center, Nashville, Tennessee

Paula Kim Translating Research across Communities, California

Stella K. Kim, MD Departments of Ophthalmology and Radiation Oncology, M.D. Anderson Cancer Center, The University of Texas, Houston, Texas

Carrie Kitko, MD Departments of Pediatrics and Internal Medicine, Blood and Marrow Transplant Program, University of Michigan, Ann Arbor, Michigan

Stephanie J. Lee, MD Fred Hutchinson Cancer Research Center, University of Washington, Seattle, Washington

Li Li, MD Rehabilitation Medicine Department, Warren G Magnuson Clinical Research Center, National Institutes of Health, Bethesda, Maryland

Paul J. Martin, MD Division of Clinical Research, Fred Hutchinson Cancer Research Center, Departments of Medicine and Pediatrics, University of Washington, Seattle, Washington

George B. McDonald, MD Gastroenterology/Hepatology Section, Fred Hutchinson Cancer Research Center, University of Washington School of Medicine, Seattle, Washington

Timothy R. McGuire, PharmD, FCCP Department of Pharmacy Practice, College of Pharmacy, University of Nebraska Medical Center, Omaha, Nebraska

Sandra A. Mitchell, CRNP, MScN, AOCN Clinical Center, National Institutes of Health, Bethesda, Maryland, National Cancer Institute, Bethesda, Maryland, Cancer Research, University of Utah College of Nursing, Salt Lake City, Utah

Mohamad Mohty, MD Hematology Department, CHU Hotel-Dieu, University of Nantes, Nantes, France

Carina Moravec, ARNP, MA Fred Hutchinson Cancer Research Center, Seattle, Washington

Harry Openshaw, MD Department of Neurology, City of Hope National Medical Center, Duarte, California

Steven Z. Pavletic, MD Graft-versus-Host and Auto-Immunity Unit, National Cancer Institute, Center for Cancer Research, Bethesda, Maryland

Donna Przepiorka, MD Center for Biologics, Evaluation Research, U.S. Food and Drug Administration, Rockville, Maryland

Bryce B. Reeve, PhD National Cancer Institute, National Institutes of Health, Bethesda, Maryland

Douglas J. Rizzo, MD, MS Department of Medicine, Division of Neoplastic Diseases and Related Disorders, Center for International Blood and Marrow Transplant Research, Medical College of Wisconsin, Milwaukee, Wisconsin

Miwa Sakai, MD Gastroenterology/Hepatology Section, Fred Hutchinson Cancer Research Center, University of Washington School of Medicine, Seattle, Washington

Jean E. Sanders, MD Pediatric Clinical Hematopoietic Cell Transplantation, Fred Hutchinson Cancer Research Center, Seattle, Washington

Mark M. Schubert, DDS, MSD Department of Oral Medicine, University of Washington, Oral Medicine, Seattle Cancer Care Alliance, Seattle, Washington

Kirk R. Schultz, MD Division of Oncology/BMT Faculty of Medicine – Pediatrics, University of British Columbia, Vancouver, British Columbia, Canada

Warren D. Shlomchik, MD Department of Immunology, Yale School of Medicine, New Haven, Connecticut

Howard M. Shulman, MD Fred Hutchinson Cancer Research Center, Seattle Cancer Care Alliance, Department of Pathology, University of Washington, Seattle, Washington

Janine A. Smith, MD Division of Epidemiology and Clinical Research, National Eye Institute, National Institutes of Health, Bethesda, Maryland

Gérard Socié, MD, PhD Department of Transplantation and Hematology, University Paris VII: Hospital Saint Louis, Paris, France

Susan Stewart BMT InfoNet, Highland Park, Illinois

Pamela Stratton, MD Reproductive Biology and Medicine Branch, National Institute of Child Health and Human Development, National Institutes of Health, Bethesda, Maryland

Karen L. Syrjala, MD Clinical Research Division, Fred Hutchinson Cancer Research Center, University of Washington, Department of Medicine, Seattle, Washington

Nathaniel S. Treister, DMD, DMSc Harvard School of Oral Medicine, Cambridge, Massachusetts, Division of Oral Medicine and Dentistry, Brigham & Women's Hospital, Boston, Massachusetts

Maria L. Turner, MD Dermatology Branch, National Cancer Institute, National Institutes of Health, Bethesda, Maryland

Georgia B. Vogelsang, MD Department of Oncology, Johns Hopkins University School of Medicine, Baltimore, Maryland

Alan S. Wayne, MD Pediatric Oncology Branch, Center for Cancer Research, National Cancer Institute, National Institutes of Health, Bethesda, Maryland

Loretta A. Williams, PhD, MSN, RN Department of Symptom Research, M.D. Anderson Cancer Center, The University of Texas, Houston, Texas

PREFACE

Bone marrow transplantation has changed remarkably from its earliest days. Patients were transplanted with bone marrow as a last resort for refractory leukemia or aplastic anemia. The transplant procedure required prolonged hospital stays – often months – with significant uncontrolled toxicities from the preparative regimen, limited antimicrobial success, and even more limited ability to prevent or treat acute graft versus host disease (GVHD). The lucky survivors now marvel at how different the experience is for patients receiving allografts as outpatients.

Unfortunately, the same level of improvement has not been seen in chronic GVHD. The reasons for this lack of success are varied – including the latency of chronic GVHD, lack of accepted readily reproducible animal models, and complex underlying immuno-pathology. It is no wonder that patients with this affliction felt like abandoned stepchildren.

Over the last 5 years, there has been both a resurgence of interest and progress in chronic GVHD. To a significant degree, the NIH-sponsored Consensus Conference on Chronic GVHD is responsible for this change. This conference suggested working definitions, standardized staging and response criteria, recommended supportive care measures, and suggested areas for future study. Although the indolent nature of the disease means that clinical progress is going to be time consuming, there has been remarkable progress since the initial NIH-sponsored meeting. One of the main lessons learned is that it is imperative to have transplant centers cooperate in studying this disorder. The success of NIH-sponsored multicentered trials, cooperative group–sponsored clinical studies, Clinical Trials Network proposals, and cooperation of European transplant groups all suggest that a new era has begun in which more patients will be intensely studied.

Our hope with this book is to provide a solid reference for this effort. By collecting in one book the state of the art, our hope is that it will provide a reference that will be valuable in many settings, including transplant clinics, oncology/hematology clinics, specialty clinics, and basic research laboratories. It is only by gathering all these diverse groups together that we are going to be able to understand the basic immunologic processes responsible for the disorder and to provide treatment to relieve the discomfort caused to the patients suffering with this disorder.

We wish to thank all those who have made this book possible. The book grew out of the NIH-sponsored Consensus Conference on Chronic GVHD – all participants in that meeting contributed to this book, whether or not they actually penned a chapter. Their thoughts and their efforts played a major part in the final Consensus Conference recommendations. Obviously, we are indebted to all of the contributors. Most of the chapters are group efforts and reflect the cooperative spirit that has made such a profound difference in the hope for the future for this disorder. Finally, we are indebted to our patients, who have waited many years for a book concerned with and dedicated to the burden they live with every day.

PART I: GENERAL PRINCIPLES

1

HISTORICAL ASPECTS OF CHRONIC GRAFT VERSUS HOST DISEASE

Alois Gratwohl

The scientific "discovery" of graft versus host disease (GVHD) mirrors some aspects of this devastating disease. It is based on an accurate observation but an error in interpretation. Similarly, GVHD and in particular chronic GVHD confront patients as a paradox. The symptoms appear just when he or she believes to be cured from the previously diagnosed lethal disease, that is, at engraftment of the healthy donor cells. GVHD can have devastating effects on patients, families, and transplant teams. Conversely, few "man made diseases" have provided so much insight into basic immunobiology as GVHD. It is the hope of this book, to turn the knowledge gained from chronic GVHD into benefit for all patients after a hematopoietic stem cell transplant (HSCT) and for the large population of patients with autoimmune disorders or cancer in general.

THE BEGINNING OF HSCT

The old Greek proverb that "war is the father of all goods" applies to few medical technologies as well as it does to HSCT. The recognition of late bone marrow failure from atomic bomb exposure in Hiroshima and Nagasaki had double consequences. Vast research funds were allotted to find tools to overcome this lethal late complication of high dose radiation exposure. Results came rapidly. As early as 1949, Jacobson showed in his pioneering work that mice survived otherwise lethal total body irradiation when their spleens were shielded during radiation exposure [1]. Humoral, spleen-derived products were believed to be protective. Two years later, Lorenz provided proof that cellular, not humoral factors were responsible [2]. He demonstrated that bone marrow cells from a healthy animal, given as intraperitoneal or intravenous injection, could protect mice from radiation-induced bone marrow aplasia (primary disease). The debate whether humoral

or cellular factors were key elements to protect bone marrow from the late sequelae of total body radiation was closed for the next 40 years; bone marrow transplantation was born. It is of interest to note that decades later, combinations of growth factors were proven to be radioprotective after total body irradiation even though this approach has never gained clinical application [3].

Clinicians involved in leukemia treatment quickly grasped the unique possibility given to them by the marrow lethal effects of radiation. For the first time, it became possible to "take away" a diseased bone marrow; total body irradiation was the tool. It was only necessary to replace the diseased bone marrow with normal healthy donor cells. Treatment for acute leukemia, a uniformly lethal disease was at hand. With the report by Ford of successful experimental bone marrow transplants in mice, it was evident that donor type cells indeed did repopulate the whole hematopoietic system [4]. It appeared to be only a question of time to find the adequate dose of total body irradiation, sufficient enough to kill all leukemic cells, but low enough not to induce irreversible organ damage outside the bone marrow. The concept was rapidly explored in humans [5]. Bone marrow transplantation spread as a promising investigational tool and more than 60 bone marrow transplants were reported to the International Bone Marrow Transplant Registry in 1962 [6]. However, frustration with the complications of transplantation tempered the initial enthusiasm and bone marrow transplants came to a near halt for more than a decade. Despite successful engraftment and complete remissions in some patients, no long-term survivors were observed. Early, aplasia-associated complications were high. Even worse, those few patients with successful initial engraftment did not survive long term. The transplants were either rejected, their leukemia returned, or patients died from a unique syndrome occurring after engraftment. They developed a generalized rash, became icteric, and suffered from untractable diarrhea. Similar observations were made in mice. Most animals with a bone marrow transplant did survive the initial total body irradiation–induced aplasia (primary disease) but died days to weeks later from a syndrome of wasting, rash, diarrhea,

Supported in part by a grant of the Swiss National Research Foundation Nr. 3200B0–118176 and the Horton Foundation.

and icterus, the "secondary disease." It did take years of intensive laboratory investigations to recognize the major histocompatibility antigens (human leukocyte antigens; HLA) as the key elements for graft rejection and GVHD and to establish the necessary instruments for supportive care to restart successful transplants. It was only in 1968 [7] when the successful bone marrow transplants from HLA-typed and identical sibling donors were performed for patients with severe combined immune deficiency syndromes that brought back HSCT as a viable treatment option.

THE CONCEPT OF GVHD

The first clinical and experimental HSCT were performed at the same time that solid organ transplantation was being developed. Rejection, a host versus graft reaction, was recognized as the first obstacle to success. Simonson in 1953 observed interstitial pyroninophilic lymphoid cells in the renal cortex as early as 6 days after the renal transplant. He postulated that kidney-derived donor cells reacted against host antigens in the renal circulation and brought up for the first time the idea of an immune response generated by the graft [8]. Today it is evident that he described the beginning of rejection. Still, his idea that a transplant could react against the recipient, that a graft versus host reaction could occur in parallel to a host versus graft reaction, was novel, revolutionary at that time, and highly controversial. A few years later, he could prove that GVHD indeed could occur. He injected lymphocytes into newborn mice and into chicken embryos. Both were immunologically naïve and unable to reject the transplanted living lymphocytes. Both, newborn mice and chicken embryos, died soon after the injection of the lymphocytes. These results were proof that his graft generated immunity hypothesis of GVHD was correct [9]. Two facts helped confirm this. First, it was recognized, that the phenomenon of chicken embryo death had been described more than 40 years earlier by Murphy [10]. He had observed lymphoid infiltrates in the spleen of chicken embryos when they were injected at day 7 into the allantois with adult chicken bone marrow or spleen tissue. No such reaction was observed after implantation of goose bone marrow. Chicken embryos were unable to reject chicken spleen cells but were capable of rejecting xenogeneic goose cells. The phenomenon could therefore only be explained as a graft versus host reaction. Second, several transplantation phenomena suddenly had a uniting explanation. Secondary disease after bone marrow transplantation and total body irradiation, acute killing effect, homologous disease, runting disease, parabiosis intoxication, parent versus hybrid effect, or embryo disease all had the same immunologic basis (Figure 1.1) [11–18]. It was Billingham who brought the puzzle together and who stipulated in 1966 the three basic requirements for GVHD [19]: (1) immunocompetent transplanted cells, (2) antigens in the host, which can be recognized by the transplanted cells but are lacking in the donor, and (3) sufficient time of complete engraftment to mount the immune response (security of tenure). These requirements remain valid till date.

THE CONCEPT OF CHRONIC GVHD

In all early clinical transplants before 1968, rejection and acute GVHD were the sole immunological complications. There were no long-term survivors. In the late seventies, several centers observed some peculiar clinical findings in some bone marrow transplant recipients who survived several months after the transplant [20]. These findings occurred when patients began to recover from their acute GVHD. The clinical syndrome of chronic GVHD became clear with the description of four patients from the bone marrow transplant programme at the National Institute of Health in Bethesda, MD, three after a bone marrow transplant for severe aplastic anemia, one for acute myeloid leukemia. [21–23] All had had acute GVHD, grade II to IV. Three patients showed skin changes that were very similar to known autoimmune disorders but different in each: one had scleroderma-like, one lupus erythematodes-like, and one lichen planus-like lesions. Furthermore, all four had a clinical syndrome indistinguishable from Sjögren's disease with a sicca syndrome, oral vasculitis, reduced Schirmer's test, reduced parotid flow, and characteristic lesions in lip biopsies. Furthermore, three patients had restrictive lung disease with reduced CO diffusion capacities and one had combined restrictive and obstructive lung disease. One patient showed liver pathologies similar to primary biliary cirrhosis. These observations came as a surprise at that time. It could not be a chance phenomenon – there were too few long-term survivors for these autoimmune-like changes to be due to chance. It was clear that the phenomenon was related to the transplant procedure and chronic GVHD was brought up as the most likely explanation. Similar observations were reported from other transplant centers and the concept of chronic GVHD in man was established [24–27] (Figure 1.2).

POLITICAL EFFECTS OF CHRONIC GVHD IN THE LATE SEVENTIES

The clarity of the syndrome and its high frequency, the clear correlation with the transplant procedure, and the lack of any meaningful preventive or therapeutic procedure had devastating effects on some transplant programmes. Most importantly, the deterrent pictures of some survivors through a "man-made disease" did have their impact. They did coincide with times, when immediate transplant-related mortality was still higher than survival [23]. This high mortality together with the portrayed idea that all survivors would develop severe complications with high morbidity and mortality was one reason that the bone marrow transplant programme at the National Institutes of Health in the United States was brought to an immediate stop in 1975 and remained closed for more than a decade.

Biology of graft versus host reactions

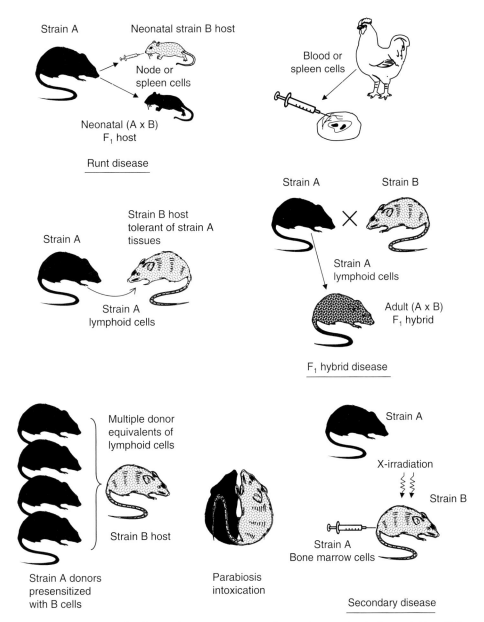

Figure 1.1 Various types of graft versus host reactions in animals, according to a drawing by van Bekkum [28].

Explanations to the illustrations:

Runt disease occurs when a neonatal animal, either strain B or offspring of strain A and B, a so called F_1 hybrid, is injected with lymphoid cells from a lymph node or spleen of type A. The neonatal animal and the neonatal F_1 hybrid cannot reject parental cells but is recognized as foreign by the parental cells. The same occurs when a neonatal (tolerant) animal of strain B is tolerized with a skin graft from an adult strain A and later injected with strain A lymphoid cells.

Adult chicken organ graft on embryo effect is observed, when adult lymphoid cells are injected into the allantois of an egg. The egg cannot reject the adult lymphoid cells; these cells recognize "the egg" as foreign and mount a reaction.

F_1 hybrid disease can occur, similar to runt disease in neonatal mice, but as well in adult F_1 A × B animals, if they are injected with either strain A or B adult lymphoid cells. An F_1 hybrid cannot reject A or B cells but is itself recognized as foreign by either parental A or B cells.

Sensitized multiple donor reaction was observed, when high numbers of lymphoid cells from multiple A animals, presensitized with strain B cells, were injected into strain B animals. The B animal cannot reject too high an amount of donor cells (high dose tolerance) but is recognized as foreign by the A cells.

Parabiosis intoxication can be observed when animals are connected with their blood circulation and one animal recognizes the other as foreign without being rejected.

Secondary disease was observed when animals survived the immediate sequelae of total body irradiation but died after engraftment of donor cells.

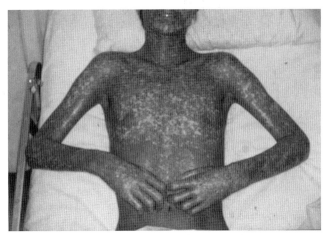

Figure 1.2 Severe chronic graft versus host disease in one of the first-described patients [22]. See Plate 1 in the color plate section.

CHRONIC GVHD AND AUTOIMMUNITY

The close similarity of the clinical syndrome of chronic GVHD and some clinical entities of autoimmune disease brought up the debate on whether chronic GVHD is an entity by its own or simply an autoimmune disease, triggered by the host versus graft–graft versus host interaction [29]. Chronic GVHD in animals, termed also as chronic allogeneic disease was already known [30] and Fialkow had shown in some elegant mice experiments in F_1 hybrid mice with chronic GVHD that host helper T cells were stimulated and were responsible for the production of autoantibodies. He believed chronic graft versus host to be a true host-derived but graft-triggered autoimmune process [31]. Still, in contrast to his mice experiments where Fialkow did find autoantibodies, none of the autoantibodies that are typical in Sjögren's disease, lupus erythematodes, or primary biliary cirrhosis were found in those four initial chronic GVHD patients [21, 22]. Obviously, the F_1 hybrid model could not explain sufficiently the human disease. The debate on the pathophysiology of chronic GVHD is ongoing.

CHRONIC GVHD AND GRAFT VERSUS LEUKAEMIA EFFECTS

As early as the first experiments by Ford, who documented the cellular replacement of donor by recipient hematopoiesis after an allogeneic HSCT, the impact of GVHD on residual leukemia was described [4]. The clinical relevance was realized by G. Mathé in 1964 when he described a patient with acute leukemia, treated for his severe pancytopenia and fever by infusions of granulocytes from a donor with chronic myeloid leukemia. The patient recovered from his neutropenia, showed defervescence, and cleared his bone marrow from all leukemic blasts. In parallel, he developed a skin rash, icterus, and diarrhea. A few weeks later all clinical signs of graft versus host disease disappeared and his leukemia returned [32]. The formal

correlation between acute and, even more so chronic GVHD, and control of leukemia was reported by Weiden [33] in 1979 in his seminal paper. The finding of a clear correlation between graft versus host disease and graft versus leukemia or graft versus tumor effects have since been confirmed repeatedly. Still, it remains a matter of debate whether the beneficial effects of increased tumor control outweigh the detrimental effects of the increased transplant-related mortality, which are invariably associated with acute and chronic GVHD [34].

CHRONIC GVHD AS LATE ALTERED IMMUNITY?

The recognition of chronic GVHD as a clinical syndrome similar to known autoimmune disorders suggested a new therapeutic approach to autoimmune disorders. If HSCT, by its transfer of hematopoietic stem cells, could induce an autoimmune-like syndrome, it should be possible to eradicate the hematopoietic (including the immune) system of a patient with a severe autoimmune disease by HSCT from a healthy donor. Debate over this concept was passionate. It was known that patients with severe aplastic anemia could be cured with a transplant from a twin donor. It was intensively debated whether they would need conditioning for treatment of their disease. If it were a true stem cell defect only, stem cells alone would be sufficient; if it were an autoimmune disease, some conditioning for eradication of the disease would be required [35]. HSCT for aplastic anemia paved the way for the concept of HSCT in autoimmune diseases. The high transplant-related mortality was prohibitive for any clinical trials in other less immediately fatal autoimmune disorders for a long time. Experimental studies in animals, however, proved the concept to be valid. They prepared the way to where we stand today [36–38].

The original work of Fialkow has been taken up again. Today, autoimmune disorders are viewed as the consequence of environmental effects and chance phenomena on a particular genetic background, resulting in skewed immune response. Increasing findings suggest today that patients after successful allogeneic HSCT might follow a similar pattern. HSCT changes the genetic background and gives an exogenous stimulus. HSCT patients indeed can have a skewed immune reconstitution and can develop a late altered immune syndrome [36–39]. It remains open and it will be fascinating to see in the future whether such late altered immunity and chronic GVHD are distinct entities or just quantitatively different subsets of the same basic underlying immune reaction.

REFERENCES

1. Jacobson LO, Marks EK, Gaston EO, Robson M, Zirkle RE. The role of the spleen in radiation injury. *Proc Soc Exp Biol Med.* 1949;70:740–742.
2. Lorenz E, Uphoff D, Reid TR, Shelton E. Modification of irradiation injury in mice and guinea pigs by bone marrow injections. *J Natl Cancer Inst.* 1951;12:197–201.

3. Gratwohl A, John L, Baldomero H, et al. FLT-3 ligand provides hematopoietic protection from total body irradiation in rabbits. *Blood*. 1998;92:765–769.

4. Ford CE, Hamerton JL, Barnes DW, Loutit JF. Cytological identification of radiation-chimaeras. *Nature*. 1956;177:452–454.

5. Thomas ED, Lochte HL Jr., Lu WC, Ferrebee JW. Intravenous infusion of bone marrow in patients receiving radiation and chemotherapy. *N Engl J Med*. 1957;257:491–496.

6. Bortin MM. A compendium of reported human bone marrow transplants (Review). *Transplantation*. 1970;9:571–587.

7. Bach FH, Albertini RJ, Joo P, Anderson JL, Bortin MM. Bone-marrow transplantation in a patient with the Wiskott-Aldrich syndrome. *Lancet*. 1968;2:1364–1366.

8. Simonsen M, Buemann J, Gammeltoft A, Jensen F, Jorgensen K. Biological incompatibility in kidney transplantation in dogs. I. Experimental and morphological investigations. *Acta Pathol Microbiol Scand*. 1953;32:1–35.

9. Simonsen M. The impact on the developing embryo and newborn animal of adult homologous cells. *Acta Pathol Microbiol Scand*. 1957;40:480–500.

10. Murphy JB. The effect of adult chicken organ graft on the chick embryo. *J Exp Med*. 1916;24:1–5.

11. Barnes DW, Loutit JF. Protective effects of implants of splenic tissue. *Proc R Soc Med*. 1953;46:251–252.

12. Schwartz EE, Upton AC, Congdon CC. A fatal reaction caused by implantation of adult parental spleen tissue in irradiated F_1 mice. *Proc Soc Exp Biol Med*. 1957;96:797–800.

13. Van Bekkum DW, Vos O, Weyzen WW. The pathogenesis of the secondary disease following foreign bone marrow transplantation in irradiated mice. *Bull Soc Int Chir*. 1959;18:302–314.

14. Trentin JJ. Mortality and skin transplantability in x-irradiated mice receiving isologous, homologous or heterologous bone marrow. *Proc Soc Exp Biol Med*. 1956;92:688–693.

15. Billingham RE, Brent L. A simple method for inducing tolerance of skin homografts in mice. *Transplant Bull*. 1957;4:67–71.

16. Sauerbruch F, Heyden M. Parabiosis. *Muench Med Wschr*. 1908;55:153–156.

17. Oliner H, Schwartz R, Dameshek W. Studies in experimental autoimmune disorders. I. Clinical and laboratory features of autoimmunization (runt disease) in the mouse. *Blood*. 1961;17:20–44.

18. Brandly CA, Thorp F, Prickett CO. *Poultry Sci*. 1949;28:486–489.

19. Billingham RE. The biology of graft-versus-host reactions. *Harvey Lect*. 1966–1967;62:21–78.

20. Thomas ED, Storb R, Clift RA, et al. Bone-marrow transplantation (second of two parts). *N Engl J Med*. 1975;292:895–902.

21. Gratwohl AA, Moutsopoulos HM, Chused TM, et al. Sjögren-type syndrome after allogeneic bone-marrow transplantation. *Ann Intern Med*. 1977;87:703–706.

22. Lawley TJ, Peck GL, Moutsopoulos HM, Gratwohl AA, Deisseroth AB. Scleroderma, Sjögren-like syndrome, and chronic graft-versus-host disease. *Ann Intern Med*. 1977;87:707–709.

23. Graw RG Jr., Lohrmann HP, Bull MI, et al. Bone-marrow transplantation following combination chemotherapy immunosuppression (B.A.C.T.) in patients with acute leukemia. *Transplant Proc*. 1974;6:349–354.

24. Kolb HJ, Wundisch GF, Bender C, et al. Chronic graft-versus-host disease (GVHD) [proceedings]. *Pathol Biol (Paris)*. 1978;26:52.

25. Shulman HM, Sale GE, Lerner KG, et al. Chronic cutaneous graft-versus-host disease in man. *Am J Pathol*. 1978;91:545–570.

26. Shulman HM, Sullivan KM, Weiden PL, et al. Chronic graft-versus-host syndrome in man. A long-term clinicopathologic study of 20 Seattle patients. *Am J Med*. 1980;69:204–217.

27. Berman MD, Rabin L, O'Donnell J, et al. The liver in long-term survivors of marrow transplant-chronic graft-versus-host disease. *J Clin Gastroenterol*. 1980;2:53–63.

28. Van Bekkum DW, de Vries MJ. *Radiation Chimeras*. New York: Academic Press; 1967.

29. Graze PR, Gale RP. Chronic graft versus host disease:a syndrome of disordered immunity. *Am J Med*. 1979;66:611–620.

30. Schwartz RS. Chronic allogeneic disease as a model of autoimmunity and malignancy. *Vox Sang*. 1969;16:325–330.

31. Fialkow PJ, Gilchrist C, Allison AC. Autoimmunity in chronic graft-versus-host disease. *Clin Exp Immunol*. 1973;13:479–486.

32. Mathé G, Amiel JL, Schwarzenberg L. *Bone Marrow. Transplantation and Leukocyte infusions*. American Lecture Series 793. Springfield, Illinois: Charles Thomas; 1971.

33. Weiden PL, Flournoy N, Thomas ED, et al. Antileukemic effect of graft-versus-host disease in human recipients of allogeneic-marrow grafts. *N Engl J Med*. 1979;300:1068–1073.

34. Gratwohl A, Hermans J, Apperley J, et al. Acute graft-versus-host disease: grade and outcome in patients with chronic myelogenous leukemia. Working Party Chronic Leukemia of the European Group for Blood and Marrow Transplantation. *Blood*. 1995;86:813–818.

35. Haak HL, Goselink HM. Mechanisms in aplastic anaemia. *Lancet*. 1977;1:194.

36. Daikeler T, Tyndall A. Autoimmunity following haematopoietic stem-cell transplantation. *Best Pract Res Clin Haematol*. 2007;20:349–360.

37. Passweg J, Tyndall A. Autologous stem cell transplantation in autoimmune diseases. *Semin Hematol*. 2007;44:278–285.

38. Tyndall A, Black C, Finke J, et al. Treatment of systemic sclerosis with autologous haemopoietic stem cell transplantation. *Lancet*. 1997;349:254.

39. Trendelenburg M, Gregor M, Passweg J, Tichelli A, Tyndall A, Gratwohl A "Altered immunity syndrome," a distinct entity in long-term bone marrow transplantation survivors? *Bone Marrow Transplant*. 2001;28:1175–1176.

2

The Pathophysiology of Acute Graft versus Host Disease

Carrie Kitko and James L. M. Ferrara

ACUTE GVHD PATHOPHYSIOLOGY: A THREE-STEP MODEL

Acute graft versus host disease (GVHD) results from complex interactions between donor T cells and host tissues in an inflammatory milieu. The pathophysiology of acute GVHD can be considered as a three-step process involving both the innate and adaptive immune systems (Figure 2.1). GVHD pathophysiology can be summarized in a three-step process. In step 1, the conditioning regimen (irradiation, chemotherapy, or both) leads to the damage and activation of host tissues, especially the intestinal mucosa. This allows the translocation of lipopolysaccharide (LPS) and other inflammatory stimuli from the intestinal lumen to the circulation, stimulating the secretion of the inflammatory cytokines such as tumor necrosis factor-alpha (TNF-α) from host tissues. These mediators increase the expression of major histocompatibility complex (MHC) antigens and adhesion molecules on host antigen-presenting cells (APC)s, enhancing the recognition of MHC and minor histocompatibility antigens (mHA) by mature donor T cells. Donor T-cell activation in step 2 is characterized by a predominance of T-helper type 1 subset (Th1) cells and the secretion of interferon-gamma (IFN-γ), which activates mononuclear phagocytes. Regulatory T cells (Treg) limit the proliferation and clonal expansion of activated donor T cells. In step 3, effector functions of activated mononuclear phagocytes are triggered by the secondary signal provided by LPS and other stimulatory molecules that leak through the intestinal mucosa damaged during steps 1 and 2. Activated macrophages, along with cytotoxic T lymphocyte (CTL), secrete inflammatory cytokines that cause target cell apoptosis. CD8+ CTL also lyse target cells directly. Damage to the GI tract in this phase, principally by inflammatory cytokines, amplifies LPS release and leads to the "cytokine storm" characteristic of severe acute GVHD. This damage results in the amplification of local tissue injury, and it further promotes an inflammatory response.

It should be noted from the outset that all these steps do not carry equal weight in the pathogenesis of acute GVHD. The pivotal interaction occurs in step 2, where host APCs activate allogeneic donor T cells. The subsequent cytokine cascade is clearly important, but blockade of individual cytokines may not reverse established GVHD when other cellular effectors such as CTL are present. GVHD can also occur when no conditioning of the host has occurred (e.g., transfusion associated GVHD).

Step 1: Effects of Hematopoietic Cell Transplantation Conditioning

The first step of acute GVHD starts before donor cells are infused. Prior to hematopoietic cell transplantation (HCT), a patient's tissues have been damaged, sometimes profoundly, by underlying disease and its treatment, infection and transplant conditioning. These important effects help explain a number of unique and seemingly unrelated aspects of GVHD. For example, a number of clinical reports have noted increased risks of GVHD associated with advanced stage leukemia, certain intensive conditioning regimens, and histories of viral infections [1]. Total-body irradiation (TBI) is particularly important in this process because it activates host tissues to secrete inflammatory cytokines, such as TNF-α and IL-1 [2], and it induces endothelial apoptosis that leads to epithelial cell damage in the gastrointestinal (GI) tract [3]. Injury to the gut is transient and self-limited after autologous HCT. However, after allogeneic HCT, further damage by GVHD effectors amplifies GI and systemic GVHD by allowing the translocation of microbial products such as LPS into systemic circulation. This scenario helps to explain the increased risk of GVHD associated with intensive conditioning regimens. The overall risk of GVHD after reduced intensity regimens is similar but usually occurs later due to the lower level tissue injury involved. The relationship between conditioning intensity, inflammatory cytokines, and GVHD severity have been confirmed by animal models [4] and by clinical observations [1].

Step 2: Donor T-cell Activation and Cytokine Secretion

Donor T-cell Activation

Donor T-cell activation occurs during the second step of acute GVHD. Murine studies have demonstrated that host

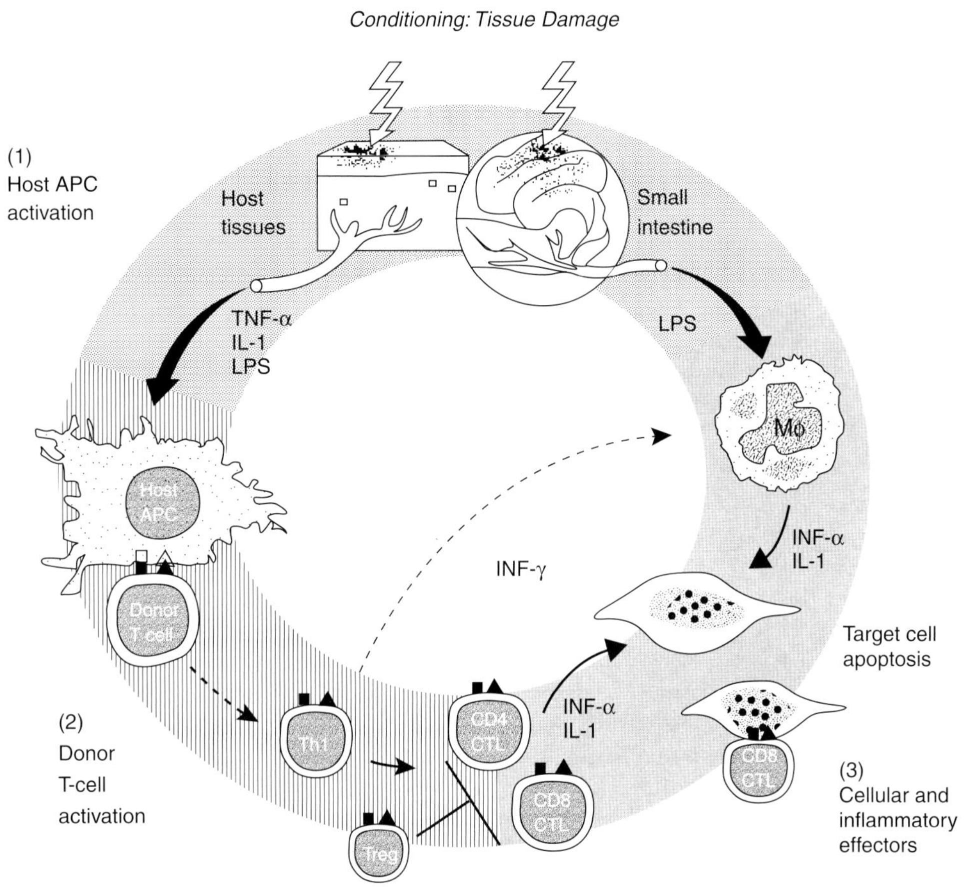

Conditioning: Tissue Damage

Figure 2.1 The pathophysiology of acute graft versus host disease (GVHD).

The three steps are (1) tissue damage to the recipient by the radiation/chemotherapy pretransplant conditioning regimen, (2) donor T-cell activation and clonal expansion by host antigen-presenting cells (APCs), and (3) cellular and inflammatory factors. This schema underscores the importance of mononuclear phagocytes and other accessory cells to the development of GVHD after complex interactions with cytokines secreted by activated donor T cells.

CTL, cytotoxic T lymphocyte; GI, gastrointestinal; IL, interleukin; IFN-γ, interferon-gamma; LPS, lipopolysaccharide; MHC, major histocompatibility complex; mHA, minor histocompatibility antigens; Treg, regulatory T cells; Th1, T-helper type 1 subset; TNF-α, tumor necrosis factor-alpha.

APCs alone are both necessary and sufficient to stimulate donor T cells [5, 6]. Donor T cells migrate to secondary lymphoid organs, such as Peyer patches, lymph nodes, and spleen where they first encounter host APCs [7]. In murine models of GVHD to MHC differences between donor and host, robust donor T-cell proliferation is observed in the spleen as early as day 3 after HCT, preceding the engraftment of donor stem cells [5, 7].

After allogeneic HCT, both host- and donor-derived APCs are present in secondary lymphoid organs. T-cell receptors (TCRs) of donor T cells can recognize alloantigens either on host APCs (direct presentation) or donor APCs (indirect presentation). During direct presentation, donor T cells recognize either the peptide bound to allogeneic MHC molecules or the foreign MHC molecules themselves [8]. During indirect presentation, T cells respond to the peptides generated by degradation of the allogeneic MHC molecules that are presented on

self MHC [9]. In GVHD to mHA, direct presentation is dominant because APCs derived from the host, rather than from the donor, are critical [6].

Several laboratories have identified that naïve (CD62L+) T cells cause experimental GVHD whereas memory (CD62L+) do not, although memory stem cells may be involved [10, 11]. In the majority of HLA-identical HCT, GVHD is induced by mHA, which are peptides derived from polymorphic cellular proteins that are presented on the cell surface by MHC molecules [12]. Because the genes for these proteins are located outside of the MHC, two siblings often will have many different peptides in the MHC groove. In this case, different peptides presented by the same MHC are recognized by donor T cells and lead to GVHD. In mice, the actual number of so-called "major minor antigens" that can potentially induce GVHD is likely to be limited. Several mHA are encoded on the male-specific Y chromosome and are associated with an increased risk of GVHD when male recipients are transplanted from female donors [13]. mHA with tissue expression limited to the hematopoietic system are potential target antigens of graft-versus-leukemia (GVL) reactivity [14], and separation of GVHD and GVL by using CTLs specific for such antigens is an area of intense research [15].

Adhesion molecules mediate the initial binding of T cells to APCs. TCR signaling after antigen recognition induces a conformational change in adhesion molecules, resulting in higher affinity binding to the APC [16]. Full T-cell activation also requires costimulatory signals provided by APCs in addition to TCR signals. Two primary costimulatory pathways signal through either CD28 or TNF receptors. The best-characterized costimulatory molecules, CD80 and CD86, deliver positive signals through CD28 that lower the threshold for T-cell activation and promote T-cell differentiation and survival, while signaling through CTLA-4 is inhibitory [17].

The most potent APCs are dendritic cells (DCs); however, the relative contribution of DCs and other semiprofessional APCs to the development of GVHD, such as monocytes/macrophages and B cells, remains to be elucidated. Donor APCs may also amplify GVHD, but in the skin, Langerhans cells of host origin appear to be essential for the activation of donor T cells [17, 18]. Signaling through Toll-like receptors (TLRs) and through other innate immune receptors such as NOD may act as "danger signals" and activate host APCs, amplifying the donor T-cell response [19, 20]. DCs can be matured and activated during HCT by (1) inflammatory cytokines; (2) microbial products such as LPS and the dinucleotide CpG entering systemic circulation from intestinal mucosa damaged by conditioning; and (3) necrotic cells that are damaged by recipient conditioning. All of these stimuli may be considered "danger signals" [19] and may make the difference between an immune response and tolerance [21]. When T cells are exposed to antigens in the presence of an adjuvant such as LPS, the migration and survival of T cells are dramatically enhanced in vivo [22]. The effect of age in enhancing allostimulatory activity of host APCs may also help explain the increased incidence of acute GVHD in older recipients [23]. The elimination of host APCs by activated natural killer (NK) cells can prevent GVHD [24]. This suppressive effect of NK cells on GVHD may have relevance in humans. HLA class I differences driving donor NK-mediated alloreactions in the graft-versus-host (GVH) direction mediate potent GVL effects and produce higher engraftment rates without causing severe acute GVHD [24, 25].

Cytokine Secretion by Donor T Cells

T-cell activation involves multiple, rapidly occurring intracellular biochemical changes, including the rise of cytoplasmic free calcium and activation of protein kinase C and tyrosine kinases [26]. These pathways in turn activate transcription of genes for cytokines, such as IL-2, IFN-γ, and their receptors. Cytokines secreted by activated T cells are often classified as Th1 (secreting IL-2 and IFN-γ) or T-helper type-2 subset (Th2) (secreting IL-4, IL-5, IL-10, and IL-13) [27]. The role of Th17 cells, a recently described functional T-cell subset, has not yet been clarified in GVHD [28]. Several factors influence the ability of DCs to instruct naive CD4+ T cells to secrete Th1 or Th2 cytokines. These factors include the type and duration of DC activation along with the DC/T-cell ratio and the proportions of DC subsets present during T-cell interactions [29]. Differential activation of Th1 or Th2 cells has been evoked in the immunopathogenesis of GVHD and the development of infectious and auto-immune diseases. Although this dichotomy has many exceptions, in both settings activated Th1 cells (1) amplify T-cell proliferation by secreting IL-2; (2) lyse target cells by Fas/Fas ligand (FasL) interactions; (3) induce macrophage differentiation in the bone marrow by secreting IL-3 and granulocyte macrophage colony-stimulating factor (GM-CSF); (4) activate macrophages by secreting IFN-γ and by their CD40-CD40 ligand interactions; (5) activate endothelium to induce macrophage binding and extravasation; and (6) recruit macrophages by secreting monocyte chemoattractant protein-1 (MCP-1) [30].

During step 2 of acute GVHD pathophysiology, IL-2 has a pivotal role in both controlling and amplifying the immune response against alloantigens. IL-2 induces the expression of its own receptor (autocrine effect) and stimulates proliferation of other cells expressing the receptor (paracrine effect). IL-2 is secreted by donor CD4+ T cells in the first several days after GVHD induction [31]. In some studies, the addition of low doses of IL-2 during the 1st week after allogeneic bone marrow transplantation (BMT) enhanced the severity and mortality of GVHD [32, 34]. The precursor frequency of host-specific IL-2 producing cells predicts the occurrence of clinical acute GVHD [33, 34]. Monoclonal antibodies (MABs) against IL-2 or its receptor can prevent GVHD when administered shortly after the infusion of T cells [35, 36], but this strategy was only moderately successful in reducing the incidence of severe GVHD [37]. Cyclosporine (CSP) and tacrolimus dramatically reduce IL-2 production and effectively prevent GVHD. IL-15 is another critical cytokine in initiating allogeneic T-cell division *in vivo* [38] and may also be important in clonal T-cell expansion.

IFN-γ is another crucial cytokine that can be implicated in the second step of the pathophysiology of acute GVHD. Increased levels of IFN-γ are associated with acute GVHD [39, 40] and a large proportion of T-cell clones isolated from GVHD patients produce IFN-γ [41]. In animals with GVHD, IFN-γ levels peak between days 4 and 7 after transplantation before clinical manifestations are apparent. Experimental data demonstrate that IFN-γ modulates several aspects of the pathophysiology of acute GVHD. First, IFN-γ increases the expression of numerous molecules involved in GVHD, including adhesion molecules, chemokines, MHC antigens, and Fas, resulting in enhanced antigen presentation and the recruitment of effector cells into target organs [42]. Second, IFN-γ alters target cells in the GI tract and skin so that they are more vulnerable to damage during GVHD; the administration of anti-IFN-γ MABs prevents GI GVHD [43] and high levels of both IFN-γ and TNF-α correlate with the most intense cellular damage in the skin [44]. Third, IFN-γ mediates GVHD-associated immunosuppression seen in several experimental HCT systems in part by the induction of nitric oxide (NO) [45–47]. Fourth, IFN-γ primes macrophages to produce proinflammatory cytokines and NO in response to LPS [48]. At early time points after HCT, IFN-γ may paradoxically reduce GVHD by enhancing Fas-mediated apoptosis of activated donor T cells [49, 50].

Both cell-mediated and inflammatory cytokine GVHD effector mechanisms can sometimes be inhibited if donor T cells produce less Th1 cytokines [51]. Furthermore, cell mixtures of Th2 donor cells with an otherwise lethal inoculum of allogeneic bone marrow and T cells also protect recipient mice from LPS-induced lethality, demonstrating the ability of Th2 cells to modulate Th1 responses after allogeneic transplantation [52]. Polarization of donor T cells toward a Th2 phenotype by pretreating HCT donors with granulocyte colony-stimulating factor (G-CSF) also results in less severe GVHD [53]. It should be noted, however, that systemic administration of Th2 cytokines IL-4 or IL-10 as experimental prophylaxis of GVHD was either ineffective or toxic [54, 55].

On the other hand, administration of Th1 cytokines can also reduce GVHD. High doses of exogenous IL-2 early after BMT protects animals from GVHD mortality [56]. It has been suggested that IL-2 mediates its protective effect via inhibition of IFN-γ [39]. But injection of IFN-γ itself can prevent experimental GVHD [57] and neutralization of IFN-γ results in accelerated GVHD in lethally irradiated recipients [58]. These paradoxes may be explained by the complex dynamics of donor T-cell activation, expansion, and contraction. Activation-induced cell death (AICD) is a chief mechanism of clonal deletion and is largely responsible for the rapid contraction of activated T cells following an initial massive expansion [59]. Thus, the complete absence of IFN-γ may result in an unrestrained expansion of activated donor T cells, leading to accelerated GVHD. Similarly, administration of IFN-γ inducing cytokines, such as IL-12 or IL-18, protects mice from GVHD in a Fas dependent fashion [50]. Thus, moderate amounts of Th1 cytokines production after donor T-cell expansion may amplify GVHD; extremes in production (either low or high), particularly during T-cell expansion, may hasten the death of activated donor T cells, aborting T-cell expansion and reducing GVHD.

Regulatory T Cells

In both humans and mice, Treg deficiency results in immune dysregulation and autoimmunity, as characterized by the human IPEX syndrome resulting from loss of function mutations of FOXP3 [60]. A similar condition occurs in scurfy mice, a strain that lacks the transcription factor FOXP3 [61]. FOXP3 appears to function as a master control gene for the development and function of natural Treg, which normally constitute ~5% to 10% of the circulating CD4+ T-cell population. Tregs suppress both innate and the adaptive immune functions [62–64] by producing inhibitory cytokines (IL-10 and TGF-B) as well as by cell contact dependent inhibition of APC function and direct cytotoxicity against antigen-presenting B cells [63–65].

Additional purified CD4+CD25+Treg populations can suppress the proliferation of conventional T cells and prevent GVHD [66, 67]. Tregs do not themselves induce GVHD and

the small numbers of Treg cells present in a graft appear to be overwhelmed by the large number of conventional donor T cells present. The use of calcineurin inhibitors (CNI) and thymic injury from GVHD may also interfere with the development of adequate numbers of Treg cells that can control GVHD [66, 68–70]. NK1.1+ T cells (NKT) may also possess regulatory function, and both peripheral blood and marrow NKT cells can prevent GVHD by their IL-4 secretion [71].

Step 3: Cellular and Inflammatory Effectors

The pathophysiology of acute GVHD culminates in the generation of multiple cytotoxic effectors that contribute to target tissue injury. Significant experimental and clinical data suggest that soluble inflammatory mediators act in conjunction with direct cell-mediated cytolysis by CTL and NK cells to cause the full spectrum of deleterious effects seen during acute GVHD. As such, the effector phase of GVHD involves aspects of both the innate and adaptive immune response and the synergistic interactions of components generated during step 1 and step 2.

Cellular Effectors

The Fas/FasL and the perforin/granzyme (or granule exocytosis) pathways are the principal effector mechanisms used by CTLs and NK cells to lyse their target cells [72, 73]. Following recognition of a target cell through TCR-MHC interaction, CTLs secrete perforin and insert it into the target cell membrane forming "perforin pores" that allow granzymes to enter the cell and induce apoptosis through various downstream effector pathways [74]. Ligation of Fas results in the formation of the death-inducing signaling complex and the subsequent activation of caspases [75]. A number of ligands on T cells also possess the capability to trimerize TNF-α receptor (TNFR)-like death receptors (DR) on their targets, such as TNF-related apoptosis inducing ligand (TRAIL:DR4,5 ligand) and TNF-like weak inducer of apoptosis (TWEAK:DR3 ligand) [76, 77].

The involvement of these pathways in GVHD has been tested by utilizing donor cells that are genetically deficient in each molecule. Lethal GVHD occurs even in the *absence* of perforin dependent killing demonstrating that the perforin/granzyme pathway plays a significant, but not exclusive, role in target organ damage. CD4+ CTLs preferentially use the Fas/FasL pathway during acute GVHD, while CD8+ CTLs primarily use the perforin/granzyme pathway, consistent with other conditions involving cell-mediated cytolysis [17].

Fas is a TNF-receptor family member that is expressed by many tissues, including GVHD target organs. Inflammatory cytokines such as IFN-γ and TNF-α can increase the expression of Fas during GVHD [78]. FasL expression on donor T cells is also increased during GVHD [79, 80]. Elevated serum levels of soluble FasL and Fas have also been observed in some patients with acute GVHD [81, 82]. The Fas/FasL pathway is particularly important in hepatic GVHD, consistent with the marked sensitivity of hepatocytes to Fas-mediated cytotoxicity in models of murine hepatitis [83]. Fas-deficient recipients are protected from hepatic GVHD, but not from GVHD in other target organs [84]. Administration of anti-FasL (but not anti-TNF) MAB significantly blocked hepatic GVHD damage occurring in one model [85] whereas the use of FasL-deficient donor T cells or the administration of neutralizing FasL MABs had no effect on the development of intestinal GVHD in several studies [86, 87].

Inflammatory Effectors

In the effector phase of acute GVHD, inflammatory cytokines synergize with CTLs resulting in the amplification of local tissue injury and the development of target organ dysfunction in the transplant recipient. The cytokines TNF-α and IL-1 are produced by an abundance of cell types involved in innate and adoptive immune responses and they have synergistic and redundant activities during several phases of acute GVHD. A central role for inflammatory cytokines in acute GVHD was confirmed by a recent murine study using bone-marrow chimeras in which either MHC class I or MHC class II alloantigens were not expressed on target epithelium but on APCs alone [5]. GVHD target organ injury was induced in these chimeras even in the absence of epithelial alloantigens and mortality and target organ injury was prevented by the neutralization of TNF-α and IL-1. These observations were particularly true for CD4-mediated acute GVHD but also applied, at least in part, for CD8-mediated disease.

A critical role for TNF-α in the pathophysiology of acute GVHD was first suggested almost 15 years ago because mice transplanted with mixtures of allogeneic bone marrow and T cells developed severe skin, gut, and lung lesions that were associated with high levels of TNF-α messenger RNA (mRNA) in these tissues [88]. Target organ damage could be inhibited by infusion of anti-TNF-α MABs, and mortality could be reduced from 100% to 50% by the administration of the soluble form of the TNF-α receptor (sTNFR) [2] Extensive experimental data further suggest that TNF-α is involved in the multistep process of GVHD pathophysiology. TNF-α can (1) cause cachexia, a characteristic feature of GVHD; (2) induce activation of DCs, thus enhancing alloantigen presentation; (3) recruit effector T cells, neutrophils, and monocytes into target organs through the induction of inflammatory chemokines; and (4) cause direct tissue damage by inducing apoptosis and necrosis [89]. TNF-α is also involved in donor T-cell activation directly through its signaling via TNFR1 and TNFR2 on T cells; TNF-TNFR1 interactions promote alloreactive T-cell responses [90], whereas TNF-TNFR2 interactions are critical for intestinal GVHD [91]. TNF-α plays a central role in intestinal GVHD in murine and human studies [92, 93]. TNF-α also seems to be an important effector molecule in GVHD in skin and lymphoid tissue [87, 93, 94] and can contribute to hepatic GVHD, probably by enhancing effector cell migration to the liver via the induction of inflammatory chemokines. Studies in animals have demonstrated that neutralization of TNF-α alone or in combination with IL-1 resulted in a significant reduction of hepatic GVHD [5, 95]. An important role for TNF-α in clinical acute GVHD has also been suggested by multiple studies.

Elevations of TNF-α protein (serum) and mRNA (peripheral blood mononuclear cells) have been measured in patients with acute GVHD and other endothelial complications, such as hepatic veno-occlusive disease now termed *sinusoidal obstructive syndrome* (SOS) [96–98].

Finally, macrophages can also produce significant amounts of NO as a result of activation during GVHD. Several studies have shown that NO contributes to the deleterious effects of GVHD on target tissues and specifically to GVHD-induced immunosuppression [47, 99]. NO also inhibits repair mechanisms of target tissue by inhibiting proliferation of epithelial stem cells in the gut and skin [100]. In humans and rats, development of GVHD is preceded by an increase of NO oxidation products in the serum [101].

Toll-like Receptors and Innate Immunity

As alluded, components of the HCT conditioning regimen (in particular TBI) and the secretion of type 1 cytokines (specifically IFN-γ) prime mononuclear phagocytes to produce inflammatory cytokines. However, the actual secretion of soluble cytokines occurs after primed macrophages are triggered or stimulated by a second signal. This stimulus may be provided through TLRs by LPS and other microbial products that have leaked though an intestinal mucosa damaged initially by HCT conditioning regimens during step 1. Since the GI tract is known to be particularly sensitive to the injurious effects of cytokines [88, 102], damage to the GI tract during the effector phase can lead to a positive feed back loop wherein increased translocation of LPS results in further cytokine production and progressive intestinal injury. Thus, the GI tract may be critical in propagating the "cytokine storm" characteristic of acute GVHD; increasing experimental and clinical evidence suggests that damage to the GI tract during acute GVHD plays a major role in the amplification of systemic disease [90].

This conceptual framework underscores the role of LPS in the development of acute GVHD as suggested by several groups [48, 102, 103]. LPS is a major structural component of Gram-negative bacteria and is a potent stimulator of cellular activation and cytokine release [104]. LPS shed from bowel flora may stimulate gut-associated lymphocytes and macrophages [48]. Following allogeneic HCT, LPS accumulates in both the liver and spleen of animals with GVHD prior to its appearance in the systemic circulation [103]. Elevated serum levels of LPS have been shown to correlate directly with the degree of intestinal histopathology occurring after allogeneic HCT [102, 105].

Donor mice with a genetic mutation in the Toll-like receptor 4 (*Tlr4*) gene makes them resistant to LPS (LPS-r) and transplantation with LPS-r donor cells resulted in a significant reduction of TNF-α levels, GI tract histopathology and systemic GVHD compared to animals receiving LPS-s HCT [102]. In addition, transplantation from donors deficient in CD14 that are insensitive to LPS stimulation *in vitro* resulted in a major reduction in GI GVHD and improved long-term survival compared to normal controls [106]. Early animal studies showed that death from GVHD could be prevented if transplanted mice were given antibiotics to decontaminate the gut [107].

Accordingly, gram-negative gut decontamination during HCT has also been shown to reduce GVHD [108] and the intensity of this decontamination can predict GVHD severity [109, 110].

Traffic of Cellular Effectors

Regulation of effector cell migration into target tissues during the development of GVHD occurs in a complex milieu of chemotactic signals where several chemokine receptors may be triggered simultaneously or successively. Inflammatory chemokines expressed in inflamed tissues are specialized to recruit effector cells, such as T cells, neutrophils, and monocytes [111]. Chemokine receptors are differentially expressed on subsets of activated/effector T cells. Upon stimulation, T cells can rapidly switch chemokine receptor expression, acquiring new migratory capacity [22, 112].

The involvement of inflammatory chemokines and their receptors in GVHD has been recently investigated in mouse models of GVHD. MIP-1a recruits CCR5+CD8$^+$ T cells into the liver, lung, and spleen during GVHD [113, 114], and levels of several chemokines are elevated in GVHD-associated lung injury [115]. DCs in the lymph node activate lymphocytes and induce a profile of adhesion molecules and chemokine receptors that direct the activated cells to migrate back to the organ of DC origin. For example, activated T cells that leave a lymph node in the skin express cutaneous lymphocyte antigen (CLA) [116]. T cells expressing CLA only home back to the skin where they may mediate cutaneous GVHD, but they do not traffic to other organs. Similarly T cells exiting mesenteric lymph nodes express α4β7 (LPAM-1) which is necessary for homing to GI tract and gut-associated lymphoid tissues (GALT) [117] but they do not express CLA. Thus, cells bearing the appropriate cell surface adhesion receptors for the GI tract (e.g., LAPM-1) and chemokine receptors (e.g., CCR25) undergo firm adhesion followed by transmigration from the vessel into the appropriate organ.

CONCLUSIONS

Complications of HCT, particularly GVHD, remain major barriers to the wider application of allogeneic HCT for a variety of diseases. Recent advances in the understanding of cytokine networks, as well the direct mediators of cellular cytotoxicity, have led to improved understanding of this complex disease process. GVHD can be considered an exaggerated, undesirable manifestation of a normal inflammatory mechanism in which donor lymphocytes encounter foreign antigens in a milieu that fosters inflammation. Tissue injury related to the conditioning regimen or infection is then amplified by direct cytotoxicity via perforin-granzyme and Fas/FasL pathways, through direct cytokine-induced damage, and by recruitment of secondary effectors such as granulocytes and monocytes. Blockade of TNF-α may represent a new treatment for acute GVHD. Thymic injury and loss of regulatory T-cell function may enhance donor cell recognition of histocompatibility antigens by both T and B cells. Moreover the production

of auto- and allo-antibodies may further result in tissue injury as well as enhancing T cell related cellular injury. The net effects of this complex system are the severe inflammatory manifestations that we recognize as clinical GVHD.

REFERENCES

1. Gale RP, Bortin MM, van Bekkum DW, et al. Risk factors for acute graft-versus-host disease. *Br J Haematol.* 1987;67:397–406.
2. Xun CQ, Thompson JS, Jennings CD, Brown SA, Widmer MB. Effect of total body irradiation, busulfan-cyclophosphamide, or cyclophosphamide conditioning on inflammatory cytokine release and development of acute and chronic graft-versus-host disease in H-2-incompatible transplanted SCID mice. *Blood.* 1994;83:2360–2367.
3. Paris F, Fuks Z, Kang A, et al. Endothelial apoptosis as the primary lesion initiating intestinal radiation damage in mice. *Science.* 2001;293:293–297.
4. Hill GR, Crawford JM, Cooke KR, Brinson YS, Pan L, Ferrara JL. Total body irradiation and acute graft-versus-host disease: the role of gastrointestinal damage and inflammatory cytokines. *Blood.* 1997;90:3204–3213.
5. Teshima T, Ordemann R, Reddy P, et al. Acute graft-versus-host disease does not require alloantigen expression on host epithelium. *Nat Med.* 2002;8:575–581.
6. Shlomchik WD, Couzens MS, Tang CB, et al. Prevention of graft versus host disease by inactivation of host antigen-presenting cells. *Science.* 1999;285:412–415.
7. Beilhack A, Schulz S, Baker J, et al. In vivo analyses of early events in acute graft-versus-host disease reveal sequential infiltration of T-cell subsets. *Blood.* 2005;106:1113–1122.
8. Newton-Nash DK. The molecular basis of allorecognition. Assessment of the involvement of peptide. *Hum Immunol.* 1994;41:105–111.
9. Sayegh MH, Perico N, Gallon L, et al. Mechanisms of acquired thymic unresponsiveness to renal allografts. Thymic recognition of immunodominant allo-MHC peptides induces peripheral T cell anergy. *Transplantation.* 1994;58:125–132.
10. Anderson BE, McNiff J, Yan J, et al. Memory CD4+ T cells do not induce graft-versus-host disease. *J Clin Invest.* 2003;112:101–108.
11. Zhang Y, Joe G, Hexner E, Zhu J, Emerson SG. Host-reactive CD8+ memory stem cells in graft-versus-host disease. *Nat Med.* 2005;11:1299–1305.
12. Goulmy E, Schipper R, Pool J, et al. Mismatches of minor histocompatibility antigens between HLA-identical donors and recipients and the development of graft-versus-host disease after bone marrow transplantation. *N Engl J Med.* 1996;334:281–285.
13. Nash RA, Pepe MS, Storb R, et al. Acute graft-versus-host disease: analysis of risk factors after allogeneic marrow transplantation and prophylaxis with cyclosporine and methotrexate. *Blood.* 1992;80:1838–1845.
14. Goulmy E. Human minor histocompatibility antigens: new concepts for marrow transplantation and adoptive immunotherapy. *Immunol Rev.* 1997;157:125–140.
15. Dickinson AM, Wang XN, Sviland L, et al. In situ dissection of the graft-versus-host activities of cytotoxic T cells specific for minor histocompatibility antigens. *Nat Med.* 2002;8:410–414.

16. Dustin ML, Springer TA. T-cell receptor cross-linking transiently stimulates adhesiveness through LFA-1. *Nature.* 1989;341:619–624.

17. Welniak LA, Blazar BR, Murphy WJ. Immunobiology of allogeneic hematopoietic stem cell transplantation. *Annu Rev Immunol.* 2006;25:139–170.

18. Merad M, Hoffmann P, Ranheim E, et al. Depletion of host Langerhans cells before transplantation of donor alloreactive T cells prevents skin graft-versus-host disease. *Nat Med.* 2004;10:510–517.

19. Matzinger P. The danger model: a renewed sense of self. *Science.* 2002;296:301–305.

20. Holler E, Rogler G, Brenmoehl J, et al. Prognostic significance of NOD2/CARD15 variants in HLA-identical sibling hematopoietic stem cell transplantation: effect on long-term outcome is confirmed in 2 independent cohorts and may be modulated by the type of gastrointestinal decontamination. *Blood.* 2006;107:4189–4193.

21. Roncarolo MG, Levings MK, Traversari C. Differentiation of T regulatory cells by immature dendritic cells. *J Exp Med.* 2001;193:F5–9.

22. Reinhardt RL, Khoruts A, Merica R, Zell T, Jenkins MK. Visualizing the generation of memory CD4 T cells in the whole body. *Nature.* 2001;410:101–105.

23. Ordemann R, Hutchinson R, Friedman J, et al. Enhanced allostimulatory activity of host antigen-presenting cells in old mice intensifies acute graft-versus-host disease. *J Clin Invest.* 2002;109:1249–1256.

24. Ruggeri L, Capanni M, Urbani E, et al. Effectiveness of donor natural killer cell alloreactivity in mismatched hematopoietic transplants. *Science.* 2002;295:2097–2100.

25. Ruggeri L, Capanni M, Martelli MF, Velardi A. Cellular therapy: exploiting NK cell alloreactivity in transplantation. *Curr Opin Hematol.* 2001;8:355–359.

26. Samelson LE, Patel MD, Weissman AM, Harford JB, Klausner RD. Antigen activation of murine T cells induces tyrosine phosphorylation of a polypeptide associated with the T cell antigen receptor. *Cell.* 1986;46:1083–1090.

27. Mosmann TR, Cherwinski H, Bond MW, Giedlin MA, Coffman RL. Two types of murine helper T cell clone. I. Definition according to profiles of lymphokine activities and secreted proteins. *J Immunol.* 1986;136:2348–2357.

28. Weaver CT, Hatton RD, Mangan PR, Harrington LE. IL-17 Family Cytokines and the Expanding Diversity of Effector T Cell Lineages. *Annu Rev Immunol.* 2007;25:821–852.

29. Rissoan MC, Soumelis V, Kadowaki N, et al. Reciprocal control of T helper cell and dendritic cell differentiation. *Science.* 1999;283:1183–1186.

30. Carvalho-Pinto CE, Garcia MI, Mellado M, et al. Autocrine production of IFN-gamma by macrophages controls their recruitment to kidney and the development of glomerulonephritis in MRL/lpr mice. *J Immunol.* 2002;169:1058–1067.

31. Via CS, Finkelman FD. Critical role of interleukin-2 in the development of acute graft-versus-host disease. *Int Immunol.* 1993;5:565–572.

32. Malkovsky M, Brenner MK, Hunt R, et al. T-cell depletion of allogeneic bone marrow prevents acceleration of graft-versus-host disease induced by exogenous interleukin 2. *Cell Immunol.* 1986;103:476–480.

33. Theobald M, Nierle T, Bunjes D, Arnold R, Heimpel H. Host-specific interleukin-2-secreting donor T-cell precursors as predictors of acute graft-versus-host disease in bone marrow transplantation between HLA-identical siblings. *N Engl J Med.* 1992;327:1613–1617.

34. Schwarer AP, Jiang YZ, Brookes PA, et al. Frequency of anti-recipient alloreactive helper T-cell precursors in donor blood and graft-versus-host disease after HLA-identical sibling bone-marrow transplantation. *Lancet.* 1993;341:203–205.

35. Ferrara JL, Marion A, McIntyre JF, Murphy GF, Burakoff SJ. Amelioration of acute graft vs host disease due to minor histocompatibility antigens by in vivo administration of anti-interleukin 2 receptor antibody. *J Immunol.* 1986;137:1874–1877.

36. Herve P, Wijdenes J, Bergerat JP, et al. Treatment of corticosteroid resistant acute graft-versus-host disease by in vivo administration of anti-interleukin-2 receptor monoclonal antibody (B-B10). *Blood.* 1990;75:1017–1023.

37. Anasetti C, Martin PJ, Hansen JA, et al. A phase I-II study evaluating the murine anti-IL-2 receptor antibody 2A3 for treatment of acute graft-versus-host disease. *Transplantation.* 1990;50:49–54.

38. Li XC, Demirci G, Ferrari-Lacraz S, et al. IL-15 and IL-2: a matter of life and death for T cells in vivo. *Nat Med.* 2001;7:114–118.

39. Szebeni J, Wang MG, Pearson DA, Szot GL, Sykes M. IL-2 inhibits early increases in serum gamma interferon levels associated with graft-versus-host-disease. *Transplantation.* 1994;58:1385–1393.

40. Troutt AB, Maraskovsky E, Rogers LA, Pech MH, Kelso A. Quantitative analysis of lymphokine expression in vivo and in vitro. *Immunol Cell Biol.* 1992;70(pt 1):51–57.

41. Velardi A, Varese P, Terenzi A, et al. Lymphokine production by T-cell clones after human bone marrow transplantation. *Blood.* 1989;74:1665–1672.

42. Dufour JH, Dziejman M, Liu MT, Leung JH, Lane TE, Luster AD. IFN-gamma-inducible protein 10 (IP-10; CXCL10)-deficient mice reveal a role for IP-10 in effector T cell generation and trafficking. *J Immunol.* 2002;168:3195–3204.

43. Mowat AM. Antibodies to IFN-gamma prevent immunologically mediated intestinal damage in murine graft-versus-host reaction. *Immunology.* 1989;68:18–23.

44. Dickinson AM, Sviland L, Dunn J, Carey P, Proctor SJ. Demonstration of direct involvement of cytokines in graft-versus-host reactions using an in vitro human skin explant model. Bone Marrow *Transplant.* 1991;7:209–216.

45. Holda JH, Maier T, Claman HN. Evidence that IFN-gamma is responsible for natural suppressor activity in GVHD spleen and normal bone marrow. *Transplantation.* 1988;45:772–777.

46. Wall DA, Hamberg SD, Reynolds DS, Burakoff SJ, Abbas AK, Ferrara JL. Immunodeficiency in graft-versus-host disease. I. Mechanism of immune suppression. *J Immunol.* 1988; 140:2970–2976.

47. Krenger W, Falzarano G, Delmonte J, Jr., Snyder KM, Byon JC, Ferrara JL. Interferon-gamma suppresses T-cell proliferation to mitogen via the nitric oxide pathway during experimental acute graft-versus-host disease. *Blood.* 1996;88:1113–1121.

48. Nestel FP, Price KS, Seemayer TA, Lapp WS. Macrophage priming and lipopolysaccharide-triggered release of tumor necrosis factor alpha during graft-versus-host disease. *J Exp Med.* 1992;175:405–413.

49. Yang YG, Dey BR, Sergio JJ, Pearson DA, Sykes M. Donor-derived interferon gamma is required for inhibition of acute graft-versus-host disease by interleukin 12. *J Clin Invest.* 1998;102:2126–2135.

50. Reddy P, Teshima T, Kukuruga M, et al. Interleukin-18 regulates acute graft-versus-host disease by enhancing Fas-mediated donor T cell apoptosis. *J Exp Med*. 2001;194:1433–1440.

51. Fowler DH, Kurasawa K, Husebekk A, Cohen PA, Gress RE. Cells of Th2 cytokine phenotype prevent LPS-induced lethality during murine graft-versus-host reaction. Regulation of cytokines and CD8+ lymphoid engraftment. *J Immunol*. 1994;152:1004–1013.

52. Fowler DH, Kurasawa K, Smith R, Eckhaus MA, Gress RE. Donor CD4-enriched cells of Th2 cytokine phenotype regulate graft-versus-host disease without impairing allogeneic engraftment in sublethally irradiated mice. *Blood*. 1994;84:3540–3549.

53. Pan L, Delmonte J, Jr., Jalonen CK, Ferrara JL. Pretreatment of donor mice with granulocyte colony-stimulating factor polarizes donor T lymphocytes toward type-2 cytokine production and reduces severity of experimental graft-versus-host disease. *Blood*. 1995;86:4422–4429.

54. Krenger W, Snyder K, Smith S, Ferrara JL. Effects of exogenous interleukin-10 in a murine model of graft-versus-host disease to minor histocompatibility antigens. *Transplantation*. 1994;58:1251–1257.

55. Blazar BR, Taylor PA, Smith S, Vallera DA. Interleukin-10 administration decreases survival in murine recipients of major histocompatibility complex disparate donor bone marrow grafts. *Blood*. 1995;85:842–851.

56. Sykes M, Hoyles KA, Romick ML, Sachs DH. In vitro and in vivo analysis of bone marrow-derived CD3+, CD4-, CD8-, NK1.1+ cell lines. *Cell Immunol*. 1990;129:478–493.

57. Brok HP, Heidt PJ, van der Meide PH, Zurcher C, Vossen JM. Interferon-gamma prevents graft-versus-host disease after allogeneic bone marrow transplantation in mice. *J Immunol*. 1993;151:6451–6459.

58. Wall DA, Sheehan KC. The role of tumor necrosis factor and interferon gamma in graft-versus-host disease and related immunodeficiency. *Transplantation*. 1994;57:273–279.

59. Li XC, Strom TB, Turka LA, Wells AD. T cell death and transplantation tolerance. *Immunity*. 2001;14:407–416.

60. Bennett CL, Christie J, Ramsdell F, et al. The immune dysregulation, polyendocrinopathy, enteropathy, X-linked syndrome (IPEX) is caused by mutations of FOXP3. *Nat Genet*. 2001;27:20–21.

61. Fontenot JD, Gavin MA, Rudensky AY. Foxp3 programs the development and function of CD4+CD25+ regulatory T cells. *Nat Immunol*. 2003;4:330–336.

62. Janssen EM, Droin NM, Lemmens EE, et al. CD4+ T-cell help controls CD8+ T-cell memory via TRAIL-mediated activation-induced cell death. *Nature*. 2005;434:88–93.

63. Cederbom L, Hall H, Ivars F. CD4+CD25+ regulatory T cells down-regulate co-stimulatory molecules on antigen-presenting cells. *Eur J Immunol*. 2000;30:1538–1543.

64. Azuma T, Takahashi T, Kunisato A, Kitamura T, Hirai H. Human CD4+ CD25+ regulatory T cells suppress NKT cell functions. *Cancer Res*. 2003;63:4516–4520.

65. Powrie F, Carlino J, Leach MW, Mauze S, Coffman RL. A critical role for transforming growth factor-beta but not interleukin 4 in the suppression of T helper type 1-mediated colitis by CD45RB(low) CD4+ T cells. *J Exp Med*. 1996;183:2669–2674.

66. Hoffmann P, Edinger M. CD4+CD25+ regulatory T cells and graft-versus-host disease. *Semin Hematol*. 2006;43:62–69.

67. Edinger M, Hoffmann P, Ermann J, et al. CD4+CD25+ regulatory T cells preserve graft-versus-tumor activity while inhibiting graft-versus-host disease after bone marrow transplantation. *Nat Med*. 2003;9:1144–1150.

68. Zeiser R, Nguyen VH, Beilhack A, et al. Inhibition of CD4+CD25+ regulatory T-cell function by calcineurin-dependent interleukin-2 production. *Blood*. 2006;108:390–399.

69. Nguyen VH, Zeiser R, Dasilva DL, et al. In vivo dynamics of regulatory T-cell trafficking and survival predict effective strategies to control graft-versus-host disease following allogeneic transplantation. *Blood*. 2007;109:2649–2656.

70. Nguyen VH, Zeiser R, Negrin RS. Role of naturally arising regulatory T cells in hematopoietic cell transplantation. *Biol Blood Marrow Transplant*. 2006;12:995–1009.

71. Lan F, Zeng D, Higuchi M, Huie P, Higgins JP, Strober S. Predominance of NK1.1+TCR alpha beta+ or DX5+TCR alpha beta+ T cells in mice conditioned with fractionated lymphoid irradiation protects against graft-versus-host disease: "natural suppressor" cells. *J Immunol*. 2001;167:2087–2096.

72. Kagi D, Vignaux F, Ledermann B, et al. Fas and perforin pathways as major mechanisms of T cell-mediated cytotoxicity. *Science*. 1994;265:528–530.

73. Lowin B, Hahne M, Mattmann C, Tschopp J. Cytolytic T-cell cytotoxicity is mediated through perforin and Fas lytic pathways. *Nature*. 1994;370:650–652.

74. Shresta S, Pham CT, Thomas DA, Graubert TA, Ley TJ. How do cytotoxic lymphocytes kill their targets? *Curr Opin Immunol*. 1998;10:581–587.

75. Krammer PH. CD95's deadly mission in the immune system. *Nature*. 2000;407:789–795.

76. Chinnaiyan A, O'Rourke K, Yu G, et al. Signal transduction by DR3, a death domain-containing receptor related to TNFR-1 and CD95. *Science*. 1996;274:990–992.

77. Chicheportiche Y, Fossati-Jimack L, Moll S, Ibnou-Zekri N, Izui S. Down-regulated expression of TWEAK mRNA in acute and chronic inflammatory pathologies. *Biochem Biophys Res Commun*. 2000;279:162–165.

78. Ueno Y, Ishii M, Yahagi K, et al. Fas-mediated cholangiopathy in the murine model of graft versus host disease. *Hepatology*. 2000;31:966–974.

79. Shustov A, Nguyen P, Finkelman F, Elkon KB, Via CS. Differential expression of Fas and Fas ligand in acute and chronic graft-versus-host disease: up-regulation of Fas and Fas ligand requires CD8+ T cell activation and IFN-gamma production. *J Immunol*. 1998;161:2848–2855.

80. Wasem C, Frutschi C, Arnold D, et al. Accumulation and activation-induced release of preformed Fas (CD95) ligand during the pathogenesis of experimental graft-versus-host disease. *J Immunol*. 2001;167:2936–2941.

81. Liem LM, van Lopik T, van Nieuwenhuijze AE, van Houwelingen HC, Aarden L, Goulmy E. Soluble Fas levels in sera of bone marrow transplantation recipients are increased during acute graft-versus-host disease but not during infections. *Blood*. 1998;91:1464–1468.

82. Kayaba H, Hirokawa M, Watanabe A, et al. Serum markers of graft-versus-host disease after bone marrow transplantation. *J Allergy Clin Immunol*. 2000;106:S40-S44.

83. Kondo T, Suda T, Fukuyama H, Adachi M, Nagata S. Essential roles of the Fas ligand in the development of hepatitis. *Nat Med*. 1997;3:409–413.

84. van Den Brink MR, Moore E, Horndasch KJ, et al. Fas-deficient lpr mice are more susceptible to graft-versus-host disease. *J Immunol*. 2000;164:469–480.

85. Hattori Y, Azuma M, Kemmotsu O, Kanno M. Differential sensitivity of diabetic rat papillary muscles to negative inotropic effects of oxybarbiturates versus thiobarbiturates. *Anesth Analg*. 1992;74:97–104.

86. Baker MB, Altman NH, Podack ER, Levy RB. The role of cell-mediated cytotoxicity in acute GVHD after MHC-matched allogeneic bone marrow transplantation in mice. *J Exp Med*. 1996;183:2645–2656.

87. Hattori Y, Sakuma I, Kanno M. Differential effects of histamine mediated by histamine H1- and H2-receptors on contractility, spontaneous rate and cyclic nucleotides in the rabbit heart. *Eur J Pharmacol*. 1988;153:221–229.

88. Piguet PF, Grau GE, Allet B, Vassalli P. Tumor necrosis factor/cachectin is an effector of skin and gut lesions of the acute phase of graft-vs.-host disease. *J Exp Med*. 1987;166:1280–1289.

89. Laster SM, Wood JG, Gooding LR. Tumor necrosis factor can induce both apoptic and necrotic forms of cell lysis. *J Immunol*. 1988;141:2629–2634.

90. Hill GR, Teshima T, Rebel VI, et al. The p55 TNF-alpha receptor plays a critical role in T cell alloreactivity. *J Immunol*. 2000;164:656–663.

91. Brown GR, Lee E, Thiele DL. TNF-TNFR2 interactions are critical for the development of intestinal graft-versus-host disease in MHC class II-disparate (C57BL/6J- >C57BL/6J x bm12)F$_1$ mice. *J Immunol*. 2002;168:3065–3071.

92. Hattori K, Hirano T, Miyajima H, et al. Differential effects of anti-Fas ligand and anti-tumor necrosis factor alpha antibodies on acute graft-versus-host disease pathologies. *Blood*. 1998;91:4051–4055.

93. Piguet PF, Collart MA, Grau GE, Kapanci Y, Vassalli P. Tumor necrosis factor/cachectin plays a key role in bleomycin-induced pneumopathy and fibrosis. *J Exp Med*. 1989;170:655–663.

94. Murphy GF, Sueki H, Teuscher C, Whitaker D, Korngold R. Role of mast cells in early epithelial target cell injury in experimental acute graft-versus-host disease. *J Invest Dermatol*. 1994;102:451–461.

95. Cooke KR, Hill GR, Gerbitz A, et al. Tumor necrosis factor-alpha neutralization reduces lung injury after experimental allogeneic bone marrow transplantation. *Transplantation*. 2000;70:272–279.

96. Holler E, Kolb HJ, Moller A, et al. Increased serum levels of tumor necrosis factor alpha precede major complications of bone marrow transplantation. *Blood*. 1990;75:1011–1016.

97. Holler E, Kolb HJ, Hintermeier-Knabe R, et al. Role of tumor necrosis factor alpha in acute graft-versus-host disease and complications following allogeneic bone marrow transplantation. *Transplant Proc*. 1993;25:1234–1236.

98. Tanaka J, Imamura M, Kasai M, et al. Cytokine receptor gene expression in peripheral blood mononuclear cells during graft-versus-host disease after allogeneic bone marrow transplantation. *Leuk Lymphoma*. 1995;19:281–287.

99. Falzarano G, Krenger W, Snyder KM, Delmonte J, Jr., Karandikar M, Ferrara JL. Suppression of B-cell proliferation to lipopolysaccharide is mediated through induction of the nitric oxide pathway by tumor necrosis factor-alpha in mice with acute graft-versus-host disease. *Blood*. 1996;87:2853–2860.

100. Nestel FP, Greene RN, Kichian K, Ponka P, Lapp WS. Activation of macrophage cytostatic effector mechanisms during acute graft-versus-host disease: release of intracellular iron and nitric oxide-mediated cytostasis. *Blood*. 2000;96:1836–1843.

101. Weiss G, Schwaighofer H, Herold M, et al. Nitric oxide formation as predictive parameter for acute graft-versus-host disease after human allogeneic bone marrow transplantation. *Transplantation*. 1995;60:1239–1244.

102. Cooke KR, Hill GR, Crawford JM, et al. Tumor necrosis factor-alpha production to lipopolysaccharide stimulation by donor cells predicts the severity of experimental acute graft-versus-host disease. *J Clin Invest*. 1998;102:1882–1891.

103. Price KS, Nestel FP, Lapp WS. Progressive accumulation of bacterial lipopolysaccharide in vivo during murine acute graft-versus-host disease. *Scand J Immunol*. 1997;45:294–300.

104. Raetz CR. Biochemistry of endotoxins. *Annu Rev Biochem*. 1990;59:129–170.

105. Fegan C, Poynton CH, Whittaker JA. The gut mucosal barrier in bone marrow transplantation. *Bone Marrow Transplant*. 1990;5:373–377.

106. Cooke KR, Gerbitz A, Crawford JM, et al. LPS antagonism reduces graft-versus-host disease and preserves graft-versus-leukemia activity after experimental bone marrow transplantation. *J Clin Invest*. 2001;107:1581–1589.

107. van Bekkum DW, Roodenburg J, Heidt PJ, van der Waaij D. Mitigation of secondary disease of allogeneic mouse radiation chimeras by modification of the intestinal microflora. *J Natl Cancer Inst*. 1974;52:401–404.

108. Storb R, Prentice RL, Buckner CD, et al. Graft-versus-host disease and survival in patients with aplastic anemia treated by marrow grafts from HLA-identical siblings. Beneficial effect of a protective environment. *N Engl J Med*. 1983;308:302–307.

109. Beelen DW, Haralambie E, Brandt H, et al. Evidence that sustained growth suppression of intestinal anaerobic bacteria reduces the risk of acute graft-versus-host disease after sibling marrow transplantation. *Blood*. 1992;80:2668–2676.

110. Gerbitz A, Schultz M, Wilke A, et al. Probiotic effects on experimental graft-versus-host disease: let them eat yogurt. *Blood*. 2004;103:4365–4367.

111. Moser B, Loetscher P. Lymphocyte traffic control by chemokines. *Nat Immunol*. 2001;2:123–128.

112. Sallusto F, Lenig D, Forster R, Lipp M, Lanzavecchia A. Two subsets of memory T lymphocytes with distinct homing potentials and effector functions. *Nature*. 1999;401:708–712.

113. Murai M, Yoneyama H, Harada A, et al. Active participation of CCR5(+)CD8(+) T lymphocytes in the pathogenesis of liver injury in graft-versus-host disease. *J Clin Invest*. 1999;104:49–57.

114. Serody JS, Burkett SE, Panoskaltsis-Mortari A, et al. T-lymphocyte production of macrophage inflammatory protein-1alpha is critical to the recruitment of CD8(+) T cells to the liver, lung, and spleen during graft-versus-host disease. *Blood*. 2000;96:2973–2980.

115. Panoskaltsis-Mortari A, Strieter RM, Hermanson JR, et al. Induction of monocyte- and T-cell-attracting chemokines in the lung during the generation of idiopathic pneumonia syndrome following allogeneic murine bone marrow transplantation. *Blood*. 2000;96:834–839.

116. Kupper TS, Fuhlbrigge RC. Immune surveillance in the skin: mechanisms and clinical consequences. *Nat Rev Immunol*. 2004;4:211–222.

117. Berlin C, Berg EL, Briskin MJ, et al. Alpha 4 beta 7 integrin mediates lymphocyte binding to the mucosal vascular addressin MAdCAM-1. *Cell*. 1993;74:185–195.

3

PATHOPHYSIOLOGY OF CHRONIC GRAFT VERSUS HOST DISEASE

Kirk R. Schultz

INTRODUCTION

Chronic graft versus host disease (cGVHD) results in significant morbidity and mortality, yet, therapy for cGVHD has improved very little over the past 10 to 20 years. While limited cGVHD may convey a survival advantage through the graft-versus-leukemia effect (GVL or GVT) [1], cGVHD remains one of the major complications of allogeneic bone marrow transplantation (BMT). There are numerous potential immunosuppressant therapies available to be evaluated in cGVHD; however, our progress to improve cGVHD therapy is significantly limited by the lack of a good understanding of the pathophysiology of cGVHD.

DEFINITION OF CGVHD

The two major factors that have limited our understanding of cGVHD have been the lack of animal models that strongly correlate with human cGVHD and the heterogeneity of cGVHD. Other factors that have affected experimental approaches to cGVHD are the insidious onset of the diseases, resulting in difficulties in studying pathophysiological changes before and at the time of disease onset. Since there are no physiological markers that determine the onset or evolution of cGVHD in humans, the clinical diagnosis currently is the "gold standard" by which all biological changes are measured. While murine models have been very useful in evaluating the mechanism of acute graft versus host disease (aGVHD) [2], none of the models accurately reflect human cGVHD. While some models have a limited expression of cGVHD such as sclerodermatous skin involvement [3], lung involvement [4], or autoantibodies [5], none has the full range of clinical manifestations of human cGVHD. At this time, evaluation of human cGVHD appears to be the most accurate approach to gain new insights into the pathophysiology of cGVHD.

FACTORS THAT AFFECT THE PATHOPHYSIOLOGY OF CGVHD

While cGVHD is generally felt to have its onset after the first 3 months post BMT, there appear to be a number of factors impacting on the development of cGVHD. The graft composition may be important in the development of cGVHD. This conclusion is supported by the fact that there is a lower incidence of cGVHD after umbilical cord-blood transplantation [6] and possibly after granulocyte colony-stimulating factor (G-CSF)-stimulated marrow [7], whereas, the incidence of cGVHD after G-CSF-mobilized peripheral blood is higher [8, 9]. Possible explanations have been that there is a shift to an increased innate response in G-CSF-mobilized peripheral blood [10] or a different composition of dendritic cells (DC)2 and DC CD16+ [11]. Umbilical cord blood is characterized by higher numbers of naive T cells [12] and antigen presentation is inefficient in umbilical cord blood dendritic cells [13]. The potential differences between G-CSF stimulated bone marrow (BM) and G-CSF stimulated peripheral blood may be due to higher naive B cell and plasmacytoid dendritic cell populations in G-CSF stimulated bone marrow (BM) [14]. G-CSF treatment post BMT also affects the incidence of cGVHD with a marrow donor source [15].

Other factors present at the time of transplantation that appear to impact on the later development of cGVHD are the use of antithymocyte immunoglobulin [16] and Campath 1H treatment [17, 18, 19]. Depletion of donor T cells from the marrow before transplantation may impact on development of cGVHD [20] as shown in single center studies with relatively small numbers of patients although others have suggested it does not [21]. Thus, the impact of depletion of early developing T cells or possibly recipient T cell on cGVHD is not completely resolved. Other factors that impact on development of cGVHD are both older donor and recipient age [22, 23] and transplant from a female donor to a male recipient [24]. Whether this is due to a higher number of memory T cells or another factor remains to be elucidated [25]. Another factor that appears to impact on the development of cGVHD is the type of preparative regimen utilized. Patients receiving nonmyeloablative preparative regimens appear to have a higher rate of cGVHD along with delayed CD4+ T-cell and B-cell recovery [26]. GVHD post nonmyeloablative is further complicated by the fact that there is a high preponderance of a "late-onset acute GVHD" making interpretation of mechanisms around this form versus cGVDH difficult [27]. Infectious agents, in particular cytomegalovirus, have been associated as risk factors for development of cGVHD [28]. Lastly, aGVHD is strongly correlated with the later development of cGVHD [29]. Whether cGVHD preceded by aGVHD represents a different pathophysiology of cGVHD is not certain. Some have shown that certain organ manifestations of cGVHD, such as bronchiolitis obliterans organizing pneumonia, is associated with the previous diagnosis of aGVHD [30]. Engraftment syndrome, probably a form of aGVHD also is associated with the later development of cGVHD [31].

ROLE OF T CELLS

Direct Allogeneic Immune Responses Against Specific Antigens

Alloreactive donor T cells are primarily implicated in the pathophysiology of cGVHD. However, the recent randomized National Institutes of Health (NIH) unrelated donor trial failed to demonstrate that T-cell depletion reduced cGVHD incidence [21]. Therefore, the role of a direct allogeneic immune response in cGVHD is not clear, and there is no strong correlation between the number of minor histocompatibility antigen-specific T cells and cGVHD [32, 33]. In general, the antigens recognized by donor-derived recipient-reactive T-cell populations are not well-characterized, and the response of donor T cells against recipient alloantigens appears to be highly heterogeneous. This suggests that non–T-cell populations, such as DC or B-lymphocytes, also contribute to cGVHD.

Th1/Tc1 versus Th2/Tc2 Responses in cGVHD

Mouse models indicate that skewing toward Th1-type cytokines, such as IL-2 and interferon-gamma (IFN-γ) can reduce cGVHD, whereas skewing toward Th2-type cytokines, such as interleukin (IL) IL-4, IL-5, IL-10, and IL-13, can increase cGVHD [34]. Unfortunately, mouse models do not replicate human cGVHD as it occurs in the clinic, and both Th1- and Th2-type cells can cause mouse GVHD in distinct settings [34–36]. The role of Th1 versus Th2 cytokines in human cGVHD is not well described. Human studies have involved small numbers of subjects with only nominal correlations to cGVHD endpoints (e.g., clinical natural history). Nonetheless, reports exist to suggest that human cGVHD can be associated with either Th1 or Th2 cytokine imbalance, as it has been

reported that (i) IL-4-producing T cells may be a marker for cGVHD [37]; (ii) therapeutic response of cGVHD to extracorporeal photopheresis (ECP) is associated with Th1 cytokine induction in CD4+ T cells for a more equal Th1/Th2 balance [38, 39]; (iii) elevation of the Th1 cytokine, IFN-γ, has been associated with extensive cGVHD [40]; and (iv) IL-10 gene polymorphisms correlate with the development of cGVHD [41].

The recently concluded Children's Oncology Groups study also supports the conclusion that a lack of a Th1 shift (IFN-γ and IL-2 production) leads to the early-onset form of cGVHD. Other recent additional observations suggest that the ability to generate a Th1/Tc1 response (IFN-γ and IL-2) early post BMT is associated with no cGVHD and is supported by the findings that patients with high IFN-γ-producing polymorphisms have lower cGVHD [42]; that in mouse models, high-IFN-γ production by T cells (or possibly natural killer T [NKT] cells) results in lower cGVHD [43–45]; and by the concept that IFN-γ-dependent CD8+ T-cell contraction [46] is important in the development of early onset of cGVHD. Lack of CD8+ T-cell contraction may lead to increased lymphocyte senescence in cGVHD [47].

Chronic GVHD has been associated with a preponderance of IFN-γ, IL-4, IL-5, and IL-2 producing CD4+ effector memory cells as opposed to central memory cells [48, 49]. cGVHD is also associated with infiltration of CD8+ T cells in the skin [50] and intestine [51]. Both CD4+ and CD8+ T-cell populations are characterized by OX40 expression at the onset of cGVHD [52]. In murine models that may approximate the Th2 type of cGVHD, homing of donor CCR7-expressing T cells to lymphoid issues may also play a role in development of activated CD4+ T cells and IL-4 production [50]. Other characteristics that may play a role in both the incidence and severity of cGVHD include cytokine polymorphisms of donor and recipient *IL-1* and *IL-6* genes; donor TNF receptor type II 169RR-homozygous genotype; recipient IL-10 GG-homozygosity; and recipient IL-1Ra polymorphisms (IL1RN*2) [53–57]. While a Th2 predominant response may be part of cGVHD particularly one that has autoantibodies as a major clinical manifestation, this probably represents a subtype of cGVHD. Moreover, both murine and human data supports the hypothesis that a lack of balance between the two responses may be the predominant mechanism rather than simply a Th2 predominance.

THYMIC REGULATION

Murine models that attempt to approximate cGVHD have been used to evaluate the mechanisms of various populations in cGVHD. One model utilizes transplantation of donor DBA/2 (H-2d) spleen cells into major histocompatibility complex (MHC)-matched but minor antigen-mismatched sublethally irradiated BALB/c (H-2d) recipients as well as athymic BALB/c(nu/nu) and adult-thymectomized BALB/c recipients. In this model, in vivo-generated CD4+ T cells caused lesions characteristic of cGVHD when adoptively transferred into secondary allogeneic recipients. These pathogenic CD4+ T cells were thymopoiesis dependent and keratinocyte growth factor treatment improved the reconstitution of recipient thymic dendritic cells and prevented the development of pathogenic donor CD4+ T cells. These results suggest that thymus dependent de novo-generated donor CD4+ T cells, arising during acute graft-versus-host reactions, contributed to the evolution from acute to cGVHD [58]. Findings from the identical model have shown that GVHD is dependent on both donor CD25−CD4+ T and B cells in transplants with inhibition by donor CD25+CD4+ T regulatory (Treg) cells. In this model the host thymus was not required for induction of cGVHD [59]. Another group utilizing a separate murine model (lethally irradiated C3H/HeN (H-2^k) recipients reconstituted with T-cell-depleted bone marrow cells from MHC class II-deficient (H2-Ab1$^{−/−}$) B6 (H-2^b) mice) have shown that negative thymic selection of donor T cells is important [60].

Evaluation of thymic function in humans has been done using T-cell receptor excision circles (TRECs) on the basis of the fact that thymic function is necessary for de novo generation of T cells after hematopoietic stem cell transplantation (HSCT). They have found that TREC levels correlate with phenotypically naive T cells, indicating that such cells were not expanded progeny of naive T cells present in the donor graft. Low TREC appears to strongly correlate with cGVHD and slow naive T-cell recovery [61–63]. Others have shown that a TREC value greater than or equal to 172 was associated with a decreased incidence of cGVHD [64]. While murine models support a strong role for aberrant thymus selection as part of the pathophysiology of cGVHD, the role of thymic selection as a major mechanism in human cGVHD is less clear. A slow recovery of naïve T cells may be important in human cGVHD.

B CELLS IN CGVHD

There is strong evidence supporting the importance of activated antigen-presenting cells (APCs) in the development of cGVHD [65, 66]. While T cells are known end-effector cells in cGVHD, recent evidence suggests that B cells play a role in disease development [67]. T-cell activation in this context depends upon functional class II MHC [68], and presentation of costimulatory molecules such as CD80 and CD86 by professional antigen-presenting cells (APC) [69]. B cells, acting as APCs, appear to be instrumental in T-cell priming to minor histocompatibility antigens and development of cGVHD in mice [70] and humans [71]. After reduced-intensity conditioning regimen persistence of host B cells, but not dendritic cell origin or subset, was associated with cGVHD-like lesions and host origin autoantibodies [72]. This conclusion is supported by the observation that in vivo depletion of B cells with rituximab can suppress the progression of complicated cGVHD [73–75]. In addition to potential activity as an APC, B-cell production of autoantibodies is equally important.

The role of B cells in cGVHD appears to be through three separate pathways. It has been shown that CpG oligodeoxynucleotides (CpG ODN)s, which bind to one of the toll-like receptors, toll-like receptor 9 (TLR9), are capable of aggravating GVHD severity [76]. In addition, mice with GVHD have an exaggerated mitogenic and IL-6 response to synthetic CpG ODNs which is significantly ameliorated by chloroquine, a potent TLR9 inhibitor [77, 78]. In humans, B-cell population that responds to TLR9 agonists (CpG ODNs) appears to correlate with cGVHD [79]. These populations may be generated by B-cell receptor (BCR) signaling of naive B cells [80]. These high-TLR9 expressing B-cell populations appear to correspond with therapeutic response at 9 months post BMT [79]. A coordinated B–T response to minor histocompatibility alloantigens (mHA) is well described [71, 81], along with a significant high titer antibody response to mHA that correlates with cGVHD in patients [82]. As a marker of B-lymphocyte activation, B-cell activating factor of the TNF family (BAFF) is a cytokine produced by non-B cells (granulocytes, T cells, and bone marrow stromal cells) that has two possible effects on B cells: (i) preferentially attenuating B-cell receptor-triggered apoptosis of mature B cells and (ii) promoting differentiation of human antigen-experienced B cells into immunoglobulin (Ig)-producing plasma cells [83]. High concentrations of BAFF drive B-cell autoimmunity in well-defined mouse models (e.g., BAFF-overexpressing transgenic mice develop autoimmunity [84] and in autoimmune disorders (e.g., lupus, rheumatoid arthritis) [85, 86]. Two separate studies have now shown that soluble BAFF correlates with cGVHD [87, 88]. The third possibility relates to the immunoglobulin-like cell surface receptors expressed in B cells, Fc receptor-like 3 gene (FCRL3). FCRL3 is encoded by the IRTA1 and IRTA2 genes encode messenger RNAs expressed predominantly in the B-cell lineage within discrete B-cell compartments, IRTA1 being in the marginal zone and IRTA2 in the germinal center light zone [89]. A functional FCRL3 variant has been associated with autoimmunity [90] and in a recent study, recipient FCRL3 169C/C genotype was significantly less frequent in cGVHD patients than in those without cGVHD [91]. However, studies in Caucasians have failed to confirm a strong association of this gene with rheumatoid arthritis (RA) and systemic lupus erythematosus (SLE) making it questionable whether FCRL3 has a general function in all ethnic groups [92]. A recent observation is that immature/transitional circulating CD19+/CD21− B cells are significantly increased in active cGVHD compared to controls [93]. Whether this is a viable mechanism requires confirmation. In recent years, the role of B cells has increased in importance both as APCs and as the source of recipient reactive antibodies. Inflammatory responses through the TLRs and BAFF/Bly appear to be critical to these responses.

Role of Pathogens in Development of cGVHD

There is evidence that microbial products may potentially contribute to cGVHD development and disease maintenance as supported in animal models. Both microfloral decontamination [94] and blockade of pathogen-associated molecular pattern PAMP-inducible costimulatory molecules such as CD40 to

CD40L (CD152) [95] or B7.1 (CD80) and B7.2 (CD86) [96] to CD28 in mice are effective in decreasing GVHD. Additionally 4-aminoquinolines, such as chloroquine and hydroxychloroquine, which potently suppress the immunostimulatory activity of CpG-rich microbial DNA [78], have been successfully used clinically to treat cGVHD [97, 98]. Cytomegalovirus (CMV) infection is well established and associated with cGVHD [99], and cytotoxic antibodies against CD13 (anti-CD13) are described in a smaller series of patients following allo-BMT with both cGVHD and CMV reactivation [100]. Soderberg et al. demonstrated anti-CD13 antibodies in 15/33 bone marrow transplant patients, all of whom developed antibodies at the time of CMV reactivation or disease. CD13 is the known receptor for CMV entry into host cells. When the virus reactivates, it incorporates CD13 into the virion envelope, becoming immunogenic and resulting in antibody production [101, 102]. More recently, soluble CD13 has been shown to be a robust marker for cGVHD in children [88]. Recently, a strong association with a recipient NOD2/CARD15 variant associated with decreased TLR2/4 signaling polymorphisms has strongly correlated with bronchiolitis obliterans secondary to cGVHD [103]. This suggests that a decreased innate response allowing for increased infectious insult to lungs may be part of the pathogenesis of cGVHD of the lung. While the role of CMV as a cofactor for induction of cGVHD is established, the role of other bacterial or viral pathogens is less clear. An altered innate response to pathogen with either an inefficient response to pathogen as in deficient TLR2/4 signaling from a NOD2/CARD15 variant or increased TLR9 signaling in immune populations such as B cells may be an underlying mechanism for development of cGVHD.

cGVHD ANTIGENS

The number of self or minor histocompatibility antigens recognized in T- and B-cell responses appears to be very heterogeneous. Only a few antigens have been established as being closely linked to cGVHD. One minor histocompatibility antigen that may be associated with cGVHD is the histocopatibility antigen, HA-1. HA-1-reactive T cells are present in patients with GVHD and their frequencies decrease as GVHD improves during therapy, although primarily in aGVHD [104, 105]. Moreover, the frequency of HA-1 is low, suggesting that it is not the primary immune target for cGVHD in most transplants [106]. Another possible antigen is CD31: disparities of the three codons 125, 563, and 670 are associated with a trend toward increased risk of cGVHD [107]. Probably the best-documented autoantibody association with cGVHD is H-Y antigen. Males who have received sex-mismatched allogeneic HSCT from female donors (F→M BMT) are at high risk for both aGVHD and cGVHD compared to other donor and recipient sex combinations [108–110]. Male BMT recipients who had male donors (M→M BMT) had 35% less extensive cGVHD than did F→M BMT recipients [110]. Five H-Y antigens (DBY, UTY, ZFY, RPS4Y, and EIF1AY) have been identified with the development of allogeneic H-Y antibodies in 4 to 12 months after BMT in approximately 50% of F→M BMT patients [111, 112]. Because the H-Y antibodies are present 4 to 12 months after BMT there appears to be a strong role for them in cGVHD with a cumulative incidence of cGVHD reaching 89% at 5 years after transplantation [111, 112].

Chronic GVHD in humans has nonspecific associations with autoantibody-mediated diseases such as Myasthenia Gravis, but the mechanisms that account for autoantibody production remain obscure. Autoantibodies that have been described in association with cGVHD in previous smaller studies include antinuclear antibody (ANA) [113–115], anti-dsDNA antibody [115–117], antimitochondrial antibody [115], anticardiolipin antibody [115], antismooth muscle antibody (ASMA), platelet antibodies, and antineutrophil antibodies [116–120]. More recent data show that autoantibodies against platelet-derived growth factor (PDGF) receptor play a role in sclerodermatous cGVHD and should be evaluated for validation in future studies [121]. These platelet-derived growth factor receptor-alpha (PDGFR-α) autoantibodies induce tyrosine phosphorylation, accumulation of reactive oxygen species (ROS), and stimulate *type 1 collagen* gene expression through the Ha-Ras-ERK1/2-ROS signaling pathway, all processes implicated in inflammation and fibrosis. In other studies, PDGFR-α antibodies have been demonstrated to be the driving force behind the fibrosis in scleroderma, a disease with many clinical features similar to those of classic cGVHD [122].

REGULATORY IMMUNE POPULATIONS IN cGVHD

Tregs in cGVHD

Various regulatory populations appear to play important roles in the pathogenesis of cGVHD. There has been intensive investigation of CD4+CD25+ Treg cells, characterized by their constitutive expression of the IL-2 receptor α chain (CD25). Recently, FOXP3, a member of the forkhead family of transcription factors, was shown to be highly expressed in Treg cells; FOXP3 is the most widely accepted marker of this Treg cell subset. Mouse models show that Treg cells play an important role in prevention of GVHD [123] and that adoptive transfer of freshly isolated or *ex vivo* expanded CD4+CD25+ T cells can prevent GVHD [124, 125]. In humans, however, it has been difficult to establish a strong and reproducible correlation between the numbers and/or function of Tregs and GVHD severity. Some studies have shown that patients with cGVHD have markedly *elevated* numbers of Treg cells [126]; whereas, others reported *decreased* Treg numbers in cGVHD [127, 128]. Finally, others have failed to find any significant correlation between Treg numbers and cGVHD [129, 130]. Moreover, all activated T cells (not just Treg cells) express FOXP3, calling into question the results of any studies whose conclusions were exclusively based on analysis of FOXP3 expression [131]. Also measurement of Treg cells in the peripheral blood may not be the most reflective of the pathophysiology of cGVHD as evidenced by correlation of the lack of tissue Treg cells ad the presence of cGVHD [132]. Thus, the role of Tregs as a biomarker for cGVHD is not yet resolved. CD4+ effector T cell activation is associated with FOXP3 upregulation and may be a potential reason as to why this may be higher in patients with cGVHD [131]. Future studies are required to evaluate more specifically the role of Tregs and of FOXP3 upregulation in development of cGVHD.

Antigen-Presenting Cells in cGVHD

Although B cell has at least two important functions both of which contribute to cGVHD (production of antibodies and presentation of antigens to T cells), there are other populations that may regulate cGVHD through antigen presentation. It is still unclear whether plasmacytoid (IFN-α producing) DCs (pDCs) play any role in cGVHD. Increased numbers of peripheral blood donor- or host-derived pDCs have been associated with cGVHD in humans [133, 134]. This has been contradicted by other studies showing a lower incidence of cGVHD with the presence of pDCs [135, 136]. Murine models suggest that although either donor or host APCs are sufficient to stimulate skin cGVHD, donor APCs play a dominant role in intestinal cGVHD and that there are target tissue–specific differences in APC requirements. They also suggest that there are differences in APC requirements between CD8-mediated aGVHD and CD4-mediated cGVHD [137]. This difference may explain some of the conflicting findings in humans.

Role of Macrophages, Neutrophils, and Eosinophils

Other myeloid populations have both antigen presentation and potential regulatory functions. Macrophages may have a role especially at the local tissue injury level. Cutaneous and oral cGVHD have an association of CD8+ T cells and increased macrophages and CD1a+ Langerhans cells [138, 139] possible with IL-18 as an important cytokine [140]. Increased peripheral blood eosinophils have had a long-term association with cGVHD [141] although variable in presentation. Use of a cysteinyl leukotriene receptor-1 (cysLT1R) antagonist, Montelukast that specifically targets eosinophils resulted in improvement of skin, liver, and gastrointestinal cGVHD [142].

Role of NK and NKT Cells

There is some murine data supporting that alpha-Gal-Cer responsive–NKT cells may inhibit development of cGVHD in murine models by shifting a Th2 predominant cGVHD model to increased IFN-γ [143]. CD8+ NKT cells that produce IFN-γ may decrease murine GVHD, although the models are most consistent with aGVHD [144]. The role of NKT cells in human cGVHD is uncertain. NK cells may also have a regulatory role in human cGVHD in that a higher donor marrow NK cell dose is associated with an increased speed of neutrophil recovery and a decreased incidence of cGVHD [145].

Inflammatory Responses in cGVHD

Chronic GVHD is associated with a number of inflammatory responses, including alloreactive helper and cytotoxic T (Tc) cells, nonspecific suppressor cells, TNF-α-secreting macrophages, and autoreactive T-cell [146, 147] alterations in the balance of Th1/Tc1 and Th2/Tc2 populations; CD8+/CD28− T cells [34–40] and a decreased proportion of NK (CD3−/CD16+/CD56+) cells in the blood [148]. Cytokines also play a role. cGVHD-associated sclerosis is associated with high concentrations of transforming growth factor-beta (TGF-β), fatigue and wasting with high concentrations of TNF-α, and immunodeficiency with high concentrations of IL-10 and TGF-β [149]. Upon activation in cGVHD, DC and B-lymphocytes secrete inflammatory cytokines after recognition of their cognate antigen. DC and macrophages produce inflammatory cytokines implicated in both autoimmune disease and GVHD, including monocyte chemoattractant protein-1 (MCP-1) [150, 151], IL-6 [51, 52], TGF-β [152] and IFN-α [153]. As a marker of activated T cells, soluble interleukin-2 receptor alpha (sIL-2Rα) has been reported to correlate with severity of aGVHD [154–156], and cGVHD [157, 158] as well as with other autoimmune diseases [159]. It has also been suggested that cutaneous cGVHD may be associated with PDGF elevation [160, 161].

Biomarkers in cGVHD

With improved understanding of the pathophysiology of cGVHD, there has been an increased focus on identifying biomarkers in cGVHD to use therapeutically as well as in increasing the understanding of the pathophysiology of cGVHD in humans. In 2005, at the National Institutes of Health Consensus Development Project on Criteria for Clinical Trials in Chronic Graft-versus-Host Disease: a Biomarkers Working Group identified seven areas in which cGVHD biomarkers may have a role, including the ability to (i) predict response to therapy; (ii) measure disease activity and distinguish irreversible damage from continued disease activity; (iii) predict risk for developing cGVHD; (iv) diagnose cGVHD; (v) assess prognosis of cGVHD; (vi) evaluate GVHD versus GVL or GVT; and (vii) act as surrogate end points for therapeutic response. The group also recommended that the ultimate goal for biomarker identification would be for use as a surrogate end point in clinical management and trials of patients [162].

The biomarkers working group identified five biological categories of potential biomarkers that may play a role in cGVHD:

a. Allogeneic disparity – including HLA A, B, and DRB1 disparities
b. Direct allogeneic immune responses against specific antigens – including minor histocompatibility T-cell and B-cell responses (H-Y and HA-1) and nonspecific autoantibodies (ANA)
c. Inflammatory responses (Th1/Tc1 vs. Th2/Tc2, CpG B-cell responses)

d. Regulatory immune cell populations (Tregs and APC)
e. The immune-modulatory consequences of cGVHD (TREC and TCR Vβ repertoire)

To date, there have been very few large phase III clinical trials evaluating therapy in cGVHD and existing trials suffered from a number of limitations [163]. Biomarker studies are limited by a lack of common consensus on which clinical criteria are the best for evaluation of cGVHD at diagnosis [164] or for therapeutic response [165]. Ideally, biomarker validation would occur in the context of a large multicenter clinical trial that has evaluation of the clinical diagnosis and therapeutic response as one of its primary goals. As noted previously, in 2002, the Children's Oncology Group (COG) undertook a large **National Cancer Institute** (NCI)-funded phase III multicenter pediatric cGVHD therapeutic trial study. This trial evaluated 54 cGVHD patients and 28 controls for a broad simultaneous evaluation of multiple markers was performed to directly compare the relative value of multiple biomarkers in an identical population. The marker had to meet the following two criteria: (i) level had to be significantly different from control and (ii) level was either 100% ± 5% higher or 50% ± 5% lower than the control level. In the COG study, multiple plasma markers that had been identified by single center studies were evaluated [88]. cGVHD has been shown to be associated with alloreactive T-cells, B cells, and DC. As a marker of activated T cells, IL-2Rα has been correlated with cGVHD [25]. DCs and macrophages also produce inflammatory cytokines, such as IFN-γ, TGF-β, MCP-1, and IL-6, which appear to be associated with GVHD and cutaneous cGVHD may be associated with PDGF elevation [166, 167]. To investigate whether these eight soluble factors (including sBAFF) in plasma correlate with cGVHD, compared to matched control without cGVHD, patients' plasma samples were evaluated by enzyme-linked immunosorbent assay (ELISA). They confirmed that an increased level of sBAFF in cGVHD patients with both early- and late-onset cGVHD compared with controls. Soluble IL-2Rα was elevated in early onset of cGVHD but not in late-onset cGVHD. PDGF-BB was elevated in early-onset cGVHD [93] However, the difference did not reach the criteria (100% ± 5% higher) to make PDGF-BB a biomarker for early cGVHD. TGF-β, IFN-α, IL-6, and MCP-1 had no differences [93]. Since production of autoantibodies, especially ANA, had been previously found in 60% to 65% of cGVHD patients, ANA and other autoantibodies were analyzed [33, 34] Although ANA was found in 44.1% of cGVHD patients, control patients without cGVHD also have ANA (32.1%), and the level of ANA did not differ between cGVHD patient and control [88]. Although anti-ds-DNA concentrations were considered to be in the normal range, they were >10 times higher in both early- and late-cGVHD compared to non-cGVHD controls. Antimitochondrial antibody was elevated in early-onset cGVHD, but the difference did not meet our criteria for biomarkers (2-fold increase). Anticardiolipin antibody did not correlate with new-onset cGVHD. The studies also performed exploratory proteomic analyses of plasma obtained from children with and without cGVHD. The analysis identified that sCD13 was elevated in patients with cGVHD.

They found that ~50% of early cGVHD had a >2-fold increase of CD13 enzyme activity compared to controls [88]. The study evaluated NK, NKT, plasmacytoid, and myeloid dendritic cell populations and could not identify any correlation of these peripheral blood populations with cGVHD. By contrast, the study did identify that a TLR9 responsive B-cell population was strongly characteristic of cGVHD [89]. Thus, the study identified five plasma markers (TLR-9 high expressing B cells, sBAFF, sCD13, anti-dsDNA, and IL2R) that had significant correlation with the diagnosis of cGVHD.

Evaluation of factors that may impact on the expression of these biomarkers demonstrated that all were specific for cGVHD and were not markers for aGVHD and that anti-dsDNA antibody was higher than those who did not have a previous history of aGVHD over those who did. Only sBAFF is impacted by previous treatment with steroids [87, 88]. Fibrotic changes associated with ocular, joint, or sclerodermatous skin changes were associated with sBAFF and anti-dsDNA antibody as markers. Soluble CD13 was associated with hepatic involvement.

Each of the markers were evaluated by receiver operating characteristic (ROC) analysis to identify a cutoff value and sensitivity that corresponded to a >90% specificity for the plasma markers. There were not sufficient numbers to perform this for the CpG B cell response. Analysis of the area under the curve (AUC) for the early cGVHD group showed that all were close to or over 0.70 for anti-dsDNA (0.66), IL2Rα (0.83), sCD13 (0.86), and sBAFF (0.70). Sensitivity was relatively low, ranging between 42% and 56% for the four plasma biomarkers. On the basis of the biomarker concentration and sensitivity values at 90% sensitivity for each biomarker conservative cutoff values were anti-dsDNA (2.0 IU/mL), IL2Rα (10 ng/mL), sCD13 (1.8 units/mL), and sBAFF (7.5 ng/mL) at 90% specificity. The sBAFF cutoff in children appears lower than in adults (>10.0 ng/mL) [87]. Analysis of the four plasma biomarkers (sBAFF, anti-dsDNA, sCD13, and IL2Rα) in combination revealed that the overall sensitivity was relatively high (84%) if ≥1 of the 4 markers were positive in patients with cGVHD. Specificity was high (100%). Thus, it is possible that a combination of biomarkers will give higher sensitivity, specificity, and positive predictive value for cGVHD diagnosis. Evaluation of each biomarker as a surrogate end point of therapeutic response at an earlier time point (i.e., at 1 or 2 months after start of therapy) found that sBAFF and TLR9 high expressing CpG responsive B cells have potential as a surrogate end points for therapeutic response, but validation is required.

Impact of Immune Reconstitution on the Development of cGVHD

Immune reconstitution appears to have a major impact on the development of cGVHD. One good illustration of this fact is the higher rate of cGVHD after G-CSF mobilized peripheral blood compared to marrow transplants. One major observation is that T cell recovery after peripheral blood transplantation is more rapid whereas NK cell and monocyte recovery is the same [166, 167]. This is possibly due to a slower T-cell expansion after peripheral blood transplantation due to a higher initial T-cell infusion since the T-cell recolonization is closer to the "threshold size" [168]. T cells after peripheral blood transplantation appear to have a lower T-cell activation [167]. B-cell recovery also appears to be more rapid after peripheral blood progenitor cell (PBPC) transplantation [166, 167] with a higher risk of anti-A or anti-B antibodies after PBPC transplantation in ABO-mismatched donor recipient pairs [169]. Anti-HLA antibodies are also higher after PBPC transplants [170]. That PBPC is associated with a higher level of B-cell activation as evidenced by CDR0 expressing populations and increase Ig production may also be part of the more rapid B-cell reconstitution after PBC and subsequent development of cGVHD [171, 172]. Additional support on the importance of immune reconstitution of the development of cGVHD is shown by the observation that the biology of cGVHD is time dependent after BMT and different mechanisms may be important in the development of cGVHD depending on the time that cGVHD develops. Interpretation of results should take into consideration the impact of immune reconstitution post BMT.

How cGVHD may be Classified by Pathophysiology in the Future

The COG study ASCT0031 was one of the first studies to evaluate multiple immunological markers and mechanisms simultaneously in the identical patient population. There were a number of findings that have resulted in our proposal of a tentative cGVHD model. One of the major findings from the ASCT0031 study was that there are immunological differences between cGVHD that occurs early after BMT (3–9 months) compared to late onset (≥9 months post BMT). In the early-onset cGVHD the dominant characteristics were (a) lack of IFN-γ production; (b) a higher numbers of regulatory T cells; (c) an inflammatory response with a predominance of T-cell cytokines such as IL-2Rα; and (d) T-cell activation with associated sIL2R and sBAFF (Figure 3.1). Late-onset cGVHD was associated with (a) B-cell activation including sBAFF, TLR9 high expressing B cells, autoantibodies; and (b) a lack of induction of Th2 predominance. This has led us to generate a tentative model that T-cell activation with sIL2R, sBAFF, and FOXP3 upregulation is part of early cGVHD and that IFN-γ production is required for CD8+ T-cell contraction and inhibition of B-cell expansion, and antibody production [43] (see Figure 3.2). Late-onset cGVHD (Figure 3.3) is characterized by a lack of Th2 shift and development of activated TLR9 high expressing B cells that have upregulated BAFF expression in B cells [173] and by the fact that TLR9 actvation in combination with sBAFF results in increased autoantibody production [173, 174]. It should be noted that in this proposed preliminary model, we have not included all proposed and published mechanisms but have focused on integrating the findings of the preliminary COG study that included simultaneous measurement of a large number of potential markers. Thus, we consider this the first step in a more comprehensive process to identify the relationship of various mechanisms of cGVHD.

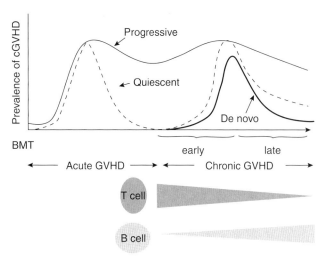

Figure 3.1 The time of onset of chronic graft versus host disease in relationship to acute GVHD.

Acute graft versus host disease (GVHD) appears to have a predominance of T-cell responses where as chronic GVHD has a B-cell predominance. There is much overlap in the two diseases and the late-onset acute GVDH probably reflects a hybrid of the two.

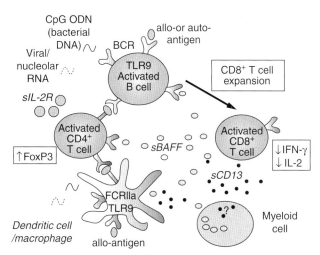

Figure 3.2 Pathophysiology of early-onset chronic graft versus host disease.

Chronic graft versus host disease (GVDH) that develops between 3 and 9 months appears to have a predominance of inflammatory responses with increase interleukin (IL2Rα), soluble CD13, CD8+ T-cell expansion, and increased B-cell activation with increased Toll-like receptor 9 (TLR9)-high expressing B cells and soluble B-cell activating factor of the TNF family (BAFF).

BCR, B-cell receptor; CpG ODN, CpG oligodeoxynucleotides; FCRIIa, Fc receptor II alpha; FOXP3, forkhead box P3; IFN-γ, interferon-gamma; RNA, ribonucleic acid.

An additional potential model that addresses the fibrotic changes associated with sclerodermatous skin cGVHD, bronchiolitis obliterans, and sicca syndrome are characterized by a two phase pathophysiology. The initial phase is based on activation of the innate pathway through the TLR pathways followed by activation of alloreactive T cells. Inflammatory signals would include infection (bacterial and viral), cytotoxic agents, and

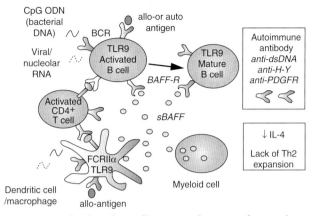

Figure 3.3. Pathophysiology of late-onset chronic graft versus host disease.

Chronic graft versus host disease (GVHD) that develops after 9 months posttransplantation appears to have a predominace of autoantibodies such as anti-dsDNA, anti-H-Y and antiplatelet-derived growth factor receptor-alpha (PDGFRα).

BAFF, B-cell activating factor of the TNF family; BCR, B-cell receptor; CpG ODN, CpG oligodeoxynucleotides; FCRIIα, Fc receptor II alpha.

aGVHD. This phase would be characterized by expression of TNFα, IFN-γ, IL-4, IL-6, IL2/IL2Ra, CD13, sBAFF, and others. The second phase is characterized by PDGF and PDGFR with secondary activation of TGF-β. Such a model would explain the findings that both recipient NOD2/CARD15 variants were associated with TLR2/4 signaling polymorphisms [175]. and PDGF [176] are associated with bronchiolitis obliterans. Since the NOD2/CARD15 variant results in defective TLR2/4 signaling, appears that these recipients have increased pulmonary infection deaths [177] in which repeated infections appear to play a role. Similarly sBAFF and TLR9 high expressing B cells [79, 87] and PDGFR antibodies [122] may be associated with sclerodermatous skin involvement with a two-phase response.

Key Points

1. The pathophysiology of cGVHD is still poorly understood and has many pathophysiological differences from aGVHD.
2. The time of onset of cGVHD appears to reflect differences in the pathophysiology of cGVHD.
3. Activation of B cells and production of autoantibodies is a major factor in many patients with cGVHD.
4. Activation through the innate pathways as controlled by the TLRs appears to be a major initial part of development of cGVHD.
5. The fibrotic changes seen as cGVHD progresses in the skin and lungs appear to be part of the evolution of cGVHD from an inflammatory response to responses mediated by PDGFRα and TGFβ.
6. Identification of biomarkers in human cGVHD is important to better understand cGVHD as animal models appears to have very limited application to cGVHD and develop better therapeutic strategies.
7. Aberrant immune reconstitution impacts on development of cGVHD.

REFERENCES

1. Ozawa S, Nakaseko C, Nishimura M, et al. Chronic graft-versus-host disease after allogeneic bone marrow transplantation from an unrelated donor: incidence, risk factors and association with relapse. A report from the Japan Marrow Donor Program. *Br J Haematol.* 2007 Apr;137(2):142–151.
2. Ferrara JL, Reddy P. Pathophysiology of graft-versus-host disease. *Semin Hematol.* 2006 Jan;43(1):3–10.
3. Zhou L, Askew D, Wu C, Gilliam AC. Cutaneous gene expression by DNA microarray in murine sclerodermatous graft-versus-host disease, a model for human scleroderma. *J Invest Dermatol.* 2007 Feb;127(2):281–292.
4. Chen W, Chatta GS, Rubin WD, et al. T cells specific for a polymorphic segment of CD45 induce graft-versus-host disease with predominant pulmonary vasculitis. *J Immunol.* 1998 Jul 15;161(2):909–918.
5. Zhang C, Todorov I, Zhang Z, et al. Donor CD4+ T and B cells in transplants induce chronic graft-versus-host disease with autoimmune manifestations. *Blood.* 2006 Apr 1;107(7):2993–3001.
6. Rocha V, Wagner JE Jr, Sobocinski KA, et al. Graft-versus-host disease in children who have received a cord-blood or bone marrow transplant from an HLA-identical sibling. Eurocord and International Bone Marrow Transplant Registry Working Committee on Alternative Donor and Stem Cell Sources. *N Engl J Med.* 2000 Jun 22;342(25):1846–1854.
7. Frangoul H, Nemecek ER, Billheimer D, et al. A prospective study of G-CSF primed bone marrow as a stem-cell source for allogeneic bone marrow transplantation in children: a Pediatric Blood and Marrow Transplant Consortium (PBMTC) study. *Blood.* 2007 Dec 15;110(13):4584–4587.
8. Eapen M, Logan BR, Confer DL, et al. Peripheral blood grafts from unrelated donors are associated with increased acute and chronic graft-versus-host disease without improved survival. *Biol Blood Marrow Transplant.* 2007 Dec;13(12):1461–1468. *Epub* 2007 Oct 10.
9. Schrezenmeier H, Passweg JR, Marsh JC, et al. Worse outcome and more chronic GVHD with peripheral blood progenitor cells than bone marrow in HLA-matched sibling donor transplants for young patients with severe acquired aplastic anemia. *Blood.* 2007 Aug 15;110(4):1397–1400. *Epub* 2007 May 2.
10. Buzzeo MP, Yang J, Casella G, Reddy V. Hematopoietic stem cell mobilization with G-CSF induces innate inflammation yet suppresses adaptive immune gene expression as revealed by microarray analysis. *Exp Hematol.* 2007 Sep;35(9):1456–1465.
11. Talarn C, Urbano-Ispizua A, Martino R, et al. G-CSF increases the number of peripheral blood dendritic cells CD16+ and modifies the expression of the costimulatory molecule CD86+. *Bone Marrow Transplant.* 2006 May;37(9):873–879.
12. Garderet L, Dulphy N, Douay C, et al. The umbilical cord blood alphabeta T-cell repertoire: characteristics of a polyclonal and naive but completely formed repertoire. *Blood.* 1998 Jan 1;91(1):340–346.
13. Canaday DH, Chakravarti S, Srivastava T, et al. Class II MHC antigen presentation defect in neonatal monocytes is not correlated with decreased MHC-II expression. *Cell Immunol.* 2006 Oct;243(2):96–106.
14. Shier LR, Schultz KR, Imren S, et al. Differential effects of granulocyte colony-stimulating factor on marrow- and blood-derived hematopoietic and immune cell populations in healthy human donors. *Biol Blood Marrow Transplant.* 2004 Sep;10(9):624–634.

15. Ringdén O, Labopin M, Gorin NC, et al. Treatment with granulocyte colony-stimulating factor after allogeneic bone marrow transplantation for acute leukemia increases the risk of graft-versus-host disease and death: a study from the Acute Leukemia Working Party of the European Group for Blood and Marrow Transplantation. *J Clin Oncol.* 2004 Feb 1;22(3):416–423. *Epub 2003 Dec 22.*

16. Bacigalupo A, Lamparelli T, Barisione G, et al; Gruppo Italiano Trapianti Midollo Osseo (GITMO). Thymoglobulin prevents chronic graft-versus-host disease, chronic lung dysfunction, and late transplant-related mortality: long-term follow-up of a randomized trial in patients undergoing unrelated donor transplantation. *Biol Blood Marrow Transplant.* 2006 May;12(5):560–565.

17. Siegal D, Xu W, Sutherland R, et al. Graft-versus-host disease following marrow transplantation for aplastic anemia: different impact of two GVHD prevention strategies. *Bone Marrow Transplant.* 2008 Mar 31. Epub ahead of print.

18. Hale G, Zhang MJ, Bunjes D, et al. Improving the outcome of bone marrow transplantation by using CD52 monoclonal antibodies to prevent graft-versus-host disease and graft rejection. *Blood.* 1998 Dec 15;92(12):4581–4590.

19. Morris E, Thomson K, Craddock C, et al. Outcomes after alemtuzumab containing reduced-intensity allogeneic transplantation regimen for relapsed and refractory non-Hodgkin lymphoma.*Blood.* 2004 Dec 15;104(13):3865–3871.

20. Pavletic SZ, Carter SL, Keman NA, et al. Influence of T-cell depletion on chronic graft-versus-host disease: results of a multicenter randomized trial in unrelated marrow donor transplantation. *Blood.* 2005;106:3308–3313.

21. Castro-Malaspina H, Jabubowski AA, Papadopoulos EB, et al. Transplantation in remission improves the disease-free survival of patients with advanced myelodysplastic syndromes treated with myeloablative T cell-depleted stem cell transplants from HLA-identical siblings. *Biol Blood Marrow Transplant.* 2008 Apr;14(4):458–468.

22. Remberger M, Kumlien G, Aschan J, et al. Risk factors for moderate-to-severe chronic graft-versus-host disease after allogeneic hematopoietic stem cell transplantation. *Biol Blood Marrow Transplant.* 2002;8(12):674–682.

23. Kollman C, Howe CW, Anasetti C, et al. Donor characteristics as risk factors in recipients after transplantation of bone marrow from unrelated donors: the effect of donor age. *Blood.* 2001;98:2043–2051.

24. Randolph SS, Gooley TA, Warren EH, Appelbaum FR, Riddell SR. Female donors contribute to a selective graft-versus-leukemia effect in male recipients of HLA-matched, related hematopoietic stem cell transplants. *Blood.* 2004;103:347–352.

25. Yamashita K, Choi U, Woltz PC, et al. Severe chronic graft-versus-host disease is characterized by a preponderance of CD4(+) effector memory cells relative to central memory cells. *Blood.* 2004 May 15;103(10):3986–3988. *Epub 2004 Feb 5.*

26. Petersen SL, Ryder LP, Björk P, et al. A comparison of T-, B- and NK-cell reconstitution following conventional or non-myeloablative conditioning and transplantation with bone marrow or peripheral blood stem cells from human leucocyte antigen identical sibling donors. *Bone Marrow Transplant.* 2003 Jul;32(1):65–72.

27. Mielcarek M, Martin PJ, Leisenring W, et al. Graft-versus-host disease after nonmyeloablative versus conventional hematopoietic stem cell transplantation. *Blood.* 2003 Jul 15;102(2):756–762. Epub 2003 Mar 27.

28. Larsson K, Aschan J, Remberger M, Ringdén O, Winiarski J, Ljungman P. Reduced risk for extensive chronic graft-versus-host disease in patients receiving transplants with human leukocyte antigen-identical sibling donors given polymerase chain reaction-based preemptive therapy against cytomegalovirus. *Transplantation.* 2004 Feb 27;77(4):526–531.

29. Wojnar J, Giebel S, Holowiecka-Goral A, et al. The incidence and risk factors for chronic graft-versus-host-disease. *Ann Transplant.* 2006;11(2):14–20; discussion 32–43.

30. Freudenberger TD, Madtes DK, Curtis JR, Cummings P, Storer BE, Hackman RC. Association between acute and chronic graft-versus-host disease and bronchiolitis obliterans organizing pneumonia in recipients of hematopoietic stem cell transplants. *Blood.* 2003 Nov 15;102(10):3822–3828. *Epub 2003 Jul 17.*

31. Schmid I, Stachel D, Pagel P, Albert MH. Incidence, predisposing factors, and outcome of engraftment syndrome in pediatric allogeneic stem cell transplant recipients. *Biol Blood Marrow Transplant.* 2008 Apr;14(4):438–444.

32. van Els CA, Bakker A, Zwinderman AH, Zwaan FE, van Rood JJ, Goulmy E. Effector mechanisms in graft-versus-host disease in response to minor histocompatibility antigens. I. Absence of correlation with cytotoxic effector cells. *Transplantation.* 1990 Jul;50(1):62–66.

33. de Bueger M, Bakker A, Bontkes H, van Rood JJ, Goulmy E. High frequencies of cytotoxic T cell precursors against minor histocompatibility antigens after HLA-identical BMT: absence of correlation with GVHD. *Bone Marrow Transplant.* 1993 May;11(5):363–368.

34. Via CS, Rus V, Gately MK, Finkelman FD. IL-12 stimulates the development of acute graft-versus-host disease in mice that normally would develop chronic, autoimmune graft-versus-host disease. *J Immunol.* 1994;153:4040–4047.

35. Nikolic B, Lee S, Bronson RT, Grusby MJ, Sykes M. Th1 and Th2 mediate acute graft-versus-host disease, each with distinct end-organ targets. *J Clin Invest.* 2000;105:1289–1298.

36. Liu J, Anderson BE, Robert ME, et al. Selective T-cell subset ablation demonstrates a role for T1 and T2 cells in ongoing acute graft-versus-host disease: a model system for the reversal of disease. *Blood.* 2001;98:3367–3375.

37. Nakamura K, Amakawa R, Takebayashi M, et al. IL-4-producing CD8(+) T cells may be an Immunological hallmark of chronic GVHD. *Bone Marrow Transplant.* 2005;36:639–647.

38. Silva MG, Ferreira Neto L, Guimaraes A, Machado A, Parreira A, Abecasis M. Long-term follow-up of lymphocyte populations and cellular cytokine production in patients with chronic graft-versus-host disease treated with extracorporeal photopheresis. *Haematologica.* 2005;90:565–567.

39. Darvay A, Salooja N, Russell-Jones R. The effect of extracorporeal photopheresis on intracellular cytokine expression in chronic cutaneous graft-versus-host disease. *J Eur Acad Dermatol Venereol.* 2004 May;18(3):279–284.

40. Ritchie D, Seconi J, Wood C, Walton J, Watt V. Prospective monitoring of tumor necrosis factor alpha and interferon gamma to predict the onset of acute and chronic graft-versus-host disease after allogeneic stem cell transplantation. *Biol Blood Marrow Transplant.* 2005;11:706–712.

41. Cavet J, Dickinson AM, Norden J, et al. Interferon-gamma and interleukin-6 gene polymorphisms associate with graft-versus-host disease in HLA-matched sibling bone marrow transplantation. *Blood.* 2001;98:1594–1600.

42. Bogunia-Kubik K, Mlynarczewska A, Wysoczanska B, Lange A. Recipient interferon-gamma 3/3 genotype contributes to the development of chronic graft-versus-host disease after allogeneic hematopoietic stem cell transplantation. *Haematologica.* 2005 Mar;90(3):425–426.

43. Puliaev R, Nguyen P, Finkelman FD, Via CS. Differential requirement for IFN-gamma in CTL maturation in acute murine graft-versus-host disease. *J Immunol.* 2004 Jul 15;173(2):910–919.

44. Asavaroengchai W, Wang H, Wang S, et al. An essential role for IFN-gamma in regulation of alloreactive CD8 T cells following allogeneic hematopoietic cell transplantation. *Biol Blood Marrow Transplant.* 2007 Jan;13(1):46–55.

45. Kim JH, Choi EY, Chung DH. Donor bone marrow type II (non-Valpha14Jalpha18 CD1d-restricted) NKT cells suppress graft-versus-host disease by producing IFN-gamma and IL-4. *J Immunol.* 2007 Nov 15;179(10):6579–6587.

46. Badovinac VP, Porter BB, Harty JT. CD8+ T cell contraction is controlled by early inflammation. *Nat Immunol.* 2004 Aug;5(8):809–817.

47. Sashida G, Ohyashiki JH, Kubota N, et al. Marked telomere fluctuation of leukocytes during graft-versus-host disease in allogeneic stem cell transplantation. *Int J Mol Med.* 2005 Nov;16(5):883–888.

48. Yamashita K, Choi U, Woltz PC, et al. Severe Chronic Graft-Versus-Host Disease is characterized by a Preponderance of CD4+ Effector Memory Cells Relative to Central Memory Cells. *Blood.* 2004;103(10):3986–3988.

49. Xystrakis E, Bernard I, Dejean AS, Alsaati T, Druet P, Saoudi A. Alloreactive CD4 T lymphocytes responsible for acute and chronic graft-versus-host disease are contained within the CD45RC high but not the CD45RC low subset. *Eur J Immunol.* 2004;34(2):408–417.

50. Biedermann BC, Sahner S, Gregor M, et al. Endothelial injury mediated by cytotoxic T lymphocytes and loss of microvessels in chronic graft versus host disease. *Lancet.* 2002 Jun 15;359(9323):2078–2083 .

51. Patey-Mariaud de Serre N, Reijasse D, Verkarre V, et al. Chronic intestinal graft-versus-host disease: clinical, histological and immunohistochemical analysis of 17 children. *Bone Marrow Transplant.* 2002 Feb;29(3):223–230.

52. Kotani A, Ishikawa T, Matsumura Y, et al. Correlation of peripheral blood OX40+(CD134+) T cells with chronic graft-versus-host disease in patients who underwent allogeneic hematopoietic stem cell transplantation. *Blood.* 2001 Nov 15;98(10):3162–3164.

53. Sasaki M, Hasegawa H, Kohno M, Inoue A, Ito MR, Fujita S. Antagonist of secondary lymphoid-tissue chemokine (CCR ligand 21) prevents the development of chronic graft-versus-host disease in mice. *J Immunol.* 2003 Jan 1;170(1):588–596.

54. Cavet J, Dickinson AM, Norden J, Taylor PR, Jackson GH, Middleton PG. Interferon-gamma and interleukin-6 gene polymorphisms associate with graft-versus-host disease in HLA-matched sibling bone marrow transplantation. *Blood.* 2001 Sep 1;98(5):1594–1600.

55. Stark GL, Dickinson AM, Jackson GH, Taylor PR, Proctor SJ, Middleton PG. Tumour necrosis factor receptor type II 196M/R genotype correlates with circulating soluble receptor levels in normal subjects and with graft-versus-host disease after sibling allogeneic bone marrow transplantation. *Transplantation.* 2003 Dec 27;76(12):1742–1749.

56. Rocha V, Franco RF, Porcher R, et al. Host defense and inflammatory gene polymorphisms are associated with outcomes after HLA-identical sibling bone marrow transplantation. *Blood.* 2002 Dec 1;100(12):3908–3918.

57. Lin MT, Storer B, Martin PJ, et al. Relation of an interleukin-10 promoter polymorphism to graft-versus-host disease and survival after hematopoietic-cell transplantation. *N Engl J Med.* 2003 Dec 4;349(23):2201–2210.

58. Zhang Y, Hexner E, Frank D, Emerson SG. CD4+ T cells generated de novo from donor hemopoietic stem cells mediate the evolution from acute to chronic graft-versus-host disease. *J Immunol.* 2007 Sep 1;179(5):3305–3314.

59. Zhang C, Todorov I, Zhang Z, et al. Donor CD4+ T and B cells in transplants induce chronic graft-versus-host disease with autoimmune manifestations. *Blood.* 2006 Apr 1;107(7):2993–3001. *Epub* 2005 Dec 13.

60. Sakoda Y, Hashimoto D, Asakura S, et al. Donor-derived thymic-dependent T cells cause chronic graft-versus-host disease. *Blood.* 2007 Feb 15;109(4):1756–1764. Epub 2006 Oct 10.

61. Weinberg K, Blazar BR, Wagner JE, et al. Factors affecting thymic function after allogeneic hematopoietic stem cell transplantation. *Blood.* 2001 Mar 1;97(5):1458–1466.

62. Fallen PR, McGreavey L, Madrigal JA, et al. Factors affecting reconstitution of the T cell compartment in allogeneic haematopoietic cell transplant recipients. *Bone Marrow Transplant.* 2003 Nov;32(10):1001–1014.

63. Wysoczanska B, Bogunia-Kubik K, Dlubek D, et al. Association with the presence of naive T cells in chronic myeloid leukemia patients after allogeneic human stem cell transplantation and the lower incidence of chronic graft-versus host disease and relapse. *Transplant Proc.* 2007 Nov;39(9):2898–2901.

64. Clave E, Rocha V, Talvensaari K, et al. Prognostic value of pretransplantation host thymic function in HLA-identical sibling hematopoietic stem cell transplantation. *Blood.* 2005 Mar 15;105(6):2608–2613.

65. Sullivan K, Storb R, Buckner D, Fefer A. Graft-versus host disease as adoptic immunotherapy in patients with advanced hematologic neoplasms. *N Engl J Med.* 1989;320:828–834.

66. Ordermann R, Hutchinson R, Friedman J, et al. Enhanced allostimulatory activity of host antigen-presenting cells in old mice intensifies acute graft-versus-host disease. *J Clin Inv.* 2002;109:1249–1256.

67. Zhang C, Todorov I, Zhang Z, et al. Donor CD4+ T and B cells in transplants induce chronic graft- versus host disease with autoimmune manifestations. *Blood.* 2006;107:2993–3001.

68. Schlomchik WD, Couzens MS, Tang CB, et al. Preventation of graft-versus host disease by inactivation of host antigen-presenting cells. *Science.* 1999;285:412–415.

69. Lang TJ, Nguyen P, Peach R, Grause WC, Via CS. In vivo CD86 blockade inhibits CD4+ T cell activation, whereas CD80 blockade potentiates CD8+ T cell activation and CTL effector function. *J Immunol.* 2002;168:3786–3792.

70. Schultz KR, Paquet J, Bader S, HayGlass KT. Requirement for B cells in T cell priming to minor histocompatibility antigens and development of graft-versus-host disease. *Bone Marrow Transplant.* 1995;16:289–295.

71. Zorn E, Miklos DB, Floyd BH, et al. Minor histocompatibility antigen DBY elicits a coordinated B and T cell response after allogeneic stem cell transplantation. *J Exp Med.* 2004;199:1133–1142.

72. Perruche S, Marandin A, Kleinclauss F, et al. Association of mixed hematopoietic chimerism with elevated circulating autoantibodies and chronic graft-versus-host disease occurrence. *Transplantation*. 2006 Feb 27;81(4):573–582.

73. Cutler C, Miklos D, Kim HT, et al. Rituximab for steroid-refractory chronic graft-versus-host disease. *Blood*. 2006 Jul 15;108(2):756–762. Epub 2006 Mar 21.

74. Ratanatharathorn V, Ayash L, Reynolds C, et al. Treatment of chronic graft-versus-host disease with anti-CD20 monoclonal antibody. *Biol Blood Marrow Transplant*. 2003;9:505–511.

75. Canninga-van Dijk MR, van der Straaten HM, Fijnheer R, Sanders CJ, van den Tweel JG, Verdonck LF. Anti-CD20 monoclonal antibody treatment in 6 patients with therapy-refractory chronic graft-versus-host disease. *Blood*. 2004 Oct 15;104(8):2603–2606.

76. Blazar BR, Krieg AM, Taylor PA. Synthetic unmethylated cytosine-phosphate-guanosine oligodeoxynucleotides are potent stimulators of antileukemia response in naïve and bone marrow transplant recipients. *Blood*. 2001;98:1217–1225.

77. Schultz KR, Su WN, Hsiao CC, et al. Chloroquine prevention of murine MHC-disparate acute graft-versus host disease correlates with inhibition of splenic response to CpG oligodeoxynucleotides and alterations in T cell cytokine production. *Biol Blood and Marrow Transplant*. 2002;8:648–655.

78. MacFarlane DE, Manzel L. Antagonism of immunostimulatory CpG-oligodeoxynucleotides by quinacrine, chloroquine, and structurally related compounds. *J Immunol*. 1998;160:1122–1131.

79. She K, Gilman AL, Aslanian S, et al. Altered Toll-like receptor 9 responses in circulating B cells at the onset of extensive chronic graft-versus-host disease. *Biol Blood Marrow Transplant*. 2007 Apr;13(4):386–397. Epub 2007 Feb 15.

80. Bernasconi NL, Onai N, Lanzavecchia A. A role for Toll-like receptors in acquired immunity: upregulation of TLR9 by BCR triggering in naïve B cells and constitutive expression in memory B cells. *Blood*. 2003;101:4500–4504.

81. Miklos DB, Kim HT, Zorn E, et al. Antibody response to DBY minor histocompatibility antigen is induced after allogeneic stem cell transplantation and in healthy female donors. *Blood*. 2004;103:353–359.

82. Miklos DB, Kim HT, Miller KH, et al. Antibody responses to H-Y minor histocompatibility antigens correlate with chronic graft-versus-host disease and disease remission. *Blood*. 2005;105:2973–2978.

83. Brink R. 2006. Regulation of B cell self-tolerance by BAFF. *Semin Immunol* 18:276–283.

84. Tangye SG, Bryant VL, Cuss AK, Good KL 2006. BAFF, APRIL and human B cell disorders. *Semin Immunol* 18:305–317.

85. Zhang J, Roscke V, Baker KP, et al. Cutting edge: a role for B lymphocyte stimulator in systemic lupus erythematosus. *J. Immunol*. 2001;166:6–10.

86. Cheema GS, Roschke V, Hilbert DM, Stohl W. Elevated serum B lymphocyte stimulator levels in patients with systemic immune-based rheumatic diseases. *Arthritis Rheum*. 2001;44:1313–1319.

87. Sarantopoulos S, Stevenson KE, Kim HT, et al. High levels of B-cell activating factor in patients with active chronic graft-versus-host disease. *Clin Cancer Res*. 2007 Oct 15;13(20):6107–6114.

88. Fujii H, Cuvelier G, She K, et al. Biomarkers in newly diagnosed pediatric-extensive chronic graft-versus-host disease: a report from the Children's Oncology Group. *Blood*. 2008 Mar 15;111(6):3276–3285. *Epub* 2007 Oct 9.

89. Miller I, Hatzivassiliou G, Cattoretti G, Mendelsohn C, Dalla-Favera R. IRTAs: a new family of immunoglobulin-like receptors differentially expressed in B cells. *Blood*. 2002 Apr 15;99(8):2662–2669.

90. Kochi Y, Yamada R, Suzuki A, et al. A functional variant in FCRL3, encoding Fc receptor-like 3, is associated with rheumatoid arthritis and several autoimmunities [Erratum in: Nat Genet. 2005 Jun;37(6):652] *Nat Genet*. 2005 May;37(5):478–485. *Epub* 2005 Apr 17.

91. Shimada M, Onizuka M, Machida S, et al. Association of autoimmune disease-related gene polymorphisms with chronic graft-versus-host disease. *Br J Haematol*. 2007 Nov;139(3):458–463. *Epub* 2007 Sep 14.

92. Chistiakov DA, Chistiakov AP. Is FCRL3 a new general autoimmunity gene? *Hum Immunol*. 2007 May;68(5):375–383. *Epub* 2007 Feb 15. Review.

93. Greinix HT, Pohlreich D, Kouba M, et al. Elevated numbers of immature/transitional CD21- B lymphocytes and deficiency of memory CD27+ B cells identify patients with active chronic graft-versus-host disease. *Biol Blood Marrow Transplant*. 2008 Feb;14(2):208–219.

94. Vossen JM, Heidt PJ, van den Berg H, Hermans J, Dooren LJ. Prevention of infection and graft-versus host disease by suppression of intestinal microflora in children treated with allogeneic bone marrow transplantation. *Eur J Clin Microbiol Infect Dis*. 1990;9:14–23.

95. Taylor PA, Friedman TM, Korngold R, Noelle R, Blazar BR. Tolerance induction of alloreactive T cells via ex vivo blockade of CD40:CD40L co-stimulatory pathway results in the generation of potent immune regulatory cell. *Blood*. 2002;99:4601–4609.

96. Lang TJ, Nguyen P, Peach R, Gause WC, Via CS. In vivo CD86 blockade inhibits CD4+ T cell activation, whereas CD80 blockade potentiates CD8+ T cell activation and CTL effector function. *J Imm*. 2002;168:3786–3792.

97. Gilman AL, Chan KW, Mogul M, et al. Hydroxychloroquine for the treatment of chronic graft-versus-host disease. *Biol Blood Marrow Transplant*. 2000;6:327–334.

98. Schultz KR, Bader S, Paquet J, Li W. Chloroquine treatment affects T-cell priming to minor histocompatibility antigens and graft-versus-host disease. *Blood*. 1995 Dec 1;86(11):4344–4352.

99. Lönnqvist B, Ringdén O, Wahren B, Gahrton G, Lundgren G. Cytomegalovirus infection associated with and preceding chronic graft-versus-host disease. *Transplantation*. 1984 Nov;38(5):465–458.

100. Soderberg C, Sumitran-Karuppan S, Ljungman P, Moller E. CD13-specific autoimmunity in cytomegalovirus-infected immunocompromised patients. *Transplantation*. 1996 Feb 27;61(4):594–600.

101. Soderberg C, Larsson S, Rozell BL, Sumitran-Karuppan S, Ljungman P, Moller E. Cytomegalovirus-induced CD13-specific autoimmunity-a possible cause of chronic graft-vs-host disease. *Transplantation*. 1996 Feb 27;61(4):600–609.

102. Naucler CS, Larsson S, Moller E. A novel mechanism for virus-induced autoimmunity in humans. *Immunol Rev*. 1996; 152: 175–92.74a.

103. Hildebrandt GC, Granell M, Urbano-Ispizua A, et al. Recipient NOD2/CARD15 variants: a novel independent risk factor for the development of bronchiolitis obliterans after allogeneic

stem cell transplantation. *Biol Blood Marrow Transplant*. 2008 Jan;14(1):67–74.

104. Mutis T, Gillespie G, Schrama E, Falkenburg JH, Moss P, Goulmy E. Tetrameric HLA class I-minor histocompatibility antigen peptide complexes demonstrate minor histocompatibility antigen-specific cytotoxic T lymphocytes in patients with graft-versus-host disease. *Nat Med*. 1999 Jul;5(7):839–842.

105. Gallardo D, Arostegui JI, Balas A, et al. GvHD Subcommittee of the Grupo Espanol de Trasplante Hemapoyetico (GETH). Disparity for the minor histocompatibility antigen HA-1 is associated with an increased risk of acute graft-versus-host disease (GvHD) but it does not affect chronic GvHD incidence, disease-free survival or overall survival after allogeneic human leucocyte antigen-identical sibling donor transplantation. *Br J Haematol*. 2001 Sep;114(4):931–936

106. Lin MT, Gooley T, Hansen JA, et al. Absence of statistically significant correlation between disparity for the minor histocompatibility antigen-HA-1 and outcome after allogeneic hematopoietic cell transplantation. *Blood*. 2001 Nov 15;98(10):3172–3173.

107. Grumet FC, Hiraki DD, Brown BWM, et al. D31 mismatching affects marrow transplantation outcome. *Biol Blood Marrow Transplant*. 2001;7(9):503–512.

108. Flowers ME, Pepe MS, Longton G, et al. Previous donor pregnancy as a risk factor for acute graft-versus-host disease in patients with aplastic anaemia treated by allogeneic marrow transplantation. *Br J Haematol*. 1990;74:492–496.

109. Kollman C, Howe CW, Anasetti C, et al. Donor characteristics as risk factors in recipients after transplantation of bone marrow from unrelated donors: the effect of donor age. *Blood*. 2001;98:2043–2051.

110. Randolph SS, Gooley TA, Warren EH, Appelbaum FR, Riddell SR. Female donors contribute to a selective graft-versus-leukemia effect in male recipients of HLA-matched, related hematopoietic stem cell transplants. *Blood*. 2004;103:347–352.

111. Miklos DB, Kim HT, Zorn E, et al. Antibody response to DBY minor histocompatibility antigen is induced after allogeneic stem cell transplantation and in healthy female donors. *Blood*. 2004;103:353–359.

112. Miklos DB, Kim HT, Miller KH, et al. Antibody Responses to H-Y Minor Histocompatibility Antigens Correlate with Chronic Graft versus Host Disease and Disease Remission. *Blood*. 2005;105:2973–2978.

113. Patriarca F, Skert C, Sperotto A, et al. The development of autoantibodies after allogeneic stem cell transplantation is related with chronic graft-vs-host disease and immune recovery. *Exp Hematol*. 2006;34:389–396.

114. Rouquette-Gally AM, Boyeldieu D, Prost AC, Gluckman E. Autoimmunity after allogeneic bone marrow transplantation. A study of 53 long-term-surviving patients. *Transplantation*. 1988;46:238–240.

115. Quaranta S, Shulman H, Ahmed A, et al. Autoantibodies in human chronic graft-versus-host disease after hematopoietic cell transplantation. *Clin Immunol*. 1999; 91:106–116.

116. Wechalekar A, Cranfield T, Sinclair D, Ganzckowski M. Occurrence of autoantibodies in chronic graft vs. host disease after allogeneic stem cell transplantation. *Clin. Lab. Haem*. 2005;27:247–249.

117. Graze PR, Gale RP. Chronic graft versus host disease: a syndrome of disordered immunity. *Am J Med*.1979 Apr;66(4):611–620.

118. Shulman HM, Sullivan KM, Weiden PL, et al. Chronic graft-versus-host syndrome in man. A long-term clinico-pathologic study of 20 Seattle patients. *Am J Med*. 1980 Aug;69(2):204–217.

119. Quaranta S, Shulman H, Ahmed A, et al. Autoantibodies in human chronic graft-versus-host disease after hematopoietic cell transplantation. *Clin Immunol*. 1999 Apr;91(1):106–116.

120. Vogelsang GB. How I treat chronic graft-versus-host disease. *Blood*. 2001 Mar 1;97(5):1196–1201.

121. Svegliati S, Olivieri A, Campelli N, et al. Stimulatory autoantibodies to PDGF receptor in patients with extensive chronic graft-versus-host disease. *Blood* 2007:110, 237–241.

122. Baroni SS, Santillo M, Bevilacqua F, et al. Stimulatory autoantibodies to the PDGF receptor in systemic sclerosis. *N Engl J Med*. 2006;354:2667–2676.

123. Sambo P, Baroni SS, Luchetti M, et al. Oxidative stress in scleroderma: maintenance of scleroderma fibroblast phenotype by the constitutive up-regulation of reactive oxygen species generation through the NADPH oxidase complex pathway. *Arthritis Rheum*. 2001;44:2653–2664.

124. Taylor PA, Lees CJ, Blazar, BR. The infusion of ex vivo activated and expanded CD4(+)CD25(+) immune regulatory cells inhibits graft-versus-host disease lethality. *Blood*. 2002;99(10):3493–3499.

125. Hoffmann P, Ermann J Edinger M, Fathman CG, Strober S. Donor-type CD4(+)CD25(+) regulatory T cells suppress lethal acute graft-versus-host disease after allogeneic bone marrow transplantation. *J Exp Med*. 2002;196(3):389–399.

126. Young KJ, DuTemple B, Phillips MJ, Zhang L. Inhibition of graft-versus-host disease by double-negative regulatory T cells. *J Immunol*. 2003 Jul;171(1):134–41.

127. Clark FJ, Gregg R, Piper K, et al. Chronic graft-versus-host disease is associated with increased numbers of peripheral blood CD4+CD25 high regulatory T cells. *Blood*. 2004;103(6):2410–2416.

128. Miura Y, Thoburn CJ, Bright EC, et. al. Association of Foxp3 regulatory gene expression with graft-versus-host disease. *Blood*. 2004;104(7):2187–2193.

129. Zorn E, Kim HT, Lee SJ, et al. Reduced frequency of FOXP3+ CD4+CD25+ regulatory T cells in patients with chronic graft-versus-host disease. *Blood*. 2005;106(8):2903–2911.

130. Sanchez J, Casano J, Alvarez MA, et al. Kinetic of regulatory CD25 high and activated CD134+ (OX40) T lymphocytes during acute and chronic graft-versus-host disease after allogeneic bone marrow transplantation. *Br J Haematol*. 2004;126(5):697–703.

131. Meignin V, Peffault de Latour R, Zuber J, et al. Numbers of Foxp3-expressing CD4+CD25 high T cells do not correlate with the establishment of long-term tolerance after allogeneic stem cell transplantation. *Exp Hematol*. 2005;33(8):894–900.

132. Allan SE, Crome SQ, Crellin NK, et al. Activation induced FOXP3 in human T effector cells does not suppress proliferation or cytokine production. *Int Immunol*. 2007 Apr;19(4):345–354.

133. Rieger K, Loddenkemper C, Maul J, et al. Mucosal FOXP3+ regulatory T cells are numerically deficient in acute and chronic GvHD. *Blood*. 2006 Feb 15;107(4):1717–1723. Epub 2005 Nov 8.

134. Chan GW, Gorgun G, Miller KB, Foss FM. Persistence of host dendritic cells after transplantation is associated with graft-versus-host disease. *Biol Blood Marrow Transplant*. 2003 Mar;9(3):170–176.

135. Clark FJ, Freeman L, Dzionek A, et al. Origin and subset distribution of peripheral blood dendritic cells in patients with chronic graft-versus-host disease. *Transplantation*. 2003 Jan 27;75(2):221–225.

136. Waller EK, Rosenthal H, Sagar L. DC2 effect on survival following allogeneic bone marrow transplantation. *Oncology (Huntingt)*. 2002 Jan;16(1 Suppl 1):19–26.

137. Rajasekar R, Mathews V, Lakshmi KM, et al. Plasmacytoid dendritic cell count on day 28 in HLA-matched related allogeneic peripheral blood stem cell transplant predicts the incidence of acute and chronic GVHD. *Biol Blood Marrow Transplant*. 2008 Mar;14(3):344–350.

138. Anderson BE, McNiff JM, Jain D, Blazar BR, Shlomchik WD, Shlomchik MJ. Distinct roles for donor- and host-derived antigen-presenting cells and costimulatory molecules in murine chronic graft-versus-host disease: requirements depend on target organ. *Blood*. 2005 Mar 1;105(5):2227–2234. Epub 2004 Nov 2.

139. Sato M, Tokuda N, Fukumoto T, Mano T, Sato T, Ueyama Y. Immunohistopathological study of the oral lichenoid lesions of chronic GVHD. *J Oral Pathol Med*. 2006 Jan;35(1):33–36.

140. Soares AB, Faria PR, Magna LA, et al. Chronic GVHD in minor salivary glands and oral mucosa: histopathological and immunohistochemical evaluation of 25 patients. *J Oral Pathol Med*. 2005 Jul;34(6):368–373.

141. Park HJ, Kim JE, Lee JY, et al. Increased expression of IL-18 in cutaneous graft-versus-host disease. *Immunol Lett*. 2004 Aug 15;95(1):57–61.

142. Shulman HM, Sullivan KM, Weiden PL, et al. Chronic graft-versus-host syndrome in man. A long-term clinicopathologic study of 20 Seattle patients. *Am J Med*. 1980 Aug;69(2):204–217.

143. Or R, Gesundheit B, Resnick I, et al. Sparing effect by montelukast treatment for chronic graft versus host disease: a pilot study. *Transplantation*. 2007 Mar 15;83(5):577–581.

144. Ilan Y, Ohana M, Pappo O, et al. Alleviation of acute and chronic graft-versus-host disease in a murine model is associated with glucocerebroside-enhanced natural killer T lymphocyte plasticity. *Transplantation*. 2007 Feb 27;83(4):458–467.

145. Baker J, Verneris MR, Ito M, Shizuru JA, Negrin RS. Expansion of cytolytic CD8(+) natural killer T cells with limited capacity for graft-versus-host disease induction due to interferon gamma production. *Blood*. 2001 May 15;97(10):2923–2931.

146. Larghero J, Rocha V, Porcher R, et al. Association of bone marrow natural killer cell dose with neutrophil recovery and chronic graft-versus-host disease after HLA identical sibling bone marrow transplants. *Br J Haematol*. 2007 Jul;138(1):101–109.

147. Ferrara JLM, Deeg HJ. GVHD – review article. *N Engl Med J*. 1991,324:667–674.

148. Facon T, Jouet JP, Noel-Walter, Bloget F, Bauters F, Janin A. Involvement of TNF-alpha secreting macrophages in lethal forms of human graft-vs.-host disease. *Bone Marrow Transplant*. 1997;20:511–515.

149. Atkinson K. Chronic graft-versus-host disease. *Bone Marrow Transplant*. 1990;5:69–82.

150. Liem LM, Fibbe WE, van Houwelingen HC, Goulmy E. Serum transforming growth factor-beta1 levels in bone marrow transplant recipients correlate with blood cell counts and chronic graft-versus-host disease. *Transplantation*. 1999 Jan 15;67(1):59–65.

151. New JY, Li B, Koh WP, et al. T cell infiltration and chemokine expression: relevance to the disease localization in murine graft-versus-host disease. *Bone Marrow Transplant*. 2002;29:979–986.

152. Hildebrandt GC, Duffner UA, Olkiewicz KM, et al. A critical role for CCR2/MCP-1 interactions in the development of idiopathic pneumonia syndrome after allogeneic bone marrow transplantation. *Blood*. 2004;103:2417–2426.

153. Banovic T, MacDonald KP, Morris ES, et al. TGF-β in allogeneic stem cell transplantation: friend or foe? *Blood*. 2005;106:2206–2214.

154. Theofilopoulos AN, Baccala R, Beutler B, Kono DH. Type I interferons (alpha/beta) in immunity and autoimmunity. *Annu Rev Immunol*. 2005;23:307–336.

155. Foley R, Couban S, Walker I, et al. Monitoring soluble interleukin-2 receptor levels in related and unrelated donor allogeneic bone marrow transplantation. *Bone Marrow Transplant*. 1998;21:769–773.

156. Grimm J, Zeller W, Zander AR. Soluble interleukin-2 receptor serum levels after allogeneic bone marrow transplantations as a marker for GVHD. *Bone Marrow Transplant*. 1998;21:29–32.

157. Miyamoto T, Akashi K, Hayashi S, et al. Serum concentration of the soluble interleukin-2 receptor for monitoring acute graft-versus-host disease. *Bone Marrow Transplant*. 1996;17:185–190.

158. Kobayashi S, Imamura M, Hashino S, Tanaka J, Asaka M. Clinical relevance of serum soluble interleukin-2 receptor levels in acute and chronic graft-versus-host disease. *Leuk Lymphoma*. 1997;28:159–169.

159. Liem LM, van Houwelingen HC, Goulmy E. Serum cytokine levels after HLA-identical bone marrow transplantation. *Transplantation*. 1998;66:863–871.

160. Campen DH, Horwitz DA, Quismorio FP Jr, Ehresmann GR, Martin WJ. Serum levels of IL-2 receptor and activity of rheumatic disease characterized by immune activation. *Arthr Rheum*. 1988;31:1358–1364.

161. Hayashi T, Morishita E, Ontachi Y, et al. Effects of sarpogrelate hydrochloride in a patient with chronic graft-versus-host disease: a case report. *Am J Hematol*. 2006 Feb;81(2):121–123.

162. Chang DM, Wang CJ, Kuo SY, Lai JH. Cell surface markers and circulating cytokines in graft versus host disease. *Immunol Invest*. 1999 Jan;28(1):77–86.

163. Schultz KR, Miklos DB, Fowler D, et al. Toward biomarkers for chronic graft-versus-host disease: National Institutes of Health consensus development project on criteria for clinical trials in chronic graft-versus-host disease: III. Biomarker Working Group Report. *Biol Blood Marrow Transplant*. 2006 Feb;12(2):126–137.

164. Martin PJ, Weisdorf D, Przepiorka D, et al. Design of Clinical Trials Working Group. National Institutes of Health Consensus Development Project on Criteria for Clinical Trials in Chronic Graft-versus-Host Disease: VI. Design of Clinical Trials Working Group report. *Biol Blood Marrow Transplant*. 2006 May;12(5):491–505.

165. Filipovich A, Weisdorf D, Pavletic S, et al. Diagnosis And Scoring Of Chronic Graft Versus Host Disease NIH Consensus Development Project on Criteria for Clinical Trials in Chronic Graft-Versus-Host Disease: I. Diagnosis and Staging Working Group Report National Institutes of Health Consensus Development Project on Criteria for Clinical Trials in Chronic Graft-versus-Host Disease: I. Diagnosis and Staging Working Group Report. *Biol Blood Marrow Transplant*. 2005;11:945–956.

166. Pavletic SZ, Martin P, Lee SJ, et al. Response Criteria Working Group. Measuring therapeutic response in chronic

graft-versus-host disease: National Institutes of Health Consensus Development Project on Criteria for Clinical Trials in Chronic Graft-versus-Host Disease: IV. Response Criteria Working Group Report. *Biol Blood Marrow Transplant.* 2006 Mar;12(3):252–266.

167. Storek J, Dawson MA, Storer B, et al. Immune reconstitution after allogeneic marrow transplantation compared with blood-stem cell transplantation. *Blood.* 2001;97:3380–3389.

168. Tayebi H, Tiberghien P, Ferrand C, et al. Allogeneic peripheral blood stem cell transplantation results in less alteration of early T-cell compartment homeostasis than bone marrow transplantation.*Bone Marrow Transplant.* 2001;27:167–175.

169. Robinet E, Lapierre V, Tayebi H, Kuentz M, Blaise D, Tiberghien P. Blood versus marrow hematopoietic allogeneic graft. *Transfus Apher Sci.* 2003 Aug;29(1):53–59.

170. Lapierre V, Oubouzar N, Auperin A, et al. Influence of the hematopoietic stem cell source on early immunohematologic reconstitution after allogeneic transplantation. *Blood.* 2001;97:2580–2586.

171. Lapierre V, Auperin A, Tayebi H, et al. Increased presence of anti-HLA antibodies early after allogeneic granulocyte colony-stimulating factor-mobilized peripheral blood hematopoietic stem cell transplantation compared with bone marrow transplantation. *Blood.* 2002;100:1484–1489.

172. Tayebi H, Lapierre V, Saas P, et al. Enhanced activation of B cells in a granulocyte colony-stimulating factor-mobilized peripheral blood stem cell graft. *Br J Haematol.* 2001; 114:698–700.

173. Morikawa K, Miyawaki T, Oseko F, Morikawa S, Imai K. G-CSF enhances the immunoglobulin generation rather than the proliferation of human B lymphocytes. *Eur J Haematol.* 1993;51:144–151.

174. Ng LG, Ng CH, Woehl B, et al. BAFF costimulation of Toll-like receptor-activated B-1 cells. *Eur J Immunol.* 2006 Jul;36(7):1837–1846.

175. Katsenelson N, Kanswal S, Puig M, Mostowski H, Verthelyi D, Akkoyunlu M. Synthetic CpG oligodeoxynucleotides augment BAFF- and APRIL-mediated immunoglobulin secretion. *Eur J Immunol.* 2007 Jul;37(7):1785–1795.

176. Granell M, Urbano-Ispizua A, Aróstegui JI, et al. Effect of NOD2/CARD15 variants in T-cell depleted allogeneic stem cell transplantation. *Haematologica.* 2006 Oct;91(10):1372–1376.

177. Tikkanen JM, Hollmén M, Nykänen AI, Wood J, Koskinen PK, Lemström KB. Role of platelet-derived growth factor and vascular endothelial growth factor in obliterative airway disease. *Am J Respir Crit Care Med.* 2006 Nov 15;174(10):1145–1152. *Epub* 2006 Aug 17.

4

ANIMAL MODELS OF CHRONIC GRAFT VERSUS HOST DISEASE

Yu-Waye Chu, Ronald Gress, and Warren D. Shlomchik

INTRODUCTION

Chronic graft versus host disease (cGVHD) remains a significant barrier to successful allogeneic hematopoietic stem cell transplantation (allo-HSCT). The incidence of cGVHD following allo-HSCT ranges from 25% to 80% and is associated with significant morbidity and mortality [1]. Nonetheless, its association with a lower risk of leukemic relapse suggests an immunologically based antitumor effect [2]. Clinical manifestations of cGVHD are highly variable with respect to organ involvement and extent, and its clinical description is further complicated by different methodologies of clinical scoring to quantitate disease severity [3]. These methodologies have been addressed in a series of efforts in the clinical community through the establishment of the National Institutes of Health Consensus Project on cGVHD [3–8].

Chronic GVHD appears to be a distinct clinical and pathologic entity from acute GVHD (aGVHD) and not merely a temporal extension of the latter [9]. In aGVHD, apoptosis in target organs (skin, liver, and gastrointestinal tract) is a characteristic diagnostic hallmark. In contrast, the clinical and pathologic manifestation of cGVHD are protean, with a wide spectrum of disease including skin fibrosis (akin to scleroderma), lacrimal and salivary gland involvement (as observed in Sjörgen's syndrome), fascitis, eosinophilia, bronchiolitis with or without organizing pneumonia and perhaps a distinct form of hepatic GVHD. These features, which are at least in part specific for cGVHD versus aGVHD, have been used to judge whether a mouse model has relevance to cGVHD.

cGVHD evolves as a consequence of interactions between mature allogeneic donor T cells and host cell populations. In support of this, cGVHD does not occur, or is at least drastically reduced in incidence, in recipients of rigorously T–cell-depleted allografts and mostly does not occur in autologous hematopoietic cell transplantation (auto-HCT). Additional support for the role of donor T cells is the temporal association of aGVHD and de novo cGVHD with donor leukocyte infusions [10]. That cGVHD is directly mediated by immune cells is supported by its occurrence following withdrawal of immunosuppression and its clinical response to a variety of therapies

which in common target immune cells. However, based on human data to date, the roles of specific T-cell or B-cell subsets and the antigens targeted remain elusive. That the clinical features of cGVHD are so variable suggest that cGVHD is a consequence of many of the immune mechanisms that evolved to resist pathogens. Moreover, the observation that certain features of cGVHD share histopathology with presumed autoimmune syndromes has led some investigators to propose that cGVHD targets antigens shared between donor and host and not only minor histocompatability antigens (miHAs) [11], suggesting defects in the ability of immune system to effect self-non-self discrimination. There is little data from humans for or against this hypothesis and other explanations for the overlap are at least as plausible. These include the consequences of chronic antigen stimulation and microenvironmental factors that favor the development of these syndromes, be the antigens shared or unshared with the donor. The delayed onset of cGVHD suggests a potential contribution by events post cell infusion such as the time from cytotoxic chemo/radiotherapy, chronic immunosuppressive therapy, and infections, which may modify immunity in the host.

Defining the pathophysiology of cGVHD has been complicated by the absence of animal models that completely recapitulate the disease or the clinical settings in which it typically develops: after aGVHD, with calcineurin inhibitor-based immunosuppression and its tapering. In contrast, murine models of aGVHD in major and minor histocompatability mismatched HSCT have more accurately modeled the clinical condition (reviewed in References 12 and 13). It is not surprising that a single model using genetically uniform donors and hosts in a controlled environment would fail to recapitulate the varied manifestations in humans, who are genetically diverse and are exposed to different environments. However, the study of available models of cGVHD has provided insights into the potential pathogenic mechanisms in cGVHD, which can suggest avenues for therapeutic and mechanistic investigation in the clinic.

The purpose of this chapter is to describe murine models that have been used in the study of cGVHD, the immunologic mechanisms that underlie each of the graft versus host reactions (GVHR) that lead to the cGVHD phenotypes, and their relevancy to clinical cGVHD. These models are divided into three broad classifications, based on phenotype and immunologic mechanism. For each, descriptions on how the model is established, their salient phenotypes and pathophysiologic mechanisms, and their relevancy to clinical cGVHD are discussed. It should be emphasized that clinical cGVHD carries a highly variable presentation, involving multiple organ systems, including but not limited to the skin, eyes, oral mucosa, gastrointestinal tract, liver, and lungs. For example, features that are diagnostic of human cGVHD include skin, oral, and genitourinary findings ranging from hyperpigmentation to lichenoid changes to frank sclerosis; esophageal pathology including webs, strictures and stenosis; bronchiolitis obliterans with and without organizing pneumonia; secretory defects in lacrimal, salivary, and exocrine glands; and inflammatory and sclerotic changes to connective tissue and joints (reviewed in Reference 1). The relevance of the murine models described in the following paragraphs to clinical cGVHD should take into account their ability to recapitulate one or more of these clinical features.

PARENT→F1 MODELS

A number of experimental systems that bear the name of cGVHD have been developed to recapitulate autoantibody production and vasculitis found in human systemic lupus erythematosus (SLE) [14–18]. These are called cGVHD models not because they resemble human cGVHD but because they are induced by the infusion of donor (graft) immune cells (later found to be CD4 cells) into MHC-disparate F1 hosts; because the syndrome is not rapidly lethal the condition was termed *chronic*. It should be noted that these models predate the clear recognition and characterization of clinical cGVHD. While autoantibodies (mostly ANA [antinuclear antibodies]) are well described in allo-HSCT recipients, their correlation with cGVHD has been inconsistent [19–22]. Antibodies against Y-chromosome-encoded antigens have also been described [23–25] and can correlate with the presence of cGVHD. Whether autoantibodies or alloantibodies do or do not correlate with cGVHD, immune-complex disease or autoantibody-related pathology is certainly not a common feature of cGVHD and relative to patients with traditional autoimmune diseases, the autoantibody titers are low. Nonetheless, as we describe in the following paragraphs, these models have contributed to an understanding of how promiscuous CD4 help directed against alloantigens can overcome mechanisms that regulate B-cell tolerance and thereby promote the development of autoantibodies. Therefore the presence of such autoantibodies or antibodies against miHAs may be a marker for alloreactive CD4 cells and perhaps a role for B cells as antigen-presenting cells (APCs) rather than as their more conventionally conceived role as antibody-producing cells [26–28].

The common feature of these models is the infusion of immune cells (usually spleen cells) from one strain of mouse

into one that is MHC-mismatched. The most typical scenario is infusion of parental cells into an F1 (P→F1), which prevents immunologic rejection of the donor cells. Several strain pairings have been used, most notably DBA (H-2^d) or B6 (H-2^b) →B6 × DBAF1 (referred to as B6D2F1) [14, 17, 29–39] and B6^{bm12}→B6 × B6^{bm12}. This latter model is an MHCII-disparate strain pairing by virtue of a three amino acid difference between the conventional IA^{b}β chain and the β chain of the bm12 variant [40–43]. The resulting phenotype in both models is characterized by the generation of autoantibodies against double stranded DNA (dsDNA), single stranded DNA (ssDNA), and chromatin, and immune-complex glomerulonephritis and arteritis. Progressive idiopathic pneumonia syndrome (IPS) has also been reported in the B6→B6DB2F1 model [44, 45]. As discussed in the following paragraphs, the relevance of this model to human cGVHD is questionable given the fact that clinical renal involvement is relatively rare and in most cases manifested as nephrotic syndrome, which has clinical and pathologic features distinct from immune-complex glomerulonephritis.

CD4 Cells Interacting with Recipient B Cells That Express Allogeneic MHCII Is Crucial

Whereas the B6→B6 × B6^{bm12} model results in SLE-cGVHD, transplantation of B6 cells into B6 × B6^{bm1} F1 recipients, which harbor the allogeneic bm1 K^{bm1} MHCI allele, do not develop this syndrome [40], which implicate CD4 T cells. By using immunoglobulin (Ig) allotype congenic donor and recipient mice, Eisenberg and colleagues elegantly demonstrated that nearly all of the autoantibodies in the B6→B6^{bm12} or B6^{bm12}→B6 models are produced by recipient B cells interacting with donor allogeneic CD4 cells, and that this occurred with either B6^{bm12} CD4 cells stimulating recipient B6 B cells or B6 CD4 cells stimulating recipient B6^{bm12} B cells (Figure 4.1) [41].

Parallel mechanisms are at play in the DBA or B6→B6D2F1 model. B6D2F1 recipients of B6 or B10 splenocytes developed "aGVHD." However, depletion of Lyt-2 cells from the B10 donor inoculum (CD8 cells) allowed the induction of a "stimulatory" SLE-like syndrome with autoantibody production [33]. An analysis of Ig allotypes also implicated recipient B cells as the source of autoantibodies. This is in marked contrast to infusion of DBA splenocytes which, even without depletion of CD8 cells, induced a SLE-syndrome with autoantibodies also of the recipient allotype [14]. Subsequent studies determined that the precursor frequency of DBA anti-B6 cytolytic T cells (CTLs) was low in comparison to the frequency of B6 anti-DBA/2 CTLs, and that without such cytolytic activity, recipient B cells were maintained [46]. Similarly, promoting host B-cell persistence by transferring perforin-deficient T cells in the aGVHD model of B6 into (B6 × DBA2)F1 hosts resulted in a shift to a GVHD phenotype resembling SLE-cGVHD [47].

These systems have been utilized to investigate pathways that modulate autoantibody formation. CD4 T-cell activation in SLE-cGVHD results in the production of type 2 helper T cells (Th2) producing the cytokines interleukin (IL)-4 and

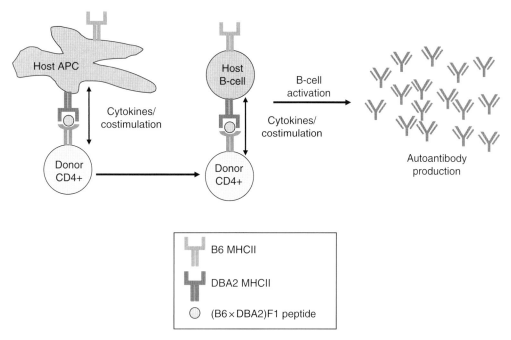

Figure 4.1 Murine SLE-cGVHD. Illustrated are the events presumed to occur in the DBA2→(B6 × DBA2) F1 model of SLE-cGVHD. Donor DBA2 CD4 T cells are stimulated by host (B6 × DBA2)F1 APCs by interactions with H-2^b allogeneic MHCII molecules bearing B6- or DBA-derived peptides. Activated CD4 T cells in turn stimulate (and likely are stimulated by) host B cells (again bearing H-2^b) to produce autoantibodies. See Plate 2 in the color plate section.

APC, antigen-presenting cells; GVHD, graft versus host disease; MHCII, major histocompatibility complex II; SLE, systemic lupus erythematosus.

IL-10 [48, 49] that contribute to polyclonal B-cell activation. As expected, blockade of CD40 ligand [50] or CD28 on donor T cells by CTLA4-Ig [51] mitigated the SLE-cGVHD phenotype. Shifting the cytokine balance from Th2 predominant to Th1 predominant using systemic administration of IL-12 at the time of adoptive transfer resulted in the suppression of autoantibody production, normalization of host splenic B and T cells, restoration of donor antihost alloreactivity [52], and decreased severity of immune-complex glomerulonephritis [53].

DOES THE P→F1 SLE-CGVHD MODEL REFLECT CLINICAL cGVHD?

The relevance of the P→F1 SLE-cGVHD model to clinical cGVHD has been called into questions for a number of reasons. First, the absence of bone-marrow-derived stem cells in the donor inoculum and the absence of any host immunodepletion prior to cell transfer is inconsistent with clinical allo-HSCT. Second, while some features of cGVHD following allo-HSCT mimic SLE, the dominance of antibody and immune complex-mediated disease is at odds with clinical cGVHD in which immune complex and autoantibody-mediated pathology is extremely rare [1, 54]. The profiles of autoantibody expression in patients with cGVHD are also more heterogeneous than in P→F1 models, and includes autoantibodies associated with other collagen vascular diseases [20, 21]. Most importantly, autoantibodies in P→F1 models arise from interactions between donor-derived CD4 T cells and *host*-derived B cells, whereas *donor*-derived B cells do not appear to be involved in the pathogenesis [41], which is contrary to the situation in human cGVHD. Similar interactions between T cells and B cells have not been observed in the clinical setting of mixed chimerism, and have not been consistently observed in other models of murine cGVHD.

On the other hand, while autoantibody production observed in these models do not reflect clinical cGVHD, they do highlight how B cells can have productive interactions with alloreactive CD4 cells, as autoantibodies in these models are class shifted, indicative of having received T cell help. These data also indicate that alloreactive follicular helper cells, which promote class-switching and AID (activation induced cytidine deaminase) activity, develop [55]. Even if autoantibodies are not pathogenic in human cGVHD, B cells may be important APCs, and this is supported by the demonstration of donor-derived antibodies against auto antigens and alloantigens in human allo-HSCT recipients and their correlation with the presence of cGVHD. Treatment of patients with refractory cGVHD with an anti-CD20 monoclonal antibody (rituximab) resulted in objective responses [54], which parallels results in a variety of other autoimmune diseases wherein B cells may also be important APCs [27]. Finally, the

SLE-cGVHD model could provide insights into interactions between host and donor immune cells that occur following reduced-intensity conditioning (RIC) where in transient or more persistent states of mixed chimerism occur [56–58].

THE B10.D2 (OR B6.C)→BALB/c MODEL

Initial Description of the Model

First described by Hamilton [59], the B10.D2→BALB/c donor:recipient pair has been well studied both as a model for cGVHD and for scleroderma. The model's characteristic skin fibrosis was first appreciated by Claman and colleagues [60], who led its early phenotypic description. Claman found that the distinctive skin (and liver) changes could be induced with lethal irradiation, donor bone marrow, and GVHD-inducing donor splenocytes, or with sublethal irradiation and only donor splenocytes [60]. Skin pathology was notable for thickening of dermal collagen with condensation, a mononuclear cell infiltrate more prominent in the dermis than in the epidermis, loss of dermal appendages and fat atrophy, which was attributed to weight loss rather than to a specific intradermal process. CD4 cells infiltrated the dermis and epidermis [61], more prominent at early time points, along with macrophages that were more numerous in the dermis than in the epidermis. Claman also described bile duct involvement in a pattern similar to human GVHD and sclerosing cholangitis [62, 63]. Salivary and lacrimal glands are also involved, which parallels human cGVHD [64, 65]. Both cellular infiltrates and fibrosis have been noted and fibrosis correlated with decreased salivary gland function. Low titer ANA was also observed in some mice [60]. GVHD of the bowel and of the lung have also been described. In sum, the B10.D2 (or B6.C, H-2^d)→BALB/c strain pairing recapitulates key histologic features of human cGVHD – skin fibrosis and salivary and lacrimal gland involvement – though bowel and liver involvement may be more typical for aGVHD.

Induction Phase

Donor CD4 cells alone are capable of inducing the characteristic skin, salivary gland, and lacrimal gland findings, along with liver and bowel GVHD [66–69]. Data have been inconsistent on whether CD8 cells alone can cause GVHD in this strain pairing, but in the study that examined this most carefully, no GVHD was induced with highly purified CD8 cells, though it is possible that when given with CD4 cells, CD8 cells are pathogenic [66–68]. Among CD4 cells, those with a naive phenotype – CD62L$^+$CD44$^-$ – induce severe disease, whereas those with an effector memory phenotype induce no disease [69]. On the other hand, CD4$^+$CD25$^+$ regulatory T cells (Tregs) of either donor or host origin infused at the time of transplantation can suppress GVHD [70].

The roles of donor and host APCs and costimulatory requirements for activating donor T cells have been examined in detail [71]. B10.D2→BALB/c BM (bone marrow) chimeras that receive a second GVHD-inducing transplant with B10.D2 BM and spleen cells develop cGVHD, though the incidence of skin GVHD was modestly but significantly reduced in comparison to control BALB/c→BALB/c recipients of a second GVHD-inducing transplant. Thus, long-term resident donor-derived APCs are sufficient and BALB/c APCs are not required. Another implication of this result is that indirectly presented miHAs of nonhematopoietic origin are also sufficient. This may be of particular relevance to human cGVHD, which occurs long after host hematopoietic cells, including APCs, have mostly been replaced with donor-derived cells.

A second approach for studying APCs was to use hosts and BM donors that lack both CD80 (B71) and CD86 (B72) [71], which in many models are critical for activating naive CD4 cells. When both donor BM and recipients were CD80/CD86$^{-/-}$, wild-type B6.C CD4 cells induced neither clinical nor histologic GVHD. Thus CD80/CD86 costimulation is absolutely essential and experiments in which donors or hosts are CD80/CD86$^{-/-}$ can validly interrogate the individual roles of donor and host APCs. If only hosts or donors were CD80/CD86$^{-/-}$, cutaneous GVHD developed. Therefore, either donor or host APCs are sufficient to mediate disease. However, the incidence of cutaneous GVHD in CD80/86$^{-/-}$ recipients was reduced, though once the disease developed it was of similar severity to that in wild-type mice. Consistent with this, adding alloreactive natural killer (NK) cells, which attack recipient hematopoietic cells including APCs, reduced the incidence of skin disease [72]. Surprisingly, GVHD of the bowel was less severe when CD80/CD86$^{-/-}$ donor BM was used and similar results were obtained with CD40$^{-/-}$ donor BM [71].

Why recipient APCs were primary for skin cGVHD and donor APCs for bowel GVHD is unresolved. Early T-cell activation on host APCs might provide optimal conditions for inducing skin GVHD, perhaps due to differences in the environments where donor T cells are initially primed, acute organ damage by irradiation, or additional drive by the molecules that promote lymphopenia-induced proliferation. However, that a reduced incidence of skin disease was seen in B10.D2→BALB/c chimeras suggests that obligate indirect presentation of antigen could also play a role. Donor APCs could be important for bowel GVHD as there is rapid turnover of gut mucosa that could shed GVHD-inducing T cells into the bowel lumen and perhaps they need to be replenished by fully competent donor APCs in order to maintain active disease. In contrast, once established, a fibrotic skin lesion may be slow to reverse and therefore be more resistant to a decline in new alloreactive T-cell immigrants.

Another consequence of using CD40 – deficient donors is that donor B cells would not be able to make class-switched antibodies [73], which makes it unlikely that the previously described autoantibodies, if they are donor-derived, are required for the cGVHD phenotype. When donor BM or hosts are B-cell deficient, and disease course was also unaffected (WDS, unpublished data and Reference 70), makes a strong argument against a pathogenic role for autoantibodies or an obligate APC function by donor or host B cells.

Effector Phase

Gilliam and colleagues have focused on the effector phase of skin GVHD in the B10.D2→BALB/c model, and in particular on mechanisms of fibrosis [74–78]. When cGVHD was induced with lethal irradiation and relatively low numbers of donor T cells, they observed early skin infiltration by CD11b⁺ cells, which by light scatter and expression of the macrophage receptor with collagenous structure (MARCO) and scavenger receptor A (ScR-A) were likely monocytes or macrophages, consistent with the early descriptions by Claman [77, 78]. RNA from affected skin analyzed by semiquantitative reverse transcriptase polymerase chain reaction (RT-PCR) or by gene chip arrays demonstrated increases in transforming growth factor-beta-(TGF-β1) RNA, without substantial increases in TGF-β2 or TGF-β3 message [75, 77, 78]. TGF-β1 RNA was specifically detected in CD4 cells and macrophages, but not in other cells in disassociated skin. An increase in collagen RNA was observed, consistent with an active fibrotic process. Treatment of mice with a pan-TGF-β blocking antibody diminished thickening of both skin and alveoli, functionally implicating TGF-β in fibrosis, though certainly the systemic administration of an anti-TGF-β1 blocking antibody could affect multiple cell types involved in the GVHD process [77, 79]. Consistent with this, skin inflammatory cell infiltration was reduced in anti-TGF-β-treated mice, which is a somewhat paradoxical result given the established role of TGF-β in suppressing T-cell responses. In the same strain pair, but with cGVHD induced with sublethal irradiation and high spleen cell doses from granulocyte-colony stimulating factor (G-CSF)-treated donors, early treatment with an anti-TGF-β1 antibody did not inhibit GVHD, but treatment after day+14 diminished skin disease as measured by the inflammatory score [80]. However, parameters measuring fibrosis were not reported. As blocking TGF-β1 would be anticipated to promote early T-cell activation, it is possible that fibrosis and inflammation are locally promoted by TGF-β1. A similar reduction in skin thickness and collagen mRNA was seen in recipients of latency-associated peptide, which inhibits free TGF-β1 [76]. IL-4 and IL-13 are not obligate inducer of fibrosis as IL-4Rα-deficient mice (used by both the IL-4 and IL-13 receptors) develop similar cutaneous cGVHD as wild-type mice (WDS, unpublished data).

The B10.D2→BALB/c cGVHD model has also been used to test the efficacy of halofuginone in blocking skin fibrosis. Halofuginone, used to treat coccidiomycosis in chickens, was incidentally found to diminish skin integrity [81] and was subsequently reported to suppress collagen α1(I) gene expression [82]. Halofuginone's mechanisms of action are not fully understood, but it has been proposed to inhibit Smad 3 phosphorylation [83], which is downstream of TGF-β receptor signaling and p38 and NF-κB activation [84, 85]. Halofuginone treatment diminished skin thickening, dermal fat atrophy, and collagen content of cGVHD mice [86]. Whether halofuginone had an effect on other histologic manifestations of cGVHD was not reported. Similar results were noted in the tight skin mouse [87–89], which develops fibrosis due to an in-frame

duplication of the *fibrillin-1* gene, which has been hypothesized to deregulate TGF-β as is the case in other *fibrillin-1* mutant mice and in patients with Marfan disease (reviewed in Reference 90).

Overall, these data are consistent with a model whereby infiltrating CD4 cells can mediate cGVHD without directly contacting nonhematopoietic host cells. MiHA-specific CD4 cells, previously activated largely in secondary lymphoid tissues [91], would enter skin and make alloantigen-specific cognate interactions with miHA-bearing MHCII⁺ hematopoietic cells, including macrophages and tissue dendritic cells (DCs). These MHCII⁺ APCs could be actived and reciprocally stimulate the CD4 cells. Proinflammatory and profibrotic mediators (such as TGF-β1) could be elaborated by APCs and CD4 cells (Figure 4.2). Consistent with these indirect mechanisms, cGVHD develops in BALB/c mice with greatly reduced recipient MHCII expression (CIITA⁻/⁻ and Ii⁻/⁻ mice [92]; and WDS, unpublished data). Also, CD4-mediated GVHD across miHAs is robust in mice with IAᵇβ⁻/⁻ and therefore MHCII-hematopoietic cells including APCs albeit in a different strain pairing [93]. While this is an attractive model, other than a role for TGF-β, the data specifically supporting this scenario are mostly observational. Experiments that directly determine if and how CD4 cells activate macrophages and which cells make TGF-β1 will be necessary to fully test this hypothesis.

Mast Cells

Early studies in the B10.D2→BALB/ model revealed evidence for mast cell degranulation in early posttransplant in cGVHD mice but not in syngeneic controls [94–96]. Mast cells are a diverse set of innate immune cells capable of releasing a wide range of molecules including histamine, cytokines, chemokines, proteases, and growth factors, which could participate in cutaneous GVHD in a number of ways. These products could promote inflammatory cell recruitment, including that of activated T cells and monocytes, and they could also directly promote fibrotic responses by acting on fibroblasts and perhaps the extracellular processing of TGF-β. Supporting the descriptive studies by Claman, treatment of BALB/c recipients with nedocromil sodium, which stabilizes mast cell granules (though not selectively in mast cells), diminished histologic cGVHD [97].

Why cGVHD in the B10.D2 (or B6.C)→BALB/c Model?

Among the many mouse models of GVHD, the clinicopathologic findings in the B10.D2 → BALB/c strain pairing are unusual. Indeed there is substantial heterogeneity in GVHD among different inbred donor-recipient pairs in mouse MHC-matched, multiple miHA mismatched allo-HSCT) [67, 68, 98, 99] and cGVHD is certainly varied in human leukocyte antigen (HLA)-matched outbred humans. Two nonexclusive hypotheses could explain the different GVHD syndromes seen in both human and murine GVHD, as epitomized by the unique form of GVHD in B10.D2→BALB/c transplants. One

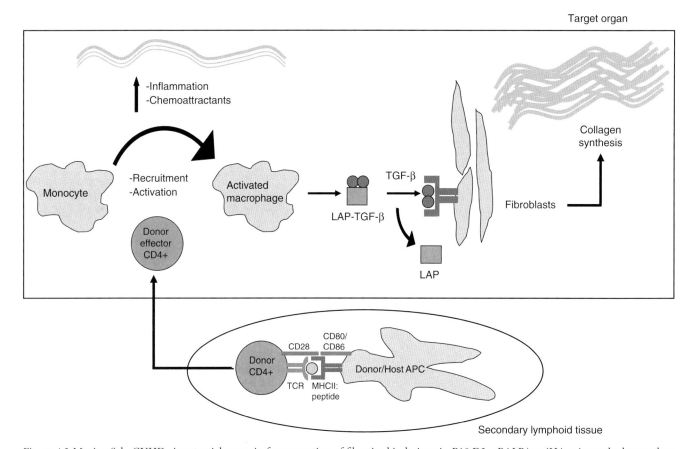

Figure 4.2 Murine Scl-cGVHD. A potential scenario for generation of fibrotic skin lesions in B10.D2→BALB/c miHA mismatched transplant model. Upon activation by donor and/or host APC, CD4 T cells are recruited into target tissue and signal macrophages to produce TGF-β. TGF-β, in turn, binds to its receptor in fibroblasts resulting in increased collagen synthesis, resulting in fibrosis. See Plate 3 in the color plate section.

APC, antigen-presenting cells; LAP, latency associated peptide; MHCII, major histocompatibility complex II; TCR, T-cell receptor; TGF-β, tumor growth factor.

possibility is that a particular GVHD phenotype results from genetic differences in "background" genes that determine the inherent nature of immune responses. For instance, levels of cytokines that determine T-cell polarization could modulate GVHD. Consistent with this, different incidences of GVHD are associated with polymorphisms in the regulatory regions of the genes for tumor necrosis factor-alpha (TNF-α), TNF receptor, IL-10, interferon-gamma (IFN-γ), IL-6, and TGF-β [100–104]. A second possibility is that the identities and tissue distribution of immunodominant target antigen(s) dictate GVHD phenotype [105, 106]. For example, in the B10.D2→BALB/c model, skin GVHD could result from cutaneous expression of immunodominant antigens while GVHD seen in other strain combinations could be the result of expression of a distinct set of immunodominant antigens, perhaps with a different tissue distribution.

To distinguish these hypotheses, GVHD was compared in three MHC-identical strain pairings in which the genetic backgrounds of all donors and all recipients were equal except for genes within the MHC loci: B10.D2→BALB/c (H-2^d), B10→BALB.B (H-2^b), and B10.BR→BALB.K (H-2^k) [68]. By

changing MHC the set of peptides presented will differ in each strain pairing, thereby creating distinct target antigens in each system. Thus by comparing GVHD in these 3 strain pairings, the impact of changing target antigens while holding constant genes that might regulate T-cell responses was tested. Each congenic pair manifested a distinct form of GVHD with unique clinical and pathologic features and different abilities of CD4$^+$ and CD8$^+$ T cells to induce disease. In particular, chronic, fibrotic, skin-targeted GVHD required H-2^d for maximal expression and was completely absent in H-2^b mice. In contrast, systemic GVHD with hunched posture and diarrhea dominated the H-2^b and H-2^k strain pairings. Transplants involving donor and recipient F1 hybrids, for example, (B10 × B10.D2) F1 (H-2^{bd}) transplanted into (BALB.B × BALB/c)F1 (H-2^{bd}) recipients, resulted in a codominant expression of the haplotype-specific GVHD phenotypes as the recipient mice developed both systemic and sclerodermatous cGVHD (Scl-cGVHD) manifestations [68]. These data argue strongly for a role of antigen in dominantly determining GVHD phenotype. These data could in part explain the heterogeneity of human cGVHD; however, the high frequency of cGVHD would suggest that there is promiscuity as to the ability of particular antigens to suffice as cGVHD target antigens, though the exact spectra of disease may differ.

CORRELATIONS OF THE B10.D2→BALB/C SCL-GVHD MODEL TO CLINICAL CGVHD

The Scl-cGVHD model shares many phenotypic features with the sclerodermatous form of clinical cGVHD, which, in combination with poor performance status, thrombocytopenia, hepatic dysfunction, and progressive cGVHD onset from prior aGVHD, is an unfavorable prognostic factor for survival post-HSCT [107, 108]. The incidence of sclerodermatous cGVHD among all long-term survivors of allo-HSCT is estimated to be 3% to 10%, and its incidence and severity could be expected to rise with the increasing numbers of unrelated donor transplants being performed and the increased use of mobilized peripheral blood as a stem cell source [109–112]. Sclerodermatous cGVHD has also been reported following donor leukocyte infusions (DLI) for relapsed disease [113], consistent with the murine models of Scl-cGVHD in which mature donor-derived postthymic T cells are required for its pathogenesis.

Fibrosis is a feature frequently observed in multiple organs in clinical cGVHD other than skin [114, 115]. There is also evidence that the mediators of fibrosis described in the murine Scl-cGVHD are similar to that observed in clinical cGVHD. *In vitro* stimulation of human mononuclear cells with allogeneic fibroblasts and IL-4, which, like IL-13 is a profibrotic cytokine, results in increased collagen synthesis. Addition of IL-12, a potent inducer of Th1 activation, suppressed this production [116]. Serum levels of TGF-β are increased in patients with cGVHD following allo-HSCT [117]. Elevations in IL-13 were observed in the bronchoalveolar lavage fluid of recipients of lung transplants with bronchiolitis obliterans [118], suggesting the importance of this cytokine in promoting fibrotic processes during cGVHD although IL-13 directly acting on host fibroblasts does not appear to play a role in the Scl-cGVHD model given the occurrence of cGVHD in IL-4Rα KO recipients. Stimulatory autoantibodies to the platelet-derived growth factor (PDGF) receptor have been found in patients with extensive sclerodermatous cGVHD as well as patients with systemic sclerosis [119, 120]. That cGVHD develops in recipient mice lacking recombination activating gene expression (RAG$^{-/-}$) and in recipients of donor RAG$^{-/-}$ or CD40-deficient bone marrow, combined with the fact that donor CD4 T cells alone are sufficient to induce cGVHD with sublethal irradiation and no donor BM, argue against the importance of stimulatory autoantibodies in the Scl-cGVHD model.

DBA/2→BALB/C WITH SUBLETHAL IRRADIATION AND NO BM RESCUE

The transfer of splenocytes derived from DBA2 (H-2^d) mice into sublethally irradiated BALB/c (H-2^d) recipients results in a cGVHD phenotype that includes both autoantibody production and glomerulonephritis observed in the DBA2 into (B6 × DBA2)F1 model of SLE-cGVHD and the fibrotic changes characteristic of the B10.D2 into BALB/c model of Scl-cGVHD [121]. In contrast to the P→F1 models, autoantibodies were of donor origin and both donor CD4 and mature B220$^+$ B cells were required to induce the cGVHD phenotype, including skin thickening, though mice still developed acute GVHD. Importantly, a similar phenotype develops in BALB/c$^{nu/nu}$ mice which excludes an essential role for radiation-resistant host CD4 cells in activating donor B cells. These data are then consistent with alloreactive donor CD4 cells stimulating donor derived B cells that indirectly present BALB/c miHAs. How B cells acquire these miHAs (via their antigen receptors or by other mechanisms) is not resolved. Also, exactly why donor B cells are important for skin thickening is unanswered, which contrasts with the B10.D2→BALB/c model (with lethal conditioning and BM rescue), which does not require donor-derived B cells (WDS, unpublished data). This suggests a role for antibody-mediated pathology and/or an obligate role for APC function by B cells specifically in the DBA/2→BALB/c strain pairing. Another question is why this phenotype occurs when DBA/2 spleen cells and not B10.D2 spleen cells are infused. A number of mechanisms could be possible, including differences in T-cell receptor (TCR) repertoires between DBA2 mice and B10.D2 mice, which could target distinct antigens, *mls* differences that could promote mls-directed activation of donor CD4 cells and then B cells, or other background genes in which DBA/2 and BIO.D2 differ that can alter immune responses.

IS CGVHD AN AUTOIMMUNE DISEASE?

While acute GVHD is clearly induced by mature αβ T cells in the donor allograft, some investigators have hypothesized that cGVHD could at least in part be induced by autoreactive T cells; that is, these T cells recognize nonpolymorphic antigens and not miHAs. One variation of this idea is that the cGVHD-inducing T cells are derived from the donor allograft and that during the alloimmune process they escape regulatory mechanisms that would otherwise prevent their full activation, expansion, and effector function. There are certainly examples of T-cell-mediated autoimmunity in mice that genetically lack molecules essential for such regulation, including CTLA-4$^{-/-}$ and FoxP3$^{-/-}$ mice [122–126]. A second variation is that autoreactive T cells are derived from donor hematopoietic progenitors that escape deletion in the recipient thymus, which is dysfunctional due to acute GVHD itself, immunosuppressive drugs and toxic damage from conditioning regimens. It is also possible that these cells are normally educated in the thymus but that peripheral tolerogenic mechanisms fail after their egress from the thymus.

Parkman analyzed T-cell clones derived from splenocytes harvested from irradiated B6 (H-2^b) mice reconstituted with LP/J (H-2^b) BM and spleen cells [127]. Recipients of 50×10^6 spleen cells are described as developing acute GVHD whereas recipients of 20×10^6 spleen cells developed "chronic" GVHD manifest by alopecia, wasting, and ear fibrosis. Clones were isolated from aGVHD mice 10 to 14 days posttransplant and from cGVHD mice 50 days post-BMT. 7/11 aGVHD clones lysed B6 and not LP/J targets and 14/23 proliferated in response to only B6 stimulators whereas 9/23 responded to both B6 and LP/J stimulators. The B6-specific cytotoxic clones were found to be D^b-restricted and at least two of the B6/LP-reactive clones were IA^b-restricted. In contrast, the cGVHD clones were not cytotoxic and 6/6 proliferated similarly to B6 or LP/J stimulators. Except for the IA^b-restricted clones, which were CD4$^+$, all the aGVHD clones were CD8$^+$, whereas cGVHD clones were CD4$^+$. These data were interpreted to indicate that aGVHD is dominated by cytotoxic alloreactive CD8$^+$ cells whereas cGVHD is dominated by autoreactive CD4$^+$ cells. However, autoreactive CD8 and CD4 clones were also found in aGVHD mice. Whether cGVHD clones were derived from infused mature αβ T cells or from the recipient thymus post-BMT was not addressed. A caveat with these experiments is that a similar clonal analysis was not performed in syngeneic recipients (that do not develop GVHD). Nonetheless, these data are provocative, and a role for CD4 cells is supported by the other miHA-directed models of cGVHD. That CD4 cells could dominate late post-BMT is in accordance with the relative efficiency of indirect presentation on MHCII relative to cross-presentation on MHCI.

The thymus is clearly a target organ in GVHD and activated T cells have ready access to it while circulating naive T cells are excluded [128]. It was therefore reasonable to suppose that alloimmune damage could disrupt the processes whereby self-reactive T cells are deleted or diverted into other lineages such as FoxP3$^+$ Tregs (reviewed in Reference 129). Several studies evaluated the efficiency of *mls*-mediated deletion of T cells bearing specific Vβ chains. *Mls* proteins are the products of mouse endogenous retrovirus (encoded in the long terminal repeats) and bind to external surfaces of TCR Vβ chains and MHCII molecules, thereby cross-linking TCRs, independent of peptides in the MHC groove. Different *mls* proteins bind to different Vβ families and distinct *mls* types breed true within mouse strains. When these *mls* proteins are presented to developing T cells in the thymus, TCRs bearing the specific Vβ are cross-linked, resulting in their near complete deletion. The efficiency of the deletion of developing donor-derived thymic T cells that express the Vβ family targeted by host-encoded mls proteins was evaluated in mice with and without GVHD. Mice with GVHD were found to have less efficient deletion of these specific families of T cells [130, 131]. However, the failure to delete these Vβ families may not be due to an intrinsic thymic defect, but rather to a GVH-induced reduction in residual host hematopoietic cells, which express both *mls* and the MHCII chain required for deletion. Nonetheless, if residual host hematopoietic cells are required for optimal tolerance to peptides only in the host (assuming indirect presentation of host antigens by DCs that migrate from the periphery to the thymus is less efficient [132]), then one would predict that full and rapid chimerism would be associated with the development of thymus-derived alloreactive T cells whereas mixed chimeras would lack these. And

if such cells are pathogenic, the prediction would be reduced cGVHD in recipients of nonmyeloablative BMT, which is not as yet supported by clinical data. However, if the mechanism for impaired deletion relates directly to thymic damage rather than to the completeness of donor chimerism, then one might predict a mix of alloreactive and autoreactive thymic emigrants. There is limited data on allo-HSCT in treatment of patients with DiGeorge syndrome, who lack thymi. These patients are usually treated in infancy and sometimes without conditioning. Little GVHD has been reported and only one case with cGVHD, which was not well documented [133].

To examine the impact of not having hematopoietically derived cells in the thymus to mediate negative selection, investigators engineered mice to express MHCI or MHCII only on thymic cortical epithelial cells. K14 promoter transgene-driven expression of MHCII (K14-IA^{b}β) on thymic cortical epithelial cells in mice that are otherwise MHCII$^-$ (K14-IA^{b}β × IA^{b}β$^{-/-}$) results in positive selection of CD4 cells but in aberrant negative selection [134]. Such mice do not develop spontaneous autoimmunity, likely because they lack MHCII$^+$ APCs in the periphery, as T cells from these mice induce autoimmunity when transferred into MHCII$^+$ syngeneic mice [135]. In parallel work examining central tolerance of CD8$^+$ T cells, K14-β2M transgenic mice crossed to β2M$^{-/-}$ mice develop CD8$^+$ T cells that can lyse syngeneic targets *in vitro* and *in vivo* [136]. Another way to create a mouse with MHC specifically expressed on thymic epithelial cells is to make MHC$^{-/-}$→wt radiation BM chimeras. In these mice, positive selection of T cells on epithelial cells can proceed but negative selection by hematopoietic cells is prevented. Such chimeras were found to have increased numbers of T cells, attributable to a failure to delete presumably autoreactive T cells [137]. With longer observation, B6 IA^{b}β$^{-/-}$ (and therefore MHCII$^-$)→B6 wt or B6IA^{b}βB2M$^{-/-}$→wt BM chimeric mice develop colitis [138]. Whether other tissues were examined and found to not have GVHD-like findings was not reported. Using somewhat different transplant conditions, B6 IA^{b}β$^{-/-}$→B6 wt mice developed a syndrome that resembles acute GVHD whereas parallel β2M$^{-/-}$→B6 recipients did not [139]. The key finding was that prior thymectomy of the recipients prevented the autoimmune syndrome, confirming a defect in central tolerance as was reported in mice with cortical epithelial cell restricted expression of MHCI or MHCII. An interesting feature of these models is a paucity of professional hematopoietically derived MHCII$^+$ APCs to prime potentially self-reactive CD4 cells. One would anticipate this would be required as single positive CD4$^+$ thymocytes had a naive phenotype. It is possible that there were small numbers of residual recipient MHCII$^+$ APCs in these chimeras, which could explain why K14-IA^{b}β × IA^{b}β$^{-/-}$ mice, which likely lacked peripheral MHCII$^+$ cells completely, did not develop spontaneous autoimmunity.

While the aforementioned models wherein central tolerance was impaired did not elicit a syndrome similar to cGVHD, an experimental system that is a variation on this theme does have features of cGVHD. When C3H (H-2^k) mice are transplanted with B6 IA^{b}β$^{-/-}$ BM, an inflammatory syndrome ensues

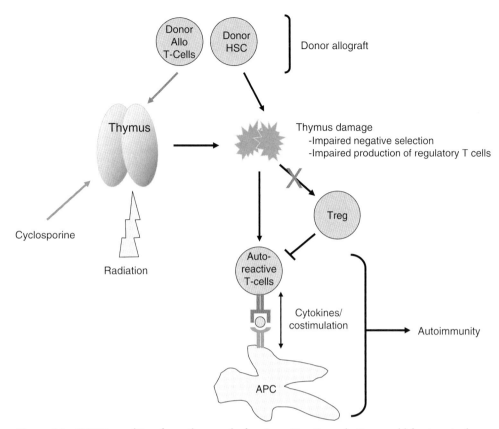

Figure 4.3 cGVHD resulting from thymus dysfunction. Negative selection could be impaired as a consequence of thymic damage by alloreactive T cells, acting in concert with irradiation. CsA may also interfere with negative selection. As a result, autoreactive T cells that would normally be deleted may escape into the periphery, where they can be activated by antigen-presenting cells. It is also possible that the thymic environment posttransplant does not favor the generation of regulatory T cells. See Plate 4 in the color plate section.

APC, antigen-presenting cells; HSC, hematopoietic stem cells; Treg, regulatory T cells.

characterized by skin thickening, biliary and hepatocyte disease, salivary gland inflammation, and death [140]. Disease was dependent on thymus-derived CD4 cells as thymectomized or CD8-depleted recipients did not develop disease. Surprisingly, T cells from these mice reacted only to B6 APCs and could induce disease when transferred to irradiated C3H recipients only if B6 BM cells were co-injected. Why these cells could be stimulated only by B6 cells ex vivo and could cause disease in the complete absence of $IA^b\beta$ in primary B6 $IA^b\beta^{-/-} \rightarrow$ C3H recipients but not in freshly transplanted C3H mice unless B6 cells were also present, was not explained. One possible mechanism would be activation by $H-2^b$ MHCI molecules, which would be present on B6 $IA^b\beta^{-/-}$ or B6 wild-type cells but not on C3H-derived cells.

A less extreme and perhaps more clinically relevant evaluation of the functional impact of an ongoing allogeneic T-cell response on central tolerance revealed the emergence of alloreactive and perhaps autoreactive CD4 cells [141]. Irradiated B6 recipients of C3H.SW ($H-2^b$) BM and purified $CD8^+$ T cells develop acute GVHD. CD4 cells recovered from aGVHD mice could induce GVHD when retransplanted into B6 mice with skin disease sharing features of fibrotic human cGVHD. When

these cells were retransplanted into C3H.SW mice, a form of GVHD developed, but without skin fibrosis. CD4 cells were few if the original transplant recipients were thymectomized indicating that it was highly likely that the CD4 cells were thymically derived, and CD4 cells recovered from irradiated thymectomized recipients of purified C3H.SW CD8 cells and $c-kit^+$ BM cells failed to induce GVHD when retransplanted.

Autologous or syngeneic GVHD (sGVHD) has been observed in syngeneic rat transplants when recipients are treated with cyclosporine [142–144]. This was shown to depend on the thymus as sGVHD cannot be initiated in thymectomized rodents, but the disease phenotype can be rescued with implantation of a fetal thymus [144]. T cells or thymocytes from rodents undergoing the sGVHD reaction can transfer the disease to irradiated secondary recipients, and cell fraction studies have implicated $CD4^+$, $CD8^+$ cells, or both [144–148]. Secondary recipients have also been described as developing a cGVHD phenotype [145]. $CD8^+$ T cells in sGVHD mice lysed autologous and allogeneic cells. Surprisingly, lysis was blocked by anti-MHCII antibodies and not by antibody against MHCI [146]. Ultimately these autoreactive CD8 cells were found largely to be $V\beta.8.5^+$ and recognized the N-terminal portion of the MHC Class II invariant chain peptide (CLIP), which is derived from the invariant chain which protects the peptide binding groove of nascent MHCII molecules until a conventional peptide can be loaded [149–151]. The *N*-terminal portion targeted by these Vβ8.5$^+$ T cells is outside of the peptide binding groove, and in this way may allow this portion of CLIP to function as a superantigen [152, 153]. Similarly reactive T cells against CLIP were demonstrated in patients with cyclosporine-induced sGVHD [154–156]. The relevance of this to human cGVHD is unknown as CsA-treatment in auto-BMT is insufficient to induce cGVHD as in allo-SCT patients [155, 157]. Nonetheless, these studies are consistent with CsA inducing defects in thymic function such that autoreactive cells can emerge (Figure 4.3) [158].

In sum it is plausible that host-reactive T cells emerge from the thymus and contribute to cGVHD pathology. The models in which there is absolutely no negative selection on hematopoietic cells would be extreme examples of a failure in negative selection, likely beyond what would occur with GVHD. Because autoreactive cells are known to emigrate from normal thymi, if newly emerging donor-derived thymic emigrants cause GVHD this could reflect a failure in peripheral tolerance as well. A prediction of the thymus damage model is that patients with human cGVHD should have donor-reactive T cells, and this could be tested by trying to raise T-cell lines and clones in patients with cGVHD by stimulating with donor-derived APCs. Against this hypothesis is apparently de novo GVHD after donor leukocyte infusions (DLI) administration though this does not exclude that thymic emigrants could cause a similar disease.

CONCLUDING REMARKS

Clinical cGVHD has diverse manifestations, which no mouse model can completely capture. Nonetheless, rodent experiments have identified pathogenic mechanisms that may contribute to specific features of GVHD, and such pathways could be targets for cGVHD treatment. They have also been pivotal in generating broader hypotheses on cGVHD pathogenesis. With renewed interest in cGVHD (of which this book is a product), hopefully the applicability of these mechanisms and hypotheses can be tested in therapeutic trials and studies into cGVHD pathogenesis in humans.

REFERENCES

1. Baird K, Pavletic SZ. Chronic graft versus host disease. *Curr Opin Hematol.* 2006;13:426–435.
2. Lee SJ, Klein JP, Barrett AJ, et al. Severity of chronic graft-versus-host disease: association with treatment-related mortality and relapse. *Blood.* 2002;100:406–414.
3. Filipovich AH, Weisdorf D, Pavletic S, et al. National Institutes of Health consensus development project on criteria for clinical trials in chronic graft-versus-host disease: I. Diagnosis and staging working group report. *Biol Blood Marrow Transplant.* 2005;11:945–956.
4. Couriel D, Carpenter PA, Cutler C, et al. Ancillary therapy and supportive care of chronic graft-versus-host disease: national institutes of health consensus development project on criteria for clinical trials in chronic Graft-versus-host disease: V. Ancillary Therapy and Supportive Care Working Group Report. *Biol Blood Marrow Transplant.* 2006;12:375–396.
5. Martin PJ, Weisdorf D, Przepiorka D, et al. National Institutes of Health Consensus Development Project on Criteria for Clinical Trials in Chronic Graft-versus-Host Disease: VI. Design of Clinical Trials Working Group report. *Biol Blood Marrow Transplant.* 2006;12:491–505.
6. Pavletic SZ, Martin P, Lee SJ, et al. Measuring therapeutic response in chronic graft-versus-host disease: National Institutes of Health Consensus Development Project on Criteria for Clinical Trials in Chronic Graft-versus-Host Disease: IV. Response Criteria Working Group report. *Biol Blood Marrow Transplant.* 2006;12:252–266.
7. Schultz KR, Miklos DB, Fowler D, et al. Toward biomarkers for chronic graft-versus-host disease: National Institutes of Health consensus development project on criteria for clinical trials in chronic graft-versus-host disease: III. Biomarker Working Group Report. *Biol Blood Marrow Transplant.* 2006;12:126–137.
8. Shulman HM, Kleiner D, Lee SJ, et al. Histopathologic diagnosis of chronic graft-versus-host disease: National Institutes of Health Consensus Development Project on Criteria for Clinical Trials in Chronic Graft-versus-Host Disease: II. Pathology Working Group Report. *Biol Blood Marrow Transplant.* 2006;12:31–47.
9. Lee SJ. New approaches for preventing and treating chronic graft-versus-host disease. *Blood.* 2005;105:4200–4206.
10. Collins RH, Jr., Shpilberg O, Drobyski WR, et al. Donor leukocyte infusions in 140 patients with relapsed malignancy after allogeneic bone marrow transplantation. *J Clin Oncol.* 1997;15:433–444.
11. Parkman R. Is chronic graft versus host disease an autoimmune disease? *Curr Opin Immunol.* 1993;5:800–803.
12. Shlomchik WD. Graft-versus-host disease. *Nat Rev Immunol.* 2007;7:340–352.
13. Ferrara JL, Levy R, Chao NJ. Pathophysiologic mechanisms of acute graft-vs.-host disease. *Biol Blood Marrow Transplant.* 1999;5:347–356.
14. Van der Veen F, Rolink AG, Gleichmann E. Diseases caused by reactions of T lymphocytes to incompatible structures of the major histocompatibility complex. IV. Autoantibodies to nuclear antigens. *Clin Exp Immunol.* 1981;46:589–596.
15. van der Veen FM, Rolink AG, Gleichmann E. Autoimmune disease strongly resembling systemic lupus erythematosus (SLE) in F1 mice undergoing graft-versus-host reaction (GVHR). *Adv Exp Med Biol.* 1982;149:669–677.
16. van Rappard-van der Veen FM, Rolink AG, Gleichmann E. Diseases caused by reactions of T lymphocytes towards incompatible structures of the major histocompatibility complex. VI. Autoantibodies characteristic of systemic lupus erythematosus induced by abnormal T-B cell cooperation across I-E. *J Exp Med.* 1982;155:1555–1560.
17. Gleichmann H, Gleichmann E, Andre-Schwartz J, Schwartz RS. Chronic allogeneic disease. 3. Genetic requirements for the induction of glomerulonephritis. *J Exp Med.* 1972;135:516–532.
18. Lewis RM, Armstrong MY, Andre-Schwartz J, Muftuoglu A, Beldotti L, Schwartz RS. Chronic allogeneic

disease. I. Development of glomerulonephritis. *J Exp Med.* 1968;128:653–679.

19. Patriarca F, Skert C, Sperotto A, et al. The development of autoantibodies after allogeneic stem cell transplantation is related with chronic graft-vs-host disease and immune recovery. *Exp Hematol.* 2006;34:389–396.

20. Rouquette-Gally AM, Boyeldieu D, Gluckman E, Abuaf N, Combrisson A. Autoimmunity in 28 patients after allogeneic bone marrow transplantation: comparison with Sjogren syndrome and scleroderma. *Br J Haematol.* 1987;66:45–47.

21. Rouquette-Gally AM, Boyeldieu D, Prost AC, Gluckman E. Autoimmunity after allogeneic bone marrow transplantation. A study of 53 long-term-surviving patients. *Transplantation.* 1988;46:238–240.

22. Wechalekar A, Cranfield T, Sinclair D, Ganzckowski M. Occurrence of autoantibodies in chronic graft vs. host disease after allogeneic stem cell transplantation. *Clin Lab Haematol.* 2005;27:247–249.

23. Zorn E, Miklos DB, Floyd BH, et al. Minor histocompatibility antigen DBY elicits a coordinated B and T cell response after allogeneic stem cell transplantation. *J Exp Med.* 2004;199:1133–1142.

24. Miklos DB, Kim HT, Miller KH, et al. Antibody responses to H-Y minor histocompatibility antigens correlate with chronic graft-versus-host disease and disease remission. *Blood.* 2005;105:2973–2978.

25. Miklos DB, Kim HT, Zorn E, et al. Antibody response to DBY minor histocompatibility antigen is induced after allogeneic stem cell transplantation and in healthy female donors. *Blood.* 2004;103:353–359.

26. Chan OT, Shlomchik MJ. Cutting edge: B cells promote CD8+ T cell activation in MRL-Fas(lpr) mice independently of MHC class I antigen presentation. *J Immunol.* 2000;164:1658–1662.

27. Shlomchik MJ, Craft JE, Mamula MJ. From T to B and back again: positive feedback in systemic autoimmune disease. *Nat Rev Immunol.* 2001;1:147–153.

28. Zhong G, Reis e Sousa C, Germain RN. Antigen-unspecific B cells and lymphoid dendritic cells both show extensive surface expression of processed antigen-major histocompatibility complex class II complexes after soluble protein exposure in vivo or in vitro. *J Exp Med.* 1997;186:673–682.

29. van der Veen JP, Rolink AG, Gleichmann E. Diseases caused by reactions of T lymphocytes to incompatible structures of the major histocompatibility complex. III. Autoantibodies to thymocytes. *J Immunol.* 1981;127:1281–1286.

30. Van Elven EH, Rolink AG, Veen FV, Gleichmann E. Capacity of genetically different T lymphocytes to induce lethal graft-versus-host disease correlates with their capacity to generate suppression but not with their capacity to generate anti-F1 killer cells. A non-H-2 locus determines the inability to induce lethal graft-versus-host disease. *J Exp Med.* 1981;153:1474–1488.

31. van Elven EH, van der Veen FM, Rolink AG, Issa P, Duin TM, Gleichmann E. Diseases caused by reactions of T lymphocytes to incompatible structures of the major histocompatibility complex. V. High titers of IgG autoantibodies to double-stranded DNA. *J Immunol.* 1981;127:2435–2438.

32. Rolink AG, Radaszkiewicz T, Pals ST, van der Meer WG, Gleichmann E. Allosuppressor and allohelper T cells in acute and chronic graft-vs-host disease. I. Alloreactive suppressor cells rather than killer T cells appear to be the decisive effector cells in lethal graft-vs.-host disease. *J Exp Med.* 1982;155:1501–1522.

33. Rolink AG, Gleichmann E. Allosuppressor- and allohelper-T cells in acute and chronic graft-vs.-host (GVH) disease. III. Different Lyt subsets of donor T cells induce different pathological syndromes. *J Exp Med.* 1983;158:546–558.

34. Rolink AG, Gleichmann H, Gleichmann E. Diseases caused by reactions of T lymphocytes to incompatible structures of the major histocompatibility complex. VII. Immune-complex glomerulonephritis. *J Immunol.* 1983;130:209–215.

35. Via CS, Sharrow SO, Shearer GM. Role of cytotoxic T lymphocytes in the prevention of lupus-like disease occurring in a murine model of graft-vs-host disease. *J Immunol.* 1987;139:1840–1849.

36. Via CS. Kinetics of T cell activation in acute and chronic forms of murine graft-versus-host disease. *J Immunol.* 1991;146:2603–2609.

37. Via CS, Rus V, Gately MK, Finkelman FD. IL-12 stimulates the development of acute graft-versus-host disease in mice that normally would develop chronic, autoimmune graft-versus-host disease. *J Immunol.* 1994;153:4040–4047.

38. Bruijn JA, Hogendoorn PC, Corver WE, van den Broek LJ, Hoedemaeker PJ, Fleuren GJ. Pathogenesis of experimental lupus nephritis: a role for anti-basement membrane and anti-tubular brush border antibodies in murine chronic graft-versus-host disease. *Clinical & Experimental Immunology.* 1990;79:115–122.

39. Bruijn JA, Van Elven EH, Corver WE, Oudshoorn-Snoek M, Fleuren GJ. Genetics of experimental lupus nephritis: non-H-2 factors determine susceptibility for renal involvement in murine chronic graft-versus-host disease. *Clin Exp Immunol.* 1989;76:284–289.

40. Rolink AG, Pals ST, Gleichmann E. Allosuppressor and allohelper T cells in acute and chronic graft-vs.-host disease. II. F1 recipients carrying mutations at H-2K and/or I-A. *J Exp Med.* 1983;157:755–771.

41. Morris SC, Cheek RL, Cohen PL, Eisenberg RA. Autoantibodies in chronic graft versus host result from cognate T-B interactions. *J Exp Med.* 1990;171:503–517.

42. Morris SC, Cheek RL, Cohen PL, Eisenberg RA. Allotype-specific immunoregulation of autoantibody production by host B cells in chronic graft-versus host disease. *J Immunol.* 1990;144:916–922.

43. Morris SC, Cohen PL, Eisenberg RA. Experimental induction of systemic lupus erythematosus by recognition of foreign Ia. *Clin Immunol Immunopathol.* 1990;57:263–273.

44. Shankar G, Bryson JS, Jennings CD, Morris PE, Cohen DA. Idiopathic pneumonia syndrome in mice after allogeneic bone marrow transplantation. *Am J Respir Cell Mol Biol.* 1998;18:235–242.

45. Shankar G, Scott Bryson J, Darrell Jennings C, Kaplan AM, Cohen DA. Idiopathic pneumonia syndrome after allogeneic bone marrow transplantation in mice. Role of pre-transplant radiation conditioning. *Am J Respir Cell Mol Biol.* 1999;20:1116–1124.

46. Via CS, Sharrow SO, Shearer GM. Role of cytotoxic T lymphocytes in the prevention of lupus-like disease occurring in a murine model of graft-vs-host disease. *J Immunol.* 1987;139:1840–1849.

47. Shustov A, Luzina I, Nguyen P, et al. Role of perforin in controlling B-cell hyperactivity and humoral autoimmunity. *J Clin Invest.* 2000;106:R39–47.

48. De Wit D, Van Mechelen M, Zanin C, et al. Preferential activation of Th2 cells in chronic graft-versus-host reaction. *J Immunol.* 1993;150:361–366.

49. Garlisi CG, Pennline KJ, Smith SR, Siegel MI, Umland SP. Cytokine gene expression in mice undergoing chronic graft-versus-host disease. *Mol Immunol.* 1993;30:669–677.

50. Durie FH, Aruffo A, Ledbetter J, et al. Antibody to the ligand of CD40, gp39, blocks the occurrence of the acute and chronic forms of graft-vs-host disease. *J Clin Invest.* 1994;94:1333–1338.

51. Via CS, Rus V, Nguyen P, Linsley P, Gause WC. Differential effect of CTLA4Ig on murine graft-versus-host disease (GVHD) development: CTLA4Ig prevents both acute and chronic GVHD development but reverses only chronic GVHD. *J Immunol.* 1996;157:4258–4267.

52. Via CS, Rus V, Gately MK, Finkelman FD. IL-12 stimulates the development of acute graft-versus-host disease in mice that normally would develop chronic, autoimmune graft-versus-host disease. *J Immunol.* 1994;153:4040–4047.

53. Okubo T, Hagiwara E, Ohno S, et al. Administration of an IL-12-encoding DNA plasmid prevents the development of chronic graft-versus-host disease (GVHD). *J Immunol.* 1999;162:4013–4017.

54. Ratanatharathorn V, Ayash L, Reynolds C, et al. Treatment of chronic graft-versus-host disease with anti-CD20 chimeric monoclonal antibody. *Biol Blood Marrow Transplant.* 2003;9:505–511.

55. Vinuesa CG, Tangye SG, Moser B, Mackay CR. Follicular B helper T cells in antibody responses and autoimmunity. *Nat Rev Immunol.* 2005;5:853–865.

56. Murphy WJ. Revisiting graft-versus-host disease models of autoimmunity: new insights in immune regulatory processes. *J Clin Invest.* 2000;106:745–747.

57. Subramaniam DS, Fowler DH, Pavletic SZ. Chronic graft-versus-host disease in the era of reduced-intensity conditioning. *Leukemia.* 2007;21:853–859.

58. Sykes M, Preffer F, McAfee S, et al. Mixed lymphohaemopoietic chimerism and graft-versus-lymphoma effects after non-myeloablative therapy and HLA-mismatched bone-marrow transplantation. *Lancet.* 1999;353:1755–1759.

59. Hamilton BL, Bevan MJ, Parkman R. Anti-recipient cytotoxic T lymphocyte precursors are present in the spleens of mice with acute graft versus host disease due to minor histocompatibility antigens. *J Immunol.* 1981;126:621–625.

60. Jaffee BD, Claman HN. Chronic graft-versus-host disease (GVHD) as a model for scleroderma. I. Description of model systems. *Cell Immunol.* 1983;77:1–12.

61. Giorno R, Choi KL, Katz HR, Claman HN. Monoclonal antibody analysis of skin in chronic murine graft vs host disease produced across minor histocompatibility barriers. *Cell Immunol.* 1987;106:76–87.

62. Howell CD, Yoder T, Claman HN, Vierling JM. Hepatic homing of mononuclear inflammatory cells isolated during murine chronic graft-vs-host disease. *J Immunol.* 1989;143:476–483.

63. Vierling JM, Ruderman WB, Jaffee BD, Fennell R, Jr., Claman HN. Hepatic lesions in murine chronic graft-versus-host disease to minor histocompatibility antigens. A reproducible model of nonsuppurative destructive cholangitis. *Transplantation.* 1989;48:717–718.

64. Nagler RM, Laufer D, Nagler A. Parotid gland dysfunction in an animal model of chronic graft-vs-host disease. *Arch Otolaryngol Head Neck Surg.* 1996;122:1057–1060.

65. Nagler RM, Laufer D, Nagler A. Parotid gland dysfunction in a murine model of acute graft versus host disease [aGVHD]. *Head Neck.* 1998;20:58–62.

66. Korngold R, Sprent J. Variable capacity of L3T4+ T cells to cause lethal graft-versus-host disease across minor histocompatibility barriers in mice. *J Exp Med.* 1987;165:1552–1564.

67. Hamilton BL. L3T4-positive T cells participate in the induction of graft-vs-host disease in response to minor histocompatibility antigens. *J Immunol.* 1987;139:2511–2515.

68. Kaplan DH, Anderson BE, McNiff JM, Jain D, Shlomchik MJ, Shlomchik WD. Target Antigens Determine Graft-versus-Host Disease Phenotype. *J Immunol.* 2004;173:5467–5475.

69. Anderson BE, McNiff J, Yan J, et al. Memory CD4+ T cells do not induce graft-versus-host disease. *J Clin Invest.* 2003;112:101–108.

70. Anderson BE, McNiff J, Matte C, Athanasiadis I, Shlomchik WD, Shlomchik MJ. Recipient CD4+ T Cells That Survive Irradiation Regulate Chronic Graft-vs.-Host Disease. *Blood.* 2004;104(5):1565–1573.

71. Anderson BE, McNiff JM, Jain D, Blazar BR, Shlomchik WD, Shlomchik MJ. Distinct roles for donor- and host-derived antigen-presenting cells and costimulatory molecules in murine chronic graft-versus-host disease: requirements depend on target organ. *Blood.* 2005;105:2227–2234.

72. Lundqvist A, McCoy JP, Samsel L, Childs R. Reduction of GVHD and enhanced antitumor effects after adoptive infusion of alloreactive Ly49-mismatched NK cells from MHC-matched donors. *Blood.* 2007;109:3603–3606.

73. DiSanto JP, Bonnefoy JY, Gauchat JF, Fischer A, de Saint Basile G. CD40 ligand mutations in x-linked immunodeficiency with hyper-IgM [see comments]. *Nature.* 1993;361:541–543.

74. Askew D, Zhou L, Wu C, Chen G, Gilliam AC. Absence of cutaneous TNFalpha-producing CD4+ T cells and TNFalpha may allow for fibrosis rather than epithelial cytotoxicity in murine sclerodermatous graft-versus-host disease, a model for human scleroderma. *J Invest Dermatol.* 2007;127:1905–1914.

75. Zhou L, Askew D, Wu C, Gilliam AC. Cutaneous gene expression by DNA microarray in murine sclerodermatous graft-versus-host disease, a model for human scleroderma. *J Invest Dermatol.* 2007;127:281–292.

76. Zhang Y, McCormick LL, Gilliam AC. Latency-associated peptide prevents skin fibrosis in murine sclerodermatous graft-versus-host disease, a model for human scleroderma. *J Invest Dermatol.* 2003;121:713–719.

77. McCormick LL, Zhang Y, Tootell E, Gilliam AC. Anti-TGF-beta treatment prevents skin and lung fibrosis in murine sclerodermatous graft-versus-host disease: a model for human scleroderma. *J Immunol.* 1999;163:5693–5699.

78. Zhang Y, McCormick LL, Desai SR, Wu C, Gilliam AC. Murine sclerodermatous graft-versus-host disease, a model for human scleroderma: cutaneous cytokines, chemokines, and immune cell activation. *J Immunol.* 2002;168:3088–3098.

79. Aoki CA, Borchers AT, Li M, et al. Transforming growth factor beta (TGF-beta) and autoimmunity. *Autoimmun Rev.* 2005;4:450–459.

80. Banovic T, MacDonald KP, Morris ES, et al. TGF-beta in allogeneic stem cell transplantation: friend or foe? *Blood.* 2005;106:2206–2214.

81. Granot I, Bartov I, Plavnik I, Wax E, Hurwitz S, Pines M. Increased skin tearing in broilers and reduced collagen

synthesis in skin in vivo and in vitro in response to the coccidiostat halofuginone. *Poult Sci.* 1991;70:1559–1563.

82. Granot I, Halevy O, Hurwitz S, Pines M. Halofuginone: an inhibitor of collagen type I synthesis. *Biochim Biophys Acta.* 1993;1156:107–112.

83. McGaha TL, Phelps RG, Spiera H, Bona C. Halofuginone, an inhibitor of type-I collagen synthesis and skin sclerosis, blocks transforming-growth-factor-beta-mediated Smad3 activation in fibroblasts. *J Invest Dermatol.* 2002;118: 461–470.

84. Leiba M, Cahalon L, Shimoni A, et al. Halofuginone inhibits NF-kappaB and p38 MAPK in activated T cells. *J Leukoc Biol.* 2006;80:399–406.

85. Popov Y, Patsenker E, Bauer M, Niedobitek E, Schulze-Krebs A, Schuppan D. Halofuginone induces matrix metalloproteinases in rat hepatic stellate cells via activation of p38 and NFkappaB. *J Biol Chem.* 2006;281:15090–15098.

86. Pines M, Snyder D, Yarkoni S, Nagler A. Halofuginone to treat fibrosis in chronic graft-versus-host disease and scleroderma. *Biol Blood Marrow Transplant.* 2003;9:417–425.

87. Saito S, Nishimura H, Phelps RG, et al. Induction of skin fibrosis in mice expressing a mutated fibrillin-1 gene. *Mol Med.* 2000;6:825–836.

88. Bona CA, Murai C, Casares S, et al. Structure of the mutant fibrillin-1 gene in the tight skin (TSK) mouse. *DNA Res.* 1997;4:267–271.

89. Siracusa LD, McGrath R, Ma Q, et al. A tandem duplication within the fibrillin 1 gene is associated with the mouse tight skin mutation. *Genome Res.* 1996;6:300–313.

90. Lemaire R, Bayle J, Lafyatis R. Fibrillin in Marfan syndrome and tight skin mice provides new insights into transforming growth factor-beta regulation and systemic sclerosis. *Curr Opin Rheumatol.* 2006;18:582–587.

91. Anderson BE, Taylor PA, McNiff JM, et al. Effects of donor T cell trafficking and priming site on GVHD induction by naive and memory phenotype CD4 T cells. *Blood.* 2008, *Blood* -2007–2009;107953.

92. Anderson BE, Shlomchik W, Shlomchik M. Mechanisms of Chronic-Graft-Versus-Host Disease Induction and Pathogenesis in an MHC-Matched MiHA-Incompatible Murine Model. *Blood.* 2001;98 (Abstract 2727).

93. Matte-Martone C, Liu J, Jain D, McNiff J, Shlomchik WD. CD8+ but not CD4+ T cells require cognate interactions with target tissues to mediate GVHD across only minor H antigens, whereas both CD4+ and CD8+ T cells require direct leukemic contact to mediate GVL. *Blood.* 2008;111: 3884–3892.

94. Claman HN. Mast cell depletion in murine chronic graft-versus-host disease. *J Invest Dermatol.* 1985;84:246–248.

95. Claman HN, Jaffee BD, Huff JC, Clark RA. Chronic graft-versus-host disease as a model for scleroderma. II. Mast cell depletion with deposition of immunoglobulins in the skin and fibrosis. *Cell Immunol.* 1985;94:73–84.

96. Claman HN, Choi KL, Sujansky W, Vatter AE. Mast cell "disappearance" in chronic murine graft-vs-host disease (GVHD)-ultrastructural demonstration of "phantom mast cells". *J Immunol.* 1986;137:2009–2013.

97. Levi-Schaffer F, Goldenhersh MA, Segal V, Nagler A. Nedocromil sodium ameliorates skin manifestations in a murine model of chronic graft-versus-host disease. *Bone Marrow Transplant.* 1997;19:823–828.

98. Korngold R, Sprent J. Features of T cells causing H-2-restricted lethal graft-vs.-host disease across minor histocompatibility barriers. *J Exp Med.* 1982;155:872–883.

99. Korngold R, Sprent J. T cell subsets and graft-versus-host disease. *Transplantation.* 1987;44:335–339.

100. Hattori H, Matsuzaki A, Suminoe A, et al. Polymorphisms of transforming growth factor-beta1 and transforming growth factor-beta1 type II receptor genes are associated with acute graft-versus-host disease in children with HLA-matched sibling bone marrow transplantation. *Bone Marrow Transplant.* 2002;30:665–671.

101. Middleton PG, Taylor PRA, Jackson G, Proctor SJ, Dickinson AM. Cytokine gene polymorphisms associating with severe acute graft-versus-host disease in HLA-identical sibling transplants. *Blood.* 1998;92:3943–3948.

102. Cavet J, Middleton PG, Segall M, Noreen H, Davies SM, Dickinson AM. Recipient tumor necrosis factor-alpha and interleukin-10 gene polymorphisms associate with early mortality and acute graft-versus-host disease severity in HLA-matched sibling bone marrow transplants. *Blood.* 1999;94:3941–3946.

103. Cavet J, Dickinson AM, Norden J, Taylor PR, Jackson GH, Middleton PG. Interferon-gamma and interleukin-6 gene polymorphisms associate with graft-versus host disease in HLA-matched sibling bone marrow transplantation. *Blood.* 2001;98:1594–1600.

104. Ishikawa Y, Kashiwase K, Akaza T, et al. Polymorphisms in TNFA and TNFR2 affect outcome of unrelated bone marrow transplantation. *Bone Marrow Transplant.* 2002;29:569–575.

105. Berger M, Wettstein PJ, Korngold R. T cell subsets involved in lethal graft-versus-host disease directed to immunodominant minor histocompatibility antigens. *Transplantation.* 1994;57:1095–1102.

106. Korngold R, Wettstein PJ. Immunodominance in the graft-vs-host disease T cell response to minor histocompatibility antigens. *J Immunol.* 1990;145:4079–4088.

107. Shulman HM, Sullivan KM, Weiden PL, et al. Chronic graft-versus-host syndrome in man. A long-term clinicopathologic study of 20 Seattle patients. *Am J Med.* 1980;69:204–217.

108. Wingard JR, Piantadosi S, Vogelsang GB, et al. Predictors of death from chronic graft-versus-host disease after bone marrow transplantation. *Blood.* 1989;74:1428–1435.

109. Fimiani M, De Aloe G, Cuccia A. Chronic graft versus host disease and skin. *J Eur Acad Dermatol Venereol.* 2003;17:512–517.

110. Skert C, Patriarca F, Sperotto A, et al. Sclerodermatous chronic graft-versus-host disease after allogeneic hematopoietic stem cell transplantation: incidence, predictors and outcome. *Haematologica.* 2006;91:258–261.

111. Flowers ME, Parker PM, Johnston LJ, et al. Comparison of chronic graft-versus-host disease after transplantation of peripheral blood stem cells versus bone marrow in allogeneic recipients: long-term follow-up of a randomized trial. *Blood.* 2002;100:415–419.

112. Mielcarek M, Martin PJ, Heimfeld S, Storb R, Torok-Storb B. CD34 cell dose and chronic graft-versus-host disease after human leukocyte antigen-matched sibling hematopoietic stem cell transplantation. *Leuk Lymphoma.* 2004;45:27–34.

113. Jones-Caballero M, Fernandez-Herrera J, Cordoba-Guijarro S, Dauden-Tello E, Garcia-Diez A. Sclerodermatous graft-versus-host disease after donor leucocyte infusion. *Br J Dermatol.* 1998;139:889–892.

114. Ogawa Y, Kodama H, Kameyama K, et al. Donor fibroblast chimerism in the pathogenic fibrotic lesion of human chronic graft-versus-host disease. *Invest Ophthalmol Vis Sci.* 2005;46:4519–4527.

115. Wolff D, Reichenberger F, Steiner B, et al. Progressive interstitial fibrosis of the lung in sclerodermoid chronic graft-versus-host disease. *Bone Marrow Transplant.* 2002;29:357–360.

116. Banning U, Krutmann J, Korholz D. The role of IL-4 and IL-12 in the regulation of collagen synthesis by fibroblasts. *Immunol Invest.* 2006;35:199–207.

117. Liem LM, Fibbe WE, van Houwelingen HC, Goulmy E. Serum transforming growth factor-beta1 levels in bone marrow transplant recipients correlate with blood cell counts and chronic graft-versus-host disease. *Transplantation.* 1999;67:59–65.

118. Keane MP, Gomperts BN, Weigt S, et al. IL-13 is pivotal in the fibro-obliterative process of bronchiolitis obliterans syndrome. *J Immunol.* 2007;178:511–519.

119. Gabrielli A, Svegliati S, Moroncini G, Luchetti M, Tonnini C, Avvedimento EV. Stimulatory autoantibodies to the PDGF receptor: a link to fibrosis in scleroderma and a pathway for novel therapeutic targets. *Autoimmun Rev.* 2007;7:121–126.

120. Svegliati S, Olivieri A, Campelli N, et al. Stimulatory autoantibodies to PDGF receptor in patients with extensive chronic graft-versus-host disease. *Blood.* 2007;110:237–241.

121. Zhang C, Todorov I, Zhang Z, et al. Donor CD4+ T and B cells in transplants induce chronic graft-versus-host disease with autoimmune manifestations. *Blood.* 2006;107:2993–3001.

122. Tivol EA, Borriello F, Schweitzer AN, Lynch WP, Bluestone JA, Sharpe AH. Loss of CTLA-4 leads to massive lymphoproliferation and fatal multiorgan tissue destruction, revealing a critical negative regulatory role of CTLA-4. *Immunity.* 1995;3:541–547.

123. Williams LM, Rudensky AY. Maintenance of the Foxp3-dependent developmental program in mature regulatory T cells requires continued expression of Foxp3. *Nat Immunol.* 2007;8:277–284.

124. Kim JM, Rasmussen JP, Rudensky AY. Regulatory T cells prevent catastrophic autoimmunity throughout the lifespan of mice. *Nat Immunol.* 2007;8:191–197.

125. Fontenot JD, Gavin MA, Rudensky AY. Foxp3 programs the development and function of CD4(+)CD25(+) regulatory T cells. *Nat Immunol.* 2003;4:330–336.

126. Khattri R, Cox T, Yasayko SA, Ramsdell F. An essential role for Scurfin in CD4(+)CD25(+) T regulatory cells. *Nat Immunol.* 2003;4:337–342.

127. Parkman R. Clonal analysis of murine graft-vs-host disease. I. Phenotypic and functional analysis of T lymphocyte clones. *J Immunol.* 1986;136:3543–3548.

128. Agus DB, Surh CD, Sprent J. Reentry of T cells to the adult thymus is restricted to activated T cells. *J Exp Med.* 1991;173:1039–1046.

129. Hogquist KA, Baldwin TA, Jameson SC. Central tolerance: learning self-control in the thymus. *Nat Rev Immunol.* 2005;5:772–782.

130. Fukushi N, Arase H, Wang B, et al. Thymus: a direct target tissue in graft-versus-host reaction after allogeneic bone marrow transplantation that results in abrogation of induction of self-tolerance. *Proc Natl Acad Sci U S A.* 1990;87:6301–6305.

131. Hollander GA, Widmer B, Burakoff SJ. Loss of normal thymic repertoire selection and persistence of autoreactive T cells in graft vs host disease. *J Immunol.* 1994;152:1609–1617.

132. Bonasio R, Scimone ML, Schaerli P, Grabie N, Lichtman AH, von Andrian UH. Clonal deletion of thymocytes by circulating dendritic cells homing to the thymus. *Nat Immunol.* 2006;7:1092–1100.

133. Goldsobel AB, Haas A, Stiehm ER. Bone marrow transplantation in DiGeorge syndrome. *J Pediatr.* 1987;111:40–44.

134. Laufer TM, DeKoning J, Markowitz JS, Lo D, Glimcher LH. Unopposed positive selection and autoreactivity in mice expressing class II MHC only on thymic cortex. *Nature.* 1996;383:81–85.

135. Laufer TM, Fan L, Glimcher LH. Self-reactive T cells selected on thymic cortical epithelium are polyclonal and are pathogenic in vivo. *J Immunol.* 1999;162:5078–5084.

136. Capone M, Romagnoli P, Beermann F, MacDonald HR, van Meerwijk JP. Dissociation of thymic positive and negative selection in transgenic mice expressing major histocompatibility complex class I molecules exclusively on thymic cortical epithelial cells. *Blood.* 2001;97:1336–1342.

137. van Meerwijk JP, Marguerat S, Lees RK, Germain RN, Fowlkes BJ, MacDonald HR. Quantitative impact of thymic clonal deletion on the T cell repertoire. *J Exp Med.* 1997;185:377–383.

138. Marguerat S, MacDonald HR, Kraehenbuhl JP, van Meerwijk JP. Protection from radiation-induced colitis requires MHC class II antigen expression by cells of hemopoietic origin. *J Immunol.* 1999;163:4033–4040.

139. Teshima T, Reddy P, Liu C, Williams D, Cooke KR, Ferrara JL. Impaired thymic negative selection causes autoimmune graft-versus-host disease. *Blood.* 2003;102:429–435.

140. Sakoda Y, Hashimoto D, Asakura S, et al. Donor-derived thymic-dependent T cells cause chronic graft-versus-host disease. *Blood.* 2007;109:1756–1764.

141. Zhang Y, Hexner E, Frank D, Emerson SG. CD4+ T cells generated de novo from donor hemopoietic stem cells mediate the evolution from acute to chronic graft-versus-host disease. *J Immunol.* 2007;179:3305–3314.

142. Tutschka PJ, Hess AD, Beschorner WE, Santos GW. Suppressor cells in transplantation tolerance. I. Suppressor cells in the mechanism of tolerance in radiation chimeras. *Transplantation.* 1981;32:203–209.

143. Glazier A, Tutschka PJ, Farmer ER, Santos GW. Graft-versus-host disease in cyclosporin A-treated rats after syngeneic and autologous bone marrow reconstitution. *J Exp Med.* 1983;158:1–8.

144. Sorokin R, Kimura H, Schroder K, Wilson DH, Wilson DB. Cyclosporine-induced autoimmunity. Conditions for expressing disease, requirement for intact thymus, and potency estimates of autoimmune lymphocytes in drug-treated rats. *J Exp Med.* 1986;164:1615–1625.

145. Beschorner WE, Hess AD, Shinn CA, Santos GW. Transfer of cyclosporine-associated syngeneic graft-versus-host disease by thymocytes. Resemblance to chronic graft-versus-host disease. *Transplantation.* 1988;45:209–215.

146. Fischer AC, Beschorner WE, Hess AD. Requirements for the induction and adoptive transfer of cyclosporine-induced syngeneic graft-versus-host disease. *J Exp Med.* 1989;169:1031–1041.

147. Hess AD, Fischer AC, Beschorner WE. Effector mechanisms in cyclosporine A-induced syngeneic graft-versus-host disease. Role of CD4+ and CD8+ T lymphocyte subsets. *J Immunol.* 1990;145:526–533.

148. Hess AD, Horwitz LR, Laulis MK, Fuchs E. Cyclosporine-induced syngeneic graft-vs-host disease: prevention of auto-aggression by treatment with monoclonal antibodies to

T lymphocyte cell surface determinants and to MHC class II antigens. *Clin Immunol Immunopathol*. 1993;69:341–350.

149. Fischer AC, Ruvolo PP, Burt R, et al. Characterization of the autoreactive T cell repertoire in cyclosporin-induced syngeneic graft-versus-host disease. A highly conserved repertoire mediates autoaggression. *J Immunol*. 1995;154:3713–3725.

150. Chen W, Thoburn C, Hess AD. Characterization of the pathogenic autoreactive T cells in cyclosporine-induced syngeneic graft-versus-host disease. *J Immunol*. 1998;161:7040–7046.

151. Hess AD, Thoburn C, Horwitz L. Promiscuous recognition of major histocompatibility complex class II determinants in cyclosporine-induced syngeneic graft-versus-host disease: specificity of cytolytic effector T cells. *Transplantation*. 1998;65:785–792.

152. Gold DP, Surh CD, Sellins KS, Schroder K, Sprent J, Wilson DB. Rat T cell responses to superantigens. II. Allelic differences in V beta 8.2 and V beta 8.5 beta chains determine responsiveness to staphylococcal enterotoxin B and mouse mammary tumor virus-encoded products. *J Exp Med*. 1994;179:63–69.

153. Surh CD, Gold DP, Wiley S, Wilson DB, Sprent J. Rat T cell response to superantigens. I. V beta-restricted clonal deletion of rat T cells differentiating in rat–>mouse chimeras. *J Exp Med*. 1994;179:57–62.

154. Hess AD, Bright EC, Thoburn C, Vogelsang GB, Jones RJ, Kennedy MJ. Specificity of effector T lymphocytes in autologous graft-versus-host disease: role of the major histocompatibility complex class II invariant chain peptide. *Blood*. 1997;89:2203–2209.

155. Yeager AM, Vogelsang GB, Jones RJ, et al. Induction of cutaneous graft-versus-host disease by administration of cyclosporine to patients undergoing autologous bone marrow transplantation for acute myeloid leukemia. *Blood*. 1992;79:3031–3035.

156. Jones RJ, Vogelsang GB, Hess AD, et al. Induction of graft-versus-host disease after autologous bone marrow transplantation. *Lancet*. 1989;1:754–757.

157. Bolanos-Meade J, Garrett-Mayer E, Luznik L, et al. Induction of autologous graft-versus-host disease: results of a randomized prospective clinical trial in patients with poor risk lymphoma. *Biol Blood Marrow Transplant*. 2007;13:1185–1191.

158. Gao EK, Lo D, Cheney R, Kanagawa O, Sprent J. Abnormal differentiation of thymocytes in mice treated with cyclosporin A. *Nature*. 1988;336:176–179.

5

Incidence and Trends

Sally Arai, Mukta Arora, and Douglas J. Rizzo

In 2006, approximately 50,000 hematopoietic cell transplants (HCT) were performed worldwide, and about 20,000 were allogeneic transplants [1]. Indeed, the number of allogeneic transplants performed has demonstrated an exponential increase through the 1980s and 1990s. While offering cure for many diseases, the success of allogeneic transplantation is limited by complications. One of the most significant complications associated with considerable morbidity and mortality is chronic graft versus host disease (cGVHD). The focus of this chapter will be on the incidence and trends in cGVHD over the last three decades since its first recognition in the mid-1970s.

1970–1980

In the 1980s, the Seattle group [2] reported the remarkable success of HCT in achieving long-term survival without disease recurrence in patients with hematologic malignancies. Among the long-term survivors, 60% to 75% were leading normal lives and, in particular, had no evidence of GVHD. However, between 25% and 40% of long-term survivors developed cGVHD. The Seattle group summarized the clinical manifestations of cGVHD in 20 patients who were transplanted between 1969 and 1976. Manifestations were similar to collagen vascular diseases and included debilitating skin sclerosis, generalized sicca syndrome, severe oral and esophageal mucositis, malabsorption, pulmonary insufficiency, chronic liver disease, recurrent bacterial infections, and generalized wasting. In this clinicopathologic observational study of the disease, three patterns of presentation of cGVHD were observed (1) progressive – continuously active acute graft versus host disease (aGVHD) progressing gradually into cGVHD; (2) quiescent – resolution of aGVHD, then a phase with no clinical GVHD activity, followed by the onset of cGVHD; and (3) de novo late onset – onset of cGVHD without prior aGVHD. cGVHD was also described by the organ systems involved and the distinctive features of each organ's clinical, pathologic, and laboratory abnormalities. Further proposed in this early study were the categories of limited cGVHD, with a better prognosis, and extensive cGVHD for the remaining patients. The extensive

designation, because of its broad range of severity of manifestations, had the shortcoming of being less prognostic with the more complex and variable clinical outcomes that occur with multiorgan involvement. Despite the limitations of this system, the limited and extensive designations have remained the standard-reported categorization of cGVHD.

The earliest reported estimate of the incidence of cGVHD was published in 1981 when Sullivan et al. described its development in 52 (30%) of the first 175 marrow recipients who survived longer than 150 days after transplantation [3]. Only five (3%) experienced the indolent and favorable limited cGVHD (skin and liver only), whereas 47 developed the unfavorable multiorgan extensive cGVHD. The patients in this era received transplantation for aplastic anemia and leukemia from human leukocyte antigen (HLA) identical sibling donors, utilizing myeloablative conditioning with high dose cyclophosphamide and total body irradiation, a marrow graft source, and GVHD prophylaxis with methotrexate for the first 100 days posttransplant. No immunosuppression was given after day 100 except in patients with ongoing aGVHD. These initial observations emphasized the need for early recognition of symptoms, combination immunosuppressive therapy, and a prolonged treatment course to prevent reactivation of GVHD.

1980–1990

During the 1980s, the number of allogeneic bone marrow transplantations performed worldwide increased exponentially as marrow transplantation was established as an important therapeutic option for patients with leukemia or lymphoma. Further observation of the incidence of cGVHD revealed that the disease status at transplant (remission or relapse) had little or no influence on the development of cGVHD. The incidence was reported in 30% to 50% of patients who survived 6 months or longer after HLA-identical sibling transplants [4] (Figure 5.1). With the expansion of the donor pool to include HLA-mismatched relatives and unrelated donors, differences in the probability of developing clinical extensive cGVHD by donor type became evident [5] (Figure 5.2). Compared to

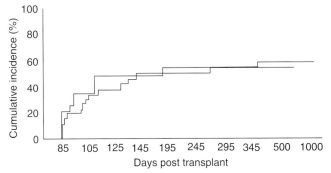

Figure 5.1 Incidence and time of onset of chronic GVHD. The data are derived from 76 recipients of non–T cell-depleted HLA-identical sibling marrow who received cyclophosphamide 120 mg/kg, fractionated total body irradiation 12 to 14 Gy and cyclosporine ($n = 59$) or methotrexate ($n = 17$). The transplant was performed in first remission of acute nonlymphoblastic leukemia (ANL) or acute lymphobalstic leukemia (ALL), or in first relapse or later phase of ANL or ALL.

Permission obtained from Nature Publishing Group [4].

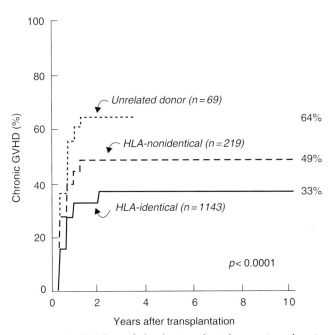

Figure 5.2 Probability of developing clinical extensive chronic GVHD in patients with hematologic malignancies transplanted through December, 1989 who survived at least 150 days after marrow transplantation from HLA-identical siblings, HLA-nonidentical family members and unrelated marrow donors. HLA-nonidentical donor recipients significantly differed from HLA-identical ($p = 0.0001$) and unrelated marrow recipients ($p = 0.0401$). Permission obtained from Elsevier Ltd [5].

patients transplanted from HLA-identical siblings who had a 33% probability of developing cGVHD by 2 years post-HCT, recipients of marrow from HLA-nonidentical family members or unrelated donors had a significantly increased probability of 49% and 64%, respectively. In addition, the reported median time for the onset of cGVHD was earlier in the mismatched

and unrelated recipients (201 vs. 159 vs. 133 days, respectively). Very few patients developed initial onset of cGVHD more than 500 days after transplantation.

Several studies published during the 1980s evaluated risk factors for the development of cGVHD. In one of the first studies conducted, involving 2534 recipients of matched sibling HCT between 1982 and 1987 reported to the International Bone Marrow Transplant Registry (IBMTR), the strongest predictor of cGVHD was the occurrence and severity of aGVHD [6]. The probabilities of cGVHD by 3 years posttransplant in persons with grade 0, I, II, III, and IV aGVHD were 28% ± 3%, 49% ± 5%, 59% ± 6%, 80% ± 9%, and 85% ± 15%, respectively (univariate $p < 0.0001$). When the analysis was restricted to cGVHD patients with no prior or grade I aGVHD only, three factors were associated with the development of cGVHD. These factors were recipient age >20 years, use of non–T-cell depleted marrow, and use of alloimmune female donors for male recipients. Patients with no prior aGVHD and without any of the adverse risk factors had a probability of developing cGVHD of 10% versus 62% ($p < 0.0001$) in those with all three risk factors. In those with grade I aGVHD, the respective probabilities were 21% versus 85% ($p < 0.0001$). These observations suggested that antihost alloreactive T cells played a role in both aGVHD and cGVHD. This implied that manipulating the method and/or duration of GVHD prophylaxis or number of T cells infused in the transplant might influence cGVHD incidence. Subsequent protocols for the prevention of GVHD would then focus primarily on reducing the incidence and severity of aGVHD with the hope of also reducing cGVHD. Prospective randomized trials comparing cyclosporine with methotrexate prophylaxis, however, showed no difference in the incidence of aGVHD (40% vs. 22%) or cGVHD (30% vs. 39%) with either agent respectively [7–8]. An additional randomized trial of combination cyclosporine and methotrexate compared to cyclosporine alone by the Seattle group [9] showed significantly reduced incidence and severity of aGVHD (grade II–IV, 33% vs. 60%, $p = 0.014$), however, no difference in cGVHD incidence (26% vs. 24%) was seen.

Another method of prophylaxis was T-cell depletion of the donor marrow. Various groups were performing T-cell depletion by physical separation (lectin agglutination) methods or by treatment with monoclonal antibodies. An early study performed by the IBMTR in 1991 compared the outcomes of 731 T-cell depleted HLA-identical sibling recipients with 2,480 non-T-cell depleted recipients. T-cell depletion did decrease aGVHD (relative risk [RR] 0.45, $p < 0.0001$) and cGVHD (RR 0.56, $p < 0.0001$) respectively when compared to unmanipulated grafts, however, this came at the expense of a higher rate of graft failure and disease relapse [10].

In contrast to the related donor setting, T-cell depletion in HLA-matched unrelated donor marrow recipients did not decrease cGVHD incidence [11]. A recent multicenter randomized trial by the National Heart, Lung, and Blood Institute (NHLBI) comparing T-cell depleted unrelated donor marrow transplants with unmanipulated grafts shows that in spite of significant reduction in aGVHD there was no difference in the incidence of cGVHD at 2 years following HCT between the two graft types (29% vs. 34%, respectively), possibly a reflection of differing pathogeneses of these two GVHD syndromes [12].

1990–2000

Despite new strategies to prevent cGVHD during the 1990s, outcomes would continue to be disappointing. Weekly administration of 500 mg/kg IV Ig through day 90 posttransplant reduced the incidence of aGVHD, however the same dose given monthly between days 90 and 360 posttransplant did not reduce the incidence of cGVHD [13, 14]. A randomized double-blind study using thalidomide prophylaxis resulted in a paradoxical outcome of higher incidence of cGVHD and lower overall survival [15]. Tacrolimus reduced the incidence of aGVHD when used for GVHD prophylaxis but did not influence the incidence of cGVHD [16, 17]. Antithymocyte globulin in the preparative regimen in unrelated marrow recipients was shown to significantly reduce grades III–IV aGVHD as well as extensive cGVHD compared to the non-ATG containing regimens (39% vs. 62% respectively), however, overall survival and nonrelapse mortality did not improve [18]. The long-term follow-up of this randomized trial with ATG had similar results (37% vs. 60%, respectively); additionally there was a protective effect in reducing chronic lung dysfunction in the ATG arm [18, 19]. Studies with Campath-1H (another type of antibody prophylaxis) for both in vivo and in vitro purging of donor T cells have reported exceptionally low incidences of cGVHD of only 4.4% compared with 56.3% in historical control groups [20] and offers some promise.

Another approach to reduce the incidence of cGVHD was to extend the course of immunosuppression with cyclosporine prophylaxis [21–23]. The basis of this approach was the clinical observation that cGVHD usually developed during or shortly after the routine 6-month taper of cyclosporine. The Seattle group provided additional insight on this observation with their trial of 103 patients given cyclosporine/methotrexate prophylaxis [24]. Those patients who had no active aGVHD by day 60 were randomized to have cyclosporine stopped at day 60 (n = 52) or continued to day 180 (n = 51) posttransplant [24]. In the group with early discontinuation, the onset of cGVHD was significantly more rapid but not significantly higher in overall incidence than in the group who continued to day 180 (43% vs. 54%, p = 0.26). Transplant-related mortality was increased in patients with preceding aGVHD in whom cyclosporine was stopped by day 60 (38% vs. 17%), thus suggesting that patients with preceding aGVHD might benefit from a longer course of cyclosporine. Another study randomized patients to receive a 24-month course compared to a 6-month course of cyclosporine prophylaxis [25]. Clinical extensive cGVHD developed in 35 of the 89 patients (39%) in the 24-month group and 37 of the 73 patients (51%) in the 6-month group. The hazard of developing cGVHD was not significantly different in the two groups (HR = 0.76; p = 0.25), and there was no significant difference in nonrelapse mortality

or survival. The study concluded there was no significant advantage for extended cyclosporine prophylaxis in reducing the incidence of clinical cGVHD.

An alternative strategy to prevent cGVHD was to prolong the treatment of aGVHD. The Minnesota group performed a randomized trial of short- versus long-term prednisone therapy for aGVHD and found the median dose of prednisone required to achieve complete resolution of aGVHD was not different between the two groups and importantly, the incidence of cGVHD and survival at 6 months was similar in the two groups [26]. Thus an effective regimen for prevention of cGVHD remains a challenge.

Donor T cells were clearly playing a central role in the immunologic attack on host tissues in both aGVHD and cGVHD. While the cytokine production pattern of aGVHD is mostly TH1 type, the TH2 cytokines predominate in patients with classic cGVHD [27, 28], with clinical manifestations consistent with TH2 elevations (e.g., associations of elevated IL-5 with eosinophilia, IL-4 with gammapathy and stimulation of collagen production by fibroblasts). This autoreactive T-cell phenotype suggested an important association between cGVHD and a damaged thymus. Experimental and clinical data would support a role for thymic regulation of autoreactive T cells in the maintenance of tolerance [29]. Thymic atrophy or damage could account for the well-recognized risk of cGVHD with advancing patient age. Among recipients of HLA-identical marrow who survived beyond day 150, the actuarial probability of developing cGVHD was 13% in patients who were 1 to 9 years old, 28% in those 10 to 19 years old and 42% to 46% in those over age 20. In recipients of HLA-nonidentical and unrelated marrow, the probability of developing cGVHD was 42% in patients who were 1 to 9 years old, increasing to 56% in those 10 to 19 years old, 50% to 52% in patients who were 20 to 49 years old, and 70% in patients over 50 years of age [5]. An interesting, but ultimately fruitless approach to overcome thymic dysfunction and prevent cGVHD in the early 1980s was unrelated thymic tissue transplants [30]. These thymic implants were likely rejected by the recipient. Recently, however, we have improved understanding of thymopoiesis from murine models, and pharmacologic approaches such as with keratinocyte growth factor (KGF), which target posttransplant thymic regeneration by restoring thymic epithelial cell function while preserving the thymic microenvironment, are now being explored [31, 32].

B cells have also been shown to play a role in the development of cGVHD [33]. In male HCT recipients of female donors, H-Y minor histocompatibility antigens are targets of donor T cells and B cells. H-Y antibodies have been found to correlate with the subsequent development of cGVHD [34]. Autoantibodies are also described in patients with cGVHD. Moreover, treatment with the anti-CD20 monoclonal antibody, rituximab, has resulted in clinical improvement in some patients with steroid-resistant cGVHD [35]. These observations have led to approaches with anti-B-cell therapy being incorporated into the transplant regimen to attempt to reduce the incidence of cGVHD.

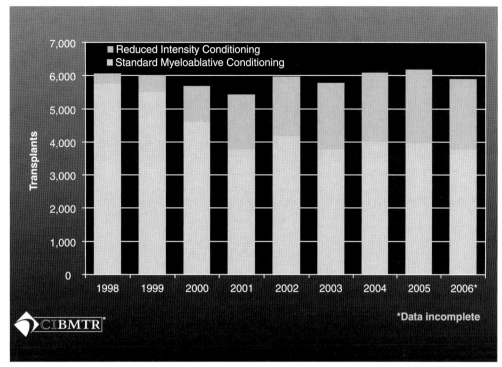

Figure 5.3 Allogeneic transplantations registered with CIBMTR by conditioning regimen intensity, 1998–2006. Pasquini M. Wang Z., Schneider L. CIBMTR summary slides, 2007. CIBMTR newsletter 2007;13:5–9. See Plate 5 in the color plate section.

Longer prospective follow-up of cGVHD patients transplanted in the early 1990s allowed for better definition of incidence and character of the GVHD. Arora et al. from the University of Minnesota reported on a prospective cohort of 159 patients undergoing related and unrelated allogeneic BMT between 1987 and 1993 who developed symptomatic cGVHD [36]. During the 4.9 years of patient enrollment, the reported incidence of cGVHD was 44%. Progressive onset of disease was seen in 45% of patients, quiescent in 43%, and de novo in 12%. Most deaths (86%) were observed within 2 years of onset, but deaths continued to occur up to 8.6 years after diagnosis. Nearly all (86%) patients died of complications related to cGVHD, the majority with infection (63%), demonstrating that cGVHD was clearly the major contributor to nonrelapse mortality.

An important correlation in this study was the determination of the prevalence of cGVHD (defined as persistence of active cGVHD among surviving patients) evaluated over time [36]. Prevalence decreases as a reflection of a clinical cure of cGVHD. In this study, the prevalence was 56% at 6 months, 60% at 1 year, and 33% at 2 years, suggesting gradual resolution of cGVHD over time with treatment.

2000–PRESENT

There have been significant shifts in graft source, conditioning regimens, immunosuppression regimens, supportive care, and degree of HLA mismatch in transplantation. Several of these changes occurred during the mid-1990s and later. The average age of allogeneic transplant recipients has increased in recent years, as has the number of transplants utilizing reduced-intensity conditioning and a peripheral blood graft source (Figures 5.3 and 5.4) [37]. These changes in practice have resulted in extending the age of transplanted patients and decreasing early nonrelapse mortality, all of which could result in increasing numbers of patients at risk of developing cGVHD. Unfortunately, there is a profound lack of epidemiology data describing the impact of these trends on the incidence and clinical presentations of cGVHD.

PERIPHERAL BLOOD VERSUS BONE MARROW GRAFTS

There are numerous reports, including randomized trials, comparing outcomes after peripheral blood stem cell (PBSC) and bone marrow (BM) transplants from HLA-matched sibling donors (Table 5.1) [38–47]. Most studies indicate a higher risk of cGVHD as well as greater severity following PBSC compared to BM grafts. In addition, a meta-analysis of nine randomized trials of matched sibling transplants that was performed by the Stem Cell Trialists' Group [48] concluded there was no difference in overall incidence of aGVHD between the two graft types (54% vs. 53%; $p = 0.49$), but a highly significant increase in the odds of developing both extensive stage

Table 5.1   Related Donors, Trials Comparing Allogeneic BM versus PBSC Grafts: Incidence of Acute and Chronic GVHD

Study	Study Design	N	Stem Cell Source	Acute GVHD Grade II–IV (%)	Acute GVHD Grade III–IV (%)	Chronic GVHD (%)
Vigorito et al., 1998 [38]	Randomized, related donor	37	PBSC	27	13	100*
			BM	19	13	50*
Blaise et al., 2000 [39]	Randomized, related donor	101	PBSC BM	44	17	50*
				42	23	28*
Heldal et al., 2000 [40]	Randomized, related donor	61	PBSC	21	NR	56
			BM	10		27
Powles et al., 2000 [41]	Randomized, related donor	39	PBSC	50	NR	44
			BM	47		40
Bensinger et al., 2001 [42]	Randomized, related donor	172	PBSC	64 (at d 100)	15 (at d 100)	46
			BM	57 (at d 100)	12 (at d 100)	35
Schmitz et al., 2002 [43] (EBMT)	Randomized, related donor	329	PBSC	52*	28	67*
			BM	39*	16	54*
Couban et al., 2002 (Canadian BMT group) [44]	Randomized, related donor	228	PBSC	44 (at d 100)	26 (at d 100)	40 (at 30 m)
			BM	44 (at d 100)	18 (at d 100)	30 (at 30 m)
Champlin et al., 2000, 2006 [45,46]**	Retrospective registry (IBMTR) related donor	824 (288-PBSC) (536-BM)	PBSC	40 (at d 100)	13 (at d 100)	65 (at 1 y)*
			BM	35 (at d 100)	19 (at d 100)	53 (at 1 y)* **update 61 (at 6 y)* 45 (at 6 y)*
Anderson et al., 2003 [47]	Prospective cohort related donor	194 (97-PBSC) (97-BM)	PBSC	46 (at d 100)	15	37 (at 1 y)
			BM	51 (at d 100)	16	28 (at 1 y)

Notes: BM, bone marrow; GVHD, d, day; graft versus host disease; m, month; NS, not significant; NR, not reported; PBSC, peripheral blood stem cell; y, year .
*Statistically significant; †2006 update results.
Adapted from Korbling M, Anderlini P. Peripheral blood stem cell versus bone marrow allotransplantation: does the source of hematopoietic stem cells matter? *Blood.* 2001;98:2900–2908, with permission from the American Society of Hematology.

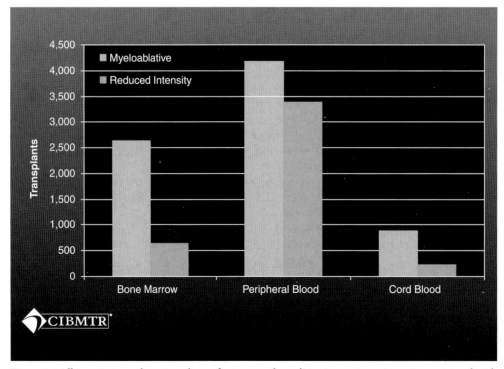

Figure 5.4 Allogeneic transplantations by graft source and conditioning regimen intensity, registered with CIBMTR, 2005–2006. Data was obtained from CIBMTR [37]. See Plate 6 in the color plate section.

Table 5.2   Unrelated Donors, Trials Comparing Allogeneic BM versus PBSC Grafts: Incidence of Acute and Chronic GVHD

Study	Study Design	N	Stem Cell Source	Acute GVHD Grade II–IV (%)	Acute GVHD Grade III–IV (%)	Chronic GVHD (%)
Ringden et al., 1999 [51]	Matched pair, unrelated donor	108 (45-PBSC) (18-PB CD34) (45-BM)	PBSC PB CD34 BM	30 18 20 (NS)	14 6 16	PBSC 59(at 1y) PB CD34 0 * BM 85 (at 1 y)
Remberger et al., 2001, (2005) [52, 53]†	Matched pair, unrelated donor	214 (107-PBSC) (107-BM)	PBSC BM	35 32	18 22	61 76 NS **extensive, PB [39] versus BM [24]*
Eapen et al., 2007 [54]	Retrospective registry, NMDP unrelated donor	331 PBSC 586 BM	PBSC BM	58 45*	28 25	56 42*

Notes: BM, bone marrow; GVHD, graft versus host disease; NMPD, National Marrow Donor Program; NS, not significant; PB, peripheral blood; PBSC, peripheral blood stem cell; y, year.
*Statistically significant; †2005 update results.
Adapted from Korbling M, Anderlini P. Peripheral blood stem cell versus bone marrow allotransplantation: does the source of hematopoietic stem cells matter? *Blood.* 2001;98:2900–2908, with permission from the American Society of Hematology.

(odds ratio [OR] = 1.89; $p < 0.00001$) and overall (OR = 1.92; $p < 0.00001$) cGVHD in patients treated with PBSC transplants. At 3 years after HCT, 47% and 68% of patients treated with PBSC transplant developed extensive or any stage cGVHD versus 31% and 52% after BM transplant, respectively. The Seattle group reported an increased severity of the cGVHD after PBSC transplants where patients experienced a more protracted course that is less responsive to treatment compared to marrow recipients [49]. A meta-analysis [50] specifically looking at incidence of cGVHD after PBSC versus BM transplant indicates the relative risk of developing clinically extensive cGVHD is 1.66 ($p < 0.001$) for PBSC grafts. The excess risk of cGVHD was possibly explained by the difference in T-cell dose delivered with the graft.

Fewer studies are available regarding outcomes of PBSC versus BM transplants for unrelated donors (Table 5.2) [51–54]. Data from the National Marrow Donor Program (NMDP) indicates that about 80% of unrelated adult donor transplants in the United States now use PBSC grafts [54]. Eapen et al. [54]. analyzed data on 331 recipients of unrelated donor PBSC and 586 recipients of unrelated donor BM transplants facilitated by the NMDP in the United States in 2000 to 2003 where allele-level HLA-typing was available. The striking finding was that despite rates of aGVHD and cGVHD, which were significantly higher for PBSC grafts than with BM grafts, there was no improvement in leukemia-free survival. Extended follow-up is warranted to better define the higher rate of cGVHD after PBSC transplants and the consequent higher rate of late adverse events. A randomized trial comparing the two graft types in unrelated donors is ongoing within the Blood and Marrow Transplant Clinical Trials Network.

HLA-MISMATCHED TRANSPLANTS

With only 30% of otherwise eligible patients with leukemia in the United States having a related histocompatible donor and only about 40% having a matched unrelated donor, the use of HLA-mismatched transplantation has increased [55]. An HLA mismatch, however, is perhaps the strongest risk factor for GVHD. Cord blood grafts from unrelated donors, which allow for a higher degree of mismatch, have been used successfully primarily in children, and now their use has increased in adults. Outcomes of one- or two-antigen mismatched cord blood transplant have recently been compared with those of HLA-mismatched and matched bone marrow in adult patients [55]. Among patients surviving ≥90 days, cGVHD developed in 86 of 243 (35%) recipients of HLA-matched bone marrow, 17 of 43 (40%) recipients of mismatched bone marrow, and 35 of 69 (51%) recipients of mismatched cord blood. The rate of cGVHD was higher among cord blood recipients than among HLA-matched marrow recipients (hazard ratio 1.62, $p = 0.02$) but similar to the rate among recipients of mismatched marrow (hazard ratio 1.12, $p = 0.69$). The proportion of extensive cGVHD was lower among cord blood recipients than among HLA-matched or mismatched marrow recipients with rates of 33%, 52%, and 71%, respectively ($p = 0.03$).

In a recent NMDP study reported by Lee et al. [56], the importance of high-resolution donor-recipient HLA matching on the outcome of 3,857 myeloablative unrelated donor transplants was examined. Mismatching at a single HLA-A, -B, -C, or DRB1 locus (7/8) was associated with lower survival and DFS, higher treatment-related mortality and more aGVHD compared with 8/8 HLA-matched pairs. There were no statistically significant differences in risk associated with single high-resolution (allele) versus single low-resolution (antigen) mismatches, so analyses in this study considered allele and antigen mismatches equivalent.

There was no statistically significant difference between 7/8 (either allele or antigen) and 8/8 matched pairs for relapse, cGVHD, and engraftment. The incidence of cGVHD at 1 year for an 8/8 match was 44% (95% CI) [41–46]; and 36% (95% CI) [33–39] for a 7/8 match. Single mismatches at HLA-B or HLA-C appear to be better tolerated than mismatches at HLA-A or HLA-DRB1 for survival. Mismatching at two or more loci compounds the risk in that each additional mismatch is associated with a 9% to 10% absolute decrease in survival. In this series, degree of high-resolution (allele-level) DNA mismatch did not seem to impact cGVHD incidence; however, in the Flomenberg series [57], HLA-A mismatches were associated with significantly higher incidence of cGVHD (RR = 1.35, $p = 0.006$) as with data from Morishima et al. (HLA-A/B mismatch with 59.6% incidence of cGVHD compared to HLA match, 44.8%) [58]. These HLA associations suggest a mechanism of cGVHD that is different from aGVHD but that is somehow regulated by disparity of HLA alleles. This better understanding of the role of high-resolution HLA matching can be incorporated in the choices made in donor selection to maximize the success of unrelated donor transplant.

NONMYELOABLATIVE OR REDUCED-INTENSITY CONDITIONING TRANSPLANTS

Nonmyeloablative (or reduced-intensity) conditioning regimens have been increasingly used, particularly in older patients and others at high risk for toxicity after conventional transplant regimens. These regimens are a spectrum of low-dose chemotherapy and/or radiation that provide sufficient immunosuppression to allow engraftment and antitumor effect without the potentially lethal effects of myeloablative conditioning. Nonmyeloablative transplants produce a less intense release of inflammatory cytokines resulting in decreased tissue damage from conditioning with a transient and potentially tolerogenic state of mixed donor/host chimerism. Frequently, novel regimens for immunosuppression (cyclosporine/mycophenolate mofetil) have been used with these transplants. These differences with myeloablative transplant might account for the lower rates of severe GVHD. The MD Anderson group [59] compared the incidence of aGVHD and cGVHD after myeloablative (busulfan/cyclophosphamide, fludarabine/melphalan) and nonmyeloablative regimens (fludarabine/cyclophosphamide and other fludarabine-containing) and found a reduced incidence of grade II–IV aGVHD (36% vs. 12%, respectively) and cGVHD (40% vs. 14%, respectively) with the nonmyeloablative regimen. This observation highlights the importance of aGVHD as a risk factor for cGVHD development and the marked impact of the nonmyeloablative regimen on GVHD outcome. The Seattle group [60] also compared the GVHD incidence after their nonmyeloablative regimen of low-dose total body irradiation (TBI) with or without fludarabine

versus their conventional regimens. They showed that the cumulative incidence of grades II–IV aGVHD was lower after nonmyeloablative transplant (64% vs. 85%, $p = 0.001$) but there was no difference in the cumulative incidence of cGVHD (73% vs. 71%, $p = 0.96$). Other groups have similarly found a lower incidence of aGVHD with the nonmyeloablative or reduced-intensity conditioning (RIC) but no statistically significant difference in incidence of cGVHD [61–64], and no difference with use of related or unrelated grafts [65]. Note should be made, however, that findings across studies are not directly comparable due to differences in the toxicities of different regimens, and the types and duration of immunosuppression utilized. This is evidenced by the frequencies of grade II–IV aGVHD ranging from 20% to 60% in reports from various studies. There are also the complexities of the impact of T-cell depletion techniques such as the use of Campath or antithymocyte globulin (ATG) on GVHD outcome in these transplants that make comparisons difficult [66–69].

The Seattle study further reported that the GVHD onset in nonmyeloablative transplant was delayed by 2 months compared to conventional transplant with clinical findings more consistent with the syndrome of aGVHD (i.e., more prevalent skin, more severe gut), favoring the term "late-onset aGVHD." [60]. This has led to the proposal of abandoning the traditional day 100 cutoff for separation of aGVHD from cGVHD and emphasizing better description of the GVHD target-organ involvement.

In summary the impact of nonmyeloablative conditioning on the incidence of cGVHD has not been evaluated systematically. The main conclusion so far seems to be that nonmyeloablative conditioning decreases the incidence and severity of aGVHD through day 100; however, there is little evidence to suggest that cGVHD is reduced [70]. Many factors are confounding in the analyses and interpretation of the data, such as short follow-up, absence of prospective comparison trials, use of a variety of RIC regimens, lack of uniform GVHD prophylaxis and lack of rigorous criteria for the diagnosis and staging of chronic GVHD [27].

FUTURE CHALLENGES

Through the history of bone marrow transplant, it can be seen how changes in transplant practice have impacted the development and severity of GVHD outcome. The failures and successes of past efforts in management and prevention of cGVHD are continually being reexamined to improve our knowledge of this disease. Reports to date on cGVHD incidence have been subject to single center bias, the variability in center assignment and grading of cGVHD (limited by the historical limited vs. extensive categories), and variabilities in immunosuppression practice (duration, type), all of which can factor into an incidence estimate. Figure 5.5 is perhaps the best published representation of an increasing trend in cGVHD incidence over the past decades but is limited by single institution data [71]. There is a profound lack of epidemiological studies addressing

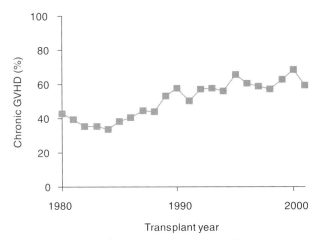

Figure 5.5 Trend of increasing cGVHD incidence/year over two decades in patients surviving at least 100 days at the Fred Hutchinson Cancer Research Center – all graft sources and regimens. Printed with permission from Elsevier, Ltd [71]. See Plate 7 in the color plate section.

the incidence and trends in chronic GVHD in the modern era. Such data are critical for both patient counseling and design and planning of clinical trials. Future trials must incorporate prospective designs, standardized means of data collection, and uniform definitions to allow interpretation of and comparison between various studies. The new efforts by the NIH Consensus Development project to standardize the diagnosis, staging, and response criteria will bring the needed structure and standards for communicating our common ideas on this important cause of late morbidity and mortality posttransplant.

KEY POINTS

Factors Having No Impact on cGVHD Incidence

Disease status at transplant [4]
T-cell depletion [12]*
IV Ig administration [13, 14]*
Prolonged immunosuppression prophylaxis [21–25]*
Prolonged steroid treatment of aGVHD [26]*
Antigen versus allele-level mismatch [56]
Nonmyeloablative (reduced-intensity) conditioning [60]

* Data derived from randomized controlled trial.

Factors Having Impact on cGVHD Incidence

Using mismatched related donor or unrelated marrow donor [5]
Occurrence and severity of prior aGVHD [6]
ATG or Campath-1H-containing preparative regimen [18–20]*
Advanced patient age, for example, thymic atrophy [5]
Use of peripheral blood stem cell grafts [38–48]*
Mismatched cord blood [55]

* Data derived from randomized controlled trial.

REFERENCES

1. Appelbaum FR. Hematopoietic-cell transplantation at 50. N Engl J Med. 2007;357:1472–1475.
2. Shulman HM, Sullivan KM, Weiden PL, et al. Chronic graft-versus-host syndrome in man: a long-term clinicopathologic study of 20 Seattle patients. Am J Med. 1980;69:204–217.
3. Sullivan KM, Shulman HM, Storb R, et al. Chronic graft-versus-host disease in 52 patients: adverse natural course and successful treatment with combination immunosuppression. Blood. 1981;57:267–276.
4. Atkinson K. Chronic graft-versus-host disease. Bone Marrow Transplant. 1990;5:69–82.
5. Sullivan KM, Agura E, Anasetti C, et al. Chronic graft-versus-host disease and other late complications of bone marrow transplantation. Sem Hematol. 1991;28:250–259.
6. Atkinson K, Horowitz MM, Gale RP, et al. Risk factors for chronic graft-versus-host disease after HLA-identical sibling bone marrow transplantation. Blood. 1990;75:2459–2464.
7. Biggs JC, Atkinson K, Gillet E, Downs K, Concannon A, Dodds A. A randomized prospective trial comparing cyclosporine and methotrexate given for prophylaxis of graft-versus-host disease after bone marrow transplantation. Transplant Proc. 1986;18:253–255.
8. Ringden O, Backman L, Lonnqvist D, et al. A randomized trial comparing the use of cyclosporine and methotrexate for graft-versus-host disease prophylaxis in bone marrow transplant recipients with haematological malignancies. Bone Marrow Transplant. 1986;1:41–51.
9. Storb R, Deeg HJ, Pepe M, et al. Methotrexate and cyclosporine alone for prophylaxis of graft-versus-host disease in patients given HLA-identical marrow grafts for leukemia: long-term follow-up of a controlled trial. Blood. 1989;73:1729–1734.
10. Marmont AM, Horowitz MM, Gale RP, et al. T-cell depletion of HLA-identical transplants in leukemia. Blood. 1991;78:2120–2130.
11. Ash RC, Casper JT, Chitambar CR, et al. Successful allogeneic transplantation of T-cell-depleted bone marrow from closely HLA-matched unrelated donors. N Engl J Med. 1990;322:485–494.
12. Pavletic SZ, Carter SL, Kernan NA, et al. Influence of T-cell depletion on chronic graft-versus-host disease: results of a multicenter randomized trial in unrelated marrow donor transplantation. Blood. 2005;106:3308–3313.
13. Sullivan KM, Kopecky KJ, Jocom J, et al. Immunomodulatory and antimicrobial efficacy of intravenous immunoglobulin in bone marrow transplantation. N Engl J Med. 1990;323:705–712.
14. Sullivan KM, Storek J, Kopecky KJ, et al. A controlled trial of long-term administration of intravenous immunoglobulin to prevent late infection and chronic graft-versus-host disease after marrow transplantation: clinical outcome and effect on subsequent immune recovery. Biol Blood Marrow Transplant. 1996;2:44–53.
15. Chao NJ, Parker PM, Niland JC, et al. Paradoxical effect of thalidomide prophylaxis on chronic graft-vs-host disease. Biol Blood Marrow Transplant. 1996;2:86–92.
16. Ratanatharathorn V, Nash RA, Przepiorka D, et al. Phase III study comparing methotrexate and cyclosporine for graft-versus-host disease prophylaxis after HLA-identical sibling bone marrow transplantation. Blood. 1998;92:2303–2314.

17. Nash RA, Antin JH, Karanes C, et al. Phase 3 study comparing methotrexate and tacrolimus with methotrexate and cyclosporine for prophylaxis of acute graft-versus-host disease after marrow transplantation from unrelated donors. *Blood.* 2000;96:2062–2068.

18. Bacigalupo A, Lamparelli T, Bruzzi P, et al. Antithymocyte globulin for graft-versus-host disease prophylaxis in transplants from unrelated donors: 2 randomized studies from Gruppo Italiano Trapianti Midollo Osseo (GITMO). *Blood.* 2001;98:2942–2947.

19. Bacigalupo A, Lamparelli T, Barisione G, et al. Thymoglobulin prevents chronic graft-versus-host disease, chronic lung dysfunction, and late transplant-related mortality: long-term follow-up of a randomized trial in patients undergoing unrelated donor transplantation. *Biol Blood Marrow Transplant.* 2006;12:560–565.

20. Chakrabarti S, MacDonald D, Hale G, et al. T-cell depletion with Campath-1H 'in the bag' for matched related allogeneic peripheral blood stem cell transplantation is associated with reduced graft-versus-host disease, rapid immune constitution and improved survival. *Br J Haematol.* 2003;121:109–118.

21. Ruutu T, Volin L, Elonen E. Low incidence of severe acute and chronic graft-versus-host disease as a result of prolonged cyclosporine prophylaxis and early aggressive treatment with corticosteroids. *Transplant Proc.* 1988;20:491–493.

22. Lonnqvist B, Aschan J, Ljungman P, Ringden O. Long-term cyclosporin therapy may decrease the risk of chronic graft-versus-host disease. *Br J Haematol.* 1990;74:547–548.

23. Bacigalupo A, Maiolino A, Van Lint MT et al. Cyclosporin A and chronic graft versus host disease. *Bone Marrow Transplant.* 1990;6:341–344.

24. Storb R, Leisenring W, Anasetti C, et al. Methotrexate and cyclosporine for graft-vs-host disease prevention: what length of therapy with cyclosporine? *Biol Blood Marrow Transplant.* 1997;3:194–201.

25. Kansu E, Gooley T, Flowers ME, et al. Administration of cyclosporine for 24 months compared with 6 months for prevention of chronic graft-versus-host disease: a prospective randomized clinical trial. *Blood.* 2001;98:3868–3870.

26. Hings IM, Filipovich AH, Miller WJ, et al. Prednisone therapy for acute graft-versus-host disease: short- versus long-term treatment. A prospective randomized trial. *Transplantation.* 1993;56:577–580.

27. Filipovich AH, Weisdorf D, Pavletic S, et al. National Institutes of Health consensus development project on criteria for clinical trials in chronic graft-versus-host disease: I. Diagnosis and staging working group report. *Biol Blood Marrow Transplant.* 2005;11:945–955.

28. Ratanatharathorn V, Ayash L, Lazarus HM, Fu J, Uberti JP. Chronic graft-versus-host disease: clinical manifestation and therapy. *Bone Marrow Transplant.* 2001;28:121–129.

29. Ferrara JLM, Deeg HJ. Graft-versus-host disease. *N Engl J Med.* 1991;324:667–674.

30. Atkinson K, Storb R, Ochs HD, et al. Thymus transplantation after allogeneic bone marrow grafting to prevent chronic graft-versus-host disease in humans. *Transplantation.* 1982;33:168–173.

31. Alpdogan O, Hubbard VM, Smith OM, et al. Keratinocyte growth factor (KGF) is required for postnatal thymic regeneration. *Blood.* 2006;107:2453–2460.

32. Min D, Panoskaltsis-Mortari A, Kuro-O M, Hollander GA, Blazar BR, Weinberg KI. Sustained thymopoiesis and improvement in functional immunity induced by exogenous KGF administration in murine models of aging. *Blood.* 2007;109:2529–2537.

33. Zhang C, Todorov I, Zhang I, et al. Donor CD4+ T and B cells in transplants induce chronic graft-versus-host disease with auto-immune manifestations. *Blood.* 2006;107:2993–3001.

34. Miklos DB, Kim HT, Miller KH, et al. Antibody responses to H-Y minor histocompatibility antigens correlate with chronic graft-versus-host disease and disease remission. *Blood.* 2005;105:2973–2978.

35. Cutler C, Miklos D, Kim HT, et al. Rituximab for steroid-refractory chronic graft-versus-host disease. *Blood.* 2006;108:756–762.

36. Arora M, Burns LJ, Davies SM, et al. Chronic graft-versus-host disease: a prospective cohort study. *Biol Blood Marrow Transplant.* 2003;9:38–45.

37. Pasquini M, Wang Z, Schneider L. CIBMTR summary slides, 2007. *CIBMTR newsletter.* 2007;13:5–9.

38. Vigorito AC, Azevedo WM, Marques JFC, et al. A randomised, prospective comparison of allogeneic bone marrow and peripheral blood progenitor cell transplantation in the treatment of haematological malignancies. *Bone Marrow Transplant.* 1998;22:1145–1151.

39. Blaise D, Kuentz M, Fortanier C, et al. Randomized trial of bone marrow versus lenograstim-primed blood cell allogeneic transplantation in patients with early-stage leukemia: a report from the Societe Francaise de Greffe de Moelle. *J Clin Oncol.* 2000;18:537–546.

40. Heldal D, Tjonnfjord G, Brinch L, et al. A randomised study of allogeneic transplantation with stem cells from blood or bone marrow. *Bone Marrow Transplant.* 2000;25:1129–1136.

41. Powles R, Mehta J, Kulkarni S, et al. Allogeneic blood and bone-marrow stem-cell transplantation in haematological malignant diseases: a randomised trial. *Lancet.* 2000;355:1231–1237.

42. Bensinger WI, Martin PJ, Storer B, et al. Transplantation of bone marrow as compared with peripheral blood cells from HLA-identical relatives in patients with hematologic cancers. *N Engl J Med.* 2001;344:175–181.

43. Schmitz N, Beksac M, Hasenclever D, et al. Transplantation of mobilized peripheral blood cells to HLA-identical siblings with standard-risk leukemia. *Blood.* 2002;100:761–767.

44. Couban S, Simpson DR, Barnett MJ, et al. A randomized multicenter comparison of bone marrow and peripheral blood recipients of matched sibling allogeneic transplants for myeloid malignancies. *Blood.* 2002;100:1525–1531.

45. Champlin RE, Schmitz N, Horowitz MM, et al. The IBMTR Histocompatibility and Stem Cell Sources Working Committee and the European Group for Blood and Marrow Transplantation (EBMT). *Blood.* 2000;95:3702–3709.

46. Schmitz N, Eapen M, Horowitz MM. et al. Long-term outcome of patients given transplants of mobilized blood or bone marrow: a report from the International Bone Marrow Transplant Registry and the European Group for Blood and Marrow Transplantation. *Blood.* 2006;108:4288–4290.

47. Anderson D, DeFor T, Burns L, et al. A comparison of related donor peripheral blood and bone marrow transplants: importance of late-onset chronic graft-versus-host disease and infections. *Biol Blood Marrow Transplant.* 2003;9:52–59.

48. Stem Cell Trialists' Collaborative Group. Allogeneic peripheral blood stem-cell compared with bone marrow transplantation in the management of hematologic malignancies: an individual patient data meta-analysis of nine randomized trials. *J Clin Oncol.* 2005;23:5074–5087.

49. Flowers MED, Parker PM, Johnston LJ, et al. Comparison of chronic graft-versus-host disease after transplantation of

peripheral blood stem cells versus bone marrow in allogeneic recipients: long-term follow-up of a randomized trial. *Blood.* 2002;100:415–419.

50. Cutler C, Giri S, Jeyapalan S, Paniagua D, Viswanathan A, Antin JH. Acute and chronic graft-versus-host disease after allogeneic peripheral-blood stem-cell and bone marrow transplantation: a meta-analysis. *J Clin Oncol.* 2001;19:3685–3691.

51. Ringden O, Remberger M, Runde V, et al. Peripheral blood stem cell transplantation from unrelated donors: a comparison with marrow transplantation. *Blood.* 1999;94:455–464.

52. Remberger M, Ringden O, Blau IW, et al. No difference in graft-versus-host disease, relapse, and survival comparing peripheral stem cells to bone marrow using unrelated donors. *Blood.* 2001;98:1739–1745.

53. Remberger M, Beelen DW, Fauser A, Basara N, Basu O, Ringden O. Increased risk of extensive chronic graft-versus-host disease after allogeneic peripheral blood stem cell transplantation using unrelated donors. *Blood.* 2005;105:548–551.

54. Eapen M, Logan BR, Confer DL, et al. Peripheral blood grafts from unrelated donors are associated with increased acute and chronic graft-versus-host disease without improved survival. *Biol Blood Marrow Transplant.* 2007;13:1461–1468.

55. Laughlin MJ, Eapen M, Rubinstein P, et al. Outcomes after transplantation of cord blood or bone marrow from unrelated donors in adults with leukemia. *N Engl J Med.* 2004;351:2265–2275.

56. Lee SJ, Klein J, Haagenson M, et al. High-resolution donor-recipient HLA matching contributes to the success of unrelated donor marrow transplantation. *Blood.* 2007;110:4576–4583.

57. Flomenberg N, Baxter-Lowe LA, Confer D, et al. Impact of HLA class I and class II high-resolution matching on outcomes of unrelated donor bone marrow transplantation: HLA-C mismatching is associated with a strong adverse effect on transplantation outcome. *Blood.* 2004;104:1923–1930.

58. Morishima Y, Sasazuki T, Inoko H, et al. The clinical significance of human leukocyte antigen (HLA) allele compatibility in patients receiving a marrow transplant from serologically HLA-A, HLA-B, and HLA-DR matched unrelated donors. *Blood.* 2002;99:4200–4206.

59. Couriel DR, Saliba RM, Giralt S, et al. Acute and chronic graft-versus-host disease after ablative and nonmyeloablative conditioning for allogeneic hematopoietic transplantation. *Biol Blood Marrow Transplant.* 2004;10:178–185.

60. Mielcarek M, Martin PJ, Leisenring W, et al. Graft-versus-host disease after nonmyeloablative versus conventional hematopoietic stem cell transplantation. *Blood.* 2003;102:756–762.

61. Perez-Simon JA, Diez-Campelo M, Martino R, et al. Influence of the intensity of the conditioning regimen on the characteristics of acute and chronic graft-versus-host disease after allogeneic transplantation. *Br J Haematol.* 2005;130:394–403.

62. Kim DH, Sohn SK, Baek JH, et al. Retrospective multicenter study of allogeneic peripheral blood stem cell transplantation followed by reduced intensity conditioning or conventional myeloablative regimen. *Acta Haematol.* 2005;113:220–227.

63. Aoudjhane M, Labopin M, Gorin RP, et al. Comparative outcome of reduced intensity and myeloablative conditioning regimen in HLA-identical sibling allogeneic haematopoietic stem cell transplantation for patients older than 50 years of age and acute myeloblastic leukaemia: a retrospective survey from the Acute Leukemia Working Party (ALWP) of the European group for Blood and Marrow Transplantation (EBMT). *Leukemia.* 2005;19:2304–2312.

64. Busca A, Rendine S, Locatelli F, et al. Chronic graft-versus-host disease after reduced-intensity stem cell transplantation versus conventional hematopoietic stem cell transplantation. *Hematology.* 2005;10:1–10.

65. Mielcarek M, Storer BE, Sandmaier BM, et al. Comparable outcomes after nonmyeloablative hamtopoietic cell transplantation with unrelated and related donors. *Biol Blood Marrow Transplant.* 2007;13:1499–1507.

66. Morris E, Thomson K, Craddock C, et al. Outcomes after alemtuzumab-containing reduced-intensity allogeneic transplantation regimen for relapsed and refractory non-Hodgkin lymphoma. *Blood.* 2004;104:3865–3871.

67. Mohty M, Bay JO, Faucher C, et al. Graft-versus-host disease following allogeneic transplantation from HLA-identical sibling with antithymocyte globulin-based reduced-intensity preparative regimen. *Blood.* 2003;102:470–476.

68. Bacigalupo A. Antithymocyte globulin for prevention of graft-versus-host disease. *Curr Opin Hematol.* 2005;6:457–462.

69. Lowsky R, Takahashi T, Liu YP, et al. Protective conditioning for acute graft-versus-host disease. *N Engl J Med.* 2005;353:1321–1331.

70. Subramaniam DS, Fowler DH, Pavletic SZ. Chronic graft-versus-host disease in the era of reduced-intensity conditioning. *Leukemia.* 2007;21:853–859.

71. Lee SJ, Vogelsang G, Flowers ME. Chronic graft-versus-host disease. *Biol Blood Marrow Transplant.* 2003;9:215–233.

6

Clinical Manifestations and Natural History

Mary Evelyn D. Flowers and Georgia B. Vogelsang

INTRODUCTION

Chronic graft versus host disease (cGVHD) is a clinical syndrome characterized by pleomorphic manifestation occurring over time with periods of exacerbation of acute manifestations or development of new clinical features in previously uninvolved or involved organs. cGVHD can affect multiple sites (Figure 6.1) and resembles manifestations of scleroderma, Sjogren syndrome, wasting syndrome, primary biliary cirrhosis, bronchiolitis obliterans, immune cytopenias, and chronic immunodeficiency disorders [1, 2]. The etiology of the variable phenotype of cGVHD is poorly understood and may depend on the type and intensity of the inflammatory and cellular process caused by immune dysregulation associated with cGVHD. Immune mechanisms leading to the diverse clinical manifestations of cGVHD have not been elucidated. Autoimmunity is thought to be involved because of the clinical similarities between cGVHD and autoimmune diseases. Dysfunctional T-cell selection in the thymus leading to a population of T_H2 self (recipient)-reactive T cells and differences in T_H1 and T_H2 responses by donor cells to recipient alloantigens may also play a role in pathogenesis. Recent studies reported that regulatory T cells (T_{reg}) are major determinants of a persistent immune imbalance that may result in cGVHD. Although T cells clearly play a central role in alloimmunity, the persistence of both T- and B-cell responses to multiple distinct **D/H Box 3, Y linked** (DBY) peptide epitopes in a patient with cGVHD and the strong correlation between the presence of antibodies to at least one H-Y mHA with cGVHD in male recipients of female hematopoietic cell transplantation (HCT) donors, support the role of B cells in cGVHD as well [3, 4]. Approximately 60% of adults who survive for more than 100 days after a non–T-depleted HCT will develop cGVHD [5]. The incidence of cGVHD is influenced by the source of stem cells, female donor into male recipient, human leukocyte antigen (HLA) matching, and age. The risk of nonrelapse mortality is higher for patients with cGVHD with direct progression from acute GVHD (aGVHD), platelet count <100,000/μL, hyperbilirubinemia, extensive skin disease, or multiple organ involvement, and low clinical performance score [2]. Mild forms of cGVHD can be manageable with local or low-dose systemic immunosuppression treatment and do not affect long-term survival. Failure to recognize early clinical manifestations of GVHD activity can result in progression to more severe forms such as sclerotic features and advanced lung involvement. Severe forms of cGVHD require prolonged and intensive medical management and adversely affect quality of life and survival.

cGVHD occurs within 3 years after HCT, with most patients diagnosed by 12 months after transplantation. Manifestations of cGVHD can occur before day 100 after the transplant and manifestations that are "classical" of acute GVHD may develop, persist, or recur long after day 100, as observed in a large proportion of patients after nonmyeloablative HCT conditioning [6]. Presentation of both acute and cGVHD manifestation can occur simultaneously especially after DLI [7]. Refinement of the diagnosis and classification of cGVHD first reported several decades ago [8, 9] have resulted from better understanding of cGVHD and advances in HCT. New criteria to differentiate late acute GVHD from cGVHD have been proposed by the National Institute of Health (NIH) cGVHD Consensus Group that take into consideration manifestations that are characteristic of cGVHD (See Chapter 9, Diagnosis and Staging) [10]. In addition, for purposes of clinical trials, a new scoring system for grading cGVHD in each organ (0–3) and a new global scoring system to assess overall severity of cGVHD (*mild, moderate, and severe*) have been developed to replace the historical "extensive/limited" classification, albeit validation of such system remains to be studied [8, 9]. This chapter provides an overview of a practical approach in the clinical assessment and monitoring of cGVHD. Each organ system is discussed in greater detail in Chapters 9 to 15 of this book.

PRACTICAL APPROACHES IN THE CLINICAL ASSESSMENT OF CGVHD

Clinical manifestations of cGVHD vary according to organ and clinical course. The clinical and the histological manifestations of cGVHD are discussed by organ system in

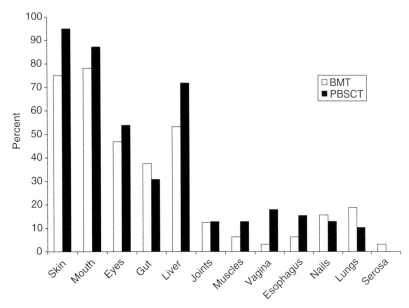

Figure 6.1 Prevalence of sites affected by chronic graft versus host disease (cGVHD) after peripheral blood stem cell transplant (PBSCT) compared to bone marrow transplant (BMT). Skin and vaginal involvement is more prevalent after PBSCT. Columns show the proportions of patients with organs affected by cGVHD at any time. Adapted with permission from Reference 14.

Part III, Organ Site or System Specific Manifestations of this book. Advanced forms of cGVHD including sclerotic/fibrotic manifestation involving the chest wall or resulting in joint contractures, severe pulmonary insufficiency or severe keratoconjunctivitis sicca [11] often result from failure to recognize early signs of disease activity or inadequate treatment.

Systematic and focused cGVHD history and physical examination are imperative to establish the initial diagnosis promptly, but also, to monitor disease course including detection of early or new signs of disease manifestations and to assess treatment response. Recognition of inflammatory type of disease activity (e.g., edema, eosinophilia, early fasciitis that may mimic "tunnel carpal syndrome") is important to guide further evaluation. Appropriate intervention should be taken to prevent the development of advanced sclerotic phenotype of cGVHD, such as joint contractures and restrictive lung defect secondary to scleroderma involving the chest wall. Conversely, not every problem posttransplant is caused by cGVHD. For instance, other conditions can be mislabeled as cGVHD, such as eczema (skin); iron overload (liver); hypothyroidism (hair loss and fatigue); joint stiffness, weight loss, nausea, and increased fatigue (adrenal insufficiency following corticosteroids discontinuation).

Recognition of early or subtle manifestations of cGVHD can help prevent the development of more severe forms of the disease, determine if further screening evaluation for disease activity in other organs is necessary, and guide monitoring and treatment. Long-term follow-up evaluation is necessary

and important for management of patients with cGVHD and should include systematic clinical monitoring with focused medical history and focused physical examination.

The cGVHD-focused medical history should always include (1) appropriate description of *both* symptoms and physical findings (positive and negative), (2) dates and reasons for initiation, changes, and discontinuation of prior treatments for *"classical, recurrent, or delayed"* onset of a acute GVHD and for *"classical"* cGVHD or "overlap syndrome"(see Chapter 9, Diagnosis and Staging), (3) list of current treatments including doses and supplements, topical treatments, and other supportive care (e.g., stretching exercise, physical therapy, massage therapy, use and frequency of ocular lubricants, punctal plugs, topical immunosuppressive medications, etc.), and (4) list of other relevant past and current diagnosis.

An easy approach for a systematic evaluation is to have patients complete a cGVHD-focused questionnaire with relevant elements of the medical history including review of systems (see Box 6.1). Such clinical questionnaires can be completed electronically as well. This approach systematically records relevant elements of the clinical assessment, can become part of the patient's medical records, helps in the patients' clinical assessment, and optimizes efficiency of clinic time.

The skin is the most frequent organ affected by cGVHD. One of the most common mistakes made by physicians and other primary care providers is that they fail to completely examine the skin which requires the patient to undress. Thus,

Box 6.1 Chronic GVHD-Focused Review of Systems and Other Relevant Medical History Elements

Seattle Long-Term follow-Up Screening History Form (completed by the patient)
Patients are asked to check "YES," "NO," OR "DON'T KNOW" as appropriate to the questions below about current symptoms and other information about their health since their LAST EVALUATION.

Please check the one phrase that best describes your level of activity during the past 2 weeks.

My Activity Level is:	v
Normal. No complaints about activities or health	☐
Normal but I am not completely healthy	☐
Normal if I make an extra effort	☐
Less than normal. I cannot work but I can take care of all my personal needs	☐
I sometimes need help with my personal needs	☐
I often need help with my personal needs	☐
Most of the time I need special care and help with my personal needs	☐
I need special care, sometimes in the hospital	☐
I am in the hospital most of the time	☐

Skin and Appendages: *Does any part of your skin*:	Yes	No	
- feel tight?	☐	☐	
- have a rash or is raw or sore?	☐	☐	
- itch or feels very dry?	☐	☐	
- look like a shiny scar or have scales or flakes?	☐	☐	
- appear lighter or darker than normal?	☐	☐	
- noticed hair loss, hair thinning (scalp, arms or legs)	☐	☐	
Do your fingernails or toenails look unusual (new changes)?	☐	☐	

Eyes: *Do your eyes*:	Yes	No	Don't Know
- feel dry or gritty, like they have sand in them?	☐	☐	
- have excessive tearing?	☐	☐	
- hurt because of wind?	☐	☐	
- have difficulty opening when you wake up?	☐	☐	
- hurt because of bright light?	☐	☐	
Have you had a Schirmer's test to measure tear formation?	☐	☐	☐
Have you had your tear ducts blocked (plugs or ligation)?	☐	☐	☐
Have you been diagnosed with cataracts?	☐	☐	☐
- Have cataracts been removed?	☐	☐	

Mouth: *Do you have*:	Yes	No
- sores inside of mouth?	☐	☐
- discomfort with hot/cold?	☐	☐
- discomfort with toothpaste?	☐	☐
- discomfort with spicy food?	☐	☐
- discomfort with soda/pop?	☐	☐
- dry feeling most of time?	☐	☐
- difficulty opening your mouth wide?	☐	☐
- sores on your lips?	☐	☐
- increased decay of teeth?	☐	☐

Sinuses: *Do you have or have you had*:	Yes	No	Don't Know
- dripping or draining liquid into your throat?	☐	☐	
- congestion or pain?	☐	☐	
- a sinus infection? Date: ___/___/___	☐	☐	☐
- your sinuses operated on? Date: ___/___/___	☐	☐	☐

Throat and Esophagus	Yes	No
Do pills or dry foods get stuck after you swallow?	☐	☐
Does it hurt to swallow solids or liquids?	☐	☐
Do you have heartburn?	☐	☐

Chest/Lungs: *Do you have or have you had*:	Yes	No
- shortness of breath when you walk uphill or climb stairs?	☐	☐
Does shortness of breath limit your usual normal activity?	☐	☐
- shortness of breath at rest?	☐	☐
- a cough?	☐	☐
- any wheezing or asthma?	☐	☐
- chest pain or heart palpitation?	☐	☐

Gut, Belly, Abdomen: *Do you have or have you had*:	Yes	No	Don't Know
- decreased appetite?	☐	☐	
- frequent nausea /vomiting? If vomiting _____times a day	☐	☐	
- diarrhea? If yes, ___ times per day	☐	☐	
- blood in your stool?	☐	☐	☐
- weight loss equal to or more than 10 lbs/5 kg without trying?	☐	☐	☐
- signs of jaundice (yellow skin, yellow eyes)?	☐	☐	☐
- pain in your stomach/belly?	☐	☐	
- gallstones?	☐	☐	☐

Muscle-skeletal: *Do you have*:	Yes	No	Don't Know
- difficulty climbing hills or stairs?	☐	☐	
- difficulty getting up from the floor because of weakness?	☐	☐	
- painful hips, knees, ankles, shoulders, elbows, or wrists?	☐	☐	
- joint stiffness or any joints that cannot move freely?	☐	☐	
- muscle pain or cramps?	☐	☐	
- any tremor or shakiness?	☐	☐	
- swollen feet or ankles?	☐	☐	
- weakness in your legs?	☐	☐	
- difficulty putting clothes on over your head?	☐	☐	
- difficulty making a fist?	☐	☐	
- swollen joints?	☐	☐	

Sexuality: *Do you*:	Yes	No
- have problems with sexual desire, erection, ejaculation or vaginal dryness or pain?	☐	☐

What do you usually do? *(Check all that apply)*:	
Full-time work or attendance in school	☐
Part-time work or attendance in school	☐
Retired	☐

Can you do your usual job, housework or school work?

Yes, doing this without limitation	☐
Yes, but limited a little	☐
Yes, but limited a lot	☐
No, unable to do these things	☐

Course Since Your Last Evaluation

Infection:	**Yes**	**No**	**Don't Know**
- *Herpes simplex virus* (HSV) or cold sores?	○	○	○
- Chicken pox, Shingles or *Varicella-Zoster* (VZV)? If yes, location:_____	○	○	○
- CMV in the blood, lungs, GI or other sites?	○	○	○
- pneumonia? Date: ___/___/___	○	○	○
- bronchitis? Date: ___/___/___	○	○	○
- Bacteria in the blood or your central line?	○	○	○
- yeast in the mouth or vagina (*women*)?	○	○	○
- fungus (yeast or mold) anywhere else?	○	○	○
- any other organisms? If yes, please indicate the type and location:	○	○	○
- warts? If yes, location _____	○	○	○
- Have you had an IVIG immunoglobulin infusion? If yes, last dose on ___/___/___	○	○	○

Hospitalization: *How many times have you been admitted to the hospital AND the reasons?*

None	○
1	○
2	○
3	○
More than 3	○

OTHERS: *Have you had*	**Yes**	**No**	
- osteoporosis or osteopenia of the hip or spine?	○	○	Don't know ○
- broken bone, or compression or collapse of spine bones?	○	○	___/___/___
- avascular necrosis of hips, knees, other? _____	○	○	Don't know ○
- diagnosed with a new type of cancer or malignancy? If yes, location:	○	○	___/___/___
- have you had any medical problems that we've not asked about?	○	○	

Transfusion: *Since last evaluation in our center:*	**Yes**	**No**	**Don't Know**
- any red cell transfusions?	○	○	○
If yes, date of last red cells transfusion: ___/___/___			
- any platelet transfusions?	○	○	○
If yes, date of last platelet transfusion: ___/___/___			
- any growth factor to stimulate cell growth (i.e., EPO, Neupogin)	○	○	○
Last dose of _____: ___/___/___			

List Current Medications and Treatments (including over-the-counters, vitamins, naturopathics)

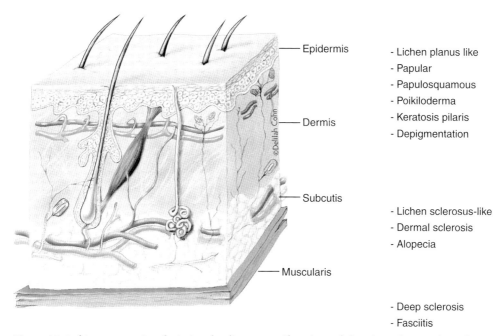

- Lichen planus like
- Papular
- Papulosquamous
- Poikiloderma
- Keratosis pilaris
- Depigmentation

- Lichen sclerosus-like
- Dermal sclerosis
- Alopecia

- Deep sclerosis
- Fasciitis

Epidermis

Dermis

Subcutis

Muscularis

Figure 6.2 A skin cross section depicting the diverse manifestations of chronic graft versus host disease (cGVHD).
The diverse manifestations of cGVHD are as follows:
Lichen planus-like, Papular, Papulosquamous, Poikiloderma, Keratosis pilaris, Depigmentation, Deep Sclerosis, Fasciitis, Lichen-sclerosus like, Dermal sclerosis, Alopecia. See Plate 8 in the color plate section.

the physical examination must always include a complete evaluation of the skin. Manifestations of GVHD vary according to phases of the disease (early or "inflammatory" vs. late or "cellular or fibrotic" types), affected skin layers, and disease course (Figure 6.2). Many cutaneous findings are easily missed without specific physical examination. The cGVHD-focused physical examination must include (1) *tactile* examination and *inspection* of the skin and appendages to detect changes in *color, texture, and surface*, (2) *range of motion* to include extension of wrists, shoulders, and ankles; ability to squat; and ability to stand up from a squat position (Figure 6.3), (3) *oral examination using an halogen lighting source* (othoscopic light) to inspect the lips, buccal mucosa, tongue, palate, teeth, and ability to open the mouth without restriction, and (4) *eyes examination* to look for signs of sicca keratoconjunctivitis, periorbital hyperpigmentation, premature gray hair of eyelashes and eyebrows. Formal examination by an ophthalmologist, including testing of tear production (Schirmer test) is also necessary along with oral medicine and gynecological evaluation periodically. Table 6.1 displays a list of specific evaluations and frequency of monitoring recommended in patients with cGVHD. Additional practical approaches of the clinical assessment of the most common organs and sites with severe forms of cGVHD are discussed in the following paragraphs.

Skin and Dermal Appendages

The skin is the most common organ affected by cGVHD. As stated in the preceding paragraphs, it is critical to have the patient undress to adequately examine the skin. A common issue is the *inadequate description of the physical examination findings* in the medical records. Systematic recording of the review of the system and physical examination findings (both positive and negatives) are necessary to make the initial diagnosis, detect early and progressive signs of disease activity, determine further evaluation and to guide appropriate treatment and monitoring.

History – The cGVHD-focused review of systems (Box 6.1) include questions related to changes in the skin *appearance* (i.e., erythematous rash, pigmentation changes, ulcers, shining appearance, scales, papular lesions, irregular surface "rippling" etc.); *texture* (i.e., thickening, less pliable); *sensation* (i.e., pruritus, decreased sweating, tightness, dryness); and questions related to appearance of derma appendages (i.e., hair loss, premature gray scalp hair, eyelashes, eye brows; loss of shining hair, thinning hair, onychodystrophy, ridging of nails).

Physical examination – The diverse clinical manifestations depends on the layers of the skin affected by GVHD (Figure 6.2) which is likely dependent on the type, severity, and duration of the allogeneic immune responses targeting the skin. For instance, when the immune process is predominantly of "inflammatory" type, the erythematous of skin rash is more likely to be the clinical manifestation of GVHD as opposed to sclerotic features when the GVHD activity is of a predominant "cellular" or "fibrotic" type. Inadequate tissue repair caused by the immune dysregulation of cGVHD may play a role in the development of sequelae observed over time. Inspections for *color changes* and, as important, *tactile* examination to look for

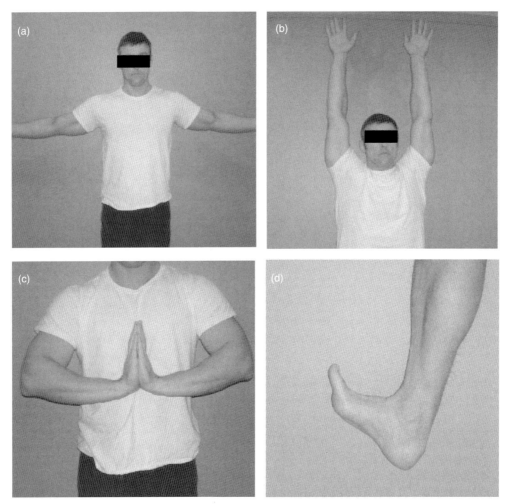

Figure 6.3 Assessment of limited range of motion (ROM).
A: extension of the arms laterally; B: extension of the arms above the head; C: Flexion of wrists "Buddha hands prayer position" with palms and fingers together; D: extension of ankles. See Plate 9 in the color plate section.

texture abnormalities and surface irregularities are necessary elements of the focused skin cGVHD examination. Complete examination of the *skin and appendages* are the most important diagnostic tool to identify manifestation of cGVHD involving this organ system.

The key elements of the skin/appendages examination include

1) Patients must be *undressed* (including no socks) for examination of the total skin surface area and appendages (no wigs or hats).
2) *Inspection* of scalp and body hair and nails to look for hair loss; thinning or premature gray hair; ridges or brittle nails, onycholysis, or pterygium of nails.
3) *Color* changes (i.e., hyper or hypopigmentation; erythematous rash including poikiloderma) should be sought.

4) *Texture abnormalities and surface irregularities* need to be assessed by inspection, tactile examination, and by direct halogen lighting (othoscopic light). Examples of manifestations with surface irregularities and texture abnormalities include *lichen-planus-like and lichen-sclerosus* (Figure 6.4); *papular or papulosquamous* rash (Figure 6.4), *dermal sclerosis* (Figure 6.5) and *ulcers* in advanced deep sclerosis. Abnormalities in the surface and texture caused by sclerosis of the subcutaneous fat tissue and fasciae can be detected on physical examination by *rippling and grooving* appearance or joint contractures (Figure 6.5).
5) To look for the presence of *rippling and grooving* in the arms, ask the patient to completely extend their arms laterally and to completely extend their shoulders above the heads. To look for the presence of *grooving and rippling* in the thighs, ask patient while lying down

Table 6.1   List of Evaluations and Frequency of Monitoring in Patients with cGVHD

Evaluation	*Frequency of Evaluation/Monitoring*	
	Organ/Site Involved or Symptomatic	
	Yes	*No*
Interval history with symptoms and list of treatments completed *by the patient* (see Box 6.1)	Every clinic visit	Every clinic visit
Physical exam by primary physician		
Complete *skin* examination	Every clinic visit	Every clinic visit
Oral exam by primary physician	Every clinic visit	Every clinic visit
Limited *range of motion* assessment (Figure 6.3)	Every clinic visit	Every clinic visit
Performance score	Every clinic visit	Every clinic visit
Nurse assessment to include		
Weight	Every clinic visit	Every clinic visit
Height: *Adults*	Yearly	Yearly
Children	3–12 months	3–12 months
Medical photographs	At initial diagnosis and every 6 months if skin/joint involved until resolution of reversible manifestation or discontinuation of treatment whichever is longer	80–100 days after transplant (baseline)
Schirmer tear test	At initial diagnosis and at least yearly or sooner in symptomatic patients	80–100 days after transplant (baseline), then yearly
Laboratory monitoring		
Complete blood counts with differential and platelet counts	Weekly for 2 months of starting or changing treatment, then twice monthly until stable, then monthly or more often as clinically indicated	
Chemistry panel including renal and liver function tests	Weekly for 2 months of starting or changing treatment, then twice monthly until stable, then monthly or more often as clinically indicated	
Magnesium levels	Weekly after starting or changing treatment that include calcineurin inhibitors agents (i.e., cyclosporine, tacrolimus) for the first month, then twice monthly until stable, then monthly	
Calcium levels	Weekly in patients receiving bisphosphanates for the first month, then twice monthly until stable, then monthly	
Therapeutic drug monitoring	Weekly after starting or changing treatment until stable levels, then twice monthly until stable, then monthly or more often as clinically indicated	
Fasting lipid profile	Every 6 months during treatment with corticosteroids or sirolimus	
Immunoglobulin IgG levels	Yearly or more often in patients with recurrent or major infections	
Cytomegalovirus blood monitoring	Monthly if receiving >1 mg/kg of corticosteroids or prior history of infection, or more, often as clinically indicated	
Iron indices	Every 6–12 months (if red cell transfusions dependent or if iron overload documented previously	
Thyroid function tests	Every 12 months	

Other Evaluations	*Organ/Site Involved or Symptomatic*	
	Yes	*No*
Pulmonary function tests (PFT)	If new significant obstructive changes* monthly × 3 or longer until FEV1 stabilizes, then at 3 months intervals for 1 year, if stable at 6 months × 2, thereafter if stable yearly	3 month intervals for the first year after transplant, then yearly if abnormal PFT in a previous time, new symptoms or continued systemic treatment

(continued)

Table 6.1 (*continued*)

Other Evaluations	Organ/Site Involved or Symptomatic	
	Yes	*No*
Nutritional assessment	As clinically indicated and yearly if receiving corticosteroids	As clinically indicated
Physiotherapy with assessment of range of motion	Every 3 months if sclerotic features affecting range of motion until resolution	As clinically indicated
Dental/Oral Medicine consultation with comprehensive soft and hard tissue examination, culture, biopsy or photographs of lesions (as clinically indicated)	3–6 month intervals or more often as indicated	Yearly
Ophthalmology consultation with Schirmer test, slit-lamp examination and intraocular pressure	3–6 month intervals or more often as indicated	Yearly
Gynecology examination for vulvar or vaginal involvement	6 month intervals or more often as indicated	Yearly
Dermatology consultation with assessment of extent and type of skin involvement, biopsy or photographs	As clinically indicated	
Neuropsychological testing	As clinically indicated	
Bone mineral assessment (DEXA scan)	Yearly if receiving corticosteroids or abnormal prior tests	

*Defined as a decrease of the % FEV$_1$ by $\geq$10% in comparison to pretransplant values AND the %FEV$_1$ is <80%, with an FEV$_1$/FVC ratio <0.7 and without response to bronchodilators. Pulmonary consultation should be obtained if significant new obstructive lung changes develop.

cGVHD, chronic graft versus host disease; FEV$_1$, forced expiratory volume in 1 second; FVC, forced vital capacity.

on the examination table, to rotate their hips internally and externally (Figure 6.5).

6) To detect early lichen-planus features (e.g., "shining horizontal silvery lines" rash) apply direct halogen lighting from an othoscopic source.

7) *Tactile inspection* is necessary for detection of early subcutaneous sclerosis that is NOT hidebound occurring in areas of excess adipose tissue (i.e., abdomen, thighs, and proximal arms). The dorsum of the fingers is more sensitive to detect the skin irregularities of this type than the palmar surface. In this early phase, the skin can appear normal by inspection alone.

8) *Tactile* examination by pinching the skin is necessary for detection of abnormalities in texture such as that caused by sclerosis and lichen-sclerosus and to differentiate hidebound from moveable sclerosis and pockets of normal skin.

9) *Medical photographs* of the skin, nails, and hair are important as supplementary documentation of the extent and type of GVHD manifestation and for future comparison. Medical photos should be filed in the patient's electronic medical records for easy access and comparison. Guidelines for obtaining photographs are provided under the "Practical Approach to Monitoring cGVHD" subsequent section . If unable to photograph, recording

Lichen planus-like

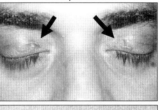
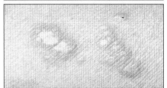

Lichen-sclerosus

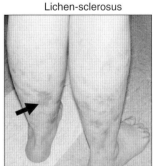

Figure 6.4 Lichen planus-like and lichen-sclerosus types of cGVHD manifestation. See Plate 10 in the color plate section.

the type of cutaneous manifestations and exact distribution using a figure of human body is extremely useful.

Mouth

History – Patients should be asked about mechanical problems (difficulty in opening mouth, difficulty talking or chewing, dry mouth, difficulty in swallowing, jaw cramps after

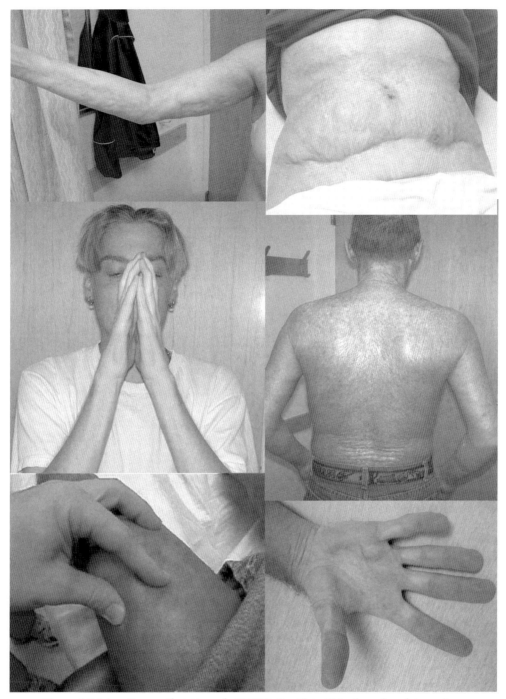

Figure 6.5 Sclerotic manifestation of cGVHD. See Plate 11 in the color plate section.

chewing or talking, etc.), oral infections (viral, bacterial, and fungal), lip problems (tightness, sores or ulcerations, sun sensitivity, thinning, discomfort, abnormality or change in color, etc.), food sensitivity and change in taste (particularly of acidic foods and tooth paste), oral pain, and oral changes (ulceration, lace-like appearance, blisters, tongue discoloration, atrophy) (see Box 6.1).

Physical Examination – The oral examination should start with inspection of the lips and mouth, including evaluating the patient for the ability to open their mouth without restriction

(i.e., rule out perioral fibrosis). If there is limitation, the size of the opening should be measured. In examining the mouth, it is important to be thorough and examine the entire mouth. The lips, entire buccal mucosa on each side, tongue, hard and soft palate, throat, gums, and teeth should be inspected using a halogen light source. The tongue blade is useful for visualization and to test for dryness. Early features of oral cGVHD include a lacey appearance (i.e., lichen or hyperkeratotic features) often in focal areas of the buccal mucosa, especially near the inside of the angles of the mouth. Also, fine white lines (keratotitic features) can be seen on the sides of the tongue detected only upon careful examination using a halogen lighting source. Other clinical signs include mucocele (clear vesicles most frequently seen in the soft palate), pseudomembrane, ulcers, erythema, and dental decay related to sicca. Oral lichen-planus features are diagnostic manifestations of cGVHD that can be mistaken as representing yeast infection or missed when focal mild signs are present. If possible, photographs are extremely helpful. Oral diagrams are available and are also very useful for recording the exact extent, distribution, and size of oral changes. As it is frequently difficult to determine if infection is present in a patient with oral GVHD, culture of the mouth is often necessary especially to rule out herpes virus (i.e., *Herpes simplex* virus [HSV], *Cytomegalovirus* [CMV], adenovirus, etc.), yeast and bacteria, especially in patients with increased symptoms with stable physical examination findings and without significant change in treatment.

Eyes

History – Patients should be asked about ocular symptoms (Box 6.1). Patients may have minimal symptoms and yet have ocular damage from dry eyes detected by complete ophthalmologic examination. In patients with symptoms, this may begin with increased or uncontrolled tearing due to lachrymal damage. More typically, patients complain of dry or gritty eyes, ocular discomfort, and/or photosensitivity (Box 6.1). While complete examination by an ophthalmologist including slit-lamp examination to look for corneal staining, filaments or corneal ulceration is necessary and Schirmer test is important, inspection of the eye for dryness, erythema, eyelid edema, periorbital hyperpigmentation and premature gray hair, or loss of eyes lashes or eye browns should be included in the physical examination by the primary physician.

Lungs

History – Patients with early obstructive lung disease are usually asymptomatic until significant damage has occurred. Patients may complain of dry cough, dyspnea on exertion, and sometimes wheezing. Patients should also be asked in detail about their infection history such as sinusitis, bronchitis, or pneumonia in the past 3 to12 months since the last visit (Box 6.1). Pulmonary function tests (PFTs) are necessary todiagnose lung involvement, to determine the severity of the process, the need for further evaluation, and to monitor the GVHD course (Table 6.1). Guidelines for obtaining PFTs, bronchoalveolar lavage, high resolution CAT scan of the chest are discussed under the "Practical Approach to Monitoring Chronic GVHD" Subsequent section. The frequency of PFTs is shown in Table 6.2.

Physical Examination – On examination, the chest wall should be inspected for sclerosis, as this process could result in pulmonary restriction. During the physical examination, besides the usual pulmonary component, chest wall movement should be examined. Rales, wheezes, or decrease breath sounds can be present on auscultation, but often are normal, except in advances cases.

Musculoskeletal/Joints

History – Patients should be asked about proximal muscle weakness, myalgias, arthralgia, joint stiffness, problems with any range of motion, joint contractures, muscle cramps, and so on (Box 6.1).

Examination – Joint contracture, an advanced manifestation of cGVHD, can be prevented or minimized by recognizing early dermal sclerosis resulting in decreased range of motion and by prompt treatment including stretching exercise. A limited range of motion of the extremities can be easily evaluated by the primary physician during the clinic visit (Figure 6.3). Palpation of subcutaneous tissue and muscles for irregularity of surface is important to detect early deep sclerosis. A simple assessment of muscle weakness of the lower extremities is to ask the patient to stand up (without the help of the arms) from a sitting position in a chair for 3 to 5 times, and to ask the patient to stand up from a squat position without using the arms.

Practical Approach to Monitoring cGVHD

The elements of the clinical evaluation for the diagnosis and monitoring of cGVHD are displayed in Table 6.1. As discussed previously, systematic clinical evaluations including at least complete skin/appendages and careful oral and eye examinations are necessary (1) to determine if a patient has developed cGVHD versus "*late, recurrent, or persistent*" a acute GVHD, (2) to recognize early clinical signs to prevent progression to a more advanced form of cGVHD, and (3) to guide duration of treatment.

Medical Evaluation and Monitoring

Patients should complete the cGVHD-focused review of the system questionnaire with other relevant medical information and provide a current list of treatment with doses at every clinic visit (Box 6.1). Physicians or other medical providers should obtain a cGVHDfocused history and physical examination (see previous section) at 80 to 100 days after allogeneic stem cell transplantation (baseline) and at least every 3 months for the first year in patients without cGVHD. The frequency of evaluation in patients diagnosed with cGVHD is displayed in Table 6.2. Complete skin/appendages, limited range of motion (see Figure 6.3), oral, and eye examinations by the primary physician should be obtained at 80 to 100 days after transplantation (baseline) and at every clinic visit (Tables 6.1 and 6.2).

Other Clinical Monitoring

Other evaluations and frequency of the monitoring are shown in Table 6.1. Ophthalmology evaluations with Schirmer test (tear test) should be obtained at 80 to 100 days after transplant (baseline) and at yearly intervals, or more often in symptomatic patients (Table 6.1). Schirmer test may be obtained by a nurse during the clinic visit. The effects of anesthesia on the Schirmer test have not been studied in cGVHD, and the formal recommendation from the NIH Consensus Conference is not to use anesthesia. However, many patients, particularly

Table 6.2 Schedule of Follow-up Visits

Situation	Frequency of Evaluations
No cGVHD	Every 3 months × 4, then every 6 months × 2, then every year
cGVHD diagnosed	Every 1–3 months or sooner as clinically indicated
Systemic treatment for GVHD discontinued	Every 1–3 months × 6 months, then every 3–6 months × 1 year, then every 6–12 months × 1 year, then every year

children and those with ocular sensitivity find this test intolerable without anesthesia. It is better to obtain the test using anesthesia, knowing the uncertainties concerning validation, than to have untreated dry eyes, and the attendant complications from this condition. Oral medicine and gynecological evaluations should also be obtained at 80 to 100 days after transplant (baseline) and at yearly intervals or sooner if clinically indicated.

Considering the significant morbidity associated with cGVHD of the lungs and the association of airway obstruction with cGVHD and high transplant-related mortality [12, 13], we recommend monitoring PFT in all allogeneic transplant recipients. Full pulmonary function tests including spirometry, lung volumes, and DLCO is preferable, but spirometry is reasonable for monitoring, and obtain full PFT when the forced expiratory volume in 1 second (FEV_1) is <80% of the predicted normal value.

Pulmonary function tests should be obtained in all patients pretransplant, at 80 to 100 days after transplant and at 3 month intervals for patients with *new significant* airflow obstruction detected at or after 3 months after transplant. Significant new obstructive change is defined by a decrease of the % FEV_1 by ≥10% in comparison to pretransplant values *AND* the % FEV_1 is <80%, with an FEV_1/forced vital capacity (FVC) ratio <0.7 and without response to bronchodilators. Definition of significant air-trapping is a residual volume (RV) >120% OR air-trapping noted on high-resolution computed tomography (HRCT). Pulmonary consultation should be obtained if significant new obstructive lung changes develop.

Table 6.1 displays the frequency of PFTs. Patients diagnosed with cGVHD within 1 year after transplantation should have PFTs obtained at 3 month intervals during the first year after transplant, then yearly if abnormal PFT in a previous time or new symptoms. For patients with new significant obstructive changes, PFT should be obtained at monthly intervals for at least 3 months or longer until % FEV_1 stabilizes, then at 3 month intervals for 1 year, then if stable at 6 month intervals for 1 year, thereafter, if stable yearly.

HRCT images (with inspiratory and expiratory images) is indicated when there is evidence of significant new obstructive changes on PFT with % FEV_1 <70%. HRCT can be used to assess for possible infectious etiologies as well as assessment of changes suggestive of bronchiolitis obliterans, such as bronchial wall thickening, bronchiectasis, and air trapping.

Medical photographs are useful for future comparison and as supportive documentation of the *type, distribution,* and *extent* of GVHD involving the skin/ appendages and joints/ fasciae. Photographs are useful to record the appearance of *rippling* and *grooving, decrease in range of motion* and *joint contractures* related to deep sclerosis of the subcutaneous fat and fasciae. Skin and major joints should be photographed at 80 to 100 days after transplantation (baseline), at the time of the initial diagnosis of cGVHD even if skin or joint are not involved, at any time during exacerbation or progression of GVHD involving the skin or joints and periodically in patients with skin or joint involvement (see Table 6.1). Procedure for obtaining medical photograph should be standardized. In the following paragraph is the standard procedure used in Seattle.

PROCEDURE

A. Obtain consent from the patient prior to shooting the first picture.
B. Patients should be photographed with their undergarments only.
C. Create a sign (8.5 × 11. inches) with the current date and the patient identification number.
D. Select the highest resolution setting on the digital camera.
E. Set a standard for shooting including the distance (4 feet away), light source(s), background, and camera settings.
F. At the end of each photograph session write in the consent form signed by the patient the number of the 1st and last image recorded in the digital camera.
G. Document in the medical records that photographs were taken.

WHAT TO PHOTOGRAPH

1. Face, neck, and upper chest. Ask the patient to hold the sign (8.5 × 11 inches) with the date and their identifier number below the neck. This first picture with the sign helps separate the different photographic sessions.
2. Hands/wrists/chest and abdomen (from the anterior neck to the hips). Ask the patient to hold the palms of their hands and fingers tight together as far below their neck as they can with the elbows extended laterally in the "Buddha" prayer hand position (Figure 6.3C). This photo is useful to document decreased range of motion of the wrists (fasciitis) caused by "deep sclerosis," which can be present in patient with normal skin examination by inspection alone.
3. Arms extension above the head. In a standing position, ask patient to extend to a *maximum* both arms above the head with the fingertips pointing toward the

ceiling and palms facing the camera without flexing the elbows, wrists, or fingers (Figure 6.3B).

4. Arms extension laterally. In a standing-up position, ask patients to extend both arms laterally to the maximum without flexing the elbows. This photo is helpful to document rippling or grooving and limited range of motion of shoulders if present (Figure 6.3A). This photo is useful to detect rippling or grooving related to deep sclerosis (fasciitis) and record decreased in range of motion.

5. Right shoulders rotation/back. This photo is taken from the posterior neck to the posterior hips. Ask patients to raise their *right hand* over their head and touch the right shoulder blade in the back while their *left hand* coming from the bottom inching up their back to reach the right shoulder blade. Ask patient to try to extend the fingers of both hands so that they touch each other.

6. Left shoulder rotation/back (same as using contralateral position). Ask patients to raise their *left hand* over their head and touch the left shoulder blade in the back while their *right hand* coming from the bottom inching up their back to reach the left shoulder blade. Ask patient to try to extend the fingers of both hands so that they touch each other.

7. Squat position. Ask patients to squat with their heels on the floor. The photo is taken on side-view of patients squatting position.

8. Nails. Close up of both thumbs resting on a flat surface. Allow camera to focus and take photo from above.

9. Nails: Close up of the fingernails resting on the same flat surface as described earlier (#8).

10. The last photograph should be taken of the consent form signed by the patient with the written first and last numbers of images taken as recorded in the digital camera for the photograph session.

11. Additional photographs including close-ups should be taken as indicated.

A. Examples of additional photographs that might be needed:

■ If sclerotic features are present, photograph the worst area with the patient pinching the skin of the affected area.

■ If sclerotic features are present in the thighs, ask patients to rotate their thighs externally while lying on an examination bed. This photo is useful to document rippling and grooving associated with deep sclerosis.

■ If fasciitis or panniculitis involves the hands or wrists, ask the patient to make a fist with the right hand and extend the left hand with the palm and fingers extended and facing up, then take the photo from above. Then, ask the patient to make a fist with the left hand and extend the right hand with the palm and fingers extended and facing up, and then take the photo from above.

■ If patient has difficulty opening their mouth wide, photograph their mouth open at its widest.

SUMMARY

cGVHD is a common complication after allogeneic HCT. Careful monitoring of allogeneic transplant recipients will identify patients at the earliest stages of the disease, ensuring the best chance for successful therapy. Once the disorder is diagnosed, diligent monitoring, as presented in this chapter, will help ensure that changes in the patient's condition are detected quickly. Although much still needs to be learned about cGVHD, meticulous patient management will significantly improve the quality of life of patients with this disorder.

REFERENCES

1. Sullivan KM. Graft-vs.-host disease. In Blume KG, Forman SJ, Appelbaum FR eds. Thomas' Hematopoietic Cell Transplantation. Third, Edition. Oxford, UK: Blackwell Publishing Ltd.; 2004: 635–664.

2. Lee SJ, Vogelsang G, Flowers MED. Chronic graft-versus-host disease. *Biol Blood Marrow Transplant*. 2003;9:215–233.

3. Miklos DB, Kim HT, Zorn E, et al. Antibody response to DBY minor histocompatibility antigen is induced after allogeneic stem cell transplantation and in healthy female donors. *Blood*. 2004;103:353–359.

4. Miklos DB, Kim HT, Miller KH, et al. Antibody responses to H-Y minor histocompatibility antigens correlate with chronic graft-versus-host disease and disease remission. *Blood*. 2005; 105:2973–2978.

5. Mielcarek M, Martin PJ, Leisenring W, et al. Graft-versus-host disease after nonmyeloablative versus conventional hematopoietic stem cell transplantation. *Blood*. 2003;102 :756–762.

6. Akpek G, Lee SJ, Flowers ME, et al. Performance of a new clinical grading system for chronic graft-versus-host disease: a multi-center study. *Blood*. 2003;102:802–809.

7. Flowers MED, Leisenring W, Beach K, et al. Granulocyte colony-stimulating factor given to donors before apheresis does not prevent aplasia in patients treated with donor leukocyte infusion for recurrent chronic myeloid leukemia after bone marrow transplantation. *Biol Blood Marrow Transplant*. 2000;6:321–326.

8. Shulman HM, Sullivan KM, Weiden PL, et al. Chronic graft-versus-host syndrome in man. A long-term clinicopathologic study of 20 Seattle patients. *Am J Med*. 1980;69:204–217.

9. Sullivan KM, Shulman HM, Storb R, et al. Chronic graft-versus-host disease in 52 patients: adverse natural course and successful treatment with combination immunosuppression. *Blood*. 1981;57:267–276.

10. Filipovich AH, Weisdorf D, Pavletic S et al. National Institutes of Health consensus development project on criteria for clinical trials in chronic graft-versus-host disease: I. Diagnosis and Staging Working Group report. *Biol Blood Marrow Transplant*. 2005;11:945–956.

11. Takahide K, Parker PM, Wu M, et al. Use of fluid-ventilated, gas-permeable scleral lens for management of severe keratoconjunctivitis sicca secondary to chronic graft-versus-host disease. *Biol Blood Marrow Transplant.* 2007;13:1016–1021.

12. Chien JW, Martin PJ, Gooley TA, et al. Airflow obstruction after myeloablative allogeneic hematopoietic stem cell transplantation. *Am J Respir Crit Care Med.* 2003;168:208–214.

13. Chien JW, Martin PJ, Flowers ME, et al. Implications of early airflow decline after myeloablative allogeneic stem cell transplantation. *Bone Marrow Transplant.* 2004;33:759–764.

14. Flowers MED, Parker PM, Johnston LJ, et al. Comparison of chronic graft-versus-host disease after transplantation of peripheral blood stem cells versus bone marrow in allogeneic recipients: long-term follow-up of a randomized trial. *Blood.* 2002;100:415–419.

7

Risk Factors and Predictive Models for Chronic Graft versus Host Disease

Görgün Akpek and Stephanie J. Lee

INTRODUCTION

Although there has been significant change in allogeneic hematopoietic cell transplantation (HCT) practice over the last four decades, chronic graft versus host disease (chronic GVHD) remains a major barrier to the ultimate success of HCT. The ability to predict who will develop chronic GVHD, how severe the organ manifestation will become, and whether the decreased relapse risk associated with chronic GVHD is offset by the increased morbidity and treatment-related mortality from chronic GVHD is of great clinical importance. Better understanding of these predictors would also aid in chronic GVHD research since appropriate patients could be targeted for prevention and treatment trials. Single arm studies would be easier to interpret if we had greater confidence in estimating the course of chronic GVHD treated with "standard care."

This chapter is intended to provide updated information for clinicians to recognize important risk factors for the occurrence and prognosis of chronic GVHD. Recently developed predictive models for prognosis of chronic GVHD are also described.

RISK FACTORS FOR THE DEVELOPMENT OF CHRONIC GVHD

Incidence

The overall chance of developing chronic GVHD is approximately 60% after allogeneic HCT [1, 2], although published estimates range from 30% to 85%. In a review of 116 human leukocyte antigen (HLA)-identical peripheral blood HCT recipients, limited chronic GVHD occurred in 6%, and clinical extensive chronic GVHD in 71% [3]. Data from the National Marrow Donor Program (NMDP) indicate that up to 70% of patients receiving adult unrelated donor marrow grafts who survive beyond day 100 develop chronic GVHD [4]. Children experience lower rates of chronic GVHD, but the major risk

factors for, organ manifestations in, and clinical impact on affected children appear similar [5].

The incidence of chronic GVHD varies in ethnic groups. The severity and death rate of Japanese patients with chronic GVHD was lower than those for populations in Western countries, which might be the result of greater genetic homogeneity among the Japanese. A recent analysis of Japanese Marrow Donor Program (JMDP) Registry data on approximately 3,000 transplant recipients who survived more than 100 days revealed the cumulative incidence of chronic GVHD (limited + extensive) and extensive chronic GVHD at 5 years posttransplant was 46% and 28%, respectively [6].

In pediatric patients with relapsed disease, second transplants are often attempted, which are also complicated by high rates of acute and chronic GVHD [7]. Donor lymphocyte infusion (DLI) given after reduced-intensity conditioning HCT or for relapse was reported to be associated with a high incidence of acute and chronic GVHD and sometimes with unusual clinical presentations [8]. This is not surprising because patients with recurrent or residual disease post-HCT are treated with repeated DLIs until GVHD occurs (hoping to achieve a graft-versus-leukemia [GVL] effect), with subsequent chronic GVHD. Collins reported that 60% of DLI recipients developed chronic GVHD, and this was highly predictive of leukemia remission [9].

Of note, the reported incidences of chronic GVHD are affected likely by the diagnostic criteria applied. In 2005, a National Institute of Health (NIH) Consensus Working Group proposed standardized minimal criteria to establish the diagnosis of chronic GVHD [10]. In the future, these criteria should allow more precise estimations of the true incidence of chronic GVHD after allografting.

Established Risk Factors

Four clinical characteristics are consistently identified as risk factors associated with increased chronic GVHD: grade II–IV acute GVHD, HLA-disparity, older recipient age, and use of allogeneic peripheral blood instead of bone marrow.

Previous Acute GVHD

Seattle reported a 44% incidence of chronic GVHD between 85 and 464 days posttransplant in 175 patients with aplastic anemia conditioned with cyclophosphamide who had sustained engraftment of marrow from HLA-identical siblings and lived for more than 6 months. Three factors predicted chronic GVHD: moderate to severe acute GVHD; increasing patient age; and the use of viable donor buffy coat cells in addition to the marrow to prevent graft rejection. The last two factors were significant only in patients without acute GVHD [11]. Subsequent studies consistently showed that the greatest risk factor for the development of chronic GVHD is the prior occurrence of acute GVHD [3, 6, 12–15]. In a recent study, severity of acute GVHD (grade III and IV), primary GVHD treatment failure and elevated alkaline phosphatase were associated with higher overall incidence of chronic GVHD in patients with any history of acute GVHD [16].

The biologic relationship between acute and chronic GVHD remains controversial since many of the same risk factors have been identified. Chronic GVHD may be a later manifestation of alloreactive acute GVHD, a result of tissue damage caused by acute GVHD [17] or treatment aimed at acute GVHD [18], or simply share the same risk factors because both acute and chronic GVHD stem from alloreactivity. The last hypothesis is supported by the observation that prevention of acute GVHD does not necessarily reduce chronic GVHD rates [19]. Some successful attempts to decrease acute GVHD may have actually increased chronic GVHD rates. Two reports have suggested that exposure to steroids as prophylaxis for acute GVHD tends to increase the rate of subsequent chronic GVHD [14, 20].

HLA Disparity between Donor and Recipient

HLA disparity is a well-known risk factor for both acute and chronic GVHD [11–13, 21]. Chronic GVHD occurs in approximately one-third of patients receiving HLA-identical sibling transplants, half of patients undergoing HLA–nonidentical-related HCT, and approximately two-thirds of those undergoing matched unrelated HCT [1, 4]. For patients receiving one-antigen mismatched unrelated marrow grafts, the cumulative incidence of chronic GVHD did not appear to be different from those recieving matched unrelated or haploidentical family donor grafts [22]. A JMDP analysis reported that HLA-A and/or -B mismatching was a risk factor for chronic GVHD [6].

Minor HLA antigen mismatches may also play a role in the development of chronic GVHD. Miklos and his colleagues showed that antibody responses to H-Y minor histocompatibility antigens correlate with chronic GVHD and disease remission [23] (see laboratory predictors in the following text for additional information).

Age of the Recipient and Donor

Risk of cGVHD increases with recipient age [11–13, 24]. Adult (>20 years old) transplant recipients tend to develop chronic GVHD more often (46%) than pediatric patients (13%) who were less than 10 years of age [1]. Similar observation was also recently reported by the JMDP [6].

Allogeneic HCT after reduced-intensity conditioning in high-risk patients (older age) also resulted in high incidences of acute and chronic GVHD [25]. However, recipient age did not appear to be associated with the development of chronic GVHD among recipients of unrelated marrow. Even in the youngest age group, the probability of chronic GVHD was 42% [1]. Older donor age (>30 years old) may be associated with increased risk of developing chronic GVHD [6, 26].

Peripheral Blood Stem Cell Transplwantation

Over the past decade, the use of peripheral blood stem cells (PBSC) has dramatically increased [27, 28]. Reasons for this increase are multifactorial including the beneficial effects of peripheral blood on engraftment and immune reconstitution as well as the convenience for both stem cell donors and health care providers. In contrast to early reports [29, 30], recent prospective studies clearly show an association between use of peripheral blood and a higher incidence of chronic GVHD. Approximately 40% to 80% of survivors transplanted with granulocyte colony-stimulating factor (G-CSF) stimulated peripheral blood from HLA-identical donors develop extensive stage chronic GVHD [3, 31–33]. Other reports suggest that chronic GVHD is also more likely to be extensive and difficult to treat in recipients of related and unrelated PBSCs compared with bone marrow [34].

A meta-analysis of all trials comparing the incidence of acute and chronic GVHD after peripheral blood and bone marrow transplantation (BMT) revealed the pooled relative risks for chronic GVHD and extensive chronic GVHD were much higher for peripheral blood compared to bone marrow [27]. The excess risk of chronic GVHD was explained by differences in the T-cell dose delivered with the graft in a metaregression model that did not reach statistical significance. There was a trend toward a decrease in the risk of relapse with peripheral blood. Sixteen studies (5 randomized controlled trials and 11 cohort studies) were included in this analysis.

Individual reports suggest that these differences are durable. The French transplant society recently published their long-term follow-up results on 101 patients [28]. After a median follow-up of 45 months, the 3-year cumulative incidence of chronic GVHD was 65% in the peripheral blood group and 36% in the bone marrow group ($p = .004$). Extensive chronic GVHD was also more frequent in the peripheral blood group (44% vs. 17%, $p = .004$). Rates of cutaneous and liver involvement were similar among marrow and peripheral blood recipients but ocular involvement was more frequent in peripheral blood recipients. Chronic GVHD occurring after peripheral blood transplantation required multiple courses of immunosuppressive therapy in addition to cyclosporine and corticosteroids for longer periods. Altogether, this translated into longer periods of hospitalization after peripheral blood transplantation, although survival was similar [28].

Another multicenter, phase III trial reported no significant difference in the cumulative incidence of chronic GVHD between peripheral blood and bone marrow recipients after 3 years [33]. However, the number of successive treatments needed to control chronic GVHD was significantly higher after peripheral blood than after BMT, and the duration of glucocorticoid treatment was also significantly longer. Involvement of skin and the female genital tract was more frequent after peripheral blood transplantation [35].

In the unrelated donor marrow setting, patients have a higher risk for chronic GVHD than HLA-matched siblings [4], but it is not clear whether PBSC further elevates this risk [36, 37]. The Karolinska group reviewed 214 patients receiving either PBSCs or bone marrow from an HLA-A, -B, and -DR compatible unrelated donor. Median follow-up was 4.4 and 5 years in the 2 groups, respectively. Although the cumulative incidence of overall cGVHD was similar in the 2 groups (78% vs. 71%), extensive chronic GVHD was significantly more common in the peripheral blood compared with the marrow group (39% vs. 24%) [38]. The 5-year transplant-related mortality, relapse, disease-free survival and overall survival were similar in both groups.

The underlying immunologic factors affecting the occurrence of GVHD in peripheral blood and bone marrow recipients are not completely understood. Data from 181 HLA-identical sibling transplants suggest that high $CD34^+$ counts may be an important factor driving this observation, since chronic GVHD did not correlate with $CD3^+$ and $CD14^+$ counts. Higher doses of CD34 cells ($>8.0 \times 10(6)$/kg) were associated with a significantly increased risk of clinical extensive chronic GVHD [39].

The use of G-CSF during stem cell collection has also been suspected of increasing chronic GVHD after peripheral blood transplantation through preferentially shifting T-helper cells to a Th-2 phenotype [40]. However, a trial performed by Morton and colleagues suggests that donor treatment *per se* with G-CSF is not the cause of the higher chronic GVHD incidence. They randomized HLA-matched sibling donors to marrow or peripheral blood collection after both groups received G-CSF stimulation. Rates of chronic GVHD were higher in the peripheral blood arm (80% vs. 22%) although overall survival was the same [41].

Other Reported Risk Factors Associated with Chronic GVHD

Male recipients with female donors, especially multiparous female donors, have an increased risk of chronic GVHD [42]. Umbilical-cord blood appears to be associated with lower rates of chronic GVHD despite greater HLA-mismatching [43]. A diagnosis of chronic myeloid leukemia and a platelet count not having reached $50 \times 10(9)$/L by day 100 have been associated with chronic GVHD [6].

Controversial Risk Factors for Development of Chronic GVHD

Viral Infections

Some investigators suggest that latent herpes virus in the marrow donor or recipient may predispose to the development of acute and chronic GVHD [44]. However, there has been no compelling evidence linking *Cytomegalovirus* (CMV) seropositivity and subsequent onset of chronic GVHD [45, 46]. A recent study suggested active CMV infection before day +60 is associated with high incidence of developing de novo chronic GVHD among 489 patients who previously had only grade 0 or 1 acute GVHD [47].

Duration of Cyclosporine A Prophylaxis

Observational studies reported that shorter duration cyclosporine A (CyA) administration was associated with increased rates of chronic GVHD [50]. However, a randomized study from Seattle did not show a statistically significant difference in the incidence of clinical-extensive chronic GVHD between recipients assigned to receive a 24-month as compared to a 6-month course of CyA prophylaxis after transplantation of allogeneic marrow from an HLA-identical sibling or alternative donor [49].

Conditioning Regimen

An earlier study reported that incidence of chronic GVHD was similar for busulfan/cyclophosphomide (BU-CY) and cyclophosphamide/total body irradiation (CY-TBI) preparative regimens [50]. A total body irradiation (TBI)-containing myeloablative conditioning regimen was recently reported to be associated with a high incidence of chronic GVHD in a large registry study from Japan [6]. Comment on the incidence and clinical manifestations of chronic GVHD after reduced-intensity conditioning regimens awaits more definitive reports.

GVHD prophylaxis

Use of either tacrolimus or cyclosporine prophylaxis resulted in similar rates of chronic GVHD although there was less "extensive" chronic GVHD in the tacrolimus group [51]. Failure to give methotrexate on day 11 was not shown to influence rates of chronic GVHD although only a small number of patients were studied [52].

Positive Screening Skin or Oral Biopsy at Day 70 to 120 Post-HCT

The value of routine chronic GVHD screening studies including skin biopsy, oral examination, lip biopsy, Schirmer's test, serum alkaline phosphatase, aspartate transaminase, immunoglobulin level, and platelet count was evaluated among 241 allograft recipients [14]. Ninety-one patients (38%) developed clinical extensive chronic GVHD. In a multivariable analysis, which adjusted for the contribution of other chronic GVHD risk factors, none of the screening tests were predictive of chronic GVHD development. Furthermore, no data suggest that the treatment of chronic GVHD in its subclinical stage would improve survival, and it is possible that preemptive treatment may blunt the GVL effect. Patients with suggestive biopsies or the other aforementioned risk factors should certainly be carefully monitored for the development of overt chronic GVHD.

PREDICTIVE MODELS FOR PROGNOSIS OF CHRONIC GVHD

Limited and Extensive

The most commonly employed clinical classification system has been the "limited/extensive" classification proposed by Seattle in 1980 on the basis of a retrospective clinical and pathological review of 20 patients with chronic GVHD [53]. This classification system was devised to distinguish patients needing system treatment (extensive GVHD) from those who did not (limited GVHD) [4, 54]. The Center for International Blood and Marrow Transplant Research (CIBMTR) reviewed data from HLA-matched sibling recipients and found many classification discrepancies, suggesting that transplant centers are not applying the formal definitions accurately, perhaps in part because many patients are unclassifiable by the strict organ criteria [4]. Nevertheless, among 2,609 Japanese patients with hematological malignancy, overall survival was found to be significantly better in patients with limited chronic GVHD but worse in patients with extensive chronic GVHD compared with those without chronic GVHD. The cumulative incidence of relapse among patients with limited or extensive chronic GVHD was significantly lower than that among patients without chronic GVHD [6]. However, the difference between limited and extensive chronic GVHD groups was not found to be statistically significant.

A large proportion of patients fall into the extensive chronic GVHD category, and there is great heterogeneity in manifestations of chronic GVHD. Within the "extensive" chronic GVHD group, mortality correlated best with Karnofsky performance status (KPS less than 70%) [53]. However, KPS alone cannot address the mortality differences among patients with KPS greater than 70%. Owing to increased knowledge about the disease over the past two decades, the majority of patients are now diagnosed long before their KPS becomes less than 70%.

Recognizing these limitations, the Seattle group has developed revised criteria for "clinical limited" and "clinical extensive" chronic GVHD to clarify ambiguities in the original definition. In the revised classification, prolonged treatment with systemic immunosuppression is indicated for patients with clinically extensive chronic GVHD or anyone with high-risk features (i.e., platelets count $<100 \times 10^9$/L, progressive onset, or receiving treatment with corticosteroids at the time of the diagnosis of chronic GVHD) [55].

Type of Onset

The majority of patients with chronic GVHD have had prior acute GVHD. Their disease may evolve directly from acute GVHD (progressive-onset), which has a grim prognosis [56, 57] or may follow a period of recovery from GVHD (quiescent), with an intermediate prognosis. In addition, about 20% to 30% of patients develop chronic GVHD with no history of prior acute GVHD (de novo) and these patients have a relatively good prognosis [53, 56, 57]. On the basis of the CIBMTR data, the distribution of chronic GVHD onset for HLA-matched siblings is 20% to 30% progressive, 30% to 40% interrupted (quiescent), and 35% de novo. Data from the NMDP for unrelated donor recipients, where the incidence of acute GVHD is higher, show the spectrum of onset as 19% progressive, 69% interrupted, and 12% de novo onset [4].

Recognition of a syndrome with mixed acute and chronic GVHD, the "overlap" syndrome, may explain the poor prognosis associated with progressive chronic GVHD. Studies are beginning to report poor survival for these types of patients.

Newer Predictive Models

Various clinical features have been associated with survival in patients with chronic GVHD. For example, "extensive" chronic GVHD [53, 56], KPS [4, 53, 56], thrombocytopenia (less than 100,000 cells/mL) [3, 56–60], progressive-type onset [57, 59, 60], lichenoid histology [57], elevated bilirubin [57, 61], older age (>20), gastrointestinal involvement, no response to therapy at 6 months [60], more than 6 months of interferon given before transplant for the treatment of chronic myelogenous leukemia [62], extensive (>50% body surface area) skin involvement [59], diarrhea and weight loss, lack of oral GVHD, and higher subjective measures of severity [4].

Thrombocytopenia (Seattle)

Thrombocytopenia (less than 100,000/mL) is the first reported and most reproducible prognostic factor that is associated with shortened survival [3, 58, 59, 63].

Progressive-Type Onset, Elevated Bilirubin and Lichenoid Histology (Johns Hopkins – I)

In an earlier study from Hopkins, baseline characteristics present at the onset of chronic GVHD (before therapy) in 85 patients with chronic GVHD treated in Baltimore were reviewed to determine the risk factors for death. Multivariate proportional hazards analysis revealed an increased risk of death in patients with progressive-type onset (HR:4.1), elevated serum bilirubin levels (HR:2.2), and lichenoid histology on skin biopsy (HR:2.1) [57]. The actuarial survival after onset of chronic GVHD in 85 patients was 42% at 10 years, but survival in the 26 patients with progressive onset was only 10%. Twenty-three patients with 0, 38 patients with 1, and 29 patients with any combination of 2 or more of these factors had a projected 6-year survival of 70%, 43%, and 20%, respectively [57].

Extensive Skin Involvement, Thrombocytopenia, Progressive Onset (Johns Hopkins – II)

Similar to the original study reported by Wingard et al., the relationship between pretreatment clinical and laboratory features of 151 consecutive patients with chronic GVHD and chronic GVHD-specific survival was studied by Akpek et al. Again, thrombocytopenia and progressive form of chronic GVHD proved to be independent risk factors at diagnosis for shortened survival with respective hazard ratios of 3.6 and 1.7. The extent of skin GVHD involvement (greater than 50% of body surface area) was identified as another independent risk factor associated with survival (HR: 7.0). Furthermore, KPS of less than 50% was identified as an additional risk factor at the time of primary treatment failure of chronic GVHD [59]. Longer follow-up of the cohort showed that the three-factor clinical grading system predicted 10-year rates of survival without recurring malignancy ranging from 9% to 90% [64].

Testing Johns Hopkins II Predictive Model in Other Data Sets

The Hopkins survival model was tested using multiple data sets that included a total of 1,105 patients from University of Nebraska ($n = 60$), CIBMTR ($n = 708$), Fred Hutchinson Cancer Research Center ($n = 188$), and University of Minnesota ($n = 149$). Despite significant heterogeneity of the data, the proposed grading system identified three prognostic groups for each data set, each with different survival outcomes although estimated hazard rates differed [63]. While thrombocytopenia itself was uniformly associated with higher risk of mortality across all test samples, extensive skin involvement and progressive-type onset showed statistically significant associations with mortality in one and two cohorts, respectively [63].

KPS, Diarrhea, Weight Loss, and Cutaneous and Oral Chronic GVHD (CIBMTR)

Lee et al. simultaneously analyzed the CIBMTR data on 1827 HLA-matched sibling allotransplant recipients and reported another set of prognostic factors for survival. KPS, diarrhea, weight loss, and cutaneous and oral involvement were independent prognostic variables, from which a grading scheme was generated. The CIBMTR scheme, the limited/extensive classification system, and a classification on the basis of clinical impression of overall chronic GVHD severity (mild/moderate/severe) was assessed in a parallel analyses of 1,092 HLA-matched sibling transplant recipients from the CIBMTR and 553 recipients of unrelated donor marrow from the NMDP. Presence of any chronic GVHD was associated with fewer relapses (relative risk [RR], 0.5–0.6) but more treatment-related mortality (RR, 1.8–2.8) in the three analyses. No grading scheme correlated chronic GVHD severity with relapse rates, but all schemes predicted treatment-related mortality. Survival and disease-free survival of the most favorable chronic GVHD group in each scheme were similar, or better, than those of patients without chronic GVHD. Notably, an overall clinical summary scale of mild, moderate, or severe chronic GVHD was the best predictor of survival [4]. However, formal definitions for the mild, moderate, and severe categories have not been established.

Summary of Available Prognostic Models

All models reported to date have limitation because of the differences in definitions, data collection methods, diagnostic criteria used and management of chronic GVHD. Factors found to be significant in one sample were not significant in other one. For example, patients within the Hopkins sample were diagnosed by clinical appearance and histology independent of time posttransplant. Thus, patients who were diagnosed before day 100 were also included. In other studies, the diagnosis of chronic GVHD was made after day 80 or 100. The internal consistency and rigor of diagnosis is the strength of the Hopkins sample and a concern for the CIBMTR study. As stated previously, 65% to 67% of CIBMTR subjects scored as limited reported organ involvement other than skin and liver – that is, were incorrectly reported. The patients were not reclassified for the analysis. Thus, the data set is limited by the expertise of those evaluating the patients and this may help explain several unexpected findings in this study – such as the significance of diarrhea [4].

Clinical and Research Needs

A new unified clinical grading or stratification system would be useful to individualize treatment plans in chronic GVHD. Patients in the favorable-risk category might be best treated with a single lympholytic agent such as corticosteroids. If patients fail to respond to steroids, combination therapies might then be instituted. Alternatively, new treatment options other than corticosteroids may be sought for initial treatment of chronic GVHD patients with favorable prognosis. In contrast, patients with limited life expectancy due to poor-risk chronic GVHD may benefit from new therapeutic approaches. Clearly, the chronic GVHD-related mortality in this group is unacceptably high with current treatment approaches and new treatment paradigms are needed. Small prospective trials evaluating any new approaches to chronic GVHD therapy may need to be appropriately stratified to ensure a balanced distribution of risk factors among groups. To improve comparability between publications, reports of chronic GVHD treatment trials should include an accurate description of the study population on the basis of the characteristics of the disease at the time of diagnosis.

NIH Consensus Classifications

The NIH Consensus recently developed a new clinical scoring system (0–3) that describes the severity of affected organ/site at any time. Chronic GVHD was also classified as mild, moderate, and severe on the basis of a global assessment method described by the same group. Also, the indications of systemic treatment were established [10]. It is unknown whether these new definitions, assessments, and groupings in chronic GVHD have any prognostic value for survival and other endpoints. The ability to predict survival, disease-free survival, nonrelapse mortality, development of functional deficits, ability to taper steroids and duration of systemic treatment awaits validation studies.

PREDICTIVE LABORATORY MARKERS

Unfortunately, there is no reliable laboratory indicator of the onset or severity of chronic GVHD possibly because of the lack of specificity. This topic is discussed separately in another chapter. The main laboratory variables that may have a role in predicting the occurrence and prognosis of chronic GVHD are described subsequently.

Expression of OX40 (CD134)

A Japanese study reported as association between expression of OX40, a member of the tumor necrosis factor receptor family, and chronic GVHD. Peripheral blood mononuclear cells from 22 patients after day 100 were subjected to multicolor flow cytometry. The percentages of both OX40 + CD4$^+$ and OX40 + CD8$^+$ T cells were significantly higher in patients with chronic GVHD than those without ($p \leq .0001$ and $p = .001$, respectively). Serial analyses showed that OX40 + CD4$^+$ T cells increased before the onset of chronic GVHD and closely correlated with the therapeutic response [65].

Soluble Biomarkers

Data from a phase III study of hydroxychloroquine added to standard cyclosporine and prednisone therapy in pediatric population were grouped into early (3–8 months) and late (≥9 months) onset chronic GVHD. Soluble BAFF (sBAFF), anti-dsDNA antibody, soluble IL-2 receptor alpha (sIL-2Ralpha), and soluble CD13 (sCD13) were elevated in early onset cGVHD compared to controls. sBAFF and anti-dsDNA were elevated in late onset cGVHD. Some of the biomarkers correlated with specific organ involvement and therapeutic response [66].

Minor Histocompatibilty Antigens

An increased risk of chronic GVHD has long been recognized when a male recipient receives a graft from a female donor, particularly one who may have been alloimmunized by pregnancy or transfusion [67]. The best explanation for this clinical observation is that mHAs encoded on the Y chromosome can elicit responses from female donors in male recipients [23]. H-Y antibodies developed 4 to 12 mos. after BMT and persist for long periods. In a study of 75 (female → male) transplants, the presence of H-Y antibodies correlated with chronic GVHD (OR = 56.5; $p < .0001$) and also maintenance of disease remission ($p < .0001$) [23]. No other minor histocompatibility antigens have been associated with chronic GVHD [68, 69].

Donor Antigen-Presenting Cells

Two studies looked at donor antigen-presenting cells (APCs), specifically plasmocytoid dendritic cells (DC2). Clark and colleagues reported that people with chronic GVHD had normal numbers of donor-derived plasmacytoid DC2s in their blood compared to reduced numbers in posttransplant controls without chronic GVHD [70]. In contrast, Waller and colleagues reported that patients receiving bone marrow grafts with higher numbers of CD3–CD4 bright, presumably DC2 cells, had a lower incidence of chronic GVHD [71]. Resolution of this controversy awaits additional studies.

Regulatory T cells

Numbers of T-regulatory cells appear to be reduced in patients with chronic GVHD although the cells seem functionally intact [72].

PREDICTIVE FACTORS IN CHILDREN WITH CHRONIC GVHD

Children experience lower rates of chronic GVHD, but the major risk factors for organ manifestations in and clinical impact on affected children appear similar [5]. Only a few studies specifically focused on children, and little information is available on the antileukemic effect of chronic GVHD and its impact on disease-free survival in children. Zecca et al. from Italy retrospectively analyzed 696 children given allogeneic HCT for malignant ($n = 450$) and nonmalignant ($n = 246$) diseases [5]. The donor was an HLA-identical sibling in 461 cases and an alternative donor in 235. Bone marrow was the stem cell source in 647 cases, peripheral blood in 17, and cord blood (CB) in 32. Chronic GVHD developed in 173 children (25%) at a median of 116 days after HCT. In multivariate analysis, variables predicting chronic GVHD were donor and recipient age, grade II to IV acute GVHD, female donor for male recipient, diagnosis of malignancy, and use of TBI; cord blood transplants had a very low risk of chronic GVHD. Chronic GVHD occurrence significantly increased transplant-related mortality. Nevertheless, in hematologic malignancies, patients with chronic GVHD had a significant reduction in relapse rate probability compared with children without chronic GVHD and a better disease-free survival (DFS). The antileukemic effect of chronic GVHD was observed mainly in patients with acute lymphoblastic leukemia [5].

In another study from Japan, data on 265 children undergoing allogeneic HCT who survived longer than 3 months post-HCT were analyzed. Fifty-five patients developed chronic GVHD between 1 and 25 months after HCT, and the 5-year cumulative incidence of chronic GVHD was 22%. By multivariate analysis, acute GVHD, malignant disease, recipient age equal or greater than 10 years and a female donor to male recipient were significant risk factors for chronic GVHD [73].

The incidence and risk factors for chronic GVHD as well as the outcome in 80 pediatric patients (36 male) (median age 13 years) who underwent allogeneic peripheral blood progenitor cell transplantation were evaluated by the Spanish Transplant group. Patients were grafted from an HLA-identical sibling after standard myeloablative conditioning and GVHD prophylaxis with cyclosporine and mini methotrexate or cyclosporine + prednisone. The median number of CD34+ cells infused was $5.8 \times 10(6)$/kg. The median follow-up was 24 months. In all, 28 patients had chronic GVHD. On multivariate analysis, only GVHD prophylaxis used was associated with a significant risk of chronic GVHD (HR:3.94). The cumulative incidence of chronic GVHD for patients receiving CyA + MTX was 41% versus 76% for patients who did not ($p = .03$). The probability of relapse was 36% for all patients (12% for patients with chronic GVHD vs. 48% without chronic GVHD). The probability of disease-free survival was better for patients with chronic GVHD (70% vs. 38%; HR: 3.6). These data suggest that the GVHD prophylaxis used is the most relevant predictor of chronic GVHD in a pediatric population. Patients with chronic GVHD had a lower risk of relapse and better survival [74].

These studies indicate that the incidence of chronic GVHD in children study appears to be lower than that observed in adults. While some of the risk factors such as diagnosis of malignancy and use of TBI increase the risk of chronic GVHD, the same association in adults has not been well demonstrated.

FUTURE DIRECTIONS

The most promising clinical and laboratory predictive models should be validated in prospective trials. To improve the success of allogeneic HCT, we must find better ways to predict the occurrence and prognosis of chronic GVHD. On the basis of this knowledge, tailored transplant approaches and targeted posttransplant immunomodulation can then be developed to maximize the GVL effect and minimize the morbidity and mortality associated with chronic GVHD.

REFERENCES

1. Sullivan KM. Agura E. Anasetti C, et al. Chronic graft-versus-host disease and other late complications of bone marrow transplantation. *Semin Hematol.* 1991;28:250–259.
2. Goerner M, Gooley T, Flowers ME, et al. Morbidity and mortality of chronic GVHD after hematopoietic stem cell transplantation from HLA-identical siblings for patients with aplastic or refractory anemias. *Biol Blood Marrow Transplant.* 2002;8:47–56.
3. Przepiorka D, Anderlini P, Saliba R, et al. Chronic graft-versus-host disease after allogeneic blood stem cell transplantation. *Blood.* 2001;98:1695–1700.
4. Lee SJ, Klein JP, Barrett AJ, et al. Severity of chronic graft-versus-host disease: association with treatment-related mortality and relapse. *Blood.* 2002;100:406–414.
5. Zecca M, Prete A, Rondelli R, et al. Chronic graft-versus-host disease in children: incidence, risk factors, and impact on outcome. *Blood.* 2002;100:1192–1200.
6. Ozawa S, Nakaseko C, Nishimura M, et al. Chronic graft-versus-host disease after allogeneic bone marrow transplantation from an unrelated donor: incidence, risk factors and association with relapse. A report from the Japan Marrow Donor Program. *Br J Haematol.* 2007;137:142–151.
7. Tomonari A, Iseki T, Ooi J, et al. Second allogeneic hematopoietic stem cell transplantation for leukemia relapse after first allogeneic transplantation: outcome of 16 patients in a single institution. *Int J Hematol.* 2002;75:318–323.
8. Akpek G, Boitnott JK, Lee LA, et al. Hepatitic-variant of graft-versus-host disease after donor lymphocyte infusion. *Blood.* 2002;100:3903–3907.
9. Collins RH, Shpilberg Jr. O, Drobyski WR, et al. Donor leukocyte infusions in 140 patients with relapsed malignancy after allogeneic bone marrow transplantation. *J Clin Oncol.* 1997;15:433–444.
10. Filipovich AH, Weisdorf D, Pavletic S, et al. National Institutes of Health consensus development project on criteria for clinical trials in chronic graft-versus-host disease: I. Diagnosis and staging working group report. *Biol Blood Marrow Transplant.* 2005;11:945–956.
11. Storb R, Prentice RL, Sullivan KM, et al. Predictive factors in chronic graft-versus-host disease in patients with aplastic anemia treated by marrow transplantation from HLA-identical siblings. *Ann Intern Med.* 1983;98:461–466.
12. Atkinson K, Horowitz MM, Gale RP, et al. Risk factors for chronic graft-versus-host disease after HLA-identical sibling bone marrow transplantation. *Blood.* 1990;75:2459–2464.
13. Ochs LA, Miller WJ, Filipovich AH, et al. Predictive factors for chronic graft-versus-host disease after histocompatible sibling donor marrow transplantation. *Bone Marrow Transplant.* 1994;13:455–460.
14. Wagner JL, Flowers ME, Longton G, Storb R, Schubert M, Sullivan KM. The development of chronic graft-versus-host disease: an analysis of screening studies and the impact of corticosteroid use at 100 days after transplantation. *Bone Marrow Transplant.* 1998;22:139–146.
15. Ochs LA, Blazar BR, Roy J, et al. Cytokine expression in human cutaneous chronic graft-versus-host disease. *Bone Marrow Transplant.* 1996;17:1085–1092.
16. Sohn SK, Kim DH, Baek JH,et al. Risk-factor analysis for predicting progressive- or quiescent-type chronic graft-versus-host disease in a patient cohort with a history of acute graft-versus-host disease after allogeneic stem cell transplantation. *Bone Marrow Transplant.* 2006;37:699–708.
17. Via CS, Shustov A, Rus V, Lang T, Nguyen P, Finkelman FD. In vivo neutralization of TNF-alpha promotes humoral autoimmunity by preventing the induction of CTL. *J Immunol.* 2001;167:6821–6826.
18. Via CS, Shearer GM. Murine graft-versus-host disease as a model for the development of autoimmunity. Relevance of cytotoxic T lymphocytes. *Ann N Y Acad Sci.* 1988;532:44–50.
19. Cutler C, Li S, Ho VT, et al. Extended follow-up of methotrexate-free immunosuppression using sirolimus and tacrolimus in related and unrelated donor peripheral blood stem cell transplantation. *Blood.* 2007;109:3108–3114.
20. Deeg HJ, Lin D, Leisenring W, et al. Cyclosporine or cyclosporine plus methylprednisolone for prophylaxis of graft-versus-host disease: a prospective, randomized trial. *Blood.* 1997;89:3880–3887.
21. Godder KT, Metha J, Chiang KY, et al. Partially mismatched related donor bone marrow transplantation as salvage for patients with AML who failed autologous stem cell transplant. *Bone Marrow Transplant.* 2001;28:1031–1036.
22. Drobyski WR, Klein J, Flomenberg N, et al. Superior survival associated with transplantation of matched unrelated versus one-antigen mismatched unrelated or highly human-leukocyte antigen disparate haploidentical family donor marrow grafts for the treatment of hematologic malignancies: establishing a treatment algorithm for recipients of alternative donor grafts. *Blood.* 2002;99:806–814.
23. Miklos DB, Kim HT, Miller KH, et al. Antibody responses to H-Y minor histocompatibility antigens correlate with chronic GVHD and disease remission. *Blood.* 2005;105:2973–2978.
24. Niederweiser D, Pepe M, Storb R, et al. Factors predicting chronic GVHD after HLA-identical sibling bone marrow transplantation for aplastic anemia. *Bone Marrow Transplant.* 1989;4:151–156.
25. Schetelig J, Kroger N, Held TK, et al. Allogeneic transplantation after reduced conditioning in high risk patients is complicated by a high incidence of acute and chronic graft-versus-host disease. *Haematologica.* 2002;87:299–305.
26. Kollman C, Howe CW, Anasetti C, et al. Donor characteristics as risk factors in recipients after transplantation of bone marrow from unrelated donors: the effect of donor age. *Blood.* 2001;98:2043–2051.
27. Cutler C, Giri S, Jeyapalan S, et al. Acute and chronic graft-versus-host disease after allogeneic peripheral-blood stem-cell and bone marrow transplantation: a meta-analysis. *J Clin Oncol.* 2001;19:3685–3691.
28. Mohty M, Kuentz M, Michallet M, et al. Chronic graft-versus-host disease after allogeneic blood stem cell transplantation: long-term results of a randomized study. *Blood.* 2002;100:3128–3134.

29. Bensinger WI, Clift R, Martin P, et al. Allogeneic peripheral blood stem cell transplantation in patients with advanced hematologic malignancies: A retrospective comparison with bone marrow transplantation. *Blood.* 1996;88:2794–2800.

30. Schmitz N, Bacigalupo A, Labopin M, et al. Transplantation of peripheral blood progenitor cells from HLA-identical sibling donors. *Br J Haematol.* 1996;95:715–723.

31. Storek J, Gooley T, Siadak M, et al. Allogeneic peripheral blood stem cell transplantation may be associated with a high risk of chronic graft-versus-host disease. *Blood.* 1997;90:4705–4709.

32. Blaise D, Kuentz M, Fortanier C, et al. Randomized trial of bone marrow versus lenograstim-primed blood cell allogeneic transplantation in patients with early-stage leukemia: a report from the Societe Francaise de Greffe de Moelle. *J Clin Oncol.* 2000;18:537–546.

33. Bensinger WI, Martin PJ, Storer B, et al. Transplantation of bone marrow as compared with peripheral-blood cells from HLA-identical relatives in patients with hematologic cancers. *N Engl J Med.* 2001;344:175–181.

34. Horowitz MM. Uses and Growth of Hematopoietic Cell Transplantation. In ED Thomas, KG Blume, SJ Forman, eds. *Hematopoietic Cell Transplantation.* Massachusetts: Blackwell Science; 1999:12–18.

35. Flowers ME, Parker PM, Johnston LJ, et al. Comparison of chronic graft-versus-host disease after transplantation of peripheral blood stem cells versus bone marrow in allogeneic recipients: long-term follow-up of a randomized trial. *Blood.* 2002;100:415–419.

36. Remberger M, O Ringden, IW Blau, et al. No difference in graft-versus-host disease, relapse, and survival comparing peripheral stem cells to bone marrow using unrelated donors. *Blood.* 2001;98:1739–1745.

37. Elmaagacli AH, Basoglu S, Peceny R, et al. Improved disease-free-survival after transplantation of peripheral blood stem cells as compared with bone marrow from HLA-identical unrelated donors in patients with first chronic phase chronic myeloid leukemia. *Blood.* 2002;99:1130–1135.

38. Remberger M, Beelen DW, Fauser A, Basara N, Basu O, Ringdén O. Increased risk of extensive chronic graft-versus-host disease after allogeneic peripheral blood stem cell transplantation using unrelated donors. *Blood.* 2005;105:548–551.

39. Zaucha JM, Gooley T, Bensinger WI, et al. CD34 cell dose in granulocyte colony-stimulating factor-mobilized peripheral blood mononuclear cell grafts affects engraftment kinetics and development of extensive chronic graft-versus-host disease after human leukocyte antigen-identical sibling transplantation. *Blood.* 2001;98:3221–3227.

40. Korbling M, Anderlini P. Peripheral blood stem cell versus bone marrow allotransplantation: does the source of hematopoietic stem cells matter? *Blood.* 2001;98:2900–2908.

41. Morton J, Hutchins C, Durrant S. Granulocyte-colony-stimulating factor (G-CSF)-primed allogeneic bone marrow: significantly less graft-versus-host disease and comparable engraftment to G-CSF-mobilized peripheral blood stem cells. *Blood.* 2001;98:3186–3191.

42. Remberger M, Kumlien G, Aschan J, et al. Risk factors for moderate-to-severe chronic graft-versus-host disease after allogeneic hematopoietic stem cell transplantation. *Biol Blood Marrow Transplant.* 2002;8:674–82.

43. Wagner JE, Barker JN, DeFor TE, et al. Transplantation of unrelated donor umbilical cord blood in 102 patients with malignant and nonmalignant diseases: influence of CD34 cell dose

and HLA disparity on treatment-related mortality and survival. *Blood.* 2002;100:1611–1618.

44. Gratama JW, Zwaan FE, Stijnen T, et al. Herpes virus immunity and acute graft-versus-host disease. *Lancet.* 1987;1:471–473.

45. Ljungman P, Niederweiser D, Pepe MS, Longton G, Storb R, Meyers JD. Cytomegalovirus infection after marrow transplantation for aplastic anemia. *Bone Marrow Transplant.* 1990;6:295–300.

46. Bostrom L, Ringden O, Jacobsen N, Zwaan F, Nilsson BA. European multicenter study of chronic graft versus host disease: the role of cytomegalovirus serology in recipients and donors, acute graft-versus-host disease, and splenectomy. *Transplantation.* 1990;49:1100–1105.

47. Wagner JL, Seidel K, Boeckh M, Storb R. De novo chronic graft-versus-host disease in marrow graft recipients given methotrexate and cyclosporine: risk factors and survival. *Biol Blood Marrow Transplant.* 2000;6:633–639.

48. Lonnqvist B, Aschan J, Ljungman P, Ringden O. Long term cyclosporine therapy may decrease then risk of chronic graft-versus-host disease. *Br J Haematol.* 1990;74:547=548.

49. Kansu E, Gooley T, Flowers ME, et al. Administration of cyclosporine for 24 months compared with 6 months for prevention of chronic graft-versus-host disease: a prospective randomized clinical trial. *Blood.* 2001;98:3868–3870.

50. Socie G, Clift RA, Blaise D, et al. Busulfan plus cyclophosphamide compared with total-body irradiation plus cyclophosphamide before marrow transplantation for myeloid leukemia: long-term follow-up of 4 randomized studies. *Blood.* 2001;98:3569–3574.

51. Ratanatharathorn V, Nash RA, Przepiorka D, et al. Phase III study comparing methotrexate and tacrolimus (prograf, FK506) with methotrexate and cyclosporine for graft-versus-host disease prophylaxis after HLA-identical sibling bone marrow transplantation. *Blood.* 1998;92:2303–2314.

52. Atkinson K, Downs K. Omission of day 11 methotrexate does not appear to influence the incidence of moderate to severe acute graft-versus-host disease, chronic graft-versus-host disease, relapse rate or survival after HLA- identical sibling bone marrow transplantation. *Bone Marrow Transplant.* 1995;16:755–758.

53. Shulman HM, Sullivan KM, Weiden PL, et al. Chronic graft-versus-host syndrome in man. A long-term clinicopathologic study of 20 Seattle patients. *Am J Med.* 1980;69:204–217.

54. Lee SJ, Vogelsang G, Gilman A, et al. A survey of diagnosis, management, and grading of chronic GVHD. *Biol Blood Marrow Transplant.* 2002;8:32–39.

55. Lee SJ, Vogelsang G, Flowers ME. Chronic graft-versus-host disease. *Biol Blood Marrow Transplant.* 2003;9:215–233.

56. Sullivan KM, Shulman HM, Storb R, et al. Chronic graft-versus-host disease in 52 patients; Adverse natural course and successfull treatment with combination immunosuppression. *Blood.* 1981;57:267–276.

57. Wingard JR, Piantadosi S, Vogelsang GB, et al. Predictors of death from chronic graft-versus-host disease after bone marrow transplantation. *Blood.* 1989;74:1428–1435.

58. Sullivan KM, Witherspoon RP, Storb R, et al. Prednisone and azathioprine compared with prednisone and placebo for treatment of chronic graft-v-host disease: prognostic influence of prolonged thrombocytopenia after allogeneic marrow transplantation. *Blood.* 1988;72:546–554.

59. Akpek G, Zahurak ML, Piantadosi S, et al. Development of a prognostic model for grading chronic graft-versus-host disease. *Blood.* 2001;97:1219–1226.

60. Arora M, Burns LJ, Davies SM, et al. Chronic graft-versus-host disease: a prospective cohort study. *Biol Blood Marrow Transplant*. 2003;9:38–45.

61. Pavletic SZ, Smith LM, Bishop MR, et al. Prognostic factors of chronic graft-versus-host disease after allogeneic blood stem-cell transplantation. *Am J Hematol*. 2005;78:265–274.

62. Morton AJ, Gooley T, Hansen JA, et al. Association between pre-transplant interferon-alpha and outcome after unrelated donor marrow transplantation for chronic myelogenous leukemia in chronic phase. *Blood*. 1998;92:394–401.

63. Akpek G, Lee SJ, Flowers ME, et al. Performance of a new clinical grading system for chronic graft-versus-host disease: a multicenter study. *Blood*. 2003;102:802–809.

64. Akpek G. Clinical grading in chronic graft-versus-host disease: is it time for change? *Leuk Lymphoma*. 2002;43:1211–1220.

65. Kotani A, Ishikawa T, Matsumura Y, et al. Correlation of peripheral blood OX40+(CD134+) T cells with chronic graft-versus-host disease in patients who underwent allogeneic hematopoietic stem cell transplantation. *Blood*. 2001;98:3162–3164.

66. Fuji H, Cuvelier G, She K, et al, Biomarkers in newly diagnosed pediatric extensive chronic graft-versus-host disease: a report from the Children's Oncology Group. Blood First Edition Paper, prepublished online October 9, 2007; DOI 10.1182/blood-2007-08-106286.

67. Randolph SS, Gooley TA, Warren EH, Appelbaum FR, Riddell SR. Female donors contribute to a selective graft-versus-leukemia effect in male recipients of HLA-matched, related hematopoietic stem cell transplants. *Blood*. 2004;103:347–352.

68. Gallardo D, Arostegui JI, Balas A, et al. Disparity for the minor histocompatibility antigen HA-1 is associated with an increased risk of acute graft-versus-host disease (GvHD) but it does not affect chronic GvHD incidence, disease-free survival or overall survival after allogeneic human leucocyte antigen-identical sibling donor transplantation. *Br J Haematol*. 2001;114:931–936.

69. Akatsuka Y, Warren EH, Gooley TA, et al. Disparity for a newly identified minor histocompatibility antigen, HA-8, correlates with acute graft-versus-host disease after haematopoietic stem cell transplantation from an HLA-identical sibling. *Br J Haematol*. 2003;123:671–675.

70. Clark FJ. Freeman L, Dzionek A, et al. Origin and subset distribution of peripheral blood dendritic cells in patients with chronic graft-versus-host disease. *Transplantation*. 2003;75:221–225.

71. Waller EK, Rosenthal H, Jones TW, et al. Larger numbers of CD4(bright) dendritic cells in donor bone marrow are associated with increased relapse after allogeneic bone marrow transplantation. [erratum appears in *Blood*. 2001;98:1677]. *Blood*. 2001;97:2948–2956.

72. Zorn E, Kim HT, Lee SJ, et al. Reduced frequency of FOXP3+ CD4+CD25+ regulatory T cells in patients with chronic graft-versus-host disease. *Blood*. 2005;106:2903–2911.

73. Kondo M, Kojima S, Horibe K, Kato K, Matsuyama T. Risk factors for chronic graft-versus-host disease after allogeneic stem cell transplantation in children. *Bone Marrow Transplant*. 2001;27:727–730.

74. Diaz MA, Vicent MG, Gonzalez ME, et al. Risk assessment and outcome of chronic graft-versus-host disease after allogeneic peripheral blood progenitor cell transplantation in pediatric patients. *Bone Marrow Transplant*. 2004;34:433–438.

8

BIOMARKERS IN CHRONIC GRAFT VERSUS HOST DISEASE

Ernst Holler and Anne Dickinson

INTRODUCTION

Graft versus host disease (GVHD) is one of the most important and potentially fatal complications of hematopoietic stem cell transplantation (HSCT). In its acute form, it can occur in 30% to 50% of patients transplanted with either a human leukocyte antigen (HLA)-matched sibling donor or matched unrelated donor, and the incidence of chronic GVHD (cGVHD) is increasing even further, affecting 40% to 70% of patients. A degree of acute GVHD (aGVHD), however, in the less severe form, grade I to II, may be beneficial and enable a graft versus leukemia (GVL) effect aiding in the destruction of residual leukemic cells. Similar to moderate aGVHD, cGVHD has been shown to be associated with a reduced relapse rate. There is a fine balance therefore between a detrimental GVHD and a beneficial GVL effect. The ability to predict GVHD and its severity or the response to therapeutic strategies would therefore enable the clinician to tailor therapy on an individual basis to improve outcome. Considering the morbidity associated with prolonged and extensive cGVHD, availability of biomarkers should improve the quality of life of patients and ultimately reduce health care costs.

The types of biomarkers for either predicting or monitoring cGVHD include the use of serum cytokines and markers indicating inflammation including cellular assays, lymphocyte subset analyses, and the use of non-HLA genotypes. Recent use and further research into the use of proteomics for predicting both GVHD and developing new biomarkers has also been described.

DEFINITION OF BIOMARKERS

A biomarker, biological or genomic, has been defined as "a characteristic that is objectively measured and evaluated as an indicator of normal biological processes, pathogenic processes, or pharmacologic responses to therapeutic intervention." [1].

Any new biomarker needs to be validated and qualified or evaluated prior to routine use, and usually needs exploratory or advanced method validation via a phase I clinical trial [1].

The emerging biomarkers must be "fit for purpose" [2] and in GVHD the biomarkers will be used as surrogate endpoints and correlated as closely as possible with the clinical endpoint [3]. In some instances, biomarkers have been substituted for clinical responses in order to improve decision making in cases of *human immunodeficiency* virus (HIV), plasma load and CD4 cell count for the evaluation of antiviral agents [4].

This chapter will review potential biomarkers for predicting the occurrence and severity of GVHD and evaluate the potential value of such markers in influencing clinical decisions.

BIOMARKERS FOR PREDICTING AND MONITORING CHRONIC GVHD

Biomarkers are derived from factors identified to be of pathophysiological relevance in experimental or clinical models. Early serum markers reflecting the extent of inflammation, utilized hepatic acute-phase proteins such as C-reactive protein (CRP), serum amyloid (SAA), alpha-1 antitrypsin (AAT), haptoglobulin, and alpha-1 antichymotrypsin and were extensively studied for predicting both GVHD and solid organ transplant rejection [5, 6]. Early activation markers such as the pteridine neopterin have correlated with CRP and levels have been used to discriminate between bacterial infection and GVHD or viral infection [7, 8]. With the characterization of cytokines as the humoral mediators of GVHD, assays analyzing cytokine levels or the capacity to produce cytokines both on a genetic and a cellular level became the focus of attention.

In addition heat shock protein 70 (Hsp70) as an early indicator of inflammation has been used in a human skin explant model of GVHD to predict both acute and chronic GVHD [9].

Serum and Cellular Cytokine Production and the Th1/Th2 Paradigm in GVHD

Serum levels of cytokines may precede clinical changes and have therefore been extensively studied as potentially better serum indictors in predicting GVHD. Several studies have investigated the role of broad inflammatory and anti-inflammatory cytokines, especially tumor necrosis factor-alpha (TNF-α), interferon-gamma (IFN-γ) and interleukin-10 (IL-10) in predicting the development of GVHD posttransplant. They have been studied most extensively in the context of aGVHD, and correlations have been reported for serum TNF-α (Holler [10, 11], Remberger [12]), and also for IL-10 and others (Visentainer, et al. [13]). Positive results in serum studies were supplemented by cellular analyses of cytokine production confirming the activation of proinflammatory cytokines such as IL-1 and IL-6 (Rowbottom, et al. [14, 15]) in aGVHD.

Several murine studies suggested aGVHD reflects a Th1 disease while chronic GVHD seemed to be driven by Th2-type responses. In line with this, cytokines like IL-4, IL-5 or tumor growth factor-beta (TGF-β) have been expected to be associated with cGVHD: Indeed, in a few studies TGF-β seemed to be a marker of cGVHD [16], and a more recent analysis of cytokine production in T-cell subpopulations identified IL-4 producing CD8 cells as markers of cGVHD [17]. However, it became quite clear, that Th1 and Th2 associated markers can be observed in any of the phases of GVHD. Thus, several studies reported a rise of TNF-α in cGVHD [18, 19], and vice versa, even classical Th2-type cytokines such as IL-5 were even more prominent in aGVHD than TNF-α [20]. In line with this, a study on cytokine RNA profiles in skin lesions of cGVHD revealed IFN-γ and TNF to be the predominant cytokines [21].

Eosinophilia has been used as an indicator of increased likelihood for development of fasciitis and sclerodermatous cGVHD [22, 23]. Eosinophils are regulated by IL-5, a classical Th2-type cytokine, and rise of eosinophils prior to cGVHD might fit again into the Th1/Th2 model [24]. However, careful analysis of biopsies from patients with aGVHD identifies eosinophilia as a general marker of immune activation in patients with GVHD and does not allow classification of eosinophilia as a biomarker specific for cGVHD.

Thus it is quite clear that there are so far no distinctive or diagnostic humoral or cellular cytokine profiles for cGVHD. This may be partially explained by the methods used so far, as there are often poor correlations between centers and between the types of assays used for measuring cytokines that have made the interpretation of data difficult and often inconsistent.

New technology may be needed to overcome these problems reflecting the pleiotropism of cytokines and the complex cascade of immunological activation: This is strongly suggested by a recent study analyzing gene profiles in donor CD4 and CD8 cells: Donors for patients who later developed severe GVHD, showed a highly significant upregulation of TGF-ß and CTLA4 related genes. Interestingly the same profile of upregulated genes could be detected in patients 1 year after transplantation suggesting a stable pattern of reaction [25].

Genetic Markers: Cytokine Gene and Inflammatory Gene Polymorphisms

Besides association and prediction of cGVHD by major and minor-HLA disparity, polymorphisms in a variety of genes directly or indirectly involved in immunoregulation have been described. As these polymorphisms frequently translate into the production of either higher or lower levels or a functionally altered relevant protein or receptor, their role in predicting aGVHD has been extensively studied (for review see Dickinson, et al. [26]): For cGVHD, the available data are rare, but focus again on a role of TNF (recipient TNFA –238, TNF 488 A [27, 28]) and the other proinflammatory cytokines (recipient IL-6 (-174) [29] and recipient IL-1 and IL-1Ra) [30, 31]. As for aGVHD, a prognostic role of the IL-10 promoter haplotypes of both, the recipient and the donor, have been observed by several groups supporting that this cytokine is a potent regulator of alloreactivity [32, 33]. An interesting and challenging observation is the fact that a recipient IFN-γ allele associated with diminished production of IFN-γ (IFN-γ 3/3) turned out to be a risk factor of extensive cGVHD [34]. These observations point to a potential immunoregulatory rather than an inflammatory role of IFN-γ, which is also confirmed by recent animal studies.

Besides cytokines, further genes of factors involved in immunoregulation have been investigated as predictors of cGVHD: These include the chemokine genes (CCL5–28 GC [35], the effector molecule Fas-L, and the Fc γ like 3 gene [36].

Infections and pulmonary complications are the main causes of morbidity and mortality in cGVHD. Among pulmonary complications, bronchiolitis obliterans has a complex pathophysiology as it seems to be triggered by infections but reflects finally a chronic obstructive inflammation related to GVHD. The demonstration of an association with polymorphisms of genes of innate immunity such as bacterial permeability increasing protein or the intracellular pathogen receptor NOD2/CARD15 [37, 38] may now explain why only certain patients develop this disabling complication.

ASSESSMENT OF T-CELL FUNCTIONS

Functional T-cell Assays

Mixed lymphocyte reactions (MLRs), limiting dilution T-cell assays and *in vitro* skin explant assays have been used to predict aGVHD but failed to demonstrate a similar role for prediction of chronic GVHD. Whereas MLRs were helpful in the HLA-different setting, limiting dilution assays have been used as more sensitive approaches in HLA-matched stem cell transplantation. By the use of host-specific IL-2 producing T-helper precursor assays Bunjes and colleagues demonstrated that these cells persist in cGVHD developing after preceding aGVHD [39, 40]. Due to the time and cellular consuming nature of these assays, however, they have not been applied in larger and further series. Antigen-specific T cells can be monitored in cGVHD if the antigen is known, as shown for the human Y chromosome (DBY) associated peptides by Zorn et al. [41].

Immunological and Molecular Characterization of T Cells

In general, immunoreconstitution following stem cell transplantation is associated with a prolonged T-cell deficiency, especially for CD4 cells and their subpopulations. This immunodeficiency is aggravated in patients suffering from cGVHD although none of the T-cell markers can be directly used for monitoring of cGVHD [42, 43]. The same holds true for more specific markers of T-cell reconstitution such as analysis of T-cell receptor excision circles representing naive T cells [44–46]. More recently, analysis of regulatory T cells as an indicator of both, acute and chronic GVHD has been postulated as biopsies showed a clear correlation between low regulatory T-cell content and GVHD [47]. Unfortunately, the studies performed so far failed to observe a clear association of peripheral blood regulatory T cells [48, 49] with cGVHD or even showed an increased proportion in these patients [50]. Whether the T-regulatory cell activation marker Ox40 may be a better marker as observed in this later study requires further confirmation.

An alternative and more sensitive method to detect T-cell subpopulations is analysis of the Vβ repertoire. In a recent Japanese study, a highly significant reduction of Vβ complexity was observed in cGVHD patients [51]. These types of assays, together with pretransplant functional analyses as reported for aGVHD clones [52], might be helpful in future approaches.

Assessment of B-cell Functions

B-cell dysfunction has raised substantial interest in the setting of cGVHD: B-cell immunodeficiency is a hallmark although not a specific marker of cGVHD as indicated by low serum and salivary immunoglobulin levels [42, 53]. More specific approaches have been developed to characterize immature B cells in patients with immunodeficiencies and these have recently been applied to patients with cGVHD [54]. In addition, and in line with the Th2 hypothesis, increased and dysregulated B-cell function is another feature of cGVHD: Autoantibodies like antinuclear, antismooth muscle, or anticytoskeleton proteins have been found in about 20% to 30% of patients with cGVHD and may be used as markers in this subgroup [55–60]. The concept of autoantibody production is in line with the recently described increased production of B-cell activating factor (BAFF) [61] and an increased reactivity of B cells from patients with cGVHD to toll-like receptor 9 (TLR9) stimulation [62]. The concept of a sequential T-cell/B-cell activation in cGVHD has been further proven by the elegant demonstration of both, T-cell and B-cell reactions against H-Y associated peptides in patients with cGVHD [63]. Hyperreactivity of B cells and autoimmune reactions is also the basis for the successful use of anti-CD20 antibodies in cGVHD that has recently been confirmed in a large multicentre study from Italy [64].

NEW APPROACHES AND CONCEPTS

Due to the complexity of the immune system and the reactions induced in the context of GVHD, identification of single and unique biomarkers may be impossible except for defined antigen-specific reactions. Therefore, methods aiming to detect patterns of RNA or translated proteins in relation to a defined clinical event seem more promising, as it is suggested by the recent results with proteomic approaches in aGVHD. Urine peptide patterns were identified which showed a sufficient specificity and sensitivity to detect aGVHD prior to clinical onset [65], and ongoing studies will apply this method to cGVHD and its specific complications.

As for the multiplex approach using gene arrays, the clinical value of this proteomic approach has been recently shown by Hori et al. After defining peptides specific for GVHD in a murine model via proteomics, they identified CCL8 as a candidate marker for GVHD and were able to confirm this by serum studies in patients [66].

Besides these multiplex techniques, biostatistics may be used to develop risk scores for cGVHD combining valid data obtained by different approaches such as genetic polymorphisms, clinical risk factors and possibly inflammatory indicators such as eosinophilia.

In addition, due to the intrinsic complexity of cGVHD, studies of biomarkers need to take into account the clinical interpretation of cGVHD to enable improved data collection and interpretation, standardization of procedures and to allow for more accurate interpretation of results. This must include standardized or agreed definitions of acute and chronic GVHD that is, acute versus late acute or classical chronic GVHD including onset posttransplant that is, 100 days posttransplant or other time frame. It should also include knowledge of high or low immunosuppression, degree of severity using the NIH consensus scoring, as well as steroid refractoriness and potential comorbidity indices. Accurate collection of this type of data is paramount to enable accurate final development of a clinical risk index for cGVHD. For example, clinical risk factors for cGVHD such as previous aGVHD, older patient age, female donors to male recipients, use of donor leukocyte infusion (DLI), and use of unrelated or mismatched donors or use of peripheral blood stem cells could all combine to provide a clinical risk score where the above types of biomarkers and genotypes (as mentioned earlier) could be used to design an prognostic index for aiding therapeutic approaches to cGVHD in the future.

This risk index would then be further improved by the addition of validated biomarkers (see Summary Table 8.1) enabling a risk score for high intermediate or low risk of cGVHD to be developed.

One important recent paper studying cGVHD in a pediatric cohort paves the way for these types of studies [67]. Data was collected from a phase III randomized, placebo controlled trial evaluating two treatments for patients with newly diagnosed extensive cGVHD. This carefully diagnosed cGVHD group was compared to a time-matched control group and plasma samples were taken throughout therapy. Several potentially important biomarkers were identified which included sBAFF, anti-dsDNA antibody, sIL-2Rα and sCD13 where sBAFF was also a potential surrogate marker for response to therapy.

Table 8.1: Potential Biomarkers Associated with cGVHD

Serum and Cellular Cytokines	Levels Associated with cGVHD	Reference
TGF-β	↑↑	Liem et al. [16]
IL-4	↑↑ CD8⁺ T cells	Nakamura et al. [17]
TNF-α	↑↑	Abdallah et al. [18] Barak et al. [19]
Gene profiling		
IFN-γ	↑↑ mRNA levels	Ochs et al. [21]
TNF-α	↑↑ mRNA levels	Ochs et al. [21]
TGF-β	↑↑	Baron et al. [25]
CTLA4	↑↑	Baron et al. [25]
SNP analysis		
Recipient TNF-238	Presence/Risk	Bogunia-Kubik et al. [27]
Recipient 488A	Presence/Risk	Mulligan et al. [28]
Recipient IL-16–174	Presence/Risk	Cavet et al. [29]
Recipient IL-1	Presence/Risk	Cullup et al. [30]
Recipient IL-1Ra	Presence/Protection	Rocha et al. [31]
Recipient IL-10 ATA/ATA haplotype	Presence ↑↑Risk	Kim et al. [32]
Donor IL-10–1064	Presence/Risk	Takahashi et al. [33]
Recipient IFN-γ 3/3	Presence/Risk	Bogunia-Kubik et al. [34]
Recipient CCL5–28CC	Presence/Risk	Kim et al. [35]
Recipient Fc receptor γ like 3 gene FCRL3–169	Presence/Protection	Shimada et al. [36]
Soluble serum factors and autoantibodies and B cells		
sBAFF	↑↑	Sarantopoulos et al. [61]
Anti dsDNA	↑↑	Fujii et al. [67]
		Kier et al. [57]
sCD13	↑↑	Fujii et al. [67]
sIL-2Ra	↑↑	Fujii et al. [67]
Immature CD21 B cells	↑↑	Greinix et al. [67]
Memory CD27 B cells	↓↓	Greinix et al. [54]
Anticytoskeleton	↑↑	Dighiero et al. [56]

A combination of these approaches should aid early prediction, diagnosis, prognosis, and monitoring of cGVHD that should allow a customized and risk adapted therapy in the future.

REFERENCES

1. Wagner JA, Williams SA, Webster CJ. Biomarkers and surrogate end points for fit-for-purpose development and regulatory evaluation of new drugs. *Clin Pharmacol Ther.* 2007;81:104–107.

2. Lee JW, Devanarayan V, Barrett YC, et al. Fit-for-purpose method development and validation for successful biomarker measurement. *Pharm Res.* 2006;23:312–328.

3. Schultz KR, Miklos DB, Fowler D, et al. Toward biomarkers for chronic graft-versus-host disease: National Institutes of Health consensus development project on criteria for clinical trials in chronic graft-versus-host disease: III. Biomarker Working Group Report. *Biol Blood Marrow Transplant.* 2006;12:126–137.

4. Lagakos SW. Surrogate markers in AIDS clinical trials: conceptual basis, validation, and uncertainties. *Clin Infect Dis.* 1993;16(Suppl 1):S22–S25.

5. Cohen J, Bayston K. Lympho`kines and the acute-phase response in clinical bone marrow transplantation. *Eur Cytokine Netw.* 1990;1:251–255.

6. Magalini SC, Nanni G, Agnes S, et al. Neopterin, amyloid A, C-reactive protein, gamma-interferon, and interleukin-2 receptor in diagnosis of posttransplantation rejection. *Transplant Proc.* 1991;23:2267–2268.

7. de Bel C, Gerritsen E, de Maaker G, Moolenaar A, Vossen J. C-reactive protein in the management of children with fever after allogeneic bone marrow transplantation. *Infection.* 1991;19:92–96.

8. Sheldon J, Riches PG, Soni N, et al. Plasma neopterin as an adjunct to C-reactive protein in assessment of infection. *Clin Chem.* 1991;37:2038–2042.

9. Jarvis M, Marzolini M, Wang XN, Jackson G, Sviland L, Dickinson AM. Heat shock protein 70: correlation of expression with degree of graft-versus-host response and clinical graft-versus-host disease. *Transplantation.* 2003;76:849–853.

10. Holler E, Ertl B, Hintermeier-Knabe R, et al. Inflammatory reactions induced by pretransplant conditioning–an alternative target for modulation of aGvHD and complications following allogeneic bone marrow transplantation? *Leuk Lymphoma.* 1997;25:217–224.

11. Holler E, Kolb HJ, Moller A, et al. Increased serum levels of tumor necrosis factor alpha precede major complications of bone marrow transplantation. *Blood.* 1990;75:1011–1016.

12. Remberger M, Ringden O, Markling L. TNF alpha levels are increased during bone marrow transplantation conditioning in patients who develop acute GVHD. *Bone Marrow Transplant.* 1995;15:99–104.

13. Visentainer JE, Lieber SR, Persoli LB, et al. Serum cytokine levels and acute graft-versus-host disease after HLA-identical hematopoietic stem cell transplantation. *Exp Hematol.* 2003;31:1044–1050.

14. Rowbottom AW, Norton J, Riches PG, Hobbs JR, Powles RL, Sloane JP. Cytokine gene expression in skin and lymphoid organs in graft versus host disease. *J Clin Pathol.* 1993;46:341–345.

15. Rowbottom AW, Riches PG, Downie C, Hobbs JR. Monitoring cytokine production in peripheral blood during acute graft-versus-host disease following allogeneic bone marrow transplantation. *Bone Marrow Transplant.* 1993;12:635–641.

16. Liem LM, Fibbe WE, van Houwelingen HC, Goulmy E. Serum transforming growth factor-beta1 levels in bone marrow transplant recipients correlate with blood cell counts and chronic graft-versus-host disease. *Transplantation.* 1999;67:59–65.

17. Nakamura K, Amakawa R, Takebayashi M, et al. IL-4-producing CD8(+) T cells may be an immunological hallmark of chronic GVHD. *Bone Marrow Transplant.* 2005;36:639–647.

18. Abdallah AN, Boiron JM, Attia Y, Cassaigne A, Reiffers J, Iron A. Plasma cytokines in graft vs host disease and complications following bone marrow transplantation. *Hematol Cell Ther.* 1997;39:27–32.

19. Barak V, Levi-Schaffer F, Nisman B, Nagler A. Cytokine dysregulation in chronic graft versus host disease. *Leuk Lymphoma.* 1995;17:169–173.

20. Imoto S, Oomoto Y, Murata K, et al. Kinetics of serum cytokines after allogeneic bone marrow transplantation: interleukin-5 as a potential marker of acute graft-versus-host disease. *Int J Hematol.* 2000;72:92–97.

21. Ochs LA, Blazar BR, Roy J, Rest EB, Weisdorf DJ. Cytokine expression in human cutaneous chronic graft-versus-host disease. *Bone Marrow Transplant.* 1996;17:1085–1092.

22. Jacobsohn DA, Schechter T, Seshadri R, Thormann K, Duerst R, Kletzel M. Eosinophilia correlates with the presence or development of chronic graft-versus-host disease in children. *Transplantation* 2004;77:1096–1100.

23. Kalaycioglu ME, Bolwell BJ. Eosinophilia after allogeneic bone marrow transplantation using the busulfan and cyclophosphamide preparative regimen. *Bone Marrow Transplant.* 1994;14:113–115.

24. Masumoto A, Sasao T, Yoshiba F, et al. Hypereosinophilia after allogeneic bone marrow transplantation. A possible role of IL-5 overproduction by donor T-cells chronic GVHD. *Rinsho Ketsueki.* 1997;38:234–236.

25. Baron C, Somogyi R, Greller LD, et al. Prediction of graft-versus-host disease in humans by donor gene-expression profiling. *PLoS Med.* 2007;4:e23.

26. Dickinson AM, Middleton PG, Rocha V, Gluckman E, Holler E, on behalf of EUROBANK members. Genetic polymorphisms predicting the outcome of bone marrow transplants. *Br J Haematol.* 2004;127:479–490.

27. Bogunia-Kubik K, Wysoczanska B, Lange A. Non-HLA gene polymorphisms and the outcome of allogeneic hematopoietic stem cell transplantation. *Curr Stem Cell Res Ther.* 2006;1:239–253.

28. Mullighan C, Heatley S, Doherty K, et al. Non-HLA immunogenetic polymorphisms and the risk of complications after allogeneic hemopoietic stem-cell transplantation. *Transplantation.* 2004;77:587–596.

29. Cavet J, Dickinson AM, Norden J, Taylor PR, Jackson GH, Middleton PG. Interferon-gamma and interleukin-6 gene polymorphisms associate with graft-versus-host disease in HLA-matched sibling bone marrow transplantation. *Blood.* 2001;98:1594–1600.

30. Cullup H, Dickinson AM, Cavet J, Jackson GH, Middleton PG. Polymorphisms of IL-1alpha constitute independent risk factors for chronic graft versus host disease following allogeneic bone marrow transplantation. *Br J Haematol.* 2003;122:778–787.

31. Rocha V, Franco RF, Porcher R, et al. Host defence and inflammatory gene polymorphisms are associated with outcomes after HLA-identical sibling bone marrow transplant. *Blood.* 2002;100:3908–3918.

32. Kim DH, Lee NY, Sohn SK, et al. IL-10 promoter gene polymorphism associated with the occurrence of chronic GVHD and its clinical course during systemic immunosuppressive treatment for chronic GVHD after allogeneic peripheral blood stem cell transplantation. *Transplantation.* 2005;79:1615–1622.

33. Takahashi H, Furukawa T, Hashimoto S, et al. Contribution of TNF-alpha and IL-10 gene polymorphisms to graft-versus-host disease following allo-hematopoietic stem cell transplantation. *Bone Marrow Transplant.* 2000;26:1317–1323.

34. Bogunia-Kubik K, Mlynarczewska A, Wysoczanska B, Lange A. Recipient interferon-gamma 3/3 genotype contributes to the development of chronic graft-versus-host disease after allogeneic hematopoietic stem cell transplantation. *Haematologica.* 2005;90:425–426.

35. Kim DH, Jung HD, Lee NY, Sohn SK. Single nucleotide polymorphism of CC chemokine ligand 5 promoter gene in recipients may predict the risk of chronic graft-versus-host disease and its severity after allogeneic transplantation. *Transplantation.* 2007;84:917–925.

36. Shimada M, Onizuka M, Machida S, et al. Association of autoimmune disease-related gene polymorphisms with chronic graft-versus-host disease. *Br J Haematol.* 2007;139:458–463.

37. Chien JW, Zhao LP, Hansen JA, Fan WH, Parimon T, Clark JG. Genetic variation in bactericidal/permeability-increasing protein influences the risk of developing rapid airflow decline after hematopoietic cell transplantation. *Blood.* 2006;107:2200–2207.

38. Hildebrandt GC, Granell M, Urbano-Ispizua A, et al. Recipient NOD2/CARD15 variants: a novel independent risk factor for the development of bronchiolitis obliterans after allogeneic stem cell transplantation. *Biol Blood Marrow Transplant.* 2008;14:67–74.

39. Bunjes D, Theobald M, Nierle T, Arnold R, Heimpel H. Presence of host-specific interleukin 2-secreting T-helper cell precursors correlates closely with active primary and secondary chronic graft-versus-host disease. *Bone Marrow Transplant.* 1995;15:727–732.

40. Nierle T, Bunjes D, Arnold R, Heimpel H, Theobald M. Quantitative assessment of posttransplant host-specific interleukin-2-secreting T-helper cell precursors in patients with

and without acute graft-versus-host disease after allogeneic HLA-identical sibling bone marrow transplantation. *Blood.* 1993;81:841–848.

41. Zorn E, Miklos DB, Floyd BH, et al. Minor histocompatibility antigen DBY elicits a coordinated B and T cell response after allogeneic stem cell transplantation. *J Exp Med.* 2004;199:1133–1142.

42. Lum LG. Immune recovery after bone marrow transplantation. *Hematol Oncol Clin North Am.* 1990;4:659–675.

43. Lum LG, Orcutt-Thordarson N, Seigneuret MC, Storb R. The regulation of Ig synthesis after marrow transplantation. IV. T4 and T8 subset function in patients with chronic graft-vs-host disease. *J Immunol.* 1982;129:113–119.

44. Fallen PR, McGreavey L, Madrigal JA, et al. Factors affecting reconstitution of the T cell compartment in allogeneic haematopoietic cell transplant recipients. *Bone Marrow Transplant.* 2003;32:1001–1014.

45. Weinberg K, Blazar BR, Wagner JE, et al. Factors affecting thymic function after allogeneic hematopoietic stem cell transplantation. *Blood.* 2001;97:1458–1466.

46. Toubert A, Clave E, Talvensaari K, Douay C, Charron D. New tools in assessing immune reconstitution after hematopoietic stem cell transplantation. *Vox Sang.* 2000;78(Suppl 2):29–31.

47. Rieger K, Loddenkemper C, Maul J, et al. Mucosal FOXP3+ regulatory T cells are numerically deficient in acute and chronic GvHD. *Blood.* 2006;107:1717–1723.

48. Arimoto K, Kadowaki N, Ishikawa T, Ichinohe T, Uchiyama T. FOXP3 expression in peripheral blood rapidly recovers and lacks correlation with the occurrence of graft-versus-host disease after allogeneic stem cell transplantation. *Int J Hematol.* 2007;85:154–162.

49. Meignin V, Peffault de Latour R, Zuber J, et al. Numbers of Foxp3-expressing CD4+CD25high T cells do not correlate with the establishment of long-term tolerance after allogeneic stem cell transplantation. *Exp Hematol.* 2005;33:894–900.

50. Sanchez J, Casano J, Alvarez MA, et al. Kinetic of regulatory CD25high and activated CD134+ (OX40) T lymphocytes during acute and chronic graft-versus-host disease after allogeneic bone marrow transplantation. *Br J Haematol.* 2004;126:697–703.

51. Tsutsumi Y, Tanaka J, Miura Y, et al. Molecular analysis of T-cell repertoire in patients with graft-versus-host disease after allogeneic stem cell transplantation. *Leuk Lymphoma.* 2004;45:481–488.

52. Michalek J, Collins RH, Hill BJ, Brenchley JM, Douek DC. Identification and monitoring of graft-versus-host specific T-cell clone in stem cell transplantation. *Lancet.* 2003;361:1183–1185.

53. Norhagen G, Engstrom PE, Bjorkstrand B, Hammarstrom L, Smith CI, Ringden O. Salivary and serum immunoglobulins in recipients of transplanted allogeneic and autologous bone marrow. *Bone Marrow Transplant.* 1994;14:229–234.

54. Greinix HT, Pohlreich D, Kouba M, et al. Elevated numbers of immature/transitional CD21- B lymphocytes and deficiency of

memory CD27+ B cells identify patients with active chronic graft-versus-host disease. *Biol Blood Marrow Transplant.* 2008;14:208–219.

55. Chan EY, Lawton JW, Lie AK, Lau CS. Autoantibody formation after allogeneic bone marrow transplantation: correlation with the reconstitution of CD5+ B cells and occurrence of graft-versus-host disease. *Pathology.* 1997;29:184–188.

56. Dighiero G, Intrator L, Cordonnier C, Tortevoye P, Vernant JP. High levels of anti-cytoskeleton autoantibodies are frequently associated with chronic GVHD. *Br J Haematol.* 1987;67:301–305.

57. Kier P, Penner E, Bakos S, et al. Autoantibodies in chronic GVHD: high prevalence of antinucleolar antibodies. *Bone Marrow Transplant.* 1990;6:93–96.

58. Patriarca F, Skert C, Sperotto A, et al. The development of autoantibodies after allogeneic stem cell transplantation is related with chronic graft-vs-host disease and immune recovery. *Exp Hematol.* 2006;34:389–396.

59. Quaranta S, Shulman H, Ahmed A, et al. Autoantibodies in human chronic graft-versus-host disease after hematopoietic cell transplantation. *Clin Immunol.* 1999;91:106–116.

60. Rouquette-Gally AM, Boyeldieu D, Prost AC, Gluckman E. Autoimmunity after allogeneic bone marrow transplantation. A study of 53 long-term-surviving patients. *Transplantation.* 1988;46:238–240.

61. Sarantopoulos S, Stevenson KE, Kim HT, et al. High levels of B-cell activating factor in patients with active chronic graft-versus-host disease. *Clin Cancer Res.* 2007;13:6107–6114.

62. She K, Gilman AL, Aslanian S, et al. Altered Toll-like receptor 9 responses in circulating B cells at the onset of extensive chronic graft-versus-host disease. *Biol Blood Marrow Transplant.* 2007;13:386–397.

63. Miklos DB, Kim HT, Miller KH, et al. Antibody responses to H-Y minor histocompatibility antigens correlate with chronic graft-versus-host disease and disease remission. *Blood.* 2005;105:2973–2978.

64. Zaja F, Bacigalupo A, Patriarca F, et al. Treatment of refractory chronic GVHD with rituximab: a GITMO study. *Bone Marrow Transplant.* 2007;40:273–277.

65. Weissinger EM, Schiffer E, Hertenstein B, et al. Proteomic patterns predict acute graft-versus-host disease after allogeneic hematopoietic stem cell transplantation. *Blood.* 2007;109:5511–5519.

66. Hori T, Naishiro Y, Sohma H, et al. CCL8 is a potential molecular candidate for the diagnosis of graft versus host disease. *Blood.* 2008;111(8):4403–4412.

67. Fujii H, Cuvelier G, She K, et al. Biomarkers in newly diagnosed pediatric-extensive chronic graft-versus-host disease: a report from the Children's Oncology Group. *Blood.* 2008;111:3276–3285.

PART II: CLINICAL MANAGEMENT

9

Diagnosis and Staging

Madan Jagasia, Howard M. Shulman, Alexandra H. Filipovich, and Steven Z. Pavletic

INTRODUCTION

Chronic graft versus host disease (cGVHD) is an alloreactive phenomenon that often complicates allogeneic stem cell transplantation (SCT) [1]. Significant progress has been made in acute graft versus host disease (aGVHD) prophylaxis and management. Similar progress in cGVHD has been elusive due to multiple factors, including lack of well defined and prognostically validated classification. This in turn leads to enrollment of a heterogeneous spectrum of cGVHD patients on clinical trials and confounds accurate interpretation of the outcome. Lack of appropriate animal models and the true pathogenesis of this clinical entity with protean manifestations have limited the progress in this field.

The spectrum of allogeneic SCT has increased to include elderly patients and alternative stem cell sources. Advances in critical care, better understanding of infectious disease post SCT and the advent of reduced-intensity and nonmyeloablative conditioning regimens has decreased early mortality after SCT. Thus, the combination of these factors, over time, has lead to an increasing number of patients post SCT at risk for developing cGVHD. Thus it is important to revisit and reaccess cGVHD in the current milleau of SCT.

This chapter focuses on the classification system for staging and grading cGVHD along with the clinicopathologic features and aspects that impact the classification of cGVHD.

CHARACTERISTICS OF AN IDEAL CLASSIFICATION SYSTEM

Any classification system that is disease specific should attempt to establish a common language, segregate diseases into biologically distinct groups, and have the ability to prognosticate. In cGVHD, a classification system should allow us to classify morphologically heterogeneous presentations with a particular natural history. It would be ideal for such different subtypes to have unique biologic basis. The classification system should allow for an accurate measure of extent of the disease in the number of organ systems that it affects and also the degree of

dysfunction in each organ. As target organ dysfunction from cGVHD can be irreversible, the ideal classification system should incorporate measures of degree of disability. A grading scheme should be able to predict survival or disablity-free survival in a clinically meaningful way even as new methodologies of transplant evolve. The system should be valid irrespective of the donor stem cell source. The system should be easy to apply in the clinic and should have a high inter- and intra-observer consistency.

Classification of cGVHD will not only allow us to better characterize various subtypes of GVHD but will also have significant impact on measuring outcome of clinical trials. Currently all forms of systemic cGVHD are treated similarly. If these various subtypes are prospectively validated to have differing outcomes, customizing treatment on the basis of subtypes would be potentially feasible.

HISTORICAL PERSPECTIVE OF cGVHD CLASSIFICATION AND PROGNOSTIC FACTORS

The first attempt to classify GVHD after day 100 was published in 1980 [1]. Any GVHD after day 100 was termed as cGVHD to contrast with aGVHD that typically occurs in the first 3 months after SCT and presents as a constellation of dermatitis, hepatitis, and enteritis. It was recognized in the 1970s that cGVHD features resembled an overlap of several collagen vascular diseases with frequent involvement of skin, liver, eyes, mouth, upper respiratory tract, esophagus and less frequent involvement of the serosal surfaces, lower gastrointestinal tract, and skeletal muscles [2, 3]. Scleroderma, dry eyes, dry mouth, pulmonary insufficiency, and wasting accounted for the major causes of morbidity. cGVHD based on the pattern of onset in relation to aGVHD was classified as progressive (continuously active aGVHD gradually progressing into cGVHD), quiescent (resolution of aGVHD, then a phase of no clinical GVHD activity, followed by development of cGVHD), and de novo late onset (onset of cGVHD without clinical or biopsy evidence of prior aGVHD).

Table 9.1: Original and Revised Seattle Classification for Limited and Extensive cGVHD

Original Seattle Classification	*Revised Seattle Classification*
Limited	*Clinical Limited*

One or both of
  Localized skin
  Hepatic dysfunction due to cGVHD
	1. Oral abnormalities consistent with cGVHD, positive biopsy (skin or lip) and no other manifestations
	2. Mild LFT abnormalities with positive biopsy (skin or lip), and no other manifestations
	3. Less than six plaques, <20% BSA rash/dyspigmentation, erythema <50%, positive skin biopsy and no other manifestations
	4. Ocular sicca, positive biopsy (skin or lip), and no other manifestations
	5. Vaginal or vulvar abnormalities, with positive biopsy, and no other manifestations

Extensive
One of
  Generalized skin involvement
OR
  Localized skin involvement and/or
  hepatic dysfunction due to cGVHD, plus
  liver histology showing chronic aggressive hepatitis, bridging necrosis, or
  cirrhosis, or Involvement of eye (Schirmer <5 mm); or
  Involvement of minor salivary glands or oral mucosa demonstrated on a labial biopsy, or:
  Involvement of any other target organ
	Clinical Extensive
	1. Involvement of two or more organs with cGVHD (signs or symptoms) with biopsy confirmation in at least one organ
	2. Kanofsky or Lansky performance scores <60%, ≥15% weight loss, recurrent infections (other causes rule out), with biopsy confirmation in at least one organ
	3. Skin involvement more than defined for clinical limited with biopsy confirmation
	4. Scleroderma or morphea
	5. Onycholysis or onychodystrophy (due to cGVHD), with cGVHD in at least one other organ
	6. Decreased range of notion in ankle or wrist due to fasciitis from cGVHD
	7. Contractures as result of cGVHD
	8. Bronchiolitis obliterans (other causes rule out)
	9. Positive liver biopsy, abnormal LFTs (other causes rule out), alkaline phosphatase ≥2 × upper limit of normal, AST or ALT ≥3 × upper limit of normal, or total bilirubin >1.6, and with cGVHD in at least one other organ
	10. Positive upper or lower gut biopsy
	11. Facsiitis or serositis due to cGVHD (other causes rule out)

ALT, alanine aminotransferase; AST, aspartate aminotransferase; BSA, body surface area; GVHD, graft versus host disease; LFT, liver function test.

The concept of limited and extensive cGVHD (Table 9.1) was introduced based on the outcome of 20 patients. Of these 20 patients, 3 had limited cGVHD and 17 had extensive cGVHD. Patients were classified into three groups based on morbidity and mortality (Group I: moderate or resolved disease, alive; Group II: severe disease, alive; Group III: severe disease, dead). The authors did make an observation that among patients with extensive cGVHD the Karnofsky performance status (KPS) score was the best prognosticator of outcome. Due to lack of other classification systems, this limited/extensive cGVHD classification has been in use since its development, realizing the limited prognostic ability for both relapse and nonrelapse mortality.

Subsequent studies identified progressive presentation, bilirubin elevation, lichenoid changes of skin histology [3], platelet less than 100×10^9/L [4], and prior steroid refractory or dependent aGVHD as markers for poor outcome.

The next major attempt to develop a prognostic model was made by Lee et al. using survival data on more than a 1,000 patients above the age of 16 years from the International Bone Marrow Transplant Registry (IBMTR) who underwent non–T-cell depleted transplant from a human leukocyte antigen (HLA) identical sibling or a matched unrelated donor (matched at HLA-A, HLA-B, and HLA-DR by serologic or molecular testing) [5]. All patients in this cohort received cyclosporine and methotrexate for GVHD prophylaxis and were disease free of their underlying hematopoietic illness for at least 100 days after SCT. The authors noted a 60%–65% incorrect designation of limited cGVHD in patients undergoing a sibling SCT and a 43% misclassification of limited cGVHD in recipients of unrelated transplants. As the data could not be verified due to the retrospective nature of the study, the classification reported by the transplant center was used. A new risk scale was developed and patients were stratified into different groups

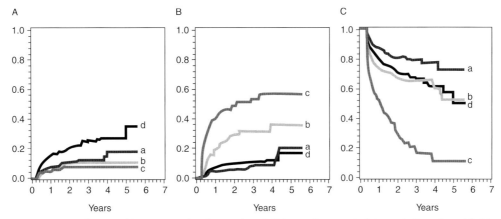

Figure 9.1 A: Relapse. B: Treatment-related mortality. C: Disease-free survival. Lines indicate low risk (a); intermediate risk (b); high risk (c); and no cGVHD (d).
Lee SJ, Klein JP, Barrett AJ et al. Severity of chronic graft-versus-host disease :association with trament-related mortality and relapse. *Blood*. 2002;100:406–414. See Plate 12 in the color plate section.

based on KPS, chronic diarrhea, weight loss, skin involvement, and oral involvement. Patients were classified as low risk (KPS ≥80%, no weight loss or chronic diarrhea), intermediate risk (KPS ≥80% with either weight loss or chronic diarrhea or KPS <80% with or without oral involvement), high risk (KPS 80% with both chronic diarrhea and weight loss or KPS <80% with chronic diarrhea, weight loss, and skin involvement or KPS <80% with oral involvement but with one or two other features). All analyses to predict disease-free survival (DFS) and transplant-related mortality (TRM) were adjusted for disease type, stage, recipient age, sex-matching, and prior aGVHD. Multivariate models were developed in an IBMTR data set and validated in an independent IBMTR data set and National Marrow Donor Program (NMDP) data set. These risk categories were able to predict DFS (low and intermediate risk) and TRM (low and intermediate risk) but were not prognostic for relapse (Figure 9.1). Interestingly no relationship between these categories and GVHD could be established.

A risk stratification system based on a retrospective review of 150 patients referred for GVHD to the Johns Hopkins Center was developed by Akpek et al. [6] The most common sites of GVHD involvement (skin and fascia, mouth and eye involvement, performance status, weight loss, and infection within 1 month before or after diagnosis of cGVHD or primary treatment failure) were coded on a scale of 1 to 3 indicating extent and severity of cGVHD. The two major statistical outcomes studied were GVHD-specific survival from onset of cGVHD and from time of primary treatment failure. According to multivariate analyses, extensive skin involvement more than 50% body surface area (hazard ratio [HR] 7.0, 95% CI 3.6–13.4), thrombocytopenia (platelet <100 × 10^9/L) (HR 3.6, 95% CI 1.9–6.8) and progressive-type onset (HR 1.7; 95% CI 0.9–3.0) significantly influenced GVHD-specific survival (Figure 9.2A). These 3 factors and KPS influenced survival from primary treatment failure. Patients were divided into 3 categories depending on their prognostic factor score (PFS) (Figure 9.2B). Patients with no adverse

prognostic factor (score 0) had a 10-year GVHD-specific survival of 82%. Patient with PFS less than 2 (extended skin involvement only or thrombocytopenia and/or progressive-type onset) had a 68% 10-year GVHD-specific survival. Patients with PFS of 2 to 3.5 (extensive skin involvement and either thrombocytopenia or progressive-type onset) had a 34% 10-year GVHD-specific survival. Patients with a prognostic factor of higher than 3.5 (presence of all 3 factors) had a 3% 10-year GVHD-specific survival (Figure 9.2B). Similarly the 5-year survival from primary treatment failure for PFSs of 0, less than 2, 2 to 3.5, and higher than 3.5 were 91%, 71%, 22%, and 4%.

The original limited and extensive classification of cGVHD was revised by the Seattle group (Table 9.1) [7]. The purpose of the revision was to guide implementation and duration of systemic immunosuppressive therapy. Patients with the revised extensive cGVHD would be candidates for prolonged immunosuppressive therapy, in contrast to the revised limited cGVHD. The prognostic impact or incidence of cGVHD using the revised Seattle classification is not known.

Thus, over the last 30 years since the first report of the limited/extensive classification, most of the prognostic systems have revolved around the same concept. More recently, the National Institute of Health (NIH) consensus criteria were developed.

NIH CONSENSUS CRITERIA FOR GRADING AND STAGING OF GVHD

The diagnostic criteria for cGVHD, its differentiation from aGVHD, and recommendations for scoring of severity in each organ system as well as the global scoring system have recently been agreed to by consensus of experts who participated in an NIH sponsored project [8].

First, the distinction between acute and chronic GVHD, traditionally defined by time of diagnosis before or after 100

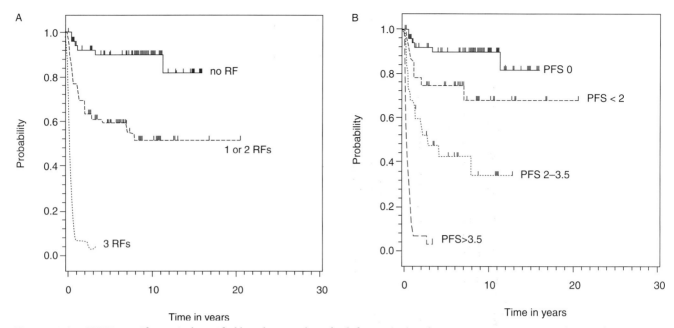

Figure 9.2 A: cGVHD-specific survival stratified based on number of risk factors (RF) at diagnosis. RF were extensive skin involvement more than 50% body surface area, thrombocytopenia (platelet $<100 \times 10^9$/L), and progressive-type onset of cGVHD. B: cGVHD-specific survival stratified based on PFS.

This research was originally published in *Blood*. Akpek G, Zahurak ML, Piantadosi S et al. Development of a prognostic model for grading chronic graft-versus-host disease. *Blood*. 2001;97:1219–1226.

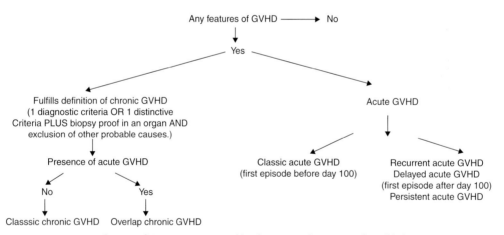

Figure 9.3. Various subtypes of GVHD as proposed by the National Institute of Health (NIH) consensus criteria.

days following a myeloablative SCT, was deemed inadequate given current treatment practices. Recent statistics from international registries indicate that the majority of SCT recipients receive products from unrelated donors, and often rely on nonmyeloablative conditioning protocols, posttransplant donor lymphocyte infusions (DLIs) and/or stem cell "boosts" and prolonged use of GVHD prophylaxes. Therefore, the NIH consensus document recognized two main categories of GVHD, each with two subcategories (Figure 9.3). aGVHD was subclassified into (1) "classic" aGVHD occurring within 100 days after hematopoietic cell transplantation (HCT) or DLI with symptoms of maculopapular rash, nausea, vomiting,

anorexia, profuse diarrhea, ileus, or cholestatic hepatitis and (2) persistent, recurrent, or late aGVHD without diagnostic or distinctive manifestations of cGVHD occurring beyond 100 days of transplantation or DLI (often seen after withdrawal of immune suppression). Characteristic skin, gastrointestinal (GI) tract, or liver abnormalities as defined above in "classic" aGVHD should be classified as aGVHD regardless of the time after transplantation. The broad category of cGVHD includes (1) classic cGVHD defined by presence of at least one diagnostic or distinctive manifestation of cGVHD (defined subsequently) without features characteristic of aGVHD and (2) an overlap syndrome in which features of chronic and acute

GVHD appear together. Onset of symptoms of classic cGVHD or overlap syndrome have no time limit post SCT or DLI.

The diagnosis of cGVHD requires the presence of at least one diagnostic clinical sign of cGVHD (described susequently) or the presence of at least one distinctive clinical manifestation confirmed by biopsy or other relevant tests in the same or another organ. Other causes may enter into the differential diagnosis of cGVHD, especially infections such as those involving the nails or mouth, and must be excluded. The list of diagnostic manifestations of cGVHD are detailed in the consensus document [8]: they can involve the skin and appendages, mouth, eyes, female genitalia, esophagus, lungs, and connective tissues. Biopsy or other testing is always encouraged to complement clinical diagnoses in these organs and tissues but is not mandatory if the patient has at least one of the diagnostic features of cGVHD, which are listed in the following text.

DIAGNOSTIC CRITERIA: SIGNS AND SYMPTOMS SUFFICIENT TO ESTABLISH THE DIAGNOSIS OF cGVHD

Skin

Manifestations include several dermatologic conditions characterized by atrophy, depigmentation, leathery consistency, or waxy appearance: *poikiloderma, lichen planus-like eruption* (e.g., erythematous/violaceous flat-topped papules or plaques with a silvery or shiny appearance), *deep sclerotic features* ("thickened or tight skin," caused by deep and diffuse sclerosis over a wide area), *morphea-like superficial sclerotic features* (e.g., localized patchy areas of moveable smooth or shiny skin with a leathery-like consistency), and *lichen sclerosus-like lesions* (discrete to coalescent gray to white moveable papules or plaques, often with a shiny appearance and leathery consistency). Severe sclerotic features characterized by thickened, tight, and fragile skin are often associated with poor wound healing, inadequate lymphatic drainage, and skin ulcers from minor trauma (Figure 9.4).

Mouth

Lichen planus-like changes (white lines and lacy-appearing lesions of the buccal mucosa, tongue, palate, or lips), hyperkeratotic plaques (**leukoplakia**), or decreased oral range of motion in patients with sclerotic features of skin GVHD.

GI Tract

Esophageal web, stricture, or concentric rings documented by endoscopy or barium contrast radiograph.

Genitalia

Lichen planus-like features and vaginal scarring or stenosis (often associated with oral GVHD).

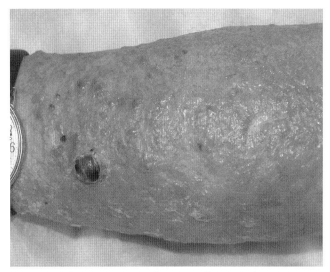

Figure 9.4 Chronic GVHD with severe sclerosis with angiomatous proliferations. (Courtesy Dr. Daniel Couriel.) See Plate 13 in the color plate section.

Lung

Biopsy proven bronchiolitis obliterans (BO). BO is characterized by the new onset of an obstructive lung defect. Clinical manifestations may include dyspnea on exertion, cough, or wheezing. Some patients may be asymptomatic early in the disease process. BO is clinically diagnosed when all of the following criteria are met: (1) Forced expiratory volume in 1 second/forced vital capacity ratio <0.7 and forced expiratory volume in 1 second <75% of predicted; (2) evidence of air trapping or small airway thickening or bronchiectasis on high-resolution chest computed tomography (with inspiratory and expiratory cuts), residual volume >120%, or pathologic confirmation of constrictive bronchiolitis; (3) absence of infection in the respiratory tract, documented with investigations directed by clinical symptoms, such as radiologic studies (radiographs or computed tomographic scans) or microbiologic cultures (sinus aspiration, upper respiratory tract viral screen, sputum culture, or bronchoalveolar lavage).

Muscles, Fascia, Joints

Fasciitis, joint stiffness, or contractures secondary to sclerosis.

DISTINCTIVE CRITERIA AND OTHER FEATURES: SEEN IN cGVHD BUT INSUFFICIENT ALONE TO ESTABLISH A DIAGNOSIS OF cGVHD

Skin

Depigmentation contributes to the diagnosis of cGVHD in combination with biopsy or laboratory confirmation of GVHD in skin or another organ. Sweat impairment and intolerance to temperature change from loss of sweat glands are seen in cGVHD. Other nondistinctive skin manifestations found with both acute and chronic GVHD include erythema, maculopapular rash, and pruritus.

Nails

Dystrophy consisting of longitudinal ridging, nail splitting or brittleness, onycholysis, pterygium unguis, and nail loss (usually symmetric and affecting most nails) are distinctive signs of cGVHD.

Hair

New scarring and nonscarring scalp alopecia (after recovery from chemotherapy or radiotherapy) and loss of body hair are a distinctive feature of cGVHD. Other characteristics seen with cGVHD include premature graying, thinning, or brittleness.

Mouth

Distinctive features of cGVHD include xerostomia (dryness), mucoceles, mucosal atrophy, pseudomembranes, and noninfectious ulcers. Manifestations common to both acute and chronic GVHD include gingivitis, mucositis, erythema, and pain.

Eyes

Distinctive manifestations of cGVHD include new onset of dry, gritty, or painful eyes; cicatricial conjunctivitis; keratoconjunctivitis sicca; and confluent areas of punctate keratopathy. New ocular sicca documented by low Schirmer test values with a mean value of both eyes ≤5 mm at 5 minutes or a new onset of keratoconjunctivitis sicca by slit-lamp examination with mean values of 6 to 10 mm on the Schirmer test is sufficient for the diagnosis of cGVHD if accompanied by distinctive manifestations in at least one other organ. Other features include photophobia, periorbital hyperpigmentation, difficulty in opening the eyes in the morning because of mucoid secretions, and blepharitis (erythema of the eye lids with edema).

Gastrointestinal Tract

Pancreatic exocrine insufficiency, anorexia, nausea, vomiting, diarrhea, weight loss, and wasting syndrome may be associated with cGVHD. Endoscopic findings of mucosal edema and erythema or focal erosions with histologic changes of apoptotic epithelial cells and crypt cell dropout are all features of GVHD per se but, with the specific diagnostic exception of esophageal webs, are not diagnostic of cGVHD unless the patient also has diagnostic or distinctive features outside the GI system.

Liver

Hepatic acute and chronic GVHD typically presents as cholestasis, with increased bilirubin or alkaline phosphatase, but it may also present as acute hepatitis. Biopsy is required to confirm GVHD involvement of the liver, which should be complemented by a distinctive manifestation in at least one other organ system.

Lungs

Restrictive pulmonary function abnormalities secondary to advanced sclerosis of the chest wall are attributable to skin GVHD. BO-organizing pneumonia not due to infections may represent a manifestation of either acute or chronic GVHD and is considered a common feature.

Musculoskeletal System

Clinical myositis with tender muscles and increased muscle enzymes is a distinctive feature of cGVHD. Evaluation of myositis involves electromyography and measurement of creatinine phosphokinase or aldolase. Arthralgia and arthritis are uncommon and are occasionally associated with the presence of autoantibodies.

Hematopoietic and Immunologic Systems

Cytopenias may result from autoimmune processes. Lymphopenia (≤500/μL), eosinophilia (≥500/μL), hypogammaglobulinemia, or hypergammaglobulinemia may be present.

Other Features

Rarely, pericardial and pleural effusions or ascites peripheral neuropathy, myasthenia gravis, nephrotic syndrome have been attributed to cGVHD.

Clinical Scoring of Individual Organ Systems

The consensus process developed a scoring system to be used at baseline (before treatment of cGVHD), which could easily be performed by primary care physicians using physical examination and readily available laboratory tests (e.g., liver function studies). A limitation of the scoring system is that it doses not distinguish between disease activity and fixed deficits.

Each organ that can be represented with diagnostic criteria of cGVHD is scored (0–3), with 0 reflecting no involvement of that organ. Performance score (according to the Karnofsky/Lansky scale) is also included. The scoring spread sheet is found in the consensus report [8].

Guidelines for Global Scoring of cGVHD

These were developed by the consensus group following confirmed diagnosis of cGVHD, and scoring of organs with diagnostic findings for cGVHD. General categories of mild, moderate, and severe cGVHD were assembled to reflect severity of individual organ involvement and functional impairment. The categories were fashioned after consideration of existing historical evidence related to prognosis of cGVHD with and without treatment.

Mild cGVHD is characterized by involvement of 1 to 2 organs or sites affected with cGVHD (except lung) that do not individually achieve a cGVHD score >1, and when clinically significant functional impairment is not seen. *Moderate cGVHD* involves (1) at least one organ or site with clinically significant but no major disability (maximum score of two in any affected organ or site) or (2) three or more organs or sites with no clinically significant functional impairment (maximum score of 1 in all affected organs or sites). A lung score of 1 will also be considered moderate cGVHD. *Severe cGVHD* indicates major disability caused by cGVHD (score of 3 in any organ or site). A lung score of 2 or greater will also be considered severe cGVHD. According to current practice, mild cGVHD usually does not require systemic immunosuppressive therapy, although topical anti-inflammatory therapy may be beneficial. Moderate and severe cGVHD should be considered for systemic therapy.

HISTOPATHOLOGICAL ASPECTS OF CGVHD

This section details pathology of target organs that are most commonly biopsied to establish a diagnosis of cGVHD. Histopathology serves as one of the several major criteria for defining the differences between aGVHD and the later-developing distinct manifestations, which came to be codified as cGVHD [9]. As detailed earlier, the original cutoff for calling any active GVHD after day 100 as chronic was predicated on experience-based clinicopathologic observations that within a few weeks of continuous activity, the GVHD manifestations developed the chronic phenotype. Today we know that GVHD active at day 100 does not inexorably progress into chronic manifestations. In the current milieu, patients may develop a sort of hybrid phenotype with features that are a composite of

acute and chronic GVHD [8]. On the other hand, there is a validated literature of histologic changes that are for specific cGVHD including certain changes in the skin, small bronchioles, tubuloalveolar glands of the lacrimal, salivary and aerodigestive tracts, joints and serosal surfaces, and mucosa of the oral, genital, and upper esophageal regions. Since the original

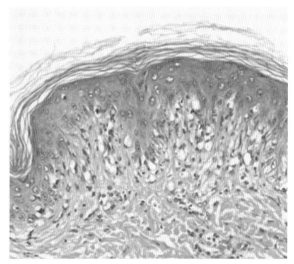

Figure 9.5 Skin, fatal acute GVHD day 30. The epidermis has an extensive interface dermatitis with continuous vacuolization along the basal, lymphocytic infiltration of the epidermis and superficial perivascular inflammation. The epidermal surface has mild basket-weave (loose) hyperkeratosis and is of normal thickness. Along the basal layer of a rete ridge are contiguous keratinocyte apoptotic bodies, clear spaces containing the contracted dense eosinophilic cytoplasm with dark membrane bound nuclear fragments. Lymphocytes partially surround the apoptotic bodies (lymphocytic satellitosis). See Plate 14 in the color plate section.

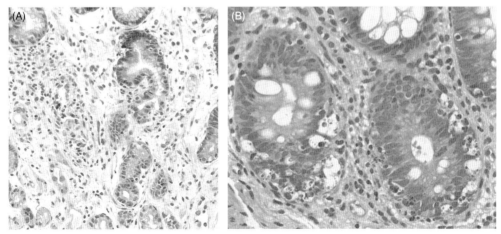

Figure 9.6 Severe, acute GVHD of gastrointestinal tract day 48. A: in the edematous gastric antrum are loosely scattered lymphocytes and a few eosinophils. The collapsed lumen of a nearly destroyed gland is filled with apoptotic debris. Many of the adjacent glands are infiltrated by lymphocytes and contain multiple contiguous apoptotic bodies in the glandular and neck regions. Apoptosis in the neck region of a gastric gland is particularly characteristic of GVHD. B: colonic biopsy shows adjacent crypts with multiple contiguous apoptotic bodies. See Plate 15 in the color plate section.

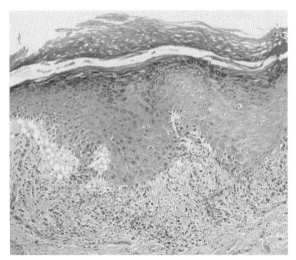

Figure 9.7 Chronic GVHD of skin with lichen planus-like appearance, day 1,267. The epidermis has compact hyperkeratosis, a thickened granular cell layer and irregular acanthosis (thickening). The rete ridges are blunted with a sawtooth shape. A band-like lymphocytic infiltrate occupies the papillary dermis and focally infiltrates the lower layers of the damaged rete ridges where there are abundant apoptotic bodies. See Plate 16 in the color plate section.

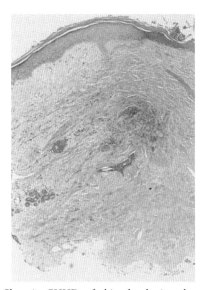

Figure 9.8 Chronic GVHD of skin developing dermal sclerosis, day 1,069. The collagen in both the papillary (upper) and reticular dermis has developed smudgy dense appearance that has replaced most of the normal collagen bundles. The entrapped dermal appendages, eccrine coils and remnants of a follicle are infiltrated by lymphocytes. The epidermis displays features of chronic GVHD with hyperkeratosis acanthosis, loss of rete ridges with and apoptosis along the straightened the dermal epidermal border. See Plate 17 in the color plate section.

descriptions of cGVHD, there are increasing reports of rare manifestations associated with cGVHD that can no longer be ignored involving the coronary arteries, kidneys [10], and the spinal cord and central nervous system [11].

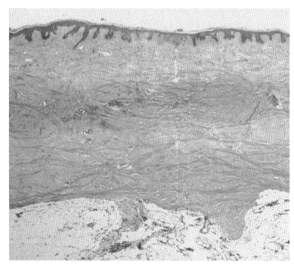

Figure 9.9 Pan-dermal sclerosis in late chronic GVHD day 1,280. Low power of skin with markedly thickened dermis composed of dense waxy collagen. The entrapped eccrine coils in the center of the dermis indicate the boundary where a normal reticular dermis would end. There was little or no inflammation or apoptotic change in the epidermis to whether the GVHD was still active. This appearance resembles progressive systemic sclerosis; hence the term sclerodermoid to describe the later skin changes of chronic GVHD. See Plate 18 in the color plate section.

The histologic criteria specific for cGVHD were derived from the National Institutes of Health Consensus Development Project on Criteria for Clinical Trials in Chronic Graft-versus-Host Disease. Criteria were developed with input from expert panels composed of dermatopathologists, surgical pathologists, and medical subspecialists familiar with the gamut of clinical and corresponding histopathologic alterations from cGVHD. The Pathology Working Group Report developed guidelines for the minimal histologic criteria for any GVHD, phase not specified, in the skin, liver, and gut, and those histologic criteria specific for cGVHD [12]. Since most histopathologic changes in the gastrointestinal tract and liver do not demonstrate a clear dichotomy between the clinical acute or chronic stages, they were not considered to be major criteria for cGVHD. Representative histopathology examples of acute and chronic GVHD are presented in the accompanying photomicrographs in Figures 9.5 to 9.18.

Overview of Histologic Studies

From the pathologist's viewpoint, cGVHD resembles a mélange of several entities; aGVHD with apoptosis and destruction of targeted epithelia (Figures 9.5 and 9.6) with variable amounts of chronic or mixed acute and chronic inflammatory cells, several autoimmune collagen vascular diseases (Figures 9.8–9.15), or rejection after solid organ transplantation (Figures 9.13–9.16).

Chronic GVHD is a dynamic process. The usual sequence evolves from an initial inflammatory state centered on the targeted epithelia (Figures 9.9, 9.10, and 9.12). Late changes

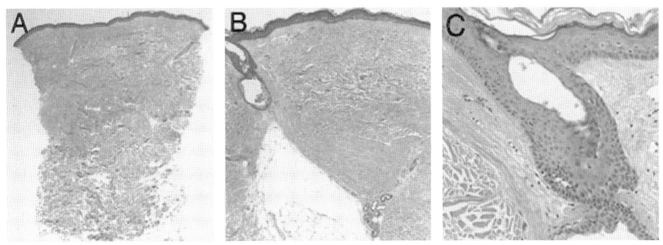

Figure 9.10 Morpheic variant of chronic GVHD day 2,028. These localized lesions on the back have a nodular focus of dermal fibrosis with dense closely packed collagen without bundles. A: is located in the mid-portion of the reticular dermis B: along the dermal subcutaneous junction shows a nodular focus of smudgy dense collagen containing an entrapped eccrine unit. In contrast, the normal collagen bundles in adjacent uninvolved reticular dermis have a curlicue pattern. C: higher power of B shows a dilated degenerative hair follicle containing a minimal focal lymphocytic infiltrate. The fibrosis appears to track along the perifollicular adventitial dermis and extend up into part of the papillary dermis. Activity is based on progression of fibrosis in serial biopsies, the development of new gross lesions or chronic inflammation. Apoptosis of the epidermis or appendages is often minimal and sometimes absent in morpheic lesions. See Plate 19 in the color plate section.

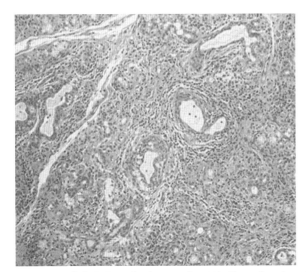

Figure 9.11 Oral GVHD early changes day 150. Extensive chronic inflammation in the corresponding minor salivary glands has resulted in subtotal destruction of the acinar tissue. The dilated and extensively infiltrated intralobular ducts display prominent vacuolization, apoptosis and segmental loss of nuclei. See Plate 20 in the color plate section.

are predominated by dropout or fibrotic obliteration of the targeted epithelia for example, skin appendages, (Figures 9.8–9.10), small bronchioles (Figure 9.13), and intralobular minor salivary gland ducts and acini (Figure 9.12). Judging activity can be difficult after treatment for GVHD is initiated. Immunosuppressive treatment of cGVHD markedly reduces or eliminates the inflammation. Minimal apoptotic change in targeted organs may only be evident by viewing multiple serial sections. Once the targeted epithelia are destroyed, activity may only be inferred by a review of previous biopsies as they may show progression of fibrosis and destruction of glands or epithelium (Figures 9.9 and 9.10).

There is confusion in the literature regarding the utility of histologic grading of acute and chronic GVHD. The histologic schema proposed for certain organs are a reflection of the timing of the biopsy in relation to the onset, duration of activity (chronicity), the influence of immunosuppression on the degree of inflammation, and the adequacy of the sample [12]. Schema that have quantified the degree of apoptosis and inflammation may facilitate the decision for immediate treatment before there is irreversible damage. However, in the current milieu such grades have not been validated to predict refractoriness or other relevant endpoints. On the other hand, stage 4/4 of various organ systems grading schema reflects cumulative damage and the expected time frame for recovery to occur. In some organs, it portends irreversibility of damage, that is, destroyed lacrimal and salivary glands means permanent keratoconjunctivitis sicca. In the liver and the gut, the time to recovery is inversely related to the degree of bile duct loss or degree of mucosal destruction, respectively.

There is a wide range of utilization of biopsies in the diagnosis and management of late acute or chronic GVHD [13]. In one tertiary center, failure to obtain prior histologic confirmation of cGVHD resulted in 7% of the referral patients being incorrectly diagnosed and treated for GVHD before their arrival [14]. Several post-HCT patients who developed Grover's transient acantholytic dermatosis were incorrectly treated for GVHD until skin biopsy was obtained [15]. Biopsies are recommended to confirm active cGVHD when alternative diagnoses are entertained, the clinical signs are confined to internal organs, or the clinical assessment of activity is obscured by prior changes.

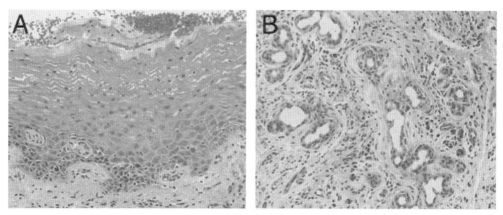

Figure 9.12 Late stage oral chronic GVHD. A: the mucosa resembles the lichenoid lesion in Figure 9.7 with sawtoothing of the rete ridges and a band-like infiltrate beneath the nonkeratinized squamous mucosa. Apoptosis is present along the basal layer though generally less marked than in cutaneous chronic GVHD. B: the destroyed glandular acinii have been completely replaced by loose fibroblastic stroma containing loosely scatted lymphocytes and plasma cells. The GVHD remains active with lymphocytic infiltration and apoptosis in the atypical proliferated ducts. The denser fibrosis in the interstitium represents more distant damage. See Plate 21 in the color plate section.

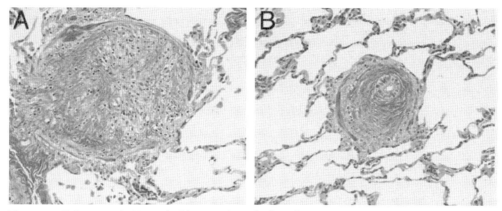

Figure 9.13 Pulmonary GVHD with obliterative bronchiolitis, day 1,822. Patient with progressive shortness of breath, worsening oxygen requirements, pulmonary function testing profile of airflow obstruction unimproved with bronchodilators, and diffuse ground glass changes on the CT scan of the lungs. Trichrome stains shows over expanded alveoli without any inflammation or consolidation. A: shows a bronchiole whose obstructed lumen contains a mixture of wispy collagen, chronic inflammatory cells and disordered respiratory epithelial cells, that is, obstructive bronchiolitis. B: is a small bronchiole with dense concentrically arranged collagen in the widened subepithelial zone surrounding the small lumen. Other small bronchioles had complete fibrous obliteration of their lumina more accurately termed *constrictive bronchiolitis*. See Plate 22 in the color plate section.

Skin

The skin is the most frequently involved site of cGVHD and readily accessible for biopsy [16]. Hymes *et al.* have provided a detailed colored glossary of the numerous gross cutaneous manifestations and the expected underlying histopathology [17]. The utilization and importance of day 80 to 100 screening biopsies from skin and oral cavity in asymptomatic patients who are being maintained on immunosuppressive drugs is highly variable. A positive skin biopsy is no longer classified as cGVHD if it lacks the specific diagnostic chronic features. Likewise a positive screening oral biopsy is not considered to be cGVHD unless there are confirmatory gross oral findings [8]. However, the diagnostic implication of marked minor salivary gland sialadentis may be upgraded in future analyses.

There are several important caveats regarding cutaneous cGVHD. Changes may not be synchronous. The different phases and types of cutaneous cGVHD lichenoid, sclerodermatous and morpheic manifestations can coexist as well as aGVHD (phase nonspecific) changes. Full thickness skin biopsies are necessary to identify changes in the dermal adnexae, reticular dermal collagen, and dermal-subcutis interface (Figures 9.8 and 9.9). Morpheic skin lesions have nodular fibrous remodeling of the deeper reticular dermal collagen with variable to no inflammation in the epidermis, dermal appendages, and subcutaneous fat (Figure 9.10). Eosinophilic fasciitis of the skin requires a deep incisional biopsy to demonstrate the characteristic edema

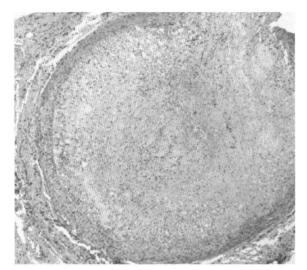

Figure 9.14 Coronary arteritis from GVHD day 615. Teenager developed severe substernal chest pain for 1 month and reduced cardiac function tests before she died suddenly with myocardial infarction. Coronary arteries were diffusely narrowed from 50% to 100%. The histology resembles the "transplant atherosclerosis" found in chronically rejected cardiac allografts. The wall and lumen of this large artery are nearly obliterated by an arteritis of chronic inflammatory cells admixed with loose extracellular matrix. See Plate 23 in the color plate section.

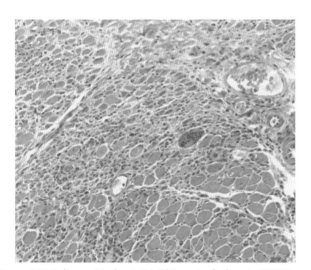

Figure 9.15 Polymyositis day 1,129. This patient's chronic GVHD, was quiescent after a complete response to treatment for histologically florid lichen-planus like skin lesions. After a hiatus, muscle tenderness with marked elevation of muscle related serum enzymes developed. This muscle biopsy from the deltoid shows a florid polymyositis. The interstitial infiltrate of macrophages, plasma cells and lymphocytes surrounds clusters of small regenerative basophilic fibers with large central nuclei. There are occasional large multinucleated fibers as well as areas of active necrosis with acute interstitial inflammation. The patient made a complete recovery and as of 2007 is status 32 years post-HCT. See Plate 24 in the color plate section.

and fibrosis of the fascia and subcutaneous septae with a mixed infiltrate of lymphocytes, histiocytes, and eosinophils. When cGVHD affects the female genitalia it leads to scarring and stricture. Histologically, it resembles lichen sclerosis atrophicus with

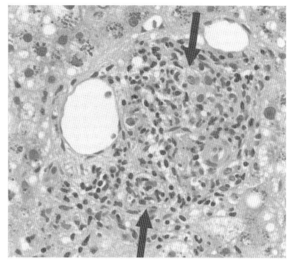

Figure 9.16 Hepatic GVHD day 454. Arrows in portal space point to damaged bile ducts that consist of a collapsed syncytium of variable sized irregularly arranged nuclei. There are segments where the nuclei are missing. Despite the marked lymphocytic ductitis with cytoplasmic vacuolization, apoptosis of bile duct epithelium is uncommon with hepatic GVHD. See Plate 25 in the color plate section.

epidermal or mucosal atrophy with basal vacuolar changes, a band-like infiltrate associated with small numbers of apoptotic cells, and subepidermal zone of pale homogenized collagen.

Flares in the skin in patients with established cGVHD, especially if the biopsy is shallow, often simply resemble aGVHD, not further classified, even if previous biopsies showed cGVHD. Since many of these patients are receiving immunosuppressive treatment, the inflammatory changes may be minimal with evidence of active GVHD limited to epithelial vacuolar degeneration or apoptosis in the basilar layers of the skin and its appendages.

Oral

Oral biopsy of mucosa and minor salivary glands is a window into the entire aerodigestive tract affected by cGVHD. The mucosal and ductular changes are similar to those in the skin epidermis and appendages with lichenoid interface inflammation, lymphocytic exocytosis, and apoptosis (Figures 9.11, 9.12A and 9.12B). There are institutional variations in how the threshold for minimal activity is defined. Active GVHD changes include lymphocytic exocytosis into the mucosa, intralobular ducts and acini, and lymphocytic periductal inflammation with or without plasma cells. Fibroblastic periductal and periacinar stroma is indicative of cGVHD activity, whereas dense fibrosis indicates only previous damage (Figure 9.12). The oral histolgic evaluation should always include an assessment for mucosal dysplasia since oral carcinoma is increased in patients with cGVHD, particularly with proliferative verrucous dysplasia [18].

Liver

Hepatic GVHD is often present in patients with cGVHD (Figure 9.16). Liver biopsies of insufficient length, obtained

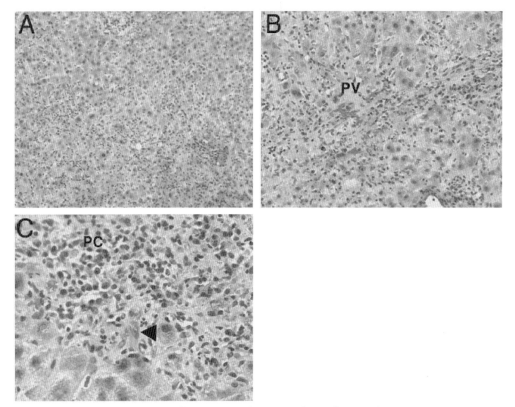

Figure 9.17 Acute hepatitic onset of liver GVHD day 757 with rapidly rising liver tests AST 1,200, ALT 2,200, bilirubin 6.5. Cultures and serologies for viruses were negative. A; low power shows a lobular and portal hepatitis. B: perivenular area (PV) shows an extensive necroinflammatory infiltrate of lymphocytes and plasma cells, hepatocyte dropout with many acidophilic bodies, and spotty hemorrhage. Endothelialitis, lymphocytic infiltration and adhesion to the venular endothelial is much less common in GVHD than orthotopic liver rejection. C: high power view shows an interface hepatitis (piecemeal necrosis) along the limiting plate of enlarged portal space. The cellular infiltrate has a prominent plasmacytic (PC) component The proliferated ductules (arrowhead) along the limiting plate appear damaged. Early in the acute hepatitic onset of GVHD the portal and lobular inflammation are the predominant features while later histologic features show more definitive bile duct injury and hepatocellular cholestasis. See Plate 26 in the color plate section.

using a narrow caliber needle, or partially crushed with a transvenous forceps may lack sufficient numbers of evaluable bile ducts for a valid assessment. Serum liver tests are the preferred tool for assessing the response to treatment of hepatic GVHD [19]. If liver biopsies are first obtained after an incomplete response to treatment, the findings can be used to verify the diagnosis and identify any other processes. The extent of bile duct injury or loss should be made using several stains besides H&E, including periodic acid Schiff with diastase, and preferably by immunostaining with cytokeratin, 7 or 19. Experience-based observations indicate that the time to recovery after immunosuppressive treatment is proportional to the degree of bile duct dropout (ductopenia). The hepatitic onset of GVHD with marked lobular and portal inflammation with damaged but preserved bile ducts can show rapid improvement within 2 months (Figure 9.17). However, with extreme ductopenia resulting in deep cholestatic jaundice, even with effective treatment, normalization of liver tests can take up to a year. Though hepatic GVHD has been compared to primary biliary cirrhosis (PBC), hepatic GVHD lacks the PBC specific autoantibodies [20] and has little propensity to cause cirrhosis [21].

Other Sites Involved in cGVHD

Some of the less common histologic manifestations of cGVHD resemble rejection after pulmonary (Figure 9.13) or cardiac solid organ transplantation (Figure 9.14), while other manifestations, such as polymyositis (Figure 9.15), resemble naturally occurring autoimmune disorders. It is of interest that both progressive systemic sclerosis and cGVHD have an autoantibody to the platelet derived growth factor receptor that stimulates the activation of skin fibroblasts in vitro [22]. This autoantibody was absent from all long-term HCT controls suggesting a direct role in the genesis of cutaneous sclerosis in both conditions.

Reporting Results of Biopsies

Unlike standardized formats used for the histopathologic staging of cancer, there is a spectrum of uncertainty when

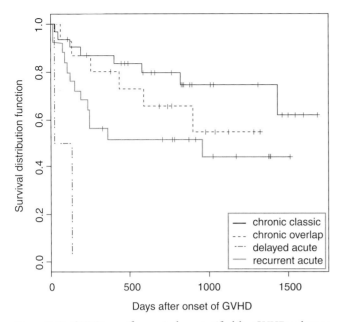

Figure 9.18. GVHD-specific survival as stratified by GVHD subtypes based on NIH Consensus Criteria.
Source: Jagasia M, Giglia J, Chinratanalab W, et al. Incidence and Outcome of Chronic Graft-versus-Host Disease Using National Institutes of Health Consensus Criteria. *Biol Blood Marrow Transplant.* 2007;13:1207–1215.

HCT biopsies are done for GVHD. Given the aforementioned factors that influence histology, it is not surprising that the final diagnostic assessment of many biopsies is equivocal, that is, neither clearly positive nor negative for active GVHD. It is important that the clinicians understand the basis for using a particular qualifier. The mitigating factors that cause the equivocal assessment and any relevant clinical data that affect the final interpretation should be included in a comment. The final diagnosis should include whether the GVHD is active and any qualifiers needed. Some quantification of the extent of abnormalities may be useful, for example, widespread destruction, marked inflammation, extensive, focal, rare, and so on.

Utility of Histopathology to Assess GVHD

The use of surgical biopsies to diagnose cGVHD and assess response to treatment is highly variable among institutions [13]. The quality of the sample has a strong bearing on the histologic interpretation. Skin biopsies should be directed at abnormal new changes. Partial thickness skin biopsies are insufficient for evaluation of dermal and fascial sclerotic changes. In patients with extensive dyspigmentation and/or dermal sclerosis recognizing response to treatment in the skin may be difficult. The selection of an informative biopsy site and the adequacy of the sample are essential. In this setting, histologic progression of dermal fibrosis and even minimal inflammatory changes without apoptosis of epithelia should be regarded as at least suggestive of active GVHD.

RETROSPECTIVE VALIDATION OF NIH STAGING AND GRADING

The prognostic value of the various subtypes of GVHD (viz classic cGVHD, overlap GVHD, recurrent, late, or persistent aGVHD) have been looked at by Jagasia et al. in retrospective study [23]. Consecutive patients ($n = 110$) at a single institute, alive at day 100 after their first allogeneic SCT for hematological malignancy, were included in the study cohort. Seventy-three patients were diagnosed with GVHD at or after day 100. Of the 73 patients with GVHD after day 100, 14 (19%) were classified as limited cGVHD, and 59 (81%) were classified as extensive cGVHD. The 3-year overall survival (OS) of the limited cGVHD cohort was significantly inferior compared to extensive cGVHD (21% vs. 63.6%, $p =.037$). Using the NIH classification, GVHD after day 100 was reclassified as persistent aGVHD (3 patients, 4%), recurrent aGVHD (22 patients, 30%), delayed aGVHD (2 patients, 3%), overlap GVHD (features of both acute and classic chronic GVHD) (15 patients, 20%), and classic cGVHD (31 patients, 42%). Patients with limited cGVHD (14 patients) were reclassified as persistent acute (one patient, 7%), recurrent acute (four patients, 29%) and classic chronic GVHD (nine patients, 64%). Patients with extensive cGVHD (59 patients) were reclassified as persistent acute (2 patients, 3%), delayed acute (2 patients, 3%), recurrent acute (18 patients, 31%), classic chronic (22 patients, 37%), and overlap GVHD (15 patients, 26%) respectively. Of the 15 patients with chronic overlap GVHD, 5 patients (33%), 9 patients (60%), and 1 patient (7%) were classified as mild, moderate, or severe GVHD. Four (13%), eighteen (58%), and nine (29%) patients with classic cGVHD were classified as mild, moderate, and severe, respectively. The overall survival for patients with persistent acute, recurrent aGVHD, delayed aGVHD, overlap cGVHD, and classic cGVHD were significantly different ($p = .0005$). Three-year overall survival for patients with persistent acute, recurrent aGVHD, delayed aGVHD, overlap cGVHD, and classic cGVHD were 100%, 45%, 0%, 57%, and 67%, respectively. This difference in survival (measured from day of SCT) was more apparent when patients with any aGVHD features (recurrent acute, delayed acute, and overlap chronic) was compared with classic cGVHD (3-year OS 47.2% vs. 66.7%, $p = .015$). This effect persisted when survival was measured from onset of GVHD and patients with chronic classic GVHD (68% vs. 46%) had a better GVHD-specific survival (calculated from onset of GVHD after day 100 to last follow-up) compared to other subtypes ($p = .0336$) (Figure 9.18). Severities were not predictive of survival in patients with either classic chronic or overlap cGVHD. Nonrelapse mortality in patients with chronic classic GVHD was not different compared to patients with other subtypes of GVHD ($p = .57$). Limited or extensive GVHD at onset had no impact on cumulative nonrelapse mortality. Among patients with overlap and chronic classic GVHD, severity at onset or at peak did not influence nonrelapse mortality. Nonrelapse mortality in patients with chronic classic GVHD was not different compared to patients with other subtypes of GVHD ($p = .57$). Among patients with overlap and chronic classic GVHD, severity at onset or at peak did not influence nonrelapse mortality. Age at transplant and donor type were adjusted for in all Cox proportional multivariable models GVHD was analyzed as a time-dependent variable.

Adjusted for donor status and age at transplant, extensive cGVHD (accounting for subtype changes) was associated with a HR of 0.36 (95% CI 0.16 to 0.91, $p = .033$). Any acute feature of GVHD (accounting for subtype changes) after day 100 (includes late acute, recurrent acute, persistent acute, overlap GVHD) was associated with a HR of 3.36 (95% CI 1.25 to 11.09, $p = .0144$) when compared to classic cGVHD. Thus the authors concluded the importance of subclassifying GVHD after day 100 as proposed by the NIH consensus criterion.

SUMMARY

The NIH consensus criterion for grading and staging cGVHD represents a significant advance in standardizing the various subtypes of cGVHD. If these criteria are prospectively validated, the various subtypes could be used as specific criteria in cGVHD clinical trials. It is likely that outcomes of therapeutic interventions may be dependent on what subtype of cGVHD is studied. Patients with features of aGVHD after day 100 represent a high-risk group for nonrelapse mortality and should be preferentially enrolled for novel therapies in cGVHD. Patients with classic cGVHD may have a better outcome due to lower nonrelapse mortality and possibly a better graft-versus-tumor effect. It would be important to differentiate the biology of the various subtypes and identify modifiable variables that can potentially be modulated to favorably impact the outcome of the patient with cGVHD.

REFERENCES

1. Shulman HM, Sullivan KM, Weiden PL, et al. Chronic graft-versus-host syndrome in man. A long-term clinicopathologic study of 20 Seattle patients. *Am J Med.* 1980;69:204–217.
2. Graze PR, Gale RP. Chronic graft versus host disease: a syndrome of disordered immunity. *Am J Med.* 1979;66:611–620.
3. Wingard JR, Piantadosi S, Vogelsang GB, et al. Predictors of death from chronic graft-versus-host disease after bone marrow transplantation. *Blood.* 1989;74:1428–1435.
4. Sullivan KM, Witherspoon RP, Storb R, et al. Prednisone and azathioprine compared with prednisone and placebo for treatment of chronic graft-v-host disease: prognostic influence of prolonged thrombocytopenia after allogeneic marrow transplantation. *Blood.* 1988;72:546–554.
5. Lee SJ, Klein JP, Barrett AJ, et al. Severity of chronic graft-versus-host disease: association with treatment-related mortality and relapse. *Blood.* 2002;100:406–414.
6. Akpek G, Zahurak ML, Piantadosi S, et al. Development of a prognostic model for grading chronic graft-versus-host disease. *Blood.* 2001;97:1219–1226.
7. Lee SJ, Vogelsang G, Flowers ME. Chronic graft-versus-host disease. *Biol Blood Marrow Transplant.* 2003;9:215–233.
8. Filipovich AH, Weisdorf D, Pavletic S, et al. National Institutes of Health consensus development project on criteria for clinical trials in chronic graft-versus-host disease: I. Diagnosis and staging working group report. *Biol Blood Marrow Transplant.* 2005;11:945–956.
9. Shulman HM, Sharma P, Amos D, Fenster LF, McDonald GB. A coded histologic study of hepatic graft-versus-host disease after human bone marrow transplantation. *Hepatology.* 1988;8:463–470.
10. Chang A, Hingorani S, Kowalewska J, et al. Spectrum of renal pathology in hematopoietic cell transplantation: a series of 20 patients and review of the literature. *Clin J Am Soc Nephrol.* 2007;2:1014–1023.
11. Kamble RT, Chang CC, Sanchez S, Carrum G. Central nervous system graft-versus-host disease: report of two cases and literature review. *Bone Marrow Transplant.* 2007;39:49–52.
12. Shulman HM, Kleiner D, Lee SJ, et al. Histopathologic diagnosis of chronic graft-versus-host disease: National Institutes of Health Consensus Development Project on Criteria for Clinical Trials in Chronic Graft-versus-Host Disease: II. Pathology Working Group Report. *Biol Blood Marrow Transplant.* 2006;12:31–47.
13. Lee SJ, Vogelsang G, Gilman A, et al. A survey of diagnosis, management, and grading of chronic GVHD. *Biol Blood Marrow Transplant.* 2002;8:32–39.
14. Jacobsohn DA, Montross S, Anders V, Vogelsang GB. Clinical importance of confirming or excluding the diagnosis of chronic graft-versus-host disease. *Bone Marrow Transplant.* 2001;28:1047–1051.
15. Bolanos-Meade J, Anders V, Wisell J, Farmer ER, Vogelsang GB. Grover's Disease after Bone Marrow Transplantation. *Biol Blood Marrow Transplant.* 2007;13:1116–1117.
16. Schaffer JV. The changing face of graft-versus-host disease. *Semin Cutan Med. Surg.* 2006;25:190–200.
17. Hymes SR, Turner ML, Champlin RE, Couriel DR. Cutaneous manifestations of chronic graft-versus-host disease. *Biol Blood Marrow Transplant.* 2006;12:1101–1113.
18. Cabay RJ, Morton TH Jr, Epstein JB. Proliferative verrucous leukoplakia and its progression to oral carcinoma: A review of the literature. *J Oral Pathol Med.* 2007;May;36(5):255–61. Review.
19. Shulman H, McDonald GB. *Hepatic complications of hematopoietic stem cell transplantation. Liver immunology: principles and practice.* Totowa, NJ: Humana Press; 2008.
20. Quaranta S, Shulman H, Ahmed A, et al. Autoantibodies in human chronic graft-versus-host disease after hematopoietic cell transplantation. *Clin Immunol.* 1999;91:106–116.
21. Strasser SI, Sullivan KM, Myerson D, et al. Cirrhosis of the liver in long-term marrow transplant survivors. *Blood.* 1999;93:3259–3266.
22. Svegliati S, Olivieri A, Campelli N, et al. Stimulatory autoantibodies to PDGF receptor in patients with extensive chronic graft-versus-host disease. *Blood.* 2007;110:237–241.
23. Jagasia M, Giglia J, Chinratanalab W, et al. Incidence and Outcome of Chronic Graft-versus-Host Disease Using National Institutes of Health Consensus Criteria. *Biol Blood Marrow Transplant.* 2007;13:1207–1215.

10

Chronic Graft versus Host Disease Pharmacology

Thomas Hughes and Timothy R. McGuire

This chapter focuses on the pharmacology, pharmacokinetics, drug interactions, and toxicity of commonly utilized immunosuppressive agents in the management of chronic graft versus host disease (cGVHD). The agents selected for review within this chapter include the corticosteroids, the calcineurin inhibitors, mycophenolate mofetil, thalidomide, and sirolimus. Table 10.1 summarizes additional pharmacologic agents that have been utilized for the systemic management of cGVHD.

CORTICOSTEROIDS

Corticosteroids and, most notably, prednisone are generally considered the mainstay and drug of choice for the initial treatment of cGVHD [1–4]. Prednisone has utility as a single agent in the initial therapy of cGVHD, particularly in standard risk patients [5] and in combination therapy with a calcineurin inhibitor, such as cyclosporine, for high-risk patients [6]. The clinical application of prednisone in the treatment of cGVHD is summarized in Chapter 12.

Pharmacology

Corticosteroids impact an extensive number of physiologic functions within the body including carbohydrate, protein, and lipid metabolism; maintenance of fluid and electrolyte balance; and preservation of a variety of organ systems including the cardiovascular, immune, skeletal muscle, renal, endocrine, and nervous systems [7]. Corticosteroids are classified according to their relative potencies in sodium retention (i.e., mineralocorticoid activity) and their effects on glucose or carbohydrate metabolism (i.e., glucocorticoid activity). The potency of a corticosteroid to impact glucose metabolism closely parallels those for anti-inflammatory activity (refer to Table 10.2). These two broad divisions of physiologic properties (sodium retention versus carbohydrate/anti-inflammatory activity) are mediated via the interaction of the corticosteroid with two specific receptor proteins – the glucocorticoid receptor (GR) and the mineralocorticoid receptor (MR) [7]. This interaction of corticosteroid with either the GR and MR receptor proteins to

either activate or inhibit gene transcription is referred to as the genomic mechanism of corticosteroid activity.

Genomic Mechanisms

The GR resides in the cell cytoplasm of target tissues and is complexed with other proteins such as the heat-shock protein (HSP) 90, HSP70, and immunophilins. Following the binding of a corticosteroid with the GR, the GR changes conformation, dissociates from its associated proteins, and translocates into the nucleus. The GR then interacts with specific DNA sequences of affected genes called *glucocorticoid responsive elements* (GREs), which provide specificity to the induction of gene transcription leading to known biologic effects [7, 8]. The impact of the GR on gene transcription may either result in the expression of certain proteins (transcriptional activation)or an inhibition of transcription (transrepression) such as with the genes for pro-opiomelanocortin, cyclooxygenase-2 (COX-2), inducible nitric oxide synthase (NOS2), and inflammatory cytokines [7]. It is generally recognized that the metabolic effects of glucocorticoids are mediated by transcriptional activation; whereas, the anti-inflammatory and immunosuppressive effects are mediated by transrepression of genes.

The MR is a similar receptor protein that again, once activated by a corticosteroid, translocates into the nucleus to interact with specific hormone responsive elements to activate transcription of specific genes. The MR is expressed within the kidney, colon, salivary glands, sweat glands, and hippocampus [7]. The mineralocorticoid effect on sodium and potassium homeostasis occurs primarily through the interaction with cells of the distal renal tubules and collecting ducts while the effects on H^+ secretion primarily occur in the intercalated cells [7].

Immunosuppression Mediated by Corticosteroids

As indicated previously, the immunosuppressive properties of corticosteroids is largely thought to be mediated by the inhibition of gene expression of a variety of inflammatory cytokines, including interleukin-1 (IL-1), interleukin-2 (IL-2), interleukin-6 (IL-6), interleukin-12 (IL-12), interferon-gamma (IFN-γ), and tumor necrosis factor-alpha (TNF-α) [9, 10]. The repression of gene transcription is also mediated through the

Table 10.1: Additional Pharmacologic Agents Utilized in cGVHD

Agents	Class	Common* Side Effects	Serious* Side Effects	Comment
Commonly used				
Pentostatin	Nucleoside analog	Nausea, vomiting	Infections, renal, CNS	–
Rituximab	Chimeric anti-CD20 MoAb	Infusional reactions	Infections	Skin and musculoskeletal respond best
Hydroxychloroquine	Antimalaric	GI symptoms	Retinal damage, myositis, polyneuropathy	Annual eye exams needed, well tolerated
Less frequent use				
Psoralen and UVA	8-metoxypsolaren and UVA irradiation	Nausea, skin phototoxicity	Nonmelanoma skin cancer	Lichen-like skin, no systemic effect
Clofazimine	Antimycobacterial	Gastrointestinal, hyperpigmentation	–	Best in sclerotic skin and oral
Rare use or new reports				
Acitretin	Retinoid	Skin flaking, dryness, cheilitis, alopecia, night blindness	Pancreatitis, hyperlipidemia	Patients with skin sclerosis, alone or as adjuvant
Azathioprine	Competitive inhibitor of purine synthesis	GI symptoms, marrow suppression	Second cancers	No formal reports in salvage
Antithymocyte globulin	Polyclonal anti–T-cell antibody	Infections	Anaphylaxis, serum sickness	No formal reports
Daclizumab	Humanized Anti IL-2 receptor MoAb	GI, dizziness, Headache, Insomnia, fatigue	Infections	Case reports, combined with other agents
Infliximab	Chimeric anti-TNFα Mo Ab	Hypersensitivity	Infections	Rare reports, combination
Etarnecept	Recombinant human soluble TNF receptor fusion protein	Infections	Infections	5/8 patients responded
Low-dose Methotrexate	Folate inhibitor, anti-inflammatory	Myelosuppression, liver toxicity	Accumulation in effusions	Can not be used in renal failure
Cyclophosphamide 200 mg/kg and stem cell rescue	Alkylating agent	Profound myelosuppression	Hemorrhagic cystitis, cardiac	Two cases reported, both responded, sclerotic skin
Cyclophosphamide pulses ~1g/m^2	Alkylating agent	Myelosuppression	Hemorrhagic cystitis	Three cases reported, all responded, liver and oral GVHD
Imatinib	Tyrosine kinase inhibitor, PDGF inhibitor	Myelosuppression, weight gain	Drug induced hepatitis	One case reported, good response in a BO patient
Montelukast	Leukotriene antagonist	Headache, nausea	–	15/19 patients responded, 3/5 with lung disease

* Only most relevant common or serious side effect that have been described with these agents in hematopoietic cell transplantation (HCT) and other patient populations are listed here. This is not an exhaustive list of all possible common or serious side effects.
BO, bronchiolitis obliterans; CNS, central nervous system; GI, gastrointestinal; Mo Ab, monoclonal antibody; PDGF, platelet-derived growth factor; UVA; ultraviolet A.

inhibitory interaction of the GR with proinflammatory transcription factors, nuclear factor κB (NFκB), and activator protein-1 (AP-1) [9, 11].

There is a demonstrated association between glucocorticoid inhibition of T-cell proliferation and glucorticoid blockade of cytokine gene expression [10]. Almawi et al. found that glucocorticoid-mediated inhibition of T-cell proliferation could be completely abrogated by the synergistic action of IL-1, IL-6, and IFN-γ implying that these cytokines play a key role in mitogen- and alloantigen-mediated cellular activation [10]. TNF-α is known to be a key cytokine in the pathophysiology of GVHD. Holler et al. demonstrated that TNF-α serum levels declined in patients treated with prednisolone for first-line treatment of acute GVHD [12].

Table 10.2: Representative Glucocorticoid Potencies and Equivalent Doses [7]

Glucocorticoid	Equivalent Dose (mg)*	Anti-inflammatory Potency*	Sodium Retaining Potency*
Short-acting (biological half-life of 8–12 hours)			
Hydrocortisone	20	1	1
Intermediate-acting (biological half-life of 12–36 hours)			
Prednisone	5	4	0.8
Prednisolone	5	4	0.8
Methylprednisolone	4	5	0.5
Triamcinolone	4	5	0
Long-acting (biological half-life of 36–72 hours)			
Dexamethasone	0.75	25	0
Betamethasone	0.75	25	0

* When converting doses, use only equivalent dose column.

This genomic-based inhibitory mechanism of cytokine gene expression appears to be the primary mechanism of action when the corticosteroid is dosed at doses in the conventional therapeutic dose range (prednisone equivalent doses up to approximately 250 mg) [9, 11].

Nongenomic Mechanisms

Nongenomic effects are thought to be the primary mechanism for corticosteroid doses that exceed a prednisone equivalent dose of approximately 250 mg. The mechanisms of high-dose or pulse corticosteroid therapy are characterized by a rapid onset of effect (<15 minutes) since no time is needed for gene transcription and translation. The nongenomic effects include both specific mechanisms mediated by the GR (independent of transcription) and some nonspecific effects. The inhibition of cytosolic phospholipase A (c PLA) activation is one known, specific nongenomic mechanism [11]. The nonspecific effects include a direct interaction with cell membranes affecting physiochemical membrane properties. This interaction with cell membranes may also subsequently affect the activity of membrane-associated proteins [11].

It has been recognized for a number of years that glucocorticoid induced lysis of activated lymphocytes may be an important mechanism for immunosuppressive activity [13]. This lympholytic effect appears to be dose related where high "pulse" doses of corticosteroids (e.g., 1 g of methylprednisolone) may induce apoptotic mechanisms of T cells, which may be an important mechanism in high-dose pulse therapy [14]. Buttgereit et al. found that high-dose pulse therapy may also lead to GR downregulation, which may be another important nongenomic effect of corticosteroids [9, 15, 16]. In the setting of severe, refractory cGVHD, Akpek et al. demonstrated that high-dose pulse methylprednisolone (10 mg/kg/day IV or PO for 4 consecutive days) could induce a clinical response in 75% of patients (48% major response; 27% minor response).

The majority of these patients had previously received a median of 11 months of systemic corticosteroid with or without other immunosuppressive agents at low doses (median prednisone dose of 0.2 mg/kg/day). The authors found that a more favorable response to high-dose pulse therapy correlated to the time of progression and thus a course of pulse therapy may also provide prognostic information [17].

Other Physiologic Effects of Corticosteroids

The diverse physiologic effects of corticosteroids on various organ and metabolic systems are summarized in Table 10.3.

Pharmacokinetics

Glucocorticoids are lipophilic and have poor water solubility. For parenteral administration, glucocorticoids are usually administered as the water soluble phosphate or succinate esters of the parent drug. These are rapidly converted to their active form within 5 to 30 minutes of administration [11].

Absorption

Prednisone is well absorbed after oral administration (84% bioavailability), which is also true of other glucocorticoids (bioavailability range of 60%–100%) [11].

Distribution

Glucocorticoids are moderately protein bound (73%–93%). Hydrocortisone, prednisone, and prednisolone bind to both the glycoprotein transcortin (corticosteroid binding globulin) and albumin. Transcortin binding has high affinity for glucocorticoid binding but is saturated at relatively low doses (hydrocortisone or prednisolone doses >20 mg). Albumin has low affinity but high capacity for glucocorticoid binding [7, 11]. Thus for these glucocorticoids, the volume of distribution (Vd) can vary with dose due to this saturable or nonlinear protein binding. Despite a dose-dependent increase in Vd and drug clearance, the elimination half-life remains constant and these changes are not reflected in free drug concentrations [11]. In contrast, methylprednisolone binds only to albumin with no binding affinity for transcortin and so it has no dose-dependent variation in Vd and clearance [11]. Since only free drug can interact with the glucocorticoid receptor, an alteration in protein binding can have the potential to be clinically relevant. For example, patients with renal failure, nephrotic syndrome, or hypoalbuminemia may have lower protein binding and in some clinical settings (renal failure, hypoalbuminemia), a higher free fraction has been noted [11].

Metabolism

The metabolism of steroid hormones generally involves the addition of oxygen or hydrogen atoms at hepatic and extrahepatic sites, followed by glucuronide or sulfate conjugation to form water soluble derivatives, which are cleared by renal elimination [7, 11]. Synthetic steroids with an 11-keto substituent, such as prednisone, must be enzymatically reduced by

Table 10.3: Physiologic Effects of Corticosteroids [7]

Organ/Metabolic System	Physiologic Effect	Clinical Manifestations/Toxicity of Pharmacologic Corticosteroid Therapy
Carbohydrate and protein metabolism	Promote gluconeogenesis Inhibit glucose utilization in peripheral tissues Increase protein breakdown	Hyperglycemia Glycosuria
Lipid metabolism	Activate lipolysis	Hyperlipidemia Redistribution of body fat
Electrolyte and water balance	Sodium retention Increased urinary excretion of K^+ and H^+ Maintainance of extracellular fluid volume	Hypokalemic acidosis Edema
Cardiovascular system	Influences blood pressure through mineralocorticoid activity Enhance vascular activity Induce interstitial cardiac fibrosis	Hypertension
Skeletal muscle	Maintain skeletal muscle activity	Proximal skeletal muscle wasting (steroid myopathy) with prolonged therapy
Central nervous system	Influence mood, behavior and brain excitability	Mood elevation, behavioral changes, psychosis
Blood cells	Redistribution of lymphocytes, eosinophils, monocytes, basophils Increased marrow release, decreased removal and demargination of polymorphonuclear leukocytes	Lymphocytopenia Leukocytosis
Immune system	Multiple (see text)	Immunosuppression, increased risk of infection

11β-hydroxysteroid dehydrogenase (11β-HSD1) to become the biologically active form (prednisolone) at the glucocorticoid and mineralocorticoid receptors. Type 1 dehydrogenase (11β-HSD1) is widely distributed in target tissues but is found predominately in the liver [7, 11]. In patients with severe hepatic failure or the rare condition of cortisone reductase deficiency, this conversion may be impaired necessitating the use of steroids that do not require activation such as hydrocortisone or prednisolone [7].

Drug Interactions

Glucocorticoids are substrates of the cytochrome p450 3A4 (CYP 3A4) isoenzyme and thus are susceptible to drug interactions with both inducers and inhibitors of CYP 3A4 to varying degrees. For example, concomitant use of glucocorticoids with potent 3A4 inducers (e.g., barbiturates, phenytoin, carbamazepine, rifampin) significantly increases the clearance and decreases the half-life of prednisone and methylprednisolone, [11, 18] which has been documented to result in adverse clinical outcomes in settings such as kidney transplantation [11, 19, 20]. However, drug interactions involving glucocorticoids with known CYP 3A4 inhibitors are not consistent or well characterized among all the glucocorticoids. For example, ketoconazole and clarithromycin (potent CYP 3A4 inhibitors) have been shown to decrease clearance and increase half-life of

methylprednisolone and dexamethasone but not prednisolone [11]. Likewise, grapefruit juice has been shown to increase the half-life of methylprednisolone but not prednisolone [11].

Toxicity

Refer to Table 10.4 for a summary of potential corticosteroid toxicities and related prevention and management strategies.

CALCINEURIN INHIBITORS

Introduction

The modern era of transplantation began with the development of cyclosporine A (CSA). This cyclic polypeptide was isolated from the soil fungus *Beauveria nivea* and initially received interest as an antifungal molecule. In the early 1970s, CSA was found to have immunosuppressive activity in various animal transplant models [22]. From the outset, the water insolubility of CSA was one of the challenges in bringing this interesting compound to clinical trials; however, after an acceptable formulation was developed in the late 1970s, the drug began to be administered to solid organ and bone marrow transplant patients. There are numerous CSA molecules that can be

Table 10.4: Corticosteroid Toxicity and Prevention/Management Strategies [7,21]

Toxicity	Monitoring	Prevention/Management	Comments
Hyperglycemia	Blood glucose	Pharmacologic management with insulin or oral hypoglycemics	Consideration of endocrine consult
Edema	Weight, physical exam	Diuretics	
Hyperlipidemia	Lipid profile	Antihyperlipidemics	
Hypertension	Blood pressure	Diuretics, antihypertensives	
Steroid myopathy	Physical exam, range of motion assessment	Physical and occupational therapy; strengthening exercises	
Behavioral changes (mood elevation, neurosis, pyschosis)	History, review of systems	Consultation with psychiatry; antipsychotics	Consideration of psychiatry consult
Osteoporosis	Calcium, 25-OH vitamin D Bone densiometry	Calcium and vitamin D replacement bisphosphonates	Alternative antiresportive therapy may include hormonal replacement, raloxifene or calcitonin
Osteonecrosis	History, review of systems	Physical and occupational therapy, strengthening and aerobic exercises	
Immunosuppression	Fever Review of systems Imaging studies when clinically indicated	Vaccination Prophylaxis for encapsulated organisms (e.g., Penicillin VK) Pneumocystis prophylaxis (e.g., SMX/TMP) Consideration of antifungal agent with mold coverage Consideration of HSV/VZV prophylaxis (e.g., acyclovir or valacyclovir)	
Peptic Ulcer Disease	History, review of systems	Consideration of prophylaxis with proton pump inhibitor or H_2 receptor antagonist	The association between corticosteroid use and PUD and the value of prophylaxis is controversial
Cataracts	Slit-lamp examination		Consider ophthalmology consult
Growth retardation (children)	Height, weight, physical exam, Tanner score, developmental assessment		

HSV, *Herpes simplex virus*; PUD, peptic ulcer disease; SMX, sulfamethoxazole; TMP, trimethoprim; VZV *Varicella zoster virus*.

isolated from its fungal source with CSA being the major compound with immunosuppressive activity [23].

Tacrolimus (TAC) is a macrolide and chemically distinct from CSA. TAC was isolated in 1984 from *Streptomyces tsukubaensis* in a soil sample obtained from outside of Tokyo. The drug was approved and moved into clinical practice in 1994 after benefit was shown in several preclinical models for immunosuppression and subsequently in clinical trials in transplant patients [24].

Pharmacology

Mechanism of Action

While the target signaling pathway for CSA and TAC are the same, they have different binding proteins. CSA binds to cyclophilin while TAC binds to FK-binding protein. Figure 10.1 illustrates the mechanism of action of CSA and TAC. Briefly, CSA forms a binary complex with its intracellular binding protein, cyclophilin. This binary complex binds to calcineurin and inhibits its phosphatase activity leading to an inhibition of nuclear factor of activated T cells (NFAT) dephosphorylation. This inhibits NFAT nuclear translocation and IL-2 gene transcription. Inhibition of IL-2 gene transcription blocks T-cell activation [25]. In addition, CSA is able to increase the expression of transforming growth factor-beta (TGF-β), which also inhibits IL-2 gene expression. As a result, CSA is a potent inhibitor of antigen-related T-lymphocyte signaling and thus prevents the early immune changes associated with graft versus host disease.

Similar to CSA, TAC inhibits calcineurin mediated T-lymphocyte activation. TAC binds to FK-506 binding protein-12 (FKBP-12), which while related to cyclophilin is structurally distinct. A complex of calcium-calmodulin, TAC, and

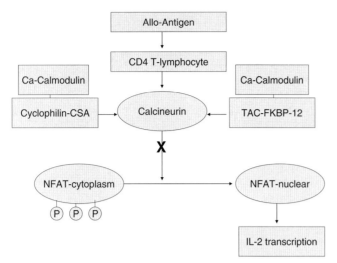

Figure 10.1 CSA and TAC inhibit calcineurin catalyzed de phosphorylation of NFAT and it's subsequent translocation into the nucleus. Net effect is inhibition of lymphokine (IL-2) transcription.

CSA, cyclosporine A; IL, interleukin; NFAT, nuclear factor of activated T cells; TAC, tacrolimus. See Plate 27 in the color plate section.

FKBP-12 inhibits calcineurin activity and like CSA, prevents nuclear translocation of NFAT and reduces IL-2 gene expression. There are several subtle effects on T and B lymphocytes seen with TAC and not with CSA. The mechanism or clinical significance of these differences is unclear. For example, there is some evidence that TAC has posttranscriptional effects on various cytokine receptors and may better inhibit cytokine-mediated responses [26]. TAC is approximately 100 times more potent then CSA [27].

Clinical Pharmacology

CSA and TAC are commonly used in combination with other therapies to treat cGVHD because these drugs usually produce low response rates as single agents. The mechanism of action of CSA and TAC, inhibiting the early steps in T-lymphocyte activation, makes them more useful agents in the prevention of acute GVHD. The major benefit of CSA and TAC in cGVHD may be the indirect benefit of reducing the rates of acute GVHD due to their inclusion in immunoprophylaxis. Generally, it is viewed that acute GVHD is the major risk for subsequent development of cGVHD. However, recently this has been questioned because reduced-intensity transplant, which seems to lower acute GVHD rates, may not result in lower cGVHD rates [28]. In support of using aggressive calcineurin inhibitor therapy, Mengarelli et al. reported that extending CSA immunoprophylaxis beyond the usual 6 months to 12 months led to reduced rates of cGVHD [29].

Chronic GVHD, predominantly, is caused by T-effector cells and mature B cells, which are relatively unresponsive to IL-2 inhibiting agents. This is supported clinically by a number of studies that suggest that the addition of calcineurin inhibitors to corticosteroids does not add benefit in patients with cGVHD outside of a possible reduction in corticosteroid toxicity [30]. This steroid sparing benefit of the calcineurin inhibitors and the

benefit reported in an older study comparing every-other-day CSA and prednisone to prednisone alone is the basis for the common practice of using alternate day combinations of CSA and prednisone as the initial treatment of cGVHD [6]. Refer to Chapter 12 for additional discussion on the clinical application of CSA and TAC in the management of cGHVD.

Pharmacokinetics

CSA pharmacokinetics have been well described [31, 32]. Historically, the differences in the biologic matrix and assays used to perform therapeutic drug monitoring (TDM) complicate the interpretation of the clinical pharmacokinetics of CSA. Various transplant programs selected from, radioimmunoassay (RIA) using a polyclonal antibody, RIA using a monoclonal antibody, monoclonal TDx, and high performance liquid chromatography (HPLC). Each assay had varying specificity for parent drug and metabolites giving very different concentrations and therefore different therapeutic target levels. The complexity of TDM required knowledge of both the biologic matrix being analyzed (blood vs. plasma vs. serum) and characteristics of the assay being used. This variability has been reduced by clinical laboratories settling on the use of the monoclonal TDx assay in whole blood. TAC is a macrolide drug and distinct from the polypeptide drug, CSA [33]. However, like CSA, the relationship between dose and blood concentrations is poor and the therapeutic window is narrow, which results in the need for TDM to optimize therapy. Similar to CSA, TAC is bound to red blood cells, and in order to reduce variability of measuring TAC concentrations whole blood concentrations are usually measured.

Absorption

CSA was originally developed as an oral solution in an olive oil diluent because of its lipophilicity. The oral dosing of this Sandimmune® product reflected the highly variable and incomplete oral absorption of the product. Because of this variability, TDM was used to optimally dose CSA. In addition to incomplete and variable absorption, CSA has interesting partitioning characteristics in the blood with approximately half of the drug being bound to red blood cells. The extent of binding is temperature dependent. The Sandimmune® liquid has largely been replaced by a microemulsion formulation in both a capsule and liquid dosage forms (Neoral®, Gengraf®, others), which have improved absorption characteristics compared to Sandimmune®. Practically, this leads to a different conversion ratio when going from intravenous CSA to oral CSA. The conversion factor when converting from intravenous to oral dosing utilizing the newer microemulsion formulations is in the range of 1:1 to at most 1:2 compared to a 1:3–4 conversion with Sandimmune® [32]. In comparison, the bioavailability of oral TAC is approximately 17%–30% and an intravenous to oral dosing ratio of 1:3 is generally employed [27].

Distribution

CSA and TAC are highly lipophilic and distribute widely with CSA having a larger Vd in whole blood compared to TAC

(4–5 L/kg vs. 1L/kg). As stated previously, both CSA and TAC are bound to red blood cells. TAC more extensively distributes into red blood cells than does CSA. In addition, CSA binds to plasma liproproteins and TAC is bound by alpha-1 acid glyco-protein and albumin in the plasma. Hematocrit, liproprotein profiles and alpha-1 acid glycoprotein concentrations may affect the free fraction of CSA and TAC and potentially their pharmacokinetics and pharmacodynamics. The distribution characteristics of these drugs are complex and give further sup-port for aggressive TDM measuring concentrations in whole blood and using a specific assay.

Metabolism

Both CSA and TAC undergo extensive metabolism in the liver and, to a lesser extent, in the intestinal mucosa through the CYP p450 isoenzyme 3A4 to multiple metabolites, which are then eliminated in the bile. Depending on the patient population stud-ied, the half-lives of CSA and TAC range between 6 to 24 hours and 12 to 35 hours, respectively [27, 31]. Steady state after initia-tion of a dosing regimen generally takes 3 to 5 days. The effect of inhibitors and inducers of CYP3A4 metabolism both in the gut and liver can have a profound effect on blood concentrations.

Drug Interactions

Drug interactions with the calcineurin inhibitors are often clin-ically important and a good understanding of magnitude and mechanism of these interactions can affect patient outcomes. Table 10.5 summarizes the more important drug interactions associated with the calcineurin inhibitors in stem cell trans-plant patients. Since TDM is standard of care for calcineurin inhibitors, identification of interacting agents should lead to more intense monitoring of CSA and TAC during coadminis-tration. A number of drug classes have been implicated includ-ing antibacterials, calcium channel blockers, azole antifungals, antiepileptics, and serotonin-reuptake inhibitors (SSRIs). The azole antifungals may be most clinically relevant given they are commonly coadministered with calcineurin inhibitors in patients diagnosed with cGVHD. A complete discussion of drug interactions associated with calcineurin inhibitors is beyond the scope of this chapter. However, since azole drugs can be potent inhibitors of CSA and TAC metabolism and are frequently administered concomitantly, these interactions will be highlighted.

Ketoconazole, while no longer used with any frequency in stem cell transplant patients, was the initial represen-tative of the azole drug class. Its interaction with CSA is relatively well described with CSA area under the concentration–time curve increasing 3 to 4 times after the institution of ketoconazole. This interaction can occur within the first 24 to 48 hours of instituting ketoconazole and requires 1 to 2 weeks or more after stopping ketoconazole for the effect to resolve [34, 35]. The mechanism relates to the high binding affinity of ketoconazole to CYP3A4, which is the drug metabolizing enzyme for both CSA and TAC. In addition, the azole drugs are *pgp* substrates and since *pgp* efflux of CSA and TAC from brush border cells

Table 10.5:   Drug Interactions with Calcineurin inhibitors

Calcineurin Inhibitor	Interacting Agent	Mechanism/Comments
Cyclosporine	*Inhibitors (Increased CSA concentrations)*	
	Azole Antifungals	
	Ketoconazole	
	Intraconazole	
	Voriconazole	
	Posaconazole	
	Fluconazole	
	Macrolide Antibiotics	
	Erythromycin	
	Clarithromycin	
	Calcium Channel Blockers	
	Verapamil	
	Diltiazem	
	Nicardipine	
	Inducers (Decreased CSA concentrations)	
	Antiepileptics	
	Phenobarbital	
	Phenytoin	
	Carbamazepine	
	SSRI	
	Nefazodone	
	Fluvoxamine	
	Antibiotics	
	Rifampin	
	Nafcillin	
	Rifabutin	
	Miscellaneous	
	Grapefruit Juice	
	St John's Wort	
Tacrolimus	**Similar to CSA**	
	Interactions more poorly described	

CSA, cyclosporine A; SSRI, serotonin-reuptake inhibitor.

of the gut reduce bioavailability, competitive inhibition of *pgp* by azole drugs leads to elevated blood concentrations.

Itraconazole is a commonly used azole in the outpatient management of patients with GVHD. It has been studied in an in vitro micosomal enzyme system and was found to inhibit CYP3A4 metabolism nearly as well as ketoconazole [36]. A recent study using intravenous itraconzole with intra-venous CSA or TAC reported a 24% to 149% and 49% to 117% increase in serum concentrations, respectively [37]. The interaction of CSA with intravenous itraconazole is clinically important but may be lower than reported with oral itracon-azole and oral CSA or oral TAC [24]. These data raise the pos-sibility that these clinically important interactions are greatest when each drug is administered orally. This may relate to the fact that many of the azoles are *pgp* substrates and can inhibit CSA and TAC efflux from gastrointestinal epithelial cells thus

Table 10.6: Relative Toxicities of Cyclosporine and Tacrolimus

Toxicity	Cyclosporine	Tacrolimus
Renal	††	††
Hypertension	††	†
Diabetes	*	†
Neurologic	†	†
Hypercholesterolemia	†	*
Hirsutism	††	*
Gum Hyperplasia	††	*
Gingivitis	††	*

* Incidence generally less than 10%.
† Incidence generally 10% to 30%.
†† Incidence generally >30%.

increasing the oral bioavailability of the calcineurin inhibitors [36]. In addition, CYP3A4 is found in the small bowel, which can reduce bioavailability on the basis of presystemic metabolism. The oral administration of azoles and CSA or TAC may maximize the inhibitory effect of the azole drugs on presystemic metabolism [36]. It is interesting that fluconazole, which only produces clinically important interactions with CSA or TAC when both are administered orally, is not a potent CYP3A4 inhibitor and is a relatively poor *pgp* substrate [38, 40].

In summary, the importance of the route of administration remains unclear but a reasonable interpretation of the data suggests that fluconazole only produces clinically relevant drug interactions when given orally at doses greater than 200 mg per day. In comparison, ketoconazole produces large and important elevations in CSA and TAC levels. Itraconazole interactions are clinically important in a magnitude that is only slightly less than ketoconazole. Newer azole entries into the market include voriconazole and posaconazole. Limited data suggest that voriconazole produces elevations in CSA and TAC that are higher than fluconzole but less than itraconazole while the effect of posaconazole is similar to fluconazole [35].

Toxicity

The toxicity profile for CSA and TAC are similar and include nephrotoxicity, neurotoxicity, hypertension, and changes in glucose metabolism. However, the degree to which each agent causes toxicity varies. TAC does appear to have less effect on cholesterol levels and causes less hypertension than does CSA. Also, hirsutism, gum hyperplasia, and gingivitis, which are common with CSA, are uncommon with TAC. On the other hand, TAC may cause more diabetes and may cause more neurotoxicity then CSA [39]. TAC may be associated with lower rates of clinically important nephrotoxicity compared to CSA. Table 10.6 lists the relative toxicities of CSA and TAC.

MYCOPHENOLATE MOFETIL

Mycophenolate mofetil (MMF) has become a commonly used agent in steroid resistant cGVHD [40]. MMF has a more beneficial toxicity profile compared to methotrexate (MTX) and is often substituted for MTX as part of acute GVHD immunoprohylaxis. Its major toxicities are gastrointestinal and relatively mild to moderate bone marrow suppression. This improved toxicity profile is beneficial in steroid-refractory cGVHD patients who often have declining performance status. In a large retrospective study evaluating the use of MMF in de novo or refractory cGVHD, patients who received MMF combined with corticosteroids or calcineurin inhibitor as primary therapy for newly diagnosed cGVHD obtained a 90% response [41]. In patients who received MMF as salvage therapy, there was a 75% response rate. Other smaller uncontrolled studies have supported a similar response rate of 60% to 80% in patients with steroid-refractory cGVHD [42–45]. Unfortunately, the responses associated with MMF in patients who respond poorly to steroids are usually partial responses and long-term outcome for these patients remain poor due to the negative effects of active cGVHD and the need for long-term immunosuppression.

Pharmacology and Pharmacokinetics

MMF is a prodrug of mycophenolic acid (MPA), which inhibits inosine monophosphate dehydrogenase. This results in reduced purine nucleoside synthesis and apoptosis of lymphocytes. MPA is rapidly absorbed from the gut with peak MPA levels occurring 1 hour after administering MMF. MPA is metabolized to the glucuronide by uridine diphosphate gluconosyltransferase (UGT). The glucuronide metabolite is excreted in the bile and undergoes entero-hepatic recirculation producing a second peak 6 to 12 hours after dosing [46]. The glucuronide metabolites while not active immunosuppressives may be involved in toxicity. The acyl MPA-glucuronide is implicated in cytokine release *in vitro*. This raises the interesting possibility that the occasional weight loss unrelated to diarrhea seen with chronic MMF dosing is related to this cytokine release particularly TNF, which is a known cause of cachexia [47, 48].

MPA is highly albumin bound and one of its renally eliminated metabolites can displace MPA from its albumin binding site. When this displacement occurs, it produces higher free MPA concentrations thus producing higher effective concentrations. The importance of diminished renal function or hypoalbuminemia on MMF efficacy and toxicity are not well described in patients with cGVHD but may be two of the major reasons to institute a TDM program for MMF. Measuring MPA concentrations in the blood is not the standard of care currently despite having shown that low free concentrations of MPA are associated with higher rates of GVHD [49, 50].

Drug Interactions

There are a number of drug interactions reported with MMF and several of the major interactions are highlighted in

Table 10.7: Drug Interactions Associated with MMF

Interacting Drug	Comments
Cyclosporine	↓ AUC MPA due to inhibition of biliary secretion and entero-hepatic recirculation
Norfloxacin	See CSA comments previously
Metronidazole	
Antacids	↓ AUC of MPA due to ↓ absorption
Cholestyramine	See antacids
Corticosteroids	↓ AUC of MPA due to UGT induction
Rifampin	See corticosteroids

AUC, area under curve; CSA, cyclosporine A; MMF, mycophenolate mofetil; MPA, mycophenolic acid; UGT, uridine diphosphate gluconosyltransferase.

Table 10.7. One of the more important interactions is that associated with CSA. CSA and MMF combinations for acute GVHD are common and the use of the combination in the setting of cGVHD is also common. CSA decreases MPA concentrations in the blood because of a reduction in the transport of MPA-glucuronide into the bile leading to reduced entero-hepatic recirculation of MPA [51]. It is interesting that in a recent pharmacokinetic study in hematopoietic stem cell transplantation (HSCT) patients, the majority did not have a second MPA peak that corresponds to entero-hepatic recirculation. The authors proposed this was an effect of CSA included in the immunoprophylaxis regimen. Norfloxacin and metronidazole, two antibacterials, also inhibit entero-hepatic recirculation leading to reduced MPA blood concentrations [52]. Antacids and cholestyramine decrease the absorption of MMF leading to a decline in drug concentrations. Unlike the interactions described in the preceding text that either affect absorption or transport of drug into the bile, rifampin reduces MPA concentrations as a result of induction of UGT and more rapid glucuronidation and elimination [53].

Polymorphisms in the UGT enzyme and mrp-2 have been identified and may be relevant to the elimination of MMF and may in part be responsible for the high interpatient variability seen in blood concentrations. More work will be required to describe the importance of these single nucleotide polymorphisms in a HSCT. While TDM of MMF is not established, evidence that trough concentrations correlate with response in cGVHD, interactions with other drugs, and genetic variability in drug elimination suggests a benefit to establishing a target concentration and performing TDM in HSCT patients.

Toxicity

As stated previously, the toxicity profile of MMF is one of its strengths in salvage regimens. MMF is associated with a dose dependent myelosuppression that is usually mild to moderate in severity. One of the underrated toxicities associated with MMF in these patients is opportunistic infections. In one series approximately 50% of patients with acute or chronic GVHD being treated with MMF had serious infections including *Aspergillus*, *Cytomegalovirus*, *Herpes simplex* and zoster, and some serious bacterial infections [54].

SIROLIMUS

Sirolimus (originally referred to as rapamycin) is a macrocyclic lactone originally isolated from *Streptomyces hygroscopicus*, a soil actinomycete removed from Rapa Nui (Easter Island). Once isolated, sirolimus was found to have antifungal activity but was subsequently discovered to have potent antitumor/proliferative and immunosuppressive properties [55–60]. Sirolimus has been extensively evaluated for the prophylaxis of organ rejection following renal transplantation. It was approved for this indication by the U.S. Food and Drug Administration in 1999. In allogeneic HSCT, sirolimus has been evaluated both for the prophylaxis of acute GVHD [61, 62] and in the treatment of steroid-refractory acute GHVD [64]. For cGVHD, sirolimus has been evaluated in the treatment of refractory or relapsed disease in combination with other immunosuppressive agents including calcineurin inhibitors, corticosteroids, and MMF [64–66]. These studies are discussed in Chapter 12.

Pharmacology

Sirolimus is structurally similar to other macrocyclic lactones, such as TAC and erythromycin. However, despite the structural similarity to TAC (FK-506), sirolimus has a distinct mechanism that does not include inhibition of calcineurin and the subsequent inhibitory effects on T-cell activation.

Sirolimus is a lipophilic molecule that readily penetrates the cellular plasma membrane. Once sirolimus enters the cell, it binds to the intracellular binding protein FK-binding protein-12 (FKBP-12). The formation of this immunophilin–drug complex is necessary to then modulate the activity of other specific intracellular targets. However, unlike TAC, the sirolimus–FKBP-12 complex does not inhibit calcineurin but instead inhibits the mammalian target of rapamycin (mTOR). Through inhibition of mTOR, sirolimus inhibits multiple signal-transduction pathways resulting in the arrest of the cell cycle in G1 phase in various cell types [56, 58].

The cell signaling pathways that are impacted through the inhibitory effects of sirolimus on the mTOR include the following:

1. **p70^{S6} (70-kD ribosomal S6) kinase phosphorylation:** Through inhibition of mTOR, sirolimus inhibits p70^{S6} kinase and the resulting phosphorylation of the ribosomal S6 protein and synthesis of endosomal structural proteins. In addition, p70^{S6} kinase mediates activation of CREMτ, a transcription factor necessary to the transcription of proliferating nuclear cell antigen (PNCA). Sirolimus thus inhibits PNCA transcription [56, 58].

2. **eIF-4E (eukaryotic initiation factor 4E) binding protein phosphorylation:** Through inhibition of mTOR, sirolimus inhibits the phosphorylation of eIF-4E binding protein that leads to an inhibition of the translation of specific mRNAs necessary for cell growth and proliferation [56, 58, 59].

3. **p27[kip1] (p27 kinase inhibitory protein-1):** Through mTOR inhibition, sirolimus blocks the degradation of p27[kip1], which is a negative regulatory factor for cyclin dependent kinases (cdks). Sirolimus thus decreases the kinase activity of the cdk/cyclin complexes that peak in the G1 phase of the cell cycle and are necessary for entry into the S phase [56, 58].

4. **CD28-mediated downregulation of IκBα:** Costimulation of CD28 in T lymphocytes and p70[S6] kinase leads to the downregulation of the inhibitory protein IκBα. The downregulation of IκBα allows the translocation of c-Rel (a member of the Rel family of transcription factors) to the nucleus of cells and transcription activation of several lymphokine genes, including IL-2. Thus by inhibiting the downregulation of IκBα (possibly through its downstream inhibitory effects on p70[S6] kinase), sirolimus prevents the CD28-mediated upregulation of IL-2 transcription in T cells [58, 67].

Pharmacokinetics

Absorption

Sirolimus is available in two oral formulations; an oral solution (concentration 1 mg/mL) and tablets (1 mg and 2 mg). The systemic availability of the oral solution is estimated to be approximately 15% whereas the mean bioavailability of the tablets is approximately 27% higher [57, 60, 68]. The two formulations are not bioequivalent but clinical equivalence has been demonstrated at the 2 mg dose level [68]. The low bioavailability of sirolimus is secondary to extensive intestinal and hepatic first-pass metabolism by the CYP 450, CYP 3A4 isoenzyme and countertransport by the multidrug efflux pump, intestinal p-glycoprotein [60]. The time to peak concentration (tmax) after oral administration is approximately 1 hour (range 0.5–3 hours) [57, 60, 68]. Administration of sirolimus with a high-fat meal results in greater bioavailability but the difference is small, relative to known inter- and intra-subject variabilities demonstrated for sirolimus. It is recommended that sirolimus be administered consistently in regards to meals [68, 69].

Distribution

Sirolimus is distributed in human whole blood among red blood cells (94.5%), plasma (3.1%), lymphocytes (1.01%), and granulocytes (1.0%). Distribution is not temperature or concentration dependent. The sequestration of sirolimus by red blood cells is believed to be partially due to the high content of immunophilins. In the plasma compartment, sirolimus is bound to lipoproteins (40%), although this percentage increases with increasing sirolimus concentrations. Among the fraction not bound to lipoproteins, only 4% is bound to plasma proteins. Therefore, utilizing whole blood for TDM is most appropriate. Sirolimus has a large Vd (5.6–16.7 L/kg) due to its lipophilic nature and is widely distributed in lipid membranes of body tissues as well as erythrocytes. [57, 60]

Metabolism and Elimination

Sirolimus is extensively metabolized by the CYP3A4 isoenzyme by both enterocytes in the intestinal wall as well is in the liver. It also undergoes countertransport from the enterocytes into the gut lumen by the p-glycoprotein drug efflux pump and is potentially recycled to allow continued metabolism by CYP3A4. Thus, absorption as well as metabolism/elimination of systemically absorbed sirolimus can be heavily influenced by drugs and food that affect these proteins [68]. Sirolimus is metabolized by O-demethylation and/or hydroxylation forming multiple metabolites. However, these metabolites appear to display less than 10% of the immunosuppressive activity of sirolimus [57, 60, 68]. The primary clearance route for sirolimus metabolites is biliary with 91% demonstrated recovery in the feces of healthy volunteers [57, 68]. The mean terminal elimination half-life of sirolimus in adults is approximately 62 hours. The long half-life necessitates that a loading dose (generally 3 times the maintenance dose) be given to achieve a therapeutic drug concentration within the first day of administration. The long half-life also allows for once daily administration [57, 60, 68]. Dose reductions should be considered in patients with mild to moderate hepatic impairment [68]. Pediatric patients appear to have a higher clearance and shorter half-life compared to adult patients and may require higher doses on the basis of body weight to achieve a similar area under curve (AUC) [70–72].

Therapeutic Drug Monitoring

Data from both animal studies and human clinical trials have shown good correlation between sirolimus blood concentrations and both immunosuppressive efficacy and toxicity. In addition, significant intra- and inter-subject variability in apparent clearance would suggest the need for therapeutic drug monitoring. Trough concentrations (minimum plasma concentration at steady state) have shown good correlation to AUC. For this reason, trough concentrations are a simple and useful index for therapeutic monitoring of sirolimus [57, 60]. Since parent drug concentrations correlate best to clinical effects, analytical assays that measure parent drug with minimal contamination of metabolites is preferable. HPLC with detection by either tandem mass spectroscopy (LC-MS/MS) or by ultraviolet detection (LC-UV) allow specific measurement of parent drug concentrations and provide comparable results [57, 60]. An immunoassay (microparticle enzyme immunoassay) is also available but overestimates HPLC results by 42.5% as a result of cross-reactivity with sirolimus metabolites and does not have the sensitivity suggested for sirolimus drug monitoring (2 µg/L) [57, 60]. Generally, sirolimus trough concentrations in the range of 5 to 15 µg/L have shown the best correlation to both efficacy (prevention of acute rejection) and toxicity (leukopenia, thrombocytopenia,

Table 10.8: Sirolimus Drug and Food Interactions [70,73–76]

Drug/Food	Inhibitor Potency (Strong/Moderate/Low)	Management of Interaction
Inhibitors of CYP3A4 and/or p-glycoprotein		
Clarithromycin	Strong	Coadministration is not recommended by the manufacturer
Cyclosporine capsules (MODIFIED)	Moderate	Separate administration of cyclosporine and sirolimus by 4 hours to minimize interaction.
Diltiazem	Moderate	Monitor levels; dose adjustment may be necessary
Erythromycin	Strong	Coadministration is not recommended by the manufacturer (C_{max} and AUC of sirolimus increase by 4.4 and 4.2 fold, respectively)
Fluconazole	Moderate	Monitor levels
Grapefruit, grapefruit juice	Moderate	Coadministration is not recommended
Itraconazole	Strong	Coadministration is not recommended by the manufacturer
Ketoconazole	Strong	Coadministration is not recommended by the manufacturer (C_{max} and AUC of sirolimus increase by 4.3 and 10.9 fold, respectively)*
Posaconazole	Moderate	Sirolimus dose adjustment may be necessary; data lacking on degree of interaction
Tacrolimus	Moderate	Monitor levels; separation of dosing does not appear to be necessary [71]
Telithromycin	Strong	Coadministration is not recommended by the manufacturer
Verapamil	Moderate	Sirolimus dose adjustment may be necessary (C_{max} and AUC of sirolimus increase by 2.3 and 2.2 fold, respectively); monitor levels; the AUC of verapamil is also increased by 1.5 fold
Voriconazole	Strong	Coadministration is not recommended by the manufacturer*
Inducers of CYP3A4 and/or p-glycoprotein		
Anticonvulsants: carbamazepine, phenobarbital, phenytoin	Strong	Monitor levels; Significant induction of metabolism is anticipated and maintaining therapeutic levels of sirolimus may be very difficult
St. John's Wart	Moderate	Monitor levels
Rifampin	Strong	Coadministration is not recommended by the manufacturer; (C_{max} and AUC of sirolimus decrease by 71% and 82%, respectively)

Note: This is not a comprehensive list of all potential interactions with sirolimus. Refer to product labeling and standard drug references for known or suspected drug interactions (all CYP3A4 inducers/inhibitors and p-gp inhibitors).
* Case reports have been published documenting safe coadministration with some potent CYP3A4 inhibitors and sirolimus albeit with significant sirolimus dose reductions. For example, for ketoconazole and voriconazole, an approximate 90% dose reduction (10% of the original dose) has been suggested as a potential dose adjustment [70–73].
AUC, area under curve; C_{max}, maximum plasma drug concentration.

or hypertriglyceridemia) in studies involving renal transplant patients [57, 60]. Therapeutic drug concentrations generally within this range have also been utilized in clinical trials of sirolimus for the treatment of cGVHD [64–66].

Drug Interactions

As indicated in the pharmacokinetics section previously, sirolimus is a substrate for both CYP3A4 and p-glycoprotein and subsequently is quite susceptible to drug–drug and drug–food interactions. Potential drug and food interactions are summarized in Table 10.8.

Toxicity

Refer to Table 10.9 for a summary of potential sirolimus toxicities and related prevention and management strategies.

THALIDOMIDE

Thalidomide has a long but complex history of development as a therapeutic agent. Originally synthesized in 1954, thalidomide was initially developed as a sedative, tranquilizer, and antiemetic for morning sickness. The well-described teratogenic effects of thalidomide surfaced in the late 1950s and early 1960s after over 5,000 babies from 46 countries had been born with various external and internal malformations. It was withdrawn from the European markets in 1961 and from other worldwide markets in the following years [77–79]. Thalidomide reemerged as an effective agent in the treatment of erythema nodosum leprosum (ENL) in 1965 and it subsequently was evaluated as an investigational agent for a variety of malignancies and various inflammatory and immune diseases. Thalidomide was eventually approved by the U.S. Food and Drug Association (FDA) in 1998 for the treatment of ENL

Table 10.9: Sirolimus Toxicity and Prevention/Management Strategies [61–66,68]

Toxicity	Monitoring	Prevention/Management	Comments
Myelosuppression (leucopenia, thrombocytopenia, anemia)	CBC	Monitor trough levels and maintain within therapeutic range	
Hyperlipidemia and Hypertriglyceridemia	Lipid panel, triglycerides	Diet, exercise and lipid-lowering agents as indicated	Common toxicity; coadministration with HMG-CoA reductase inhibitors and fibrates can be safely combined but if cyclosporine is also utilized, monitor for creatine kinase elevations and rhabdomyolysis
Renal impairment	Serum creatinine		More common when used in combination with calcineurin inhibitors
Thrombotic microangiopathy (HUS/TTP)	Hemoglobin, hematocrit, LDH, Bilirubin, peripheral blood smear	Value of plasmapheresis unclear	Appears to be more common when sirolimus is combined with calcineurin inhibitors
Angioedema			Concomitant use with other drugs known to cause angioedema (e.g., ACE inhibitors) may increase risk
Fluid accumulation (peripheral edema, pleural effusions, pericardial effusions			
Impaired wound healing (wound dehiscence, lymphocele)			Noted in renal transplantation patients; may be dose related and more likely to occur in obese patients
Mucosal ulceration			
Hepatic transaminase elevations	Hepatic transaminases		
Interstitial lung disease (e.g., pneumonitis, bronchiolitis obliterans organizing pneumonia, pulmonary fibrosis)			Risk may be increased with high serum trough levels

ACE, angiotensin-converting enzyme; CBC, complete blood count; HUS, hemolytic uremic syndrome; LDH, lactate dehydrogenase; TTP thrombotic thrombocytopenic purpura.

under a restricted distribution program. The research conducted since the reemergence of thalidomide in the mid-1960s have shown it to have a variety of mechanisms including antiangiogenic, immunomodulatory, and anti-inflammatory activity [77, 78]. Following promising experiments by Vogelsang et al. in a rat bone marrow transplant model [80, 81], thalidomide was subsequently evaluated for the treatment of acute and chronic GVHD beginning in the late 1980s. The utilization of thalidomide in the management of cGVHD has largely gone out of favor in more recent years due to its toxicity profile, its relatively narrow therapeutic window, and the emergence of alternative therapies. The clinical experience of thalidomide in the treatment of cGVHD is summarized in Chapter 13.

Pharmacology

Thalidomide is a racemic analog of glutamic acid and consists of equimolar amounts of (+)-(R)- and (−)-(S)-enantiomers.

These enantiomers interconvert under physiologic conditions. The (S)-enantiomer is responsible for the immunomodulatory as well as the teratogenic and antiangiogenic effects. The (R)-enantiomer is responsible for the sedative effects of thalidomide probably mediated by activation of sleep receptors in the forebrain. Thalidomide undergoes spontaneous hydrolysis in aqueous solution at a pH of 6.0 or higher forming at least 12 hydrolysis products [77, 78].

The immunomodulatory and anti-inflammatory actions of thalidomide appear to be closely related through the modulation of a number of cytokines, including TNF-α, IL-2, IL-4, IL-6, IL-12, IFN-γ, and COX-2 [77, 82]. One of the primary mechanisms of thalidomide appears to be the inhibition of TNF-α production by monocytes and macrophages by enhancing the degradation of TNF-α mRNA. This inhibition of TNF-α may then lead to a reduction of other inflammatory cytokines [83, 84]. Thalidomide also has been shown to modulate T cells, although these effects are complex and not totally understood.

Table 10.10: Thalidomide Toxicity and Prevention/management Strategies [77,89,91,92]

Toxicity	Monitoring	Prevention/Management	Comments
Sedation		Dose at bedtime; dose titration	Tolerance may develop with continued dosing
Fatigue			
Dizziness		Dose at bedtime; dose titration	
Constipation		Prophylactic stool softeners/ laxatives	
Headache			
Peripheral neuropathy	Total neuropathy score; Neurophysiologic testing	Avoid thalidomide in patients with preexisting neuropathies	Primarily a sensory neuropathy; Neuropathy is more likely to result in discontinuation of drug therapy than other toxicities
Skin rash		Discontinue if symptomatic skin rash appears; for nonsevere skin rash, may restart at lower dose after clearance[21]	More common when combined with corticosteroids; severe dermatologic reactions have been reported (e.g., Stevens-Johnson syndrome, EM, TEN)
Neutropenia			May necessitate interruption in drug therapy and potentially discontinuation
Xerostomia			
Deep vein thrombosis			More common when combined with chemotherapeutic agents or corticosteroids in cancer patients
Teratogenicity	Pregnancy testing mandatory in women of childbearing age	Abstinence or two method contraception is mandatory in females; condoms in males	Drug is under a restricted distribution program (STEPS) as a risk reduction strategy

EM, erythema multiforme; TEN, toxic epidermal necrolysis.

It has been demonstrated *in vitro* that thalidomide induces T-helper cell type 2 (Th2) and inhibits Th1 cytokine production [85]. Thalidomide has also been shown to increase proliferation of T cells by acting as a costimulator, predominantly for cytotoxic (CD8+) T cells as opposed to helper T cells (CD4+) [86]. In multiple myeloma cell lines, thalidomide induced natural killer (NK) cell-mediated lysis by increasing IL-2 and IFN-γ secretion [87].

The mechanism of thalidomide also appears to be related to its ability to block NF-κB activity [88]. NF-κB is a DNA-binding factor that can regulate the expression of genes for a variety of cytokines including TNF-α, IL-8, and IL-12. NF-κB is also known to be a key regulator of oncogenes, such as those involved in cell growth, suppression of apoptosis, and metastasis. In unstimulated cells, the majority of NF-κB is localized to the cytoplasm where it is tightly bound to inhibitory proteins of the IκB family. Upon stimulation by inducers such as TNF-α or IL-1β, the inhibitory protein IκB is phosphorylated by the IκB kinase, which subsequently leads to its degradation and allows the nuclear translocation of NF-κB. Thalidomide has been shown to suppress the activity of the IκB kinase, which subsequently blocks the activity of NF-κB [88].

Pharmacokinetics

Absorption

The bioavailability of the commercially available oral formulation of thalidomide has not been characterized in human subjects although a study evaluating the (R)- and (S)-enantiomers suggested that the bioavailability of the (R)-enantiomer was close to 100% and 50% for the (S)-enantiomer [78]. The rate of absorption is relatively slow; the time to maximum plasma concentration after oral administration ranges between 3.32 and 4.71 hours [78]. The relatively slow rate of absorption is likely due to its low aqueous solubility and poor dissolution in the gastrointestinal tract. The pharmacokinetics of thalidomide can be described as absorption rate limited elimination since the elimination rate of thalidomide exceeds the absorption rate. This rate difference results in an absorption time lag of 20 to 40 minutes [78].

Distribution

Thalidomide is moderately protein bound, with the mean plasma protein binding of 55% and 66% for the (+)–(R)- and (–)–(S)-enantiomer, respectively [89].

Metabolism and Elimination

In vitro studies have shown that thalidomide is metabolized by the CYP p450 subfamily 2C19 to form active 5-hydroxy metabolites. However, human studies indicate that the CYP metabolism is minimal and the role of the 5-hydroxy metabolite in the clinical effects of thalidomide is debatable [78, 82]. Thus it appears that thalidomide is primarily broken down through nonenzymatic hydrolytic cleavage. This hydrolysis is spontaneous at physiologic pH and the subsequent hydrolytic products are assumed to be predominantly cleared by passive renal elimination based on animal studies [78]. The terminal elimination half-life has been determined to range from 6.5 to 18.3 hours in various patient populations. Clearance differs between the two enantiomers, with the (−)-(S)-enantiomer eliminated twice as fast as the (+)-(R)-enantiomer. Multiple oral dose studies have demonstrated that drug accumulation does not occur. Steady state is achieved within 2 to 3 days. Because of the slow absorption rate, there is less than proportional increase in C_{max} with increasing dose; however, there is a dose proportional increase in AUC [78]. Dosage adjustments are not required in patients with hepatic or renal impairment [78, 90].

Drug Interactions

Drug–drug interaction studies involved with thalidomide are limited in number. Two interaction studies have been conducted with oral contraceptives and no pharmacokinetic interactions were observed. Since the predominant form of metabolism is through nonenzymatic hydrolysis, interactions mediated through the hepatic CYP system are not likely to be significant [78]. Additive sedative effects may be seen when thalidomide is combined with other agents that have sedative properties [89].

Toxicity

Refer to Table 10.10 for a summary of potential thalidomide toxicities and related prevention and management strategies.

REFERENCES

1. Vogelsang GB. How I treat chronic graft-versus-host disease. *Blood.* 2001;97:1196–1201.
2. Lee SJ, Vogelsang G, Flowers MED. Chronic graft-versus-host disease. *Biol Blood Marrow Transplant.* 2003;9:215–233.
3. Akpek G, Via CS, Vogelsang GB. Clinical spectrum and therapeutic approaches to chronic graft-vs.-host disease. In: Ferrara JLM, Cooke KR, Deeg HJ, eds. Graft-vs-Host Disease, 3rd ed. *Informa Health Care.* 2004;555–608.
4. Shlomchik WD, Lee SJ, Couriel D, Pavletic SZ. Transplantation's greatest challenges: advances in chronic graft-versus-host disease. *Biol Blood Marrow Transplant.* 2007;13:2–10.
5. Koc S, Leisenring W, Flowers MED, et al. Therapy for chronic graft-versus-host disease: a randomized trial comparing cyclosporine plus prednisone versus prednisone alone. *Blood.* 2002;100:48–51.
6. Sullivan KM, Witherspoon RP, Storb R, et al. Alternating-day cyclosporine and prednisone for treatment of high-risk chronic graft-v-host disease. *Blood.* 1988;72:555–561.
7. Schimmer BP, Parker KL. Adrenocorticotropic hormone; adrenocortical steroids and their synthetic analogs; inhibitors of the synthesis and actions of adrenocortical hormones. In: Brunton LL, Lazo JS, Parker KL, eds. *Goodman & Gilman's the pharmacologic basis of therapeutics.* 11th ed. McGraw-Hill Companies, Inc., 2006:1587–1611.
8. Chao NJ. Pharmacology and the use of immunosuppressive agents after hematopoietic cell transplantation. In: Blume KG, Forman SJ, Appelbaum FR, eds. *Thomas' Hematopoietic Cell Transplantation,* 3rd ed. Blackwell Publishing, Ltd. 2004; 209–220.
9. Buttgereit F, Wehling M, Burmester GR. A new hypothesis of modular glucocorticoid actions; steroid treatment of rheumatic diseases revisited. *Arthritis Rheum.* 1998;41:761–67.
10. Almawi WY, Lipman ML, Stevens AC, Zanker B, Hadro ET, Strom TB. Abrogation of glucocorticosteroid-mediated inhibition of T cell proliferation by the synergistic action of IL-1, IL-6, and IFN-γ. *J Immunol.* 1991;146:3523–3527.
11. Czock D, Keller F, Rasche FR, Haussler U. Pharmacokinetics and pharmacodynamics of systemically administered glucocorticoids. *Clin Pharmacokinet.* 2005;44:61–98.
12. Holler E, Kolb HJ, Wilmanns W. Treatment of GVHD – TNF-antibodies and related antagonists. *Bone Marrow Transplant.* 1993;12(Suppl 3):S29-S31.
13. Cupps TR, Fauci AS. Corticosteroid-mediated immunoregulation in man. *Immunological Rev.* 1982;65:133–155.
14. Migita K, Eguchi K, Kawabe Y, et al. Apoptosis induction in human peripheral blood T lymphocytes by high-dose steroid therapy. *Transplantation.* 1997;63:583–587.
15. Sanden S, Tripmacher R, Weltrich R, et al. Glucocorticoid dose dependent down regulation of glucocorticoid receptors in patients with rheumatic diseases. *J Rheum.* 2000;27:1265–1270.
16. Andreae J, Tripmacher R, Weltrich R, et al. Effect glucocorticoid therapy on glucocorticoid receptors in children with autoimmune diseases. *Ped Research.* 2001;49:130–135.
17. Akpek G, Lee SM, Anders V, Vogelsang GB. A high-dose pulse steroid regimen for controlling active chronic graft-versus-host disease. *Biol Blood Marrow Transplant.* 2001;7:495–502.
18. Bartoszek M, Brenner AM, Szefler SJ. Prednisolone and methylprednisolone kinetics in children receiving anticonvulsant therapy. *Clin Pharmacol Ther.* 1987;42:1180–1194.
19. Wassner SJ, Malekzadeh MH, Pennisi AJ, et al. Allograft survival in patients receiving anticonvulsant medications. *Clin Nephrol.* 1977;8:293–297.
20. Buffington GA, Dominguez JH, Piering WF, et al. Interaction of rifampin and glucocorticoids: adverse effect on renal allograft function. *JAMA.* 1976;236:1958–1960.
21. Couriel D, Carpenter PA, Cutler C, et al. Ancillary therapy and supportive care of chronic graft-versus-host disease: National Institutes of Health consensus development project on criteria for clinical trials in chronic graft-versus-host disease: V. Ancillary therapy and supportive care working group report. *Biol Blood Marrow Transplant.* 2006;12:375–396.
22. Heusler K, Pletscher A. The controversial early history of cyclosporine. *Swiss Med Weekly.* 2001;131:299–302.
23. Kahan BD. Cyclosporine. *N Eng J Med.* 1989;321:1725–1738.
24. Fung JJ. Tacrolimus and transplantation: a decade in review. *Transplantation.* 2004;77:S41-S43.

25. Sieber M, Karanik M, Brandt C, et al. Inhibition of calcineurin-NFAT signaling by the pyrazolopyrimidine compound NCI3. *Eur J Immunol.* 2007;37:2617–2626.

26. Almawi W, Melemedjian O. Clinical and mechanistic differences between FK506 (Tacrolimus) and cyclosporine A. *Nephrol Dial Transplant.* 2000;15:1916–1918.

27. Scott LJ, McKeage K, Keam SJ, et al. Tacrolimus: a further update of its use in the management of organ transplantation. *Drugs.* 2003;63:1247–1297.

28. Subramaniam DS, Fowler DH, Pavletic SZ. Chronic graft versus host disease in the era of reduced intensity conditioning. *Leukemia.* 2007;21:853–859.

29. Mengarelli A, Lori AP, Romano A, et al. One year cyclosporine prophylaxis reduces the risk of developing extensive chronic graft versus host disease after allogeneic peripheral blood stem cell transplantation. *Haematologica.* 2003;88:315–323.

30. Koc S, Leisenring W, Flowers ME, et al. Therapy for chronic graft-versus-host disease: a randomized trial comparing cyclosporine plus prednisone versus prednisone alone. *Blood.* 2002;100:48–51.

31. Ptachcinski RJ, Venkataramenan R, Burckart GJ. Clinical pharmacokinetics of cyclosporine. *Clin Pharmacokinet.* 1986;2:107–132.

32. Parquet N, Reigneau O, Humbert H, et al. New oral formulation of cyclosporine A (Neoral) pharmacokinetics in allogeneic bone marrow transplant patients. *Bone Marrow Transplant.* 2000;25:965–968.

33. Fung JJ. Tacrolimus and transplantation: a decade in review. *Transplantation.* 2004;9:S41-S43.

34. Leather HL. Drug interactions in the hematopoietic stem cell transplant recipient: what every transplanter needs to know. *Bone Marrow Transplant.* 2004;33:137–152.

35. Saad AH, DePestel DD, Carver PL. Factors influencing the magnitude and clinical significance of drug interactions between azole antifungals and select immunosuppressants. *Pharmacotherapy.* 2006;26:1730–1744.

36. Back DJ, Tjia JF. Comparative effects of the antimycotic drugs ketoconazole, fluconazole, itraconazole, and terbinafine on the metabolism of cyclosporine by human liver microsomes. *Br J Clin Pharmacol.* 1991;32:624–626.

37. Leather H, Boyette RM, Tian L, Wingard JR. Pharmacokinetic evaluation of the drug interaction between intravenous intraconazole and intravenous tacrolimus or intravenous cyclosporin A in allogeneic hematopoietic stem cell transplant recipients. *Biol Blood Marrow Transplant.* 2006;12:325–334.

38. Kazuto Y, Lan L, Sanglard D, et al. Interaction of cytochrome P4503A inhibitors with p-glycoprotein. *J Exp Pharmacol Experimental Ther.* 2002;303:323–332.

39. Canafax DM, Graves NM, Hilligoss DM, et al. Interaction between cyclosporine and fluconazole in renal allograft recipients. *Transplantation.* 1991;51:1014 1018.

40. Cutler C, Antin JH. Chronic graft versus host disease. *Curr Opin Oncol.* 2006;18:126–131.

41. Lopez F, Parker P, Nademanee A, et al. Efficacy of mycophenolate mofetil in the treatment of chronic graft-versus-host disease. *Biol Blood Marrow Transplant.* 2005;11:307–313.

42. Krejci M, Doubek M, Buchler T, et al. Mycophenolate mofetil for the treatment of acute and chronic steroid refractory graft versus host disease. *Ann Hematol.* 2005;84:681–685.

43. Kim JG, Sohn SK, Kim DH, et al. Different efficacy of mycophenolate mofetil as salvage treatment for acute and chronic GVHD after allogeneic stem cell transplant *Eur J Haematol.* 2004; 73:56–61.

44. Busca A, Locatelli F, Marmont F, et al. Response to mycophenolate mofetil therapy in refractory chronic graft-versus-host disease. *Haematologica.* 2003;88:837–839.

45. Mookerjee B, Altomonte V, Vogelsang G. Salvage therapy for refractory chronic graft versus host disease with mycophenolate mofetil and tacrolimus. *Bone Marrow Transplant.* 1999; 24:517–520.

46. van Hest RM, Doorduijn JK, de Winter B, et al. Pharmacokinetics of mycophenolate mofetil in hematopoietic stem cell transplant recipients. *Ther Drug Monitor.* 2007;29:353–360.

47. Laskin B, Goebel J. Clinically silent weight loss associated with mycophenolate mofetil in pediatric renal transplant patients. *Pediatr Transplant.* 2008;12:113–116.

48 Wielan E, Shipkova M, Schellhaasu, et al. Induction of cytokine release by the acyl-glucuronide of mycophenolic acid: a link to side-effects? *Clin Biochem.* 2000; 33:107–113.

49. Jacobson P, Rogoshesku J, Barker JN, et al. Relationship of mycophenolate exposure to clinical outcome after hematopoietic cell transplant. *Clin Pharmacol Ther.* 2005;78:486–500.

50. Oellerich M, Hon MD, Armstrong VW. The role of therapeutic drug monitoring in individualizing immunosuppressive drug therapy: recent developments. *Ther Drug Monit.* 2006;28:720–725.

51. Hesselink DA, VanHest RM, Mathot RA, et al. Cyclosporine interacts with mycophenolic acid by inhibiting the multi-drug resistance-associated protein-2. *Am J Transplant.* 2005;5:987–994.

52. Shaw LM, Pawinski T, Korecka M, et al. Monitoring of mycophenolic acid in clinical transplant. *Ther Drug Monitor.* 2002;24:68–73.

53. Kuypers DF, Verleden G, Naesens M, et al. Drug interaction between MMF and rifampin: possible induction of uridine diphosphate glucuronsyltransferase. *Clin Pharmacol Ther.* 2005;78:81–88.

54. Baudard M, Vincent A, Moreau P, et al. Mycophenolate mofetil for the treatment of acute and chronic GVHD is effective and well tolerated but induces a high risk of infectious complications: a series of 21 BM or PBSC transplant patients. *Bone Marrow Transplant.* 2002;30:287–295.

55. MacDonald A, Scarola J, Burke JT, Zimmerman JJ. Clinical pharmacokinetics and therapeutic drug monitoring of sirolimus. *Clin Ther.* 2000;22 (Suppl B):B101-B121.

56. Kahan BD. Sirolimus: a comprehensive review. *Expert Opin Pharmacother.* 2001;2:1903–1917.

57. Mahalati K, Kahan BD. Clinical pharmacokinetics of sirolimus. *Clin Pharmacokinet.* 2001;40:573–585.

58. Sehgal SN. Sirolimus: its discovery, biological properties, and mechanism of action. *Transplant Proc.* 2003;35 (Suppl 3A):7S-14S.

59. Huang S, Bjornsti MA, Houghton PJ. Rapamycins: mechanism of action and cellular resistance. *Cancer Biol Ther.* 2003;2:222–232.

60. Stenton SB, Partovi N, Ensom MHH. Sirolimus: the evidence for clinical pharmacokinetic monitoring. *Clin Pharmacokinet.* 2005;44:769–786.

61. Antin JH, Kim HT, Cutler C, et al. Sirolimus, tacrolimus, and low-dose methotrexate for graft-versus-host disease prophylaxis in mismatched related donor or unrelated donor transplantation. *Blood.* 2003;102:1601–1605.

62. Cutler C, Antin JH. Sirolimus for GVHD prophylaxis in allogeneic stem cell transplantation. *Bone Marrow Transplant.* 2004;34:471–476.

63. Benito AI, Furlong T, Martin PJ, et al. Sirolimus (rapamycin) for the treatment of steroid-refractory acute graft-versus-host disease. *Transplantation.* 2001;72:1924–1929.

64. Couriel DR, Saliba R, Escalon MP, et al. Sirolimus in combination with tacrolimus and corticosteroids for the treatment of resistant chronic graft-versus-host disease. *Br J Haematol.* 2005;130:409–417.

65. Johnston LJ, Brown J, Shizuru JA, et al. Rapamycin (sirolimus) for treatment of chronic graft-versus-host disease. *Biol Blood Marrow Transplant.* 2005;11:47–55.

66. Jurado M, Vallejo C, Perez-Simon, JA. Sirolimus as part of immunosuppressive therapy for refractory chronic graft-versus-host disease. *Biol Blood Marrow Transplant.* 2007;13:701–706.

67. Lai JH, Tan TH. CD28 signaling causes a sustained down-regulation of IκBα which can be prevented by the immunosuppressant rapamycin. *J Biol Chem.* 1994;269:30077–30080.

68. Product label. Rapamune® (sirolimus). Philadelphia, PA. Wyeth Pharmaceuticals, Inc. 2007.

69. Zimmerman JJ, Ferron GM, Lim HK, Parker V. The effect of a high-fat meal on the oral bioavailability of the immunosuppressant sirolimus (rapamycin). *J Clin Pharmacol.* 1999;39:1155–1161.

70. Schubert M, Venkataramanan R, Holt DW, et al. Pharmacokinetics of sirolimus and tacrolimus in pediatric transplant patients. *Am J Transplant.* 2004;767–773.

71. Schachter AD, Meyers KE, Spaneas LD, et al. Short sirolimus half life in pediatric renal transplant recipients on a calcineurin inhibitor-free protocol. *Pediatr Transplant.* 2004;8:171–177.

72. Schachter AD, Benfield MR, Wyatt RJ, et al. Sirolimus pharmacokinetics in pediatric renal transplant recipients receiving calcineurin inhibitor co-therapy. *Pediatr Transplant.* 2006;10:914–919.

73. McAlister VC, Mahalati K, Peltekian KM, Fraser A, MacDonald AS. A clinical pharmacokinetic study of tacrolimus and sirolimus combination immunosuppression comparing simultaneous to separated administration. *Ther Drug Monit.* 2002;24:346–350.

74. Mathis AS, Shah NK, Friedman GS. Combined use of sirolimus and voriconazole in renal transplantation: a report of two cases. *Transplant Proc.* 2004;36:2708–2709.

75. Thomas PP, Manivannan J, John GT, et al. Sirolimus and ketoconazole co-prescription in renal transplant recipients. *Transplantation.* 2004;77:474–475.

76. Sadaba B, Campanero MA, Quetglas EG, Azanza Jr. Clinical relevance of sirolimus drug interactions in transplant patients. *Transplant Proc.* 2004;36:3226–3228.

77. Franks ME, Macpherson GR, Figg WD. Thalidomide. *Lancet.* 2004;363:1802–1811.

78. Teo SK, Colburn WA, Tracewell WG, et al. Clinical pharmacokinetics of thalidomide. *Clin Pharmacokinet.* 2004;43:311–327.

79. Lenz W. A short history of thalidomide embryopathy. *Teratology.* 1988;38:203–215.

80. Vogelsang GB, Hess AD, Friedman KJ, Santos GW. Therapy of chronic graft-v-host disease in a rat model. *Blood.* 1989;74:507–511.

81. Vogelsang GB, Hess AD, Gordon G, Santos GW. Treatment and prevention of acute graft-versus-host disease with thalidomide in a rat model. *Transplantation.* 1986;41:644–647.

82. Lepper ER, Smith NF, Cox MC, Scripture CD, Figg WD. Thalidomide metabolism and hydrolysis: mechanisms and implications. *Curr Drug Metab.* 2006;7:677–685.

83. Sampaio EP, Sarno EN, Galilly R, Cohn ZA, Kaplan G. Thalidomide selectively inhibits tumor necrosis factor α production by stimulated human monocytes. *J Exp Med.* 1991;173:699–703.

84. Moreira AL, Sampaio EP, Zmuidzinas A, Frindt P, Smith KA, Kaplan G. Thalidomide exerts its inhibitory action on tumor necrosis factor α by enhancing mRNA degradation. *J Exp Med.* 1993;177:1675–1680.

85. McHugh SM, Rifkin IR, Deighton J, et al. The immunosuppressive drug thalidomide induces T helper cell type 2 (Th2) and concomitantly inhibits Th1 cytokine production in mitogen- and antigen-stimulated human peripheral blood mononuclear cell cultures. *Clin Exp Immunol.* 1995;99:160–167.

86. Haslett PAJ, Corral LG, Albert M, Kaplan G. Thalidomide costimulates primary human T lymphocytes, preferentially inducing proliferation, cytokine production, and cytotoxic responses in the CD8+ subset. *J Exp Med.* 1998;11:1885–1892.

87. Davies FE, Raje N, Hideshima T, et al. Thalidomide and immunomodulatory derivatives augment natural killer cell cytotoxicity in multiple myeloma. *Blood.* 2001;98:210–216.

88. Keifer JA, Guttridge DC, Ashburner BP, Baldwin AS. Inhibition of NF-κB activity by thalidomide through suppression of IκB kinase activity. *J Biol Chem.* 2001;276:22382–22387.

89. Product label. Thalomid® (thalidomide). Summit, NJ: Celgene Corporation, 2007.

90. Eriksson T, Hoglund P, Turesson I, et al. Pharmacokinetics of thalidomide in patients with impaired renal function and while on and off dialysis. *J Pharm Pharmacol.* 2003;55:1701–1706.

91. Parker PM, Chao N, Nademanee A, et al. Thalidomide as salvage therapy for chronic graft-versus-host disease. *Blood.* 1995;86:3604–3609.

92. Kumar S, Witzig TE, Rajkumar SV. Thalidomide: current role in the treatment of non-plasma cell malignancies. *J Clin Oncol.* 2004;22:2477–2488.

11

PREVENTION OF CHRONIC GRAFT VERSUS HOST DISEASE

Andrea Bacigalupo and Nelson J. Chao

INTRODUCTION

Chronic graft versus host disease (GVHD) is the major complication in long-term survivors of an allogeneic hematopoietic stem cell transplant (HSCT): its detrimental effect on quality of life, especially when extensive or severe, together with its protective role on leukemia relapse are well documented. This chapter will outline programs designed to prevent GVHD, including the use of agents capable of modulating T-cell function. Recent developments in our understanding of the sclerodermatous form of chronic GVHD (cGVHD) and its clinical implications will also be discussed.

TIMING OF CHRONIC GVHD

This division on day 100 between acute and cGVHD is currently considered artificial [1]. With the advent of nonmyeloablative hematopoietic cell transplantation (HCT) regimens and the use of unrelated donor stem cells, there is a need to drop this arbitrary time point from the definition of these disease entities. Current studies are more likely to utilize the clinical manifestations of these diseases rather than the arbitrary cutoff of a particular date post transplantation. This has been the conclusion of an international group of experts [1].

A continuum of clinical findings (i.e., "overlap syndrome") may be observed in patients with acute and cGVHD, as both disorders commonly affect similar organs, principally the skin, liver, and gastrointestinal tract [1]. However, the target organs affected by and the clinical and histologic features associated with cGVHD may differ from those observed with acute disease. As an example, autoimmune phenomena, such as autoantibody formation, are more common with chronic disease. Clinical aspects of cGVHD may also mimic features frequently observed with systemic lupus erythematosus, scleroderma, sicca syndrome, eosinophilic fasciitis, rheumatoid arthritis, and primary biliary sclerosis [2].

Another important aspect of cGVHD is that the disease leads to marked immunodeficiency due to both direct immunosuppressive effects and the consequences of the agents administered to treat the disease. Since cGVHD also causes a delay in the recovery of immune function, patients remain immunodeficient as long as the disease is active [3]. Dysregulation of T and B lymphocyte control may be observed [4].

Chronic GVHD is the single major factor determining long-term outcome and quality of life following HCT. Because of the profound immunosuppression observed with this disorder, recurrent infections occur in almost all affected patients. These complications account for most of the morbidity and mortality associated with cGVHD.

Clearly, the most optimal method to avoid cGVHD would be to prevent it from occurring in the first place. Since the development of acute GVHD leads to a significant increase in the incidence of cGVHD, a more efficacious regimen for the prevention of acute GVHD would be the most optimal method for prevention of cGVHD.

PROPHYLAXIS BY REMOVING OR INACTIVATING DONOR T CELLS

Acute and cGVHD can be prevented by removal of T cells from the graft, referred to as T-cell depletion (TCD). There are two distinct types of TCD, which are not mutually exclusive: ex vivo TCD and in vivo TCD.

T-cell Depletion Ex Vivo

This procedure is accomplished by physical and/or immunologic means. In the early 1980s and 1990s the preferred method was E-rosetting and density separation [5], or treatment of the graft with a cocktail of anti-T monoclonal antibodies [6]. Current methods of TCD include the use a single monoclonal antibody targeting several cell subpopulations (CAMPATH), or immunomagnetic devices allowing the selective removal of T, B, natural killer (NK) cells, as well as the positive selection of CD34 or CD133 progenitors [7–11].

The advantage of this last method is that one can actually count the residual T cells in the graft, and assess the degree of T-cell depletion, whereas this is not possible if one adds an antibody to the cell suspension before infusion, such as the so-called CAMPATH-in-the-bag method [12]. One can also cryopreserve cells that have been removed, such as T or NK cells, and eventually manipulate and expand them for further infusion to the patient in due time [9, 13]. If the graft contains less than 1×10^4/kg CD3+ cells, acute and cGVHD will be practically abrogated, both in the human leukocyte antigen (HLA) matched and mismatched setting [14]: in this case it is possible to avoid the administration of immunosuppressive drugs post transplant. Unfortunately T-cell reconstitution after TCD grafts has been found to similar if not inferior to unmanipulated grafts [15] because the former depends entirely on maturation from lymphoid progenitors in the graft and cannot rely on mature CD3+ cells infused with the unmanipulated graft. This is one problem of patients receiving a TCD graft. The second problem is relapse of the original disease [1]: because GVHD plays a major role in controlling leukemia (and possibly also lymphoma and myeloma), the almost total abrogation of both acute and cGVHD removes this important immunologic antitumor component of the transplant, which then relies more on the intensity of the conditioning regimen. In this important report from the International Transplant Registry (IBMTR) it was shown that leukemia relapse was two times higher in TCD transplants than in unmanipulated transplants; conversely the presence of acute GVHD reduced relapse (RR 0.68) and cGVHD further reduced it (RR 0.43). Syngeneic transplants, known to be free of both acute and cGVHD, had the highest risk of relapse (RR 2.09) [16]. For these two reasons, poor immune reconstitution and relapse, the abrogation of GVHD does not translate in superior outcome of TCD transplants: actually long-term overall and leukemia free survival has been inferior to patients receiving unmanipulated grafts, in almost all large clinical data sets: in the 1990 and 1991 IBMTR analysis, the relative risk of overall treatment failure for TCD grafts was higher than for unmanipulated grafts [16, 17]. TCD should be performed in a center with a dedicated program, where different forms of T-cell removal can be explored and improved [2, 3]. TCD cannot be recommended as a standard procedure because the number of variables is too large, and because our understanding of what should or should not be in the graft is limited. Some programs of partial or selective T-cell depletion have been conducted and have produced encouraging initial results [18].

T-cell Depletion In Vivo

Treatment of the patient with T-cell antibodies before the transplant (usually intravenously) is referred to as in vivo TCD and has two targets: it reduces the host immune response, favoring engraftment, and it down regulates the incoming donor T cells, thus preventing GVHD. The latter is possible because the antibody, usually given in the week prior to transplantation, is still in circulation at the time the cells are infused, and for several weeks thereafter: this could be formally proven in a recent study, showing that the level of circulating rabbit immunoglobulin on the day of transplant is predictive of GVHD, that is the higher the level of circulating rabbit IgG the lower the incidence of acute GVHD [19]. In vivo TCD is used in many but not all centers performing transplants with a greater risk of acute and cGVHD, including family mismatched and unrelated transplants. Some of these studies are outlined in Table 11.1, which summarizes major outcomes, such as graft failure, acute GVHD grade II to IV and III to IV, cGVHD, and transplant-related mortality. From the data it can be seen that ex vivo TCD results in very little acute and cGVHD, whereas in vivo TCD still allows for a significant proportion of patients to have both acute and some form of cGVHD.

Comparison of T-cell Depletion and Unmanipulated Transplants

This is a difficult task that should be performed on a prospective basis to account for the large number of variables in patient populations. These include donor and recipient age, disease phase, donor type, stem-cell source, as all of these are known to impact on GVHD. However in review on in vivo TCD with antithymocyte globulin (ATG), an effort to account for these variables was made [20, 21]: it turns out that results of three small prospective randomized trials, including 176 patients, and a large number of retrospective trials, including 1,069 patients, show confirmatory results. In the prospective randomized trials, acute GVHD grade II to IV is reduced from 72% to 37%, grade III to IV from 36% to 11%, and cGVHD from 62% to 40%, all statistically significant ($p < 0.001$). In the retrospective trials, with many more patients, acute GVHD grade II to IV is reduced from 51% to 20%, grade III to IV from 22% to 10%, and cGVHD from 65% to 41%, all statistically significant ($p < 0.001$). Therefore acute GVHD grade II to IV is reduced by 30%, grade III to IV is reduced by 20%, and cGVHD by 20%. Does this translate in improved survival? Not to a great extent, but there is a trend for improved survival both in the prospective trials (43% vs. 55%) and in the retrospective studies (55% to 64%). Therefore broad specificity antibodies, such as (ATG), can provide significant protection against acute and cGVHD thus shortening the time to come off immunosuppression and can improve quality of life. With longer follow-up exceeding 7 years, patients receiving ex vivo TCD may also have a survival advantage.

PROPHYLAXIS WITH COMBINED IMMUNOSUPPRESSION

Although T-cell depletion may help decrease the incidence and severity of cGVHD, chronic disease frequently develops in those receiving pharmacologic therapy, even if the patient did not develop significant acute GVHD. Various regimens have been used to prevent the development of cGVHD; none appears to be highly effective at this time (see Table 11.2).

The HCT programs at City of Hope and Stanford evaluated thalidomide as preventive therapy based upon its efficacy in

Table 11.1: Selected Studies Of Ex vivo and In vivo T-cell Depletion

Method	Reference	N.Pts	Type of Donor	GF (%)	aGVHD II–IV (%)	aGVHD III–IV (%)	GVHD Chronic (%)	TRM (%)
Ex vivo TCD								
CD34 sel	Urbano [1]	50	HLA id sibs	4	16	6	22	18
CAMP bag	Barge [6]	73	HLA id sibs	0	22	0	19	8
CAMP bag	Chakrab [3]	24	HLA id sibs	0	8	0	4	19
CD34 sel	Aversa [5]	101	Haploidentical	1*	8	0	5	38
In vivo TCD								
CAMP 1G i.v.	Hale [98]	50	HLA id sibs	31	20	NA	21	53
ATG	Baciga [2]	160	UD + fam mism	0	51	14	28	33
ATG	Remberg [19]	52	UD	0	12	0	NA	NA
ATG–G	Basara [5]	87	UD	NA	NA	15	17	42
CAMP 1G i.v.	Rizzieri [7]	49	Fam. Haplo	1	NA	8	NA	10
ATG	LU [6]	135	Fam. Haplo	NA	40	NA	55	22
Ex vivo + in vivo TCD								
CAMP bag + CAMP i.v.	Hale [98]	70	HLA id sibs	6	4	0	3	15

aGVHD, acute graft versus host disease; ATG, antithymocyte globulin; CAMP bag, CAMPATH 1H given in the bag (alemtuzumba); CMAP i.v., CAMPATH given intravenously; CD34 sel, selection of CD34 cells by immunomagnetic beads; fam mism, family mismatched donors; fam haplo, family haploidentical donors; GF, graft failure; HLA id sibs, human leukocyte antigen identical siblings; N pts., number of patients; NA, not available; TRM, transplant-related mortality; UD, unrelated donors. Six out of seven primary graft failure were rescued with a second transplant.

Table 11.2: Trials of Combination Immunosuppression after Marrow Transplantation: Chronic GVHD Studies

Author	Patients (n)	Regimens compared	Chronic GVHD (%)	GVHD response (%)	Non-relapse mortality (%)	Overall survival (%)
Prevention						
Kansu et al. (2001)	73	6 month CSP	51			84
		versus	(n.s.)			(n.s.)
	89	24 month CSP	39			88
Treatment						
Sullivan et al. (1988) (Standard risk)	63	PSE + placebo		62	21	61
		versus		(n.s.)	(p = 0.003)	(p = 0.03)
	63	PSE + AZ		64	40	47
Koc et al. (2002) (Standard risk)	145	PSE		53	13	54
		versus		(n.s.)	(n.s.)	(n.s.)
	142	PSE + CSP		54	17	66
Arora et al. (2001) (Standard and high risk)	27	PSE + CSP		73		72
		versus		(n.s.)		(n.s.)
	27	PSE + CSP + Thal		88		67
Sullivan et al. (1988) (High risk)	38	PSE (placebo) (thrombocytopenia)		32	58	26
Sullivan et al. (1988) (High risk)	40	PSE + CSP		56	40	52
Koc et al. (2000) (High risk)	26	PSE + [CSP or TACR] + placebo		23		47
		versus		(n.s.)		(n.s.)
	26	PSE + [CSP or TACR] + Thal		39		49
Bolwell et al. (2004)	21	CSP + MMF	63			52
		versus	(n.s.)			(n.s.)
	19	CSP + MTX	64			68
Neumann et al. (2005)	26	CSP + MMF	50		17	76
		versus	(n.s.)			(n.s.)
		CSP + MTX	45		27	55

AZ, azathioprine; CSP, cyclosporine; GVHD, graft-versus-host disease; n.s., not significant; PSE, prednisone; TACR, tacrolimus; Thal, thalidomide.

patients with established cGVHD [22]. At 80 days post transplantation, 59 patients were randomly assigned to treatment with thalidomide (200 mg BID) or placebo. The study was terminated early because the first interim analysis revealed a higher mortality and incidence of cGVHD among the group receiving thalidomide. The reasons for this seemingly paradoxical observation are unclear (since thalidomide appeared to be effective in the treatment of cGVHD). The hypothesis was that thalidomide might have interfered with normal regulatory mechanisms perhaps abrogating the effects of regulatory T cells.

In another study, thymus tissue implants, thymic endothelial cells, or thymic hormones (thymosin fraction five and thymopentin) were administered to recipients of HLA-matched sibling HCT [23]. No difference in the incidence of cGVHD was observed in patients receiving thymic tissue or thymic hormones compared with concurrent or historic controls.

Many studies have examined the efficacy of glucocorticoids, cyclosporine, and intravenous immune globulin (either alone or in combination) in preventing both acute and chronic disease. In a randomized prospective study, for example, the prophylactic efficacy of cyclosporine alone versus cyclosporine plus methylprednisolone was evaluated in 122 patients in whom HCT was performed from a HLA-identical sibling [24]. An increased incidence of cGVHD was observed in patients receiving combination therapy versus cyclosporine alone (44% vs. 21%, $p = 0.02$), suggesting that the addition of methylprednisolone to cyclosporine therapy may enhance the probability of developing cGVHD. At a median follow-up of 6.1 years, there was also the suggestion that more patients receiving the combination developed other complications, such as aseptic necrosis of the bone and chronic pulmonary disease, and have required immunosuppressive therapy for a longer duration [25].

To test the ability of prolonged use of cyclosporine in preventing cGVHD, patients who had received allogeneic HCT and had acute GVHD or histologic evidence of subclinical GVHD were randomly assigned to receive either 6 or 24 months of oral cyclosporine [26]. Clinical extensive cGVHD developed in 39% and 51% of those in the 6 and 24 month treatment groups, respectively ($p = 0.25$).

It is interesting that acute GVHD is the major predictor of cGVHD; however, combination immunosuppressive regimens showing reduced acute GVHD in prospective trials and have not had the same protective effect on cGVHD: there has been often a reduction of cGVHD in the arm with less acute GVHD, but not statistically significant. This suggests that cGVHD observed in some patients is independent from clinical acute GVHD.

STEM CELL SOURCE

It is now well documented that peripheral blood transplants (PBT) produce more cGVHD as compared to bone marrow transplants (BMT) [27–29]; recipients of a BMT have more cGVHD as compared to cord blood transplants (CBT) [30]. This is thought to be due to the larger number of T cells infused in PBT as compared to BMT and CBT, and this is in keeping with the observation that physical removal of T cells from the graft prevents both acute and cGVHD [11], also if the donor is HLA mismatched. Chronic GVHD after PBT is more frequent, more severe and less sensitive to treatment [31]. In some nonneoplastic disorders, such as aplastic anemia, cGVHD can only be harmful, and one may decide against using PBT, as suggested by a recent IBMTR/**The European Group for Blood and Marrow Transplantation** (EBMT) contribution [30]. In other diseases, one may want to maximize the antileukemic effect of the transplant: in this setting PBT are usually preferred, although strong evidence for an increased antileukemic effect of PBT is missing [32]. Cord blood transplants is probably the fastest growing type of transplant from unrelated donors: this is because the search is fast and the chance of finding at least one cord blood unit for a given patient is close to 100%: CBT produce significantly less cGVHD as compared to BMT, and the relapse rate in leukemia patients is not different [28, 29]. This interesting observation suggests that some of the antileukemic effect of the graft is either due to subclinical cGVHD or to some other mechanism: the correlation of cGVHD with RR remains very strong, in almost all disease categories, but CBTs suggest that there may be more than one way to prevent leukemia relapse.

In conclusion, the choice of the stem-cell source will have an impact on cGVHD: but sometimes we cannot choose, as we have only one option, and one may then modulate the transplant programs according to the stem-cell source.

RECENT DEVELOPMENTS

T Cells

An increase in suppressor T cells may be observed in cGVHD. These cells suppress T-cell proliferation and polyclonal immunoglobulin synthesis induced by various antigens [33, 34]. This may be one explanation for the increased immunosuppressive state found in patients with cGVHD and impaired immunologic tolerance.

Regulatory T Cells

A population of CD4+/CD25high T cells (T regulatory cells [Treg]) has been described in cGVHD [35]. Treg cells are able to prevent proliferation of a mixed leukocyte reaction and prevent acute GVHD in vivo. In one study, these Treg cells were hyporesponsive to polyclonal stimulation in vitro and suppressed the proliferation and cytokine synthesis of CD4+CD25- cells, an effect that was independent of IL-10 [35]. These results indicate that cGVHD injury does not occur as a result of Treg-cell deficiency. However, conflicting data have been reported with regards to the role of Treg cells in the development of cGVHD in humans [35, 36]. In one study, flow cytometry was used to measure the size of the Treg pool in the peripheral blood of 40 patients who survived more than 100 days following allogeneic HCT. Patients with cGVHD had significantly increased Treg cells, expressed both as a percentage of CD4+ T cells or as absolute counts, compared to patients without cGVHD. The authors also purified Treg cells from patients with cGVHD and used an in vitro functional assay to demonstrate that these cells display suppressive capabilities comparable to Treg cells isolated from healthy individuals.

Two additional studies [37, 38] further addressed the role of Treg cells in human cGVHD using both flow cytometry and quantitative PCR analysis of FoxP3 expression. One study found no significant difference between patients with or without cGVHD, in terms of both absolute FoxP3-expressing CD4+/CD25high cell counts as well as the frequency of these cells within the CD4+ T-cell compartment [37]. While the level of FoxP3 expression in the CD4+/CD25high population was comparable between allo-HCT patients and healthy individuals, there was a profound and persistent CD4+ T-cell lymphopenia in allo-HCT recipients compared to normal controls. A second study examined the expression of FoxP3 in total lymphocytes, rather than in the CD4+/CD25high T cells, as a method to evaluate the ratio of Treg cells relative to other immune cells [38]. The authors found a significant decrease in the frequency of Treg cells in patients with active cGVHD compared to patients who did not develop the disease or who had resolved disease following treatment.

These apparent discrepancies might reflect the varying strategies employed to measure the Treg population, including its phenotypic definition [39]. Utilization of additional cell surface marker such as CD127 may help to resolve these apparently contradictory results.

Agonistic Autoantibodies to Platelet-Derived Growth Factor Receptor

Patients with scleroderma have been shown to have autoantibodies against the platelet-derived growth factor receptor (PDGFR) that trigger an intracellular loop, involving Ha–Rasextracellular signal-regulated kinases 1 and 2 (ERK1/2) and reactive oxygen species (ROS) [39]. This leads to increased collagen gene expression and myofibroblast phenotype conversion of normal human primary fibroblasts, strongly suggesting a pathogenetic role of anti-PDGF autoantibodies in the fibrosis of patients with scleroderma. Also patients with cGVHD have been recently shown to have the same agonistic antibodies to PDGF receptor: 37 patients were reported, of whom 22 had extensive cGVHD and 15 were healthy long-term survivors after an allogeneic BMT [40]. The antibodies were found in all 22 patients with cGVHD and in no healthy long-term survivor. The stimulatory activity of the antibodies was proven by their ability to stimulate tyrosine phosphorilation of PDGFR, expression of type I collagen alpha 1 and alpha 2 gene, Ha–Ras ER –ROS signaling pathway. Therefore the antibodies found in

cGVHD cannot be distinguished from the antibodies found in scleroderma [41]. These results suggest that (1) cGVHD can be seen as a model for autoimmunity, (2) the identification of PDGFR antibodies may have practical relevance: for example the use of tyrosine kinase inhibitors, such as imatinib mesylate, may be of clinical benefit [42].

CONCLUSIONS

We have made some progress in our understanding of the pathogenesis of cGVHD, and this may lead to better prevention and treatment of this complication. For the time being, however, we are confronted with our transplant programs, some of which may reduce, some may increase, the incidence and severity of the disease.

If we use unrelated or family mismatched donors, after intensive preparative regimens, with peripheral blood as stem-cell source, and no T-cell antibodies in the conditioning, then the risk of cGVHD is going to be high. Cord blood transplants, or T-cell depletion, on the other hand, are associated with a low incidence of this complications. In the past three decades, reduction of GVHD has always been associated in the long term with increased leukemia relapse. We can design programs to produce a given risk of cGVHD: whether this will translate in a survival benefit for the patients can only be assessed in prospective randomized trials.

REFERENCES

1. Filipovich AH, Weisdorf D, Pavletic S, et al. National Institutes of Health consensus development project on criteria for clinical trials in chronic graft-versus-host disease: I. Diagnosis and staging working group report. *Biol Blood Marrow Transplant.* 2005 Dec;11(12):945–956.
2. Sullivan, KM. Acute and chronic graft-versus-host disease in man. *Int J Cell Cloning.* 1986; 4(Suppl 1):42.
3. Witherspoon RP, Storb R, Ochs HD, et al. Recovery of antibody production in human allogeneic marrow graft recipients: influence of time posttransplantation, the presence or absence of chronic graft-versus-host disease, and antithymocyte globulin treatment. *Blood* 1981 Aug;58(2):360–368.
4. Lum LG, Orcutt-Thordarson N, Seigneuret MC, Storb R. The regulation of Ig synthesis after marrow transplantation. IV. T4 and T8 subset function in patients with chronic graft-vs-host disease. *J Immunol.* 1982 Jul;129(1):113–119.
5. Reisner Y, Kapoor N, O'Reilly RJ, Good RA. Allogeneic bone marrow transplantation using stem cells fractionated by lectins: VI, in vitro analysis of human and monkey bone marrow cells fractionated by sheep red blood cells and soybean agglutinin *Lancet.* 1980 Dec 20–27;2(8208–8209):1320–1324.
6. Janossy G, Prentice HG, Hoffbrand AV, Blacklock HA, Ivory K, Gilmore MJ. The role of monoclonal antibodies in the prevention of graft versus host disease. *Med Oncol Tumor Pharmacother.* 1984;1(4):279–84.
7. Urbano-Ispizua A, Carreras E, Marin P, et al. Allogeneic transplantation of CD34(+) selected cells from peripheral blood from

human leukocyte antigen-identical siblings: detrimental effect of a high number of donor CD34(+) cells? *Blood*. 2001 Oct 15;98(8):2352–2357.

8. Schumm M, Handgretinger R, Pfeiffer M, et al. Determination of residual T- and B-cell content after immunomagnetic depletion: proposal for flow cytometric analysis and results from 103 separations. *Cytotherapy*. 2006;8(5):465–472.

9. Koehl U, Esser R, Zimmermann S, et al. Ex vivo expansion of highly purified NK cells for immunotherapy after haploidentical stem cell transplantation in children. *Klin Padiatr*. 2005 Nov–Dec;217(6):345–350.

10. Bitan M, Shapira MY, Resnick IB, et al. Successful transplantation of haploidentically mismatched peripheral blood stem cells using CD133+-purified stem cells. *Exp Hematol*. 2005 Jun;33(6):713–718.

11. Aversa F, Terenzi A, Tabilio A, et al. Full haplotype-mismatched hematopoietic stem-cell transplantation: a phase II study in patients with acute leukemia at high risk of relapse. *J Clin Oncol*. 2005 May 20;23(15):3447–3454.

12. Barge RM, Starrenburg CW, Falkenburg JH, Fibbe WE, Marijt EW, Willemze R. Long-term follow-up of myeloablative allogeneic stem cell transplantation using Campath "in the bag" as T-cell depletion: the Leiden experience. *Bone Marrow Transplant*. 2006 Jun;37(12):1129–1134.

13. McKenna DH Jr, Sumstad D, Bostrom N, et al. Good manufacturing practices production of natural killer cells for immunotherapy: a six-year single-institution experience. *Transfusion*. 2007 Mar;47(3):520–528.

14. Aversa F, Tabilio A, Velardi A, et al. Treatment of high-risk acute leukemia with T-cell-depleted stem cells from related donors with one fully mismatched HLA haplotype. *N Engl J Med*. 1998;17:1186–1193.

15. Keever CA, Small TN, Flomenberg N, et al. Immune reconstitution following bone marrow transplantation: comparison of recipients of T-cell depleted marrow with recipients of conventional marrow grafts. *Blood*. 1989 Apr;73(5):1340–1350.

16. Horowitz MM, Gale RP, Sondel PM, et al. Risk factors for chronic graft-versus-host disease after HLA-identical sibling bone marrow transplantation. *Blood*. 1990;75:2459–2464.

17. Marmont AM, Horowitz MM, Gale RP, et al. T-cell depletion of HLA-identical transplants in leukemia. *Blood*. 1991;78:2120–2130.

18. Kalaycio M, Rybicki L, Pohlman B, et al. CD8+ T-cell-depleted, matched unrelated donor, allogeneic bone marrow transplantation for advanced AML using busulfan-based preparative regimens. *Bone Marrow Transplant*. 2005 Feb;35(3):247–252.

19. Remberger M, Storer B, Ringden O, Anasetti C. Association between pre-transplant thymoglobulin and reduced non relapse mortality after unrelated marrow transplantation. *Bone Marrow Transpl*. 2002;29:391–394.

20. Bacigalupo A. Antilymphocyte/thymocyte globulin for graft versus host disease prophylaxis: efficacy and side effects. *Bone. Marrow Transplant*. 2005 Feb;35(3):225–231. Review.

21. Bacigalupo A, Lamparelli T, Barisione G, et al. Thymoglobulin prevents chronic graft-versus-host disease, chronic lung dysfunction, and late transplant-related mortality: long-term follow-up of a randomized trial in patients undergoing unrelated donor transplantation. *Biol Blood Marrow Transplant*. 2006 May;12(5):560–565.

22. Chao NJ, Parker PM, Niland JC, et al. Paradoxical effect of thalidomide prophylaxis on chronic graft-vs.-host disease. *Biol Blood Marrow Transplant* 1996 May;2(2):86–92.

23. Witherspoon RP, Sullivan KM, Lum LG, et al. Use of thymic grafts or thymic factors to augment immunologic recovery after bone marrow transplantation: brief report with 2 to 12 years' follow-up. *Bone Marrow Transplant*. 1988 Sep;3(5):425–435.

24. Deeg HJ, Lin D, Leisenring W, Boeckh M, et al. Cyclosporine or cyclosporine plus methylprednisolone for prophylaxis of graft-versus-host disease: a prospective, randomized trial. *Blood*. 1997 May 15;89(10):3880–3887.

25. Deeg, HJ, Flowers, ME, Leisenring, W, et al. Cyclosporine (CSP) or CSP plus methylprednisolone for graft-versus-host disease prophylaxis in patients with high-risk lymphohemopoietic malignancies: long-term follow-up of a randomized trial. *Blood*. 2000;96:1194.

26. Kansu E, Gooley T, Flowers ME, et al. Administration of cyclosporine for 24 months compared with 6 months for prevention of chronic graft-versus-host disease: a prospective randomized clinical trial. *Blood*. 2001;98(13):3868–3870.

27. Schmitz N, Beksac M, Bacigalupo A, et al. Filgrastim-mobilized peripheral blood progenitor cells versus bone marrow transplantation for treating leukemia: 3-year results from the EBMT randomized trial. *Haematologica*. 2005 May;90(5):643–648.

28. Champlin RE, Schmitz N, Horowitz MM, et al. Blood stem cells compared with bone marrow as a source of hematopoietic cells for allogeneic transplantation. IBMTR Histocompatibility and Stem Cell Sources Working Committee and the European Group for Blood and Marrow Transplantation (EBMT). *Blood*. 2000 Jun 15;95(12):3702–3709.

29. Schrezenmeier H, Passweg JR, Marsh JC, et al. Worse outcome and more chronic GVHD with peripheral blood progenitor cells than bone marrow in HLA-matched sibling donor transplants for young patients with severe acquired aplastic anemia: A report from the European Group for Blood and Marrow Transplantation and the Center for International Blood and Marrow Transplant Research. *Blood*. 2007 May 2; Epub ahead of print.

30. Rocha V, Labopin M, Sanz G, et al. Transplants of Umbilical-Cord Blood or Bone Marrow from Unrelated Donors in Adults with Acute Leukemia. *N Engl J Med*. 2004;351:2276–2285.

31. Storek J, Gooley T, Siadak M, et al. Allogeneic peripheral blood stem cell transplantation may be associated with a high risk of chronic graft-versus-host disease. *Blood* Dec 1997;90:4705–4709.

32. Champlin RE, Schmitz N, Horowitz MM, et al. Blood stem cells compared with bone marrow as a source of hematopoietic cells for allogeneic transplantation. *Blood*, 95;2000: 3702–3709.

33. Korsmeyer SJ, Elfenbein GJ, Goldman CK, et al. B cell, helper T cell, and suppressor T cell abnormalities contribute to disordered immunoglobulin synthesis in patients following bone marrow transplantation. *Transplantation*. 1982 Feb;33(2): 184–190.

34. Tsoi MS, Storb R, Dobbs S, et al. Nonspecific suppressor cells in patients with chronic graft-vs-host disease after marrow grafting. *J Immunol*. 1979 Nov;123(5):1970–1976.

35. Clark FJ, Gregg R, Piper K, et al. Chronic graft-versus-host disease is associated with increased numbers of peripheral blood CD4+CD25high regulatory T cells. *Blood*. 2004;103(6): 2410–2416.

36. Sanchez J, Casano J, Alvarez MA, et al. Kinetic of regulatory CD25high and activated CD134+ (OX40) T lymphocytes during acute and chronic graft-versus-host disease after

allogeneic bone marrow transplantation. *Br J Haematol.* 2004; 126:697–703.

37. Meignin V, de Latour RP, Zuber J, et al. Numbers of Foxp3-expressing CD4+CD25high T cells do not correlate with the establishment of long-term tolerance after allogeneic stem cell transplantation. *Exp Hematol.* 2005 Aug;33(8):894–900.

38. Zorn E, Kim HT, Lee SJ, et al. Reduced frequency of FOXP3+ CD4+CD25+ regulatory T cells in patients with chronic graft-versus-host disease. *Blood.* 2005;106(8):2903–2911.

39. Zorn E, Ritz J. Studying human regulatory T cells in vivo. *Clin Cancer Res.* 2006;12(18):5265–5267.

40. Svegliati-Baroni G, Santillo M, Bevilacqua F, et al. Stimulatory autoantibodies to PDGF in systemic sclerosis. *N Engl J Med.* 2006;354, 2667.

41. Svegliati S, Olivieri A, Campelli N, et al. Stimulatory autoantibodies to PDGF receptor in patients with extensive chronic graft-versus-host disease. *Blood.* 2007 Jul 1;110(1):237–241. Epub 2007 Mar 15.

42. Majhail NS, Schiffer CA, Weisdorf DJ. Improvement of pulmonary function with imatinib mesylate in bronchiolitis obliterans following allogeneic hematopoietic cell transplantation. *Biol Blood Marrow Transplant.* 2006 Jul;12(7):789–791.

12

Front Line Treatment of Chronic Graft versus Host Disease

Paul J. Martin and Andrew L. Gilman

INTRODUCTION

This chapter outlines an approach for front line therapy of chronic graft versus host disease (GVHD). High-dose glucocorticoids have served as the mainstay of treatment since the early 1980s, and the adjunctive administration of a calcineurin inhibitor may reduce the amount or duration of glucocorticoid treatment needed to control the disease. Judicious use of glucocorticoids at the lowest effective dose and alternate-day administration can minimize steroid-related side effects. Antibiotic prophylaxis to prevent infection and supportive care to minimize morbidity and prevent disability are critically important components in the management of patients with chronic GVHD. Approximately 50% of patients with chronic GVHD are able to discontinue immunosuppressive treatment within 5 years after the diagnosis, and 10% require continued treatment beyond 5 years. The remaining 40% die or develop recurrent malignancy before chronic GVHD resolves. Improved understanding of the pathogenesis of the disease will be needed in order to develop more effective therapy. The primary challenge for the future will be the discovery of targeted approaches that control chronic GVHD, while preserving graft-versus-malignancy effects mediated by immunologic activity of donor cells against neoplastic cells in the recipient and allowing reconstitution of normal immune defenses against pathogens.

Studies during the early 1980s demonstrated the importance of early diagnosis and the efficacy of glucocorticoid treatment in reducing morbidity and mortality among patients with chronic GVHD [1]. Outcomes for patients with chronic GVHD have not significantly improved since then, largely because the pathogenesis of chronic GVHD is poorly understood and because very few randomized phase III trials have been carried out. As discussed in other chapters, the disease presents with highly variable and protean clinical manifestations that may result from different pathophysiologic mechanisms. This variability of clinical manifestations makes laboratory studies and clinical trials particularly difficult.

INDICATIONS FOR SYSTEMIC TREATMENT OF CHRONIC GVHD

Untreated extensive chronic GVHD causes severe morbidity and disability with a high risk of death primarily due to immunodeficiency and infections, and to a lesser degree organ failure [1]. Prompt diagnosis and initiation of treatment are important to limit the severity of chronic GVHD, to minimize disability, and to prevent mortality.

A major decision to be made after the diagnosis of chronic GVHD is whether the manifestations require no therapy, topical therapy, or systemic therapy. The historical grading system of "limited" and "extensive" chronic GVHD was developed as a tool to determine which patients require systemic treatment. Patients with limited disease have localized skin involvement, liver involvement without chronic aggressive hepatitis, bridging necrosis or cirrhosis, or both localized skin involvement and liver involvement [2]. Limited chronic GVHD was described as having a favorable prognosis, suggesting that this presentation could be adequately treated with topical therapy [1–4]. Patients with extensive disease have more diffuse skin involvement, more aggressive liver disease, or involvement of other organs such as the eyes, mouth, gastrointestinal tract, connective tissues, lungs, or genital tract. Extensive chronic GVHD was described as having an unfavorable prognosis, suggesting that this presentation required systemic immunosuppressive treatment.

According to more recent recommendations, systemic immunosuppressive treatment is not needed for patients who have chronic GVHD with only mild abnormalities involving only one or two sites such as the mouth, liver, skin, eyes, or genital tract in the absence of thrombocytopenia (platelet count < 100,000/μL) or steroid treatment at the time of diagnosis, but systemic treatment is needed for patients who have chronic GVHD with more severe abnormalities, such as localized cutaneous sclerosis (morphea), even when a single site is involved (Table 12.1) [3–5]. Any functional impairment caused by chronic GVHD involving the eyes, mouth, or female genital tract warrants systemic treatment. Weight loss

Table 12.1: Indications for Systemic Immunosuppressive Treatment of Chronic GVHD

Involvement of ≥3 sites
Involvement of a single site with more than mild abnormalities
Lung involvement

Platelet count < 100,000/μL
Onset of chronic GVHD during Steroid treatment
Progressive onset from acute GVHD

GVHD, graft versus host disease.
The table is reprinted by courtesy of *International Journal of Hematology.*

(>15% of baseline), dysphagia, and odynophagia indicate severe gastrointestinal GVHD. Marked elevation of the alkaline phosphatase or serum bilirubin concentration or transaminase levels can indicate chronic GVHD requiring systemic immunosuppressive treatment [6]. Other severe complications such as fasciitis, contractures, serositis, and pulmonary involvement always require systemic treatment.

Systemic treatment is always indicated in patients with chronic GVHD involving multiple sites and in patients with thrombocytopenia (platelet count < 100,000/μL), since these patients have an increased risk of nonrelapse mortality [7–9]. Likewise, systemic immunosuppressive therapy is indicated for patients with a quiescent or progressive-onset who are diagnosed with chronic GVHD during treatment with prednisone, since the GVHD manifestations in these patients would almost certainly have greater severity in the absence of steroid administration. Moreover, the onset of chronic GHVD during treatment with prednisone is associated with an increased risk of nonrelapse mortality [10].

A variety of prognostic scores can be used in formulating treatment decisions. Progressive onset of chronic GVHD from acute GVHD, platelet count < 100,000/μl, diffuse skin involvement, gastrointestinal involvement, and poor performance status have been consistently associated with increased risk of nonrelapse mortality in retrospective studies of chronic GVHD [3]. Independent risk factors included in a prognostic score developed from International Blood and Marrow Transplant Registry (IBMTR) data were Karnofsky performance score, diarrhea, weight loss, rash, and oral involvement [11]. Additional unfavorable risk factors identified in other studies were higher dose of prednisone at the time of diagnosis, hyperbilirubinemia, and older age of the donor and recipient [10, 12]. The National Institutes of Health (NIH) Consensus Development Project proposed categories of mild, moderate, and severe chronic GVHD that may be predictive of response (Gilman, unpublished). As a simple algorithm, patients with progressive onset of chronic GVHD or with a platelet count < 100,000/μL may be considered to have "high-risk" chronic GVHD, and those with neither of these features may be considered to have "standard-risk" chronic GVHD.

INITIAL TREATMENT

The required intensity and duration of initial treatment for chronic GVHD is not well established. The benefit of controlling disease activity in order to prevent irreversible tissue damage must be weighed against the harm of any potential irreversible complications of treatment. Effective treatment should prevent disability caused by fibrosis in soft tissues, destruction of lacrimal and salivary glands, and obliteration of small airways, while minimizing the risk of severe complications such as avascular necrosis or life-threatening infections.

The complications of steroid treatment and the frequent occurrence of steroid-resistant or steroid-dependent disease have encouraged the evaluation of many immunosuppressive agents for treatment of chronic GVHD. Phase II studies have suggested that some of these immunosuppressive agents have activity for chronic GVHD. Favorable reports of results of open label phase II studies of immunosuppressive agents for secondary treatment of chronic GVHD, however, should not be extrapolated to support a presumption of similar benefit when the agent is used for initial treatment. For example, despite the activity of azathioprine for treatment of chronic GVHD, results of a double-blind phase III study showed inferior outcomes when azathioprine was used together with prednisone for initial treatment of patients with standard-risk chronic GVHD [7]. Similarly, no benefit was observed when thalidomide was used together with prednisone for initial treatment of chronic GVHD, despite reports that thalidomide can provide benefit for patients with steroid-refractory or steroid-resistant chronic GVHD [13–15].

Table 12.2 summarizes results of randomized studies for treatment of newly diagnosed chronic GVHD, and Table 12.3 outlines an approach to initial systemic immunosuppressive treatment [16]. Prednisone currently represents a major component of treatment for chronic GVHD [1, 3, 4]. The efficacy of prednisone is most easily demonstrated by common clinical experience that disease manifestations often improve after increasing the dose of prednisone and that an exacerbation of disease manifestations can follow a reduction in the dose of prednisone, regardless of concomitant treatment with other immunosuppressive medications.

Treatment with prednisone should begin as soon as possible after the initial diagnosis of chronic GVHD. As a general guideline, prednisone should be administered at the lowest dose sufficient to control the disease. The dose of prednisone at the beginning of treatment should not exceed 1.0 mg/kg actual body weight, except in patients who are under treatment with higher doses at the onset of the disease. Prednisone should be administered once daily as soon as possible after awakening in the morning in order to mimic the normal circadian rhythm of glucocorticoid secretion by the adrenal glands. Treatment should be continued at this dose until there is objective evidence of improvement in manifestations of chronic GVHD (see below). If there is no improvement, treatment with additional immunosuppressive medications should be initiated within 2 months or sooner

Table 12.2: Phase III Studies of Initial Treatment

Author	Arms Compared	Double-Blind	N (Number of Patients)	Results
Sullivan [7]	Prednisone ± azathioprine	Yes	179	Decreased survival
Koc [16]	Prednisone ± cyclosporine	No	287	Limited benefit
Koc [14]	Cyclosporine, prednisone ± thalidomide	Yes	51	Toxicity
Arora [15]	Cyclosporine, prednisone ± thalidomide	No	55	No benefit

The table is reprinted by courtesy of *International Journal of Hematology.*

if manifestations of disease progress (see below). Tapering of prednisone doses should begin within 2 weeks after the first evidence of improvement in manifestations of chronic GVHD, even if manifestations have not entirely resolved (Table 12.3 and Figure 12.1). Tapering should continue to a dose of 1.0 mg/kg every other day, as long as there is no exacerbation in manifestations of chronic GVHD. After reaching a dose of 1.0 mg/kg every other day, the taper schedule should be suspended, and the dose of prednisone should be held constant for 3 to 4 months and then tapered to 0.5 mg/kg every other day and continued until all reversible manifestations of chronic GVHD resolve. After all reversible manifestations of chronic GVHD resolve, the taper schedule should be resumed. Administration of prednisone may be discontinued after 2 to 4 weeks of treatment at a dose of 0.15 mg/kg every other day. Physicians and patients must be vigilant for the emergence of symptomatic adrenal insufficiency after the dose of prednisone has been reduced below 10 mg/day (or 20 mg every other day) for adults or below the equivalent physiologic maintenance dose for children. The rate of tapering should be slowed if a diagnosis of adrenal insufficiency is confirmed, and small doses of prednisone can be given on the "off" days to relieve symptoms. Stress dose replacement therapy should be given whenever necessary [17].

A physician should examine the patient before each reduction in the dose of prednisone. If there is exacerbation or recurrence of chronic GVHD at any step of the taper, the dose of prednisone should be increased by two levels, with daily administration for 2 to 4 weeks, followed by tapering again to alternate-day administration. Treatment should then be continued for at least 3 months before attempting to resume the taper. Toxicity associated with the administration of prednisone may require dose adjustments, which should be managed according to the needs of the patient.

Long-term treatment with high-dose prednisone is associated with a high risk of morbidity. Complications prominently include avascular necrosis, glucose intolerance requiring administration of insulin, infections, hypertension, weight gain, changes in body habitus, cutaneous atrophy and striae, cataracts, osteoporosis, emotional lability, interference with sleep, and growth retardation in children. Some of these complications can be ameliorated by alternate-day administration of prednisone as opposed to daily administration [18, 19].

Table 12.3: Approach to Initial Systemic Immunosuppressive Treatment for Chronic GVHD

Continue administration of calcineurin inhibitor
Administer prednisone, initially at 1 mg/kg/day
Taper to 1.0 mg/kg alternate day prednisone administration after clinical improvement
Continue prednisone at 1.0 mg/kg every other day for 3–4 months
Taper prednisone dose to 0.5 mg/kg every other day
Continue prednisone until clinical resolution
Gradual withdrawal of prednisone after resolution
Gradual withdrawal of calcineurin inhibitor
No demonstrated benefit from additional agents (studies in progress)

GVHD, graft versus host disease.
The table is reprinted by courtesy of *International Journal of Hematology.*

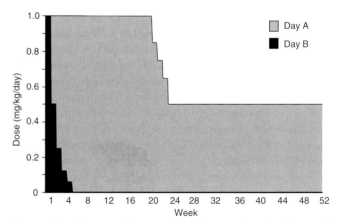

Figure 12.1 **One possible approach for tapering the doses of prednisone.** Treatment begins with daily administration of prednisone at 1 mg/kg/day. As soon as improvement occurs, doses are gradually tapered on alternate days (day B) to reach an alternate-day schedule of administration at 1.0 mg/kg every other day. This regimen is continued for another 3 months, and then the dose is gradually reduced to 0.5 mg/kg/day, provided that disease manifestations continue to improve. This dose is sustained until all readily reversible manifestations have resolved [16, 19].

Manifestations of chronic GVHD generally do not improve when steroid treatment is started as an alternate-day regimen. For this reason, daily administration of prednisone is required for initial therapy.

ROLE OF CALCINEURIN INHIBITORS FOR INITIAL TREATMENT OF CHRONIC GVHD

The use of cyclosporine for treatment of chronic GVHD was initially tested in patients with thrombocytopenia as an indicator of poor prognosis. The survival of such patients at 3 years after transplant was only 26% when prednisone was used for treatment [7]. In contrast to these results, the survival at 3 years after transplant among 40 patients treated with an alternate-day regimen of cyclosporine and prednisone was 52% [19]. These results suggested that survival of patients with newly diagnosed high-risk chronic GVHD might be improved by treatment with cyclosporine.

In a subsequent randomized trial, the efficacy of cyclosporine plus prednisone was compared to prednisone alone for treatment of clinical extensive chronic GVHD in patients who did not have thrombocytopenia [16]. Prednisone was administered initially at a dose of 1.0 mg/kg/day, followed by a prolonged taper, and cyclosporine was administered at a dose of 12 mg/kg orally every other day. The hazards of transplant-related mortality, overall mortality, recurrent malignancy, secondary systemic therapy for chronic GVHD, and discontinuation of all immunosuppressive therapy were not significantly different between the two arms, but there was a trend suggesting a lower probability of relapse-free survival in the two-drug arm. Eighteen (13%) of the 142 patients in the cyclosporine plus prednisone arm and 32 (22%) of the 145 patients in the prednisone arm developed avascular necrosis. Among patients with standard-risk chronic GVHD as indicated by a de novo or quiescent onset, there were no statistically significant differences in any of the outcome measures between the two arms, other than the incidence of avascular necrosis. The decreased incidence of avascular necrosis suggested that administration of cyclosporine reduced the amount of steroid treatment needed to control chronic GVHD in these patients. The benefit of reducing the risk of avascular necrosis must be balanced against adverse effects such as renal impairment caused by cyclosporine.

Among patients with high-risk chronic GVHD as indicated by a progressive onset from acute GVHD but with platelet counts >100,000/µL, the cumulative incidence of death from causes other than recurrent malignancy at 5 years was 38% in the cyclosporine plus prednisone arm, compared to 14% in the prednisone arm. Survival at 5 years was 43% in the cyclosporine plus prednisone arm, compared to 76% in the prednisone arm. Six of the 16 patients with high-risk chronic GVHD in the cyclosporine plus prednisone arm had fatal infections, compared to 4 of the 29 patients with high-risk chronic GVHD in the prednisone arm. The incidence of avascular necrosis was not decreased by administration of cyclosporine among patients with progressive-onset chronic GVHD. In this population, the amount of steroid treatment needed to control the disease appears to have overwhelmed any potential steroid-sparing effect of cyclosporine, at least as measured by the incidence of avascular necrosis. Since the study did not attempt to define the full spectrum of benefits and risks when using a calcineurin inhibitor as a steroid-sparing agent in patients with chronic GVHD, clinical judgments must be made for each patient on a case-by-case basis.

There was some concern that treatment with both cyclosporine and prednisone might have increased the risk of fatal infection among patients with progressive-onset chronic GVHD, but the results are difficult to interpret, since the data came from a subset analysis that was not prespecified as part of the analysis plan. In fact, survival results for the 16 patients treated with cyclosporine and prednisone were comparable to those for similarly treated patients with high-risk chronic GVHD in another study [19], while results for the 29 patients treated with prednisone alone were much better than expected, based on comparisons with a previous study [7]. These considerations suggest that results of the subset analysis cannot be taken entirely at face value, but the data emphasize the threat posed by infections and the need for antibiotic prophylaxis in patients with chronic GVHD (see below). These studies were conducted with an alternate-day regimen of cyclosporine administration, and the results might not apply with daily administration of cyclosporine, which now represents the usual clinical practice [20]. Nonetheless, the results suggest that, in the absence of a specific contraindication, it would be reasonable to consider the administration of a calcineurin inhibitor as part of the immunosuppressive regimen for patients with newly diagnosed chronic GVHD in order to decrease the need for steroid treatment as much as possible.

Cyclosporine and tacrolimus should never be given simultaneously. Dose adjustments may be made to maintain serum trough cyclosporine concentrations at 150 to 300 ng/mL or tacrolimus concentrations at 5 to 10 ng/mL. Renal function should be monitored throughout treatment, and doses of cyclosporine or tacrolimus should be reduced whenever necessary to prevent excessive renal impairment. Drug levels should be monitored in patients receiving medications that may adversely affect the concentration of cyclosporine or tacrolimus. These medications include calcium channel blockers, antimicrobials, and antiepileptic agents (Table 12.4).

ROLE OF OTHER AGENTS FOR INITIAL TREATMENT OF CHRONIC GVHD

Several studies have demonstrated activity of thalidomide for steroid-resistant chronic GVHD in adults and children. Despite the promising results from small studies, a large phase II study showed a low response rate and a high incidence of side effects including sedation, constipation, neuropathy, rash, and neutropenia[13]. Randomized phase III studies showed a high incidence of side effects and no apparent improvement

Table 12.4: Medications Affecting Blood Levels of Cyclosporine or Tacrolimus

Increase Levels	Decrease Levels
Triazole antifungals: voriconazole,* itraconazole, fluconazole, ketoconazole	*Antibiotics*: rifampin, isoniazid
Calcium channel blockers: verapamil, diltiazem, nicardipine, nifedipine	*Antiepileptics*: phenytoin, phenobarbital, carbamazepine
Antibiotics: erythromycin, clarithromycin,	
Others: sirolimus, cimetidine, metaclopromide, octreotide	

* The dose of cyclosporine or tacrolimus frequently must be reduced by 50% to 67% during concomitant therapy with voriconazole. The table is reprinted by courtesy of *International Journal of Hematology*.

in response rates when thalidomide was added to prednisone and cyclosporine for treatment of high-risk chronic GVHD [14, 15].

Several small studies have evaluated the use of mycophenolate mofetil (MMF) for treatment of steroid-resistant chronic GVHD in adults and children. MMF is a prodrug of mycophenolic acid, which inhibits T-cell proliferation by blocking the activity of inosine monophosphate dehydrogenase. In a study of MMF for 15 children with steroid-resistant chronic GVHD, improvement was observed in gastrointestinal, oral, and nonsclerotic skin manifestations, and thrombocytopenia also improved in some patients [21]. A retrospective study reported clinical improvement in 27 of 34 patients who received MMF for initial (n = 10) or secondary (n = 24) treatment of chronic GVHD [22]. Two multicenter, double-blind, randomized phase III studies of MMF or mycophenolic acid for initial systemic treatment of chronic GVHD are in progress, one in the United States and Canada and the other in Europe.

Hydroxychloroquine is an antimalarial medication that is widely used as a steroid-sparing agent for the treatment of rheumatoid arthritis and systemic lupus erythematosis. Results of a phase II study suggested that hydroxychloroquine has activity for treatment of steroid-resistant or dependent chronic GVHD, since improvement was observed in skin, oral, and hepatic manifestations, and thrombocytopenia often improved [23]. A double-blind randomized phase III study of hydroxychloroquine added to prednisone and cyclosporine for initial systemic treatment of chronic GVHD was started but could not be completed because of slow enrollment. Results of this partially completed study were not able to demonstrate clinical benefit from adding hydroxychloroquine to prednisone and a calcineurin inhibitor for the treatment of newly diagnosed chronic GVHD.

Although results of an early randomized trial did not support the use of azathioprine together with prednisone for initial treatment of chronic GVHD [7], results of a more recent retrospective study suggested that azathioprine might provide some benefit in combination with methylprednisolone and cyclosporine for initial or secondary treatment of moderate to severe chronic GVHD [24]. Cyclosporine was given daily, and methylprednisolone and azathioprine were given on alternate days. Doses of cyclosporine and azathioprine were tapered before tapering the doses of methylprednisolone. The complete

response rate for initial therapy among 18 patients was 94%, and survival at 1 year was 89%. At the time of the report, only 1 of the 16 surviving patients still had chronic GVHD requiring systemic immunosuppressive treatment. All of the patients had hematopoietic cell transplantation (HCT) for treatment of thalassemia, and all were < 26 years of age. These encouraging preliminary results have not yet been confirmed in a prospective study with older patients or for patients who have had HCT for malignant disease.

Local therapy can be useful for the treatment of some manifestations of chronic GVHD. For example, psoralen and ultraviolet A (PUVA) therapy has good activity for lichenoid skin disease but is less effective for treatment of sclerotic skin disease [25]. Topical glucocorticoid rinses are effective for management of oral manifestations [4]. High-potency inhaled steroids can help to halt the progression of bronchiolitis obliterans [26, 27].

POTENTIAL EFFECTS OF IMMUNOSUPPRESSIVE TREATMENT ON RISK OF RECURRENT MALIGNANCY

The single benefit of chronic GVHD is a reduced risk of recurrent or progressive malignancy. These observations have led to the widespread practice of withdrawing immunosuppressive treatment or giving donor lymphocytes for recurrent or progressive malignancy after HCT. In certain situations, this approach has produced durable remissions, depending on the type of the disease, the burden of malignant cells, and the duration of remission after HCT. This experience has raised the question of whether treatment for chronic GVHD should be attenuated in patients who are at high risk of recurrent or progressive malignancy after HCT.

The answer depends on whether the immunologic activity of donor cells against malignant cells in the recipient is viewed as a rapid, complete "all or none" process or a slower, gradual reduction in the number of malignant cells. Since an "all or none" graft-versus-malignancy effect is likely to have begun before the onset of treatment and might be expected to continue even after the onset of treatment, the intensity of immunosuppressive treatment for chronic GVHD might have little effect on the risk of recurrent malignancy. On the other hand, the intensity of immunosuppressive treatment would be expected to impair a gradual graft-versus-malignancy effect. A further consideration is the susceptibility of malignant cells in the recipient to immunologic effects of donor cells. The intensity of immunosuppressive treatment might be more important for indolent malignancies that are more susceptible to graft-versus-malignancy effects than for rapidly progressive diseases that are less susceptible to such effects.

Data from clinical trials are not adequate to answer this important question. The randomized trial of cyclosporine plus prednisone versus prednisone alone showed no statistically significant adverse effect of the two-drug regimen on risk of recurrent malignancy [16]. This study included patients with diverse malignancies, including acute leukemia and chronic myeloid leukemia (CML). Unfortunately, the number of patients with CML in chronic phase was too small to determine whether administration of cyclosporine together with prednisone was associated with an increased risk of recurrent malignancy for these patients. Until further results from randomized trials are available, physicians will have to use clinical judgment in weighing the risk of inadequately controlled chronic GVHD against the threat of recurrent malignancy in calibrating the intensity of immunosuppressive treatment, keeping in mind that diseases with the highest risk of recurrence typically have the lowest susceptibility to graft-versus-malignancy effects.

PREVENTION OF INFECTION DURING TREATMENT OF CHRONIC GVHD [3, 4, 28]

Recommendations for infection prophylaxis and for immunizations for patients with chronic GVHD can be obtained at the Centers for Disease Control and Prevention (CDC) web site: http://www.cdc.gov/mmwr/preview/mmwrhtml/rr4910a1.htm. Antibiotic prophylaxis to prevent *Pneumocystis* pneumonia and encapsulated bacterial infections is strongly recommended for all patients until 6 months after resolution of chronic GVHD and discontinuation of all systemic immunosuppressive treatment. Vaccination against *Pneumococci* and *Haemophilus influenzae B* at 1 year after HCT is strongly recommended, since chronic GVHD impairs splenic clearance of encapsulated organisms. Conjugate pneumococcal vaccine should be used instead of unconjugated vaccine, since the response to unconjugated vaccines is poor in patients at 1 year after HCT [29]. Intravenous administration of gamma globulin may be indicated for patients who have recurrent bacterial infections and serum immunoglobulin (Ig)G concentrations < 400 mg/dL or deficiencies of IgG2 or IgG4.

Patients who are at risk of *Cytomegalovirus* (CMV) infection should have virologic surveillance of blood and pre-emptive antiviral therapy should be instituted whenever surveillance tests become positive, before the onset of overt CMV disease [30]. If feasible, CMV-seronegative recipients with CMV-seronegative donors should receive screened or leukocyte-depleted blood products. In addition, long-term administration of valacyclovir or acyclovir is recommended to prevent reactivation of Varicella zoster in patients previously infected with this virus. Patients should not be given live virus vaccines such as MMR until at least 1 year after resolution of chronic GVHD and withdrawal of all immunosuppressive treatment. The safety and efficacy of *Varicella zoster* virus (VZV) vaccination after resolution of chronic GVHD has not yet been determined.

Glucocorticoid treatment increases the risk of fungal infections [31]. Prophylactic administration of fluconazole can prevent certain types of candida infections, but this agent is not effective for prevention of invasive mold infections. Clinical trials will be needed to determine whether newer agents such as itraconazole, voriconazole, or posaconazole can prevent invasive mold infections during glucocorticoid treatment for patients with chronic GVHD [32].

Supportive care: Site-specific therapies are an extremely important component of symptomatic management in the care of patients with chronic GVHD [4, 28]. Symptoms caused by ocular sicca can be relieved by use of artificial lubricant tears during waking hours and ointments at night. Punctal plugging can be used to decrease the need for use of artificial lubricants, while permanent punctal ligation is usually necessary for more severe cases of ocular sicca. The use of specialized moisture-chamber eyewear may be helpful. A few patients with severe sicca keratitis have reported significant relief of symptoms with the use of a newly developed scleral lens [33]. Sialogogue therapy with agents such as cevemiline or pilocarpine may improve ocular and oral sicca symptoms.

Oral cavity erythema, gingivitis, and ulcers can be managed with topical steroid rinses or ointments. Fluoride treatments and effective brushing and flossing can minimize tooth decay resulting from xerostomia [28]. Patients with chronic GVHD often experience weight loss, probably because of increased metabolic activity and decreased intestinal absorption of nutrients. Close attention should be paid to nutritional status, and protein and carbohydrate supplements provided as needed. Malabsorption can also cause deficiencies of trace elements.

Since sun exposure can activate chronic GVHD, patients should minimize time in direct sunlight. Sun block of at least SPF 30 should be applied liberally and often during sun exposure [28]. Physical therapy to maintain strength, joint mobility and range of motion can prevent the development of disability during immunosuppressive treatment for chronic GVHD. Deep tissue massage is a helpful adjunct to preserve or improve range of motion in patients with fasciitis or scleroderma. Administration of ursodeoxycholate may improve hepatic function. Vaginal GVHD may respond to topical steroids and dilator therapy. Management should also address any coexisting estrogen deficiency or yeast or bacterial infection.

Close attention must be paid to complications of glucocorticoid treatment through management of hyperglycemia and hypertension. Weight-bearing exercise together with dietary calcium and vitamin D administration should be used to retard the development of glucocorticoid-induced osteoporosis, and treatment with a bisphosphonate should be considered if loss of bone density continues despite these measures.

Measurement of response: The distinction between disease activity and damage plays a critical role in the management of chronic GVHD. Disease activity causes manifestations that would be expected to resolve promptly after pathogenic immunologic mechanisms are controlled. These manifestations generally reflect inflammation and include erythematous rash, oral erythema and lichenoid changes, diarrhea, transaminase elevations, and eosinophilia. Disease damage leads to manifestations that are generally considered to be irreversible. These manifestations reflect tissue destruction and include ocular and oral sicca and bronchiolitis obliterans. At best, an arrest of disease activity would be expected to halt progression of these manifestations. Bile duct destruction, however, is one type of damage that might be reversible. Certain disease manifestations fall between rapidly reversible and irreversible extremes. These manifestations typically reflect fibrosis and include sclerotic skin changes, fasciitis, and contractures. Control of disease activity is required in order to halt progression of these manifestations, and resolution occurs very slowly through a prolonged process of tissue remodeling.

Doses of immunosuppressive medications should be maintained at the lowest level sufficient to control disease activity. In practice, this recommendation means that periodic attempts should be made to withdraw immunosuppressive medications to a level where disease activity first becomes apparent and then increase the dose slightly to a level that suppresses manifestations of disease activity. Since chronic GVHD is a systemic disease, care should be taken not to obscure all manifestations of disease activity with the use of topical therapy in patients who have involvement at sites that are susceptible to fibrotic complications or irreversible damage. For example, patients with fasciitis and oral mucosal changes should not use dexamethasone oral rinses if there are no other manifestations that can be measured to assess whether disease activity is adequately controlled by the systemic immunosuppressive regimen.

WITHDRAWAL OF IMMUNOSUPPRESSIVE MEDICATIONS

Patients should begin withdrawal of immunosuppressive medications after resolution of all reversible manifestations of chronic GVHD. This process may be started by tapering the dose of prednisone as illustrated in Figure 12.1 without making any change in the dose of other immunosuppressive medications. If there is no recurrence of chronic GVHD within the first month after discontinuing treatment with prednisone, then the dose of cyclosporine or tacrolimus should be tapered. The daily dose of cyclosporine may be decreased by 0.5 mg/kg at weekly intervals until discontinuation of administration. The daily dose of tacrolimus may be decreased by 0.5 mg at weekly intervals until discontinuation of administration. If manifestations of chronic GVHD

recur at any step of the taper, the dose of cyclosporine or tacrolimus should be increased by two levels, and treatment should be continued for at least 3 months before attempting to resume the taper.

If possible, a biopsy of the skin should be obtained when immunosuppressive treatment is discontinued. For patients with histologic evidence of GVHD and those who do not have a biopsy, we recommend meticulous evaluation every 2 weeks during the ensuing 3 months to monitor for recurrent clinical manifestations of chronic GVHD. If histologic evidence of GVHD is absent, then monitoring at monthly intervals is adequate.

INDICATIONS FOR SECONDARY TREATMENT

In general, secondary systemic treatment is *not* indicated as long as there is continuing improvement in at least one manifestation of chronic GVHD and no progression of any other manifestations. Secondary systemic treatment should be initiated within 1 month whenever clinical manifestations of chronic GVHD show evidence of progression in a previously involved organ or whenever clinical manifestations appear in an organ that was not previously involved. Secondary systemic treatment should be initiated within 2 months whenever manifestations of chronic GVHD show no improvement during treatment with the originally prescribed medications. Secondary systemic treatment should be initiated if daily administration of prednisone cannot be tapered from a dose of 1.0 mg/kg within 2 months.

OUTCOMES AFTER INITIAL TREATMENT OF CHRONIC GVHD

Resolution of chronic GVHD occurs slowly. An early study of prednisone for chronic GVHD maintained patients on 1 mg/kg every other day until 9 months of steroid therapy had been completed. Thirty-three percent had a complete response (CR, defined as clinical and histologic resolution of GVHD) and 29% had a partial response (PR, clinical resolution but histologic evidence of active GVHD) [7]. For high-risk patients with a platelet count of < 100,000/μL, the CR rate was only 16% and the PR rate was 16%. A more recent study of patients treated with prednisone alone did not report response rates, but only 17% of patients needed secondary therapy. This study used an earlier steroid taper, with a decrease to 0.5 mg/kg of prednisone every other day starting after 22 weeks, and then continuing at the same dose until another taper began after 40 weeks of therapy. The median duration of therapy was 2.2 years, which was similar to the duration reported in the earlier study [16]. In a prospective study, Arora et al. [15] found that only 13% of patients with chronic GVHD were able to discontinue immunosuppressive treatment within 2 years after diagnosis. Among those with resolution of chronic GVHD, 18% were able to discontinue immunosuppressive treatment

Table 12.5: Five-Year Survival for Patients with "Standard-Risk" Chronic GVHD

Initial Treatment	Years	Trial Phase	N	5-Year Survival (%)	Reference
Prednisone	80–83	III	63*	65	7
Prednisone	85–92	III	116	72	16
Prednisone plus cyclosporine	85–92	III	126	70	16
Prednisone plus cyclosporine	94–00		381	71	

* Eleven patients had progressive-onset chronic graft versus host disease (GVHD).
The table is reprinted by courtesy of *International Journal of Hematology.*

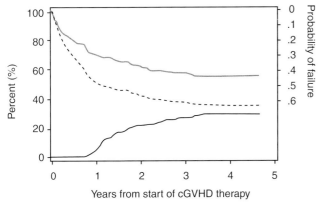

Figure 12.2 **Outcome after initial treatment for chronic GVHD.** The upper solid line and right-side scale indicates time from the beginning of treatment to failure defined as either secondary systemic treatment of chronic GVHD before recurrent malignancy or as death from causes other than recurrent malignancy during primary treatment. The upper dashed line and right-side scale indicates time from the beginning of treatment to either failure or recurrent malignancy. The lower curve and left-side scale indicates time from the beginning of treatment to discontinuation of all immunosuppressive treatment without prior secondary systemic treatment or recurrent malignancy.
The figure is reprinted by courtesy of *International Journal of Hematology.*

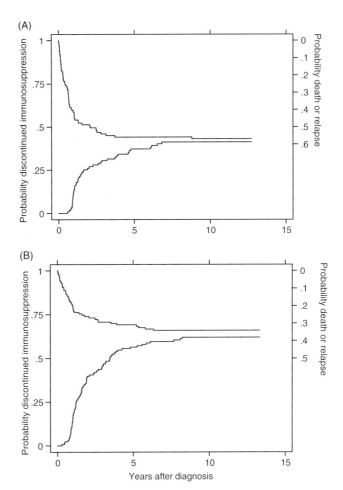

Figure 12.3 **Time to discontinuation of immunosuppressive treatment for patients with chronic GVHD** [34]. The lower curve and left-side scale represent the cumulative incidence of discontinued immunosuppressive treatment. The upper curve and right-side scale represent the cumulative incidence of death or recurrent malignancy before discontinuation of immunosuppressive treatment. The space between the two curves represents the proportion of patients who remain alive and free of recurrent malignancy with continued immunosuppressive treatment. A: shows results for patients who had "high-risk" chronic GVHD (progressive onset from acute GVHD or platelet count < 100,000/μL), and B: shows results for those with "standard-risk" chronic GVHD.

within 2 years, and 89% were able to discontinue immunosuppressive treatment within 4 years.

Koc et al. (unpublished) reviewed the outcome for 330 patients initially treated for chronic GVHD between January 1995 and December 1998 at the Fred Hutchinson Cancer Research Center (FHCRC). For most patients, marrow was used as the source of hematopoietic stem cells. Within 3 years after the diagnosis of chronic GVHD, approximately 33% of patients required secondary systemic treatment with medications other than those used for primary treatment. An

additional 10% died from causes other than recurrent malignancy during primary treatment within the first 3 years, and most of these deaths occurred during the first year. Only 5% of patients were able to discontinue treatment with all systemic immunosuppressive medications during the first year after diagnosis without the need for secondary systemic treatment. Only 27% of patients were able to discontinue treatment with all systemic immunosuppressive medications during the first 3 years after diagnosis without the need for secondary systemic treatment (Figure 12.2).

Five-year survival rates for patients with newly diagnosed "standard-risk" chronic GVHD (platelet count >100,000/μL

Table 12.6: Five-Year Survival for Patients with "High-Risk" Chronic GVHD

Initial Treatment	Years	Trial Phase	N	5-Year Survival (%)	Reference
Prednisone	80–82	II	38	26	7
Prednisone plus cyclosporine	82–85	II	40	52	19
Prednisone plus cyclosporine	85–92	III	111	40	34
Prednisone*	85–92	III	29	76	16
Prednisone plus cyclosporine*	85–92	III	16	43	16
Prednisone plus cyclosporine	94–00		366	51	

* Patients had progressive-onset chronic graft versus host disease (GVHD) without thrombocytopenia.
The table is reprinted by courtesy of *International Journal of Hematology*.

and de novo or quiescent onset) have remained at approximately 70% (Table 12.5 and Figure 12.3), and 5-year survival rates for those with "high-risk" chronic GVHD (platelet count < 100,000/μL or progressive-onset) have remained at 40% to 50% (Table 12.6 and Figure 12.3) [34]. Approximately 55% of patients with standard-risk chronic GVHD and approximately 35% of those with high-risk chronic GVHD are able to discontinue immunosuppressive treatment within 5 years after the diagnosis. Approximately 10% of all patients require continued treatment beyond 5 years, and 40% die or develop recurrent malignancy before chronic GVHD resolves. The time to resolution of chronic GVHD is longer after HCT with peripheral blood stem cells than with marrow [10, 35]. The duration of treatment is also longer for men with female donors, for patients with multiple organs affected by the disease, and for patients who are HLA-mismatched with their donors.

CHALLENGES FOR THE FUTURE

Previous studies have provided a good understanding of risk factors for development of chronic GVHD and risk factors for mortality among patients with newly diagnosed GVHD. Advances in supportive care have reduced morbidity, but survival among patients with newly diagnosed chronic GVHD has not changed since the mid-1980s. Improved understanding of the pathophysiology of chronic GVHD will be needed to develop more effective approaches for treatment. A challenge for the future will be the discovery of approaches that can target the cause of chronic GVHD while permitting reconstitution of immune defenses against pathogens and preserving immunologic effects of donor cells against malignant cells in the recipient. Broad participation in well-conducted, randomized phase III trials will be needed in order to develop more effective approaches for treatment of chronic GVHD.

REFERENCES

1. Sullivan KM, Shulman HM, Storb R, et al. Chronic graft-versus-host disease in 52 patients: Adverse natural course and successful treatment with combination immunosuppression. *Blood.* 1981;57:267–276.
2. Shulman HM, Sullivan KM, Weiden PL, et al. Chronic graft-versus-host syndrome in man: a long-term clinicopathologic study of 20 Seattle patients. *Am J Med.* 1980;69:204–217.
3. Lee SJ, Vogelsang G, Flowers MED. Chronic graft-versus-host disease. *Biol Blood and Marrow Transplantation.* 2003;9:215–233.
4. Vogelsang GB. How I treat chronic graft-versus-host disease. *Blood.* 2001;97:1196–1201.
5. Filipovich AH, Weisdorf D, Pavletic S, et al. National Institutes of Health consensus development project on criteria for clinical trials in chronic graft-versus-host disease: I. Diagnosis and Staging Working Group report. *Biol Blood Marrow Transplant.* 2005;11:945–956.
6. Strasser SI, Shulman HM, Flowers ME, et al. Chronic graft-versus-host disease of the liver: presentation as an acute hepatitis. *Hepatology.* 2000;32:1265–1271.
7. Sullivan KM, Witherspoon RP, Storb R, et al. Prednisone and azathioprine compared with prednisone and placebo for treatment of chronic graft-versus-host disease: prognostic influence of prolonged thrombocytopenia after allogeneic marrow transplantation. *Blood.* 1988;72:546–554.
8. Wingard JR, Piantadosi S, Vogelsang GB, et al. Predictors of death from chronic graft-versus-host disease after bone marrow transplantation. *Blood.* 1989;74:1428–1435.
9. Akpek G, Zahurak ML, Piantadosi S, et al. Development of a prognostic modes for grading chronic graft-versus-host disease. *Blood.* 2001;97:1219–1226.
10. Stewart BL, Storer B, Storek J, et al. Duration of immunosuppressive treatment for chronic graft-versus-host disease. *Blood.* 2004;104:3501–3506.
11. Lee SJ, Klein JP, Barrett AJ, et al. Severity of chronic graft-versus-host disease: association with treatment-related mortality and relapse. *Blood.* 2002;100:406–414.
12. Arora M, Burns LJ, Davies SM, et al. Chronic graft-versus-host disease: a prospective cohort study. *Biol Blood Marrow Transplant.* 2003;9:38–45.

13. Parker PM, Chao N, Nademanee A, et al. Thalidomide as salvage therapy for chronic graft-versus-host disease. *Blood.* 1995;86:3604–3609.

14. Koc S, Leisenring W, Flowers ME, et al. Thalidomide for treatment of patients with chronic graft-versus-host disease. *Blood.* 2000;96:3995–3996.

15. Arora M, Wagner JE, Davies SM, et al. Randomized clinical trial of thalidomide, cyclosporine, and prednisone versus cyclosporine and prednisone as initial therapy for chronic graft-versus-host disease. *Biol Blood Marrow Transplant.* 2001;7:265–273.

16. Koc S, Leisenring W, Flowers MED, et al. Therapy for chronic graft-versus-host disease: a randomized trial comparing cyclosporine plus prednisone versus prednisone alone. *Blood.* 2002;100:48–53.

17. Cooper MS, Stewart PM. Current concepts: corticosteroid insufficiency in acutely ill patients. *New Engl J Med.* 2003;348:727–734.

18. Axelrod L. Glucocorticoid therapy. *Medicine.* 1976;55:39–65.

19. Sullivan KM, Witherspoon RP, Storb R, et al. Alternating-day cyclosporine and prednisone for treatment of high-risk chronic graft-versus-host disease. *Blood.* 1988;72:555–561.

20. Flowers, MED, Lee S, Vogelsang G. An update on how to treat chronic GVHD (letter). *Blood.* 2003;102:2312.

21. Busca A, Saroglia EM, Lanino E, et al. Mycophenolate mofetil (MMF) as therapy for refractory chronic GVHD (cGVHD) in children receiving bone marrow transplantation. *Bone Marrow Transplant.* 2000;25:1067–1071.

22. Lopez F, Parker P, Nademanee A, et al. Efficacy of mycophenolate mofetil in the treatment of chronic graft-versus-host disease. *Biol Blood Marrow Transplant.* 2005;11:307–313.

23. Gilman AL, Chan KW, Mogul A, et al. Hydroxychloroquine for the treatment of chronic graft-versus-host disease. *Biol Blood Marrow Transplant.* 2000;6:327–334.

24. Gaziev D, Lucarelli G, Polchi P, et al. A three or more drug combination as effective therapy for moderate or severe chronic graft-versus-host disease. *Bone Marrow Transplant.* 2001;27:45–51.

25. Vogelsang GB, Wolff D, Altomonte V, et al. Treatment of chronic graft-versus-host disease with ultraviolet irradiation and psoralen (PUVA). *Bone Marrow Transplant.* 1996;17;1061–1067.

26. Schultz KR, Green GJ, Wensley D, et al. Obstructive lung disease in children after allogeneic bone marrow transplantation. *Blood.* 1994;84:3212–3220.

27. Dudek AZ, Mahaseth H, DeFor TE, Weisdorf DJ. Bronchiolitis obliterans in chronic graft-versus-host disease: analysis of risk factors and treatment outcomes. *Biol Blood Marrow Transplant.* 2003;9:657–666.

28. Couriel, D, Carpenter, P, Cutler C, et al. Ancillary therapy and supportive care of chronic graft-versus-host disease: National Institutes of Health consensus development project on criteria for clinical trials in chronic graft-versus-host disease: V. Ancillary therapy and supportive care working group report. *Biol Blood Marrow Transplant.* 2006;12:375–396.

29. Molrine DC, Antin JH, Guinan EC, et al. Donor immunization with pneumococcal conjugate vaccine and early protective antibody responses following allogeneic hematopoietic cell transplantation. *Blood.* 2003;101:831–836.

30. Boeckh M, Leisenring W, Riddell SR, et al. Late cytomegalovirus disease and mortality in recipients of allogeneic hematopoietic stem cell transplants: importance of viral load and T-cell immunity. *Blood.* 2003;101:407–414.

31. Marr KA, Carter RA, Boeckh M, Martin P, Corey L. Invasive Aspergillosis in allogeneic stem cell transplant recipients: changes in epidemiology and risk factors. *Blood.* 2002;100:4358–4366.

32. Ullman AJ, Lipton JH, Vasole DH, et al. Posaconazole or fluconazole for prophylaxis in severe graft-versus-host disease. *New Engl J Med.* 2007;356:335–347.

33. Kikuchi T, Parker P, Wu M, et al. Use of fluid-ventilated, gas-permeable scleral lens for management of keratoconjunctivitis sicca secondary to chronic graft-versus-host disease. *Bone Marrow Transplant.* 2006;13:1016–1021.

34. Flowers, MED. Traditional treatment of chronic graft-versus-host disease. *Blood and Marrow Transplantation Reviews.* 2002;12:5–8.

35. Flowers MED, Parker PM, Johnston LJ, et al. Comparison of chronic graft-versus-host disease after transplantation of peripheral blood stem cells versus bone marrow in allogeneic recipients: long term follow up of a randomized trial. *Blood.* 2002;100:48–51.

13

SALVAGE THERAPY IN CHRONIC GRAFT VERSUS HOST DISEASE

Hildegard T. Greinix and Joseph H. Antin

INTRODUCTION

Corticosteroids are the mainstay of therapy for chronic graft versus host disease (GVHD) [1, 2]. While calcineurin inhibitors (CNI) such as cyclosporine (CSP) and tacrolimus are active in chronic GVHD therapy, they are associated with surprisingly little additive benefit [1]. Currently, there is no standard second-line therapy for chronic GVHD and as a result, therapy for chronic GVHD often consists of prolonged administration of corticosteroids in conjunction with a CNI followed by one of several therapies with apparent, but unproven activity. In a recent randomized trial of immunosuppressive therapy for chronic GVHD, the median duration of therapy with corticosteroids and CSP was 1.6 years. Despite dual immunosuppressive therapy, only 54% of patients were successfully weaned from immunosuppressive medications at 5 years and mortality directly attributable to chronic GVHD was 17% in the combination immunosuppressive arm [1]. One problem in developing a rational set of therapies for chronic GVHD is the relatively immature nature of our understanding of this entity. We are only starting to understand the distinction between allogeneic and autologous reactivity that occurs after an allogeneic transplantation. Moreover, the importance of B cells, regulatory T cells (Treg), and dendritic cells has only started to come to light in the past few years. We can only hope that more effective approaches at prevention of chronic GVHD based on a better understanding of the physiology of chronic GVHD will make secondary therapy obsolete.

The goals of salvage or secondary therapy of chronic GVHD should be to reduce morbidity from the underlying process. In addition to immunosuppressive therapies, these treatments may include ursodeoxycholic acid to limit cholestatic liver injury, attention to dry eyes, management of dry mouth, maintenance of joint mobility, and prevention of infection. Infection is the most common cause of death in chronic GVHD, and the risk of infection may be exaggerated by the intensive immunosuppressive therapy that is often needed to ameliorate symptoms. Thus, while symptom control and establishment of a good performance status are important goals, they must be undertaken with appropriate concern for allowing some degree of immunologic recovery. Moreover, long-term corticosteroid use has well-known negative effects on metabolism, bone integrity, and so on that encourage the use of the lowest doses for the briefest time that is consistent with control of chronic GVHD. It is also critical to recognize that some manifestations of chronic GVHD may be either irreversible or require prolonged time periods. For instance, complete resolution of hyperbilirubinemia may not be feasible if all of the bile ducts are eliminated. Thus, continued high-dose therapy to treat hyperbilirubinemia must be guided by a working assessment of the underlying pathology and the likelihood of recovery. Failure to keep this in mind results in excessive prolonged use of immunosuppressants that are associated with infections, second malignancies, and drug toxicity. Ultimately, guidelines are of limited use, and the burden of judging the degree of immunosuppression that is necessary is on the clinician.

The lack of consistently effective treatment in this setting underscores the need for properly conducted clinical trials. A significant problem is the lack of agreement on the definition of "steroid-refractory" chronic GVHD. Although progression of GVHD symptoms on corticosteroids has been accepted as fulfilling the definition, lack of response has been less well defined. The pleomorphic manifestations of chronic GVHD further complicate this type of analysis. Healing of ulcerations and resolution of erythema is likely to be evaluable after a short latency, while assessing the response of scleroderma may take much longer. Moreover, as noted previously, there are some manifestations of chronic GVHD that may never resolve despite effective therapy. For instance, if lacrimal gland destruction results in keratoconjunctivitis sicca, it is unlikely that effective therapy will result in the formation of new tears. Thus, by what criterion is response determined? While the lack of response as little as 7 days, or up to 3 months, of corticosteroids has been regarded as sufficient to define refractoriness in some studies, the majority of reports have not specified any duration. In many cases, the treatment is studied after many months or years after failure of primary therapy. It is very likely that this variability in the definition of refractory chronic GVHD is an important confounding factor that could affect the reported efficacy of treatment.

Table 13.1: Tacrolimus Instead of Cyclosporine and Prednisone in Chronic GVHD

Author	Design	No. pts	CR (%)	PR (%)	ORR (%)	Comments
Tzakis [10]	Retrosp.	17	6 (35)	2 (12)	8/17 (47)	renal toxicity, hypertension
Kanamaru [11]	Phase II	26	2 (8)	10 (38)	12 /26 (46)	53% renal toxicity, 30% GI toxicity
Carnevale-Schianca [12]	Phase II	39	5 (13)	3 (8)	8/39 (21)	41% renal toxicity, 64% 3-year OS, 29% d.c. IS
Nagler [13]	Retrosp.	15	5 (33)	4 (27)	9/15 (60)	only liver involvement

CR, complete resolution; d.c., discontinued; GI, gastrointestinal; IS, immunosuppression; No, number; ORR, overall response rate; OS, overall survival; pts, eligible patients; PR, partial resolution; retrosp, retrospective study.

In many reports the criteria used to assess response are poorly defined, highlighting another difficulty in evaluating efficacy across different studies. Finally, once a satisfactory response is achieved it is clinically important to avoid immediate taper of immunosuppression that results in a saw-tooth pattern of remissions and relapses. It is a much more effective strategy to establish a remission, wait 4 to 6 months until the remission stabilizes, then begin a very slow taper of immunosuppressants.

AZATHIOPRINE

Azathioprine (AZA) was the first agent to be added to prednisone in the therapy of chronic GVHD [3]. However, its use was associated with more myelosuppression, more infections, and inferior survival [4]. In addition, there is an increased risk of developing solid tumors reported with prolonged use following hematopoietic stem cell transplantation (HSCT) [5].

CALCINEURIN INHIBITORS: CYCLOSPORINE AND TACROLIMUS

Although CSP and tacrolimus are considered standard therapy for chronic GVHD, they are incompletely effective [1]. Tacrolimus, a potent macrolide immunosuppressant, inhibits T-lymphocytes by forming a complex with FK506 binding protein 12, calcium, and calmodulin leading to decrease in the phosphatase activity of calcineurin. This prevents generation of nuclear factor of activated T cells (NFAT), a transcription factor for lymphokines like interleukin (IL)-2 and interferon-gamma (IFN-γ). Tacrolimus can also suppress IL-2 receptor (CD25) expression [6, 7] and has been used both as monotherapy as well as in combination in the treatment of steroid-refractory chronic GVHD. Although CSP binds to a different molecule, cyclophilin, the final common pathway is identical, and the drugs should have extremely similar effects. One potential limitation to the use of CNI in GVHD prevention is that they promiscuously block Treg function [8, 9]. However, sirolimus and mycophenolate mofetil (MMF) are either neutral or foster Treg growth. As data accumulate that Treg have an important role in the inhibition of autoimmunity and down-regulating the immune response, it is likely that agents that spare Treg will be more effective than more promiscuous agents.

In four reports tacrolimus was used instead of CSP and steroids resulting in modest efficacy (Table 13.1). Tzakis and colleagues treated 17 patients with extensive chronic GVHD after failure of at least 2 months of first-line therapy, persistent disease, or adverse reactions to first-line medication [10]. Six patients (35%) were judged to have had an unequivocal beneficial response. Carnevale-Schianca et al. reported on a phase II study of 39 patients who were eligible for tacrolimus either because of no improvement of chronic GVHD a minimum of 3 months on CSP and steroids or because of progression of chronic GVHD after 6 to 8 weeks on CSP and steroids [12]. At 3 years after the start of tacrolimus, 5 patients (13%) were in complete remission (CR) and had discontinued tacrolimus, and 3 (8%) were clinically stable but not able to discontinue tacrolimus. Given the similarity in mechanism of action it is possible that the response rates would have been the same if the patients had continued CSP at therapeutic doses for longer periods of time. Median duration of treatment with tacrolimus was 9 (range, 1–29) months. The Kaplan-Meier estimate of survival was 64% at 3 years. Similarly Kanamaru et al. reported on CR in 2 of 26 eligible patients (8%) and partial response in another 10 (38%) patients with localized and/or extensive chronic GVHD [11]. Patients with eye, skin, and gut involvement responded better to tacrolimus than patients having liver, mouth, and lung disease. Renal toxicity (53%), nausea, and vomiting (30%) were significant side effects of the drug. In a retrospective study Nagler et al. achieved CR in 5 of 15 (33%) patients with histologically confirmed hepatic chronic GVHD a median of 3 (range, 1–11) months after start of tacrolimus [13].

Thus, a small group of patients failing CSP may respond or stabilize with tacrolimus, but the data supporting substitution of tacrolimus for CSP are weak. CNI inhibit Treg as well as effector T cells, so theoretically alternative agents that spare Treg may be more useful.

SIROLIMUS

Sirolimus is a natural macrolide with immunosuppressive qualities that binds to the FK binding protein 12 and inhibits

Table 13.2: Sirolimus in Chronic Steroid-Refractory GVHD

Author	Design	No. pts	CR (%)	PR (%)	ORR (%)	Comments
Couriel [14]	T + P	35	6 (17)	16 (46)	22/35 (63)	66% renal toxicity, 77% infections, 41% OS at 2 yrs
Johnston [15]	CI + P	19*	15 (94)		15/16 (94)	47% d.c. drug, 37% severe toxicity, 74% infections
Jurado [16]	CI or MMF or P	47	18 (38)	20 (43)	38/47 (81)	30% renal toxicity, 8% TMA, 57% OS

CI, calcineurin inhibitor; CR, complete resolution; d.c, discontinued; GVHD, graft versus host disease; MMF, mycophenolate mofetil; No, number; ORR, overall response rate; OS, overall survival; P, prednisone; PR, partial resolution; pts, patients; T, tacrolimus; TMA, thrombotic microangiopathy; yrs, years.
* Only 16 patients evaluable for response.

cytokine-driven signaling pathways of the T cell via blockade of the mammalian target of rapamycin (mTOR). It has the advantage of having a completely different toxicity profile from the CNIs, and probably has additive or synergistic activity with those agents. Moreover, it has little effect on Treg numbers or function [9]. It has been used as a rescue therapy (Table 13.2) in a series of 35 patients with severe steroid-resistant chronic GVHD (including 12 with late acute GVHD) at a loading dose of 6 mg orally followed by a daily oral maintenance dosage of 2 mg/day. Thereafter, doses were adjusted to maintain blood concentrations between 7 and 12 ng/mL. Couriel et al. described a 63% response rate to the combination of sirolimus, tacrolimus, and corticosteroids including 6 CR and 16 PR [14]. The most important toxic effects were infectious complications in 77% of patients, renal toxicity in 66%, anemia in 63%, thrombocytopenia in 57%, and 4 cases of thrombotic microangiopathies (TMA). Median survival was 15 months, and estimated actuarial survival at 2 years was 41%. A total of 12 of 35 patients (34%) were tapered off steroids by the end of the study. Johnston et al. reported that 15 of 16 evaluable patients (94%) demonstrated a clinical response to sirolimus in combination with a CNI and prednisone in a phase II study [15]. Sirolimus was begun with a 10-mg oral loading dose followed by a daily dose of 5 mg. Doses were adjusted to have blood concentrations below 20 ng/mL. Of the 19 patients, 9 (47%) discontinued sirolimus after a median of 4 (range, 1–9) months because of renal insufficiency and hemolytic uremic syndrome (n = 2), and 7 of 19 (37%) experienced grade 3 to 4 toxicity leading to early closure of accrual. Fourteen patients (74%) had infections. Of the 15 responders, 3 had reportedly continued CR with successful tapering of immunosuppression. Of the 17 living patients (89%), 9 had continued sirolimus for a median of 20 (range, 5 to > 46) months. Renal toxicity occurs principally at supratherapeutic levels when sirolimus is used as a single agent. However, it may lower the threshold to TMA in patients receiving tacrolimus. Thus, careful attention to serum levels must be maintained and a serum trough level of 3 to 12 ng/mL is the recommended therapeutic range [17, 18].

Jurado et al. reported the results of the, so far, largest retrospective evaluation of sirolimus in combination with CNI (n = 33), MMF (n = 9), or prednisone (n = 5) in 47 patients with refractory or relapsed chronic GVHD [16]. The dosage of sirolimus was 2 mg once a day orally to maintain a level of 5 to 10 ng/mL. Of the 47 patients, 38 (81%) had clinical responses including 18 CR (38%) and 20 PR (43%). The clinical response rate was significantly lower among patients with refractory chronic GVHD as well as in those with progressive onset type of chronic GVHD. The main toxicity was mild renal function impairment in 14 patients (30%) including 3 associated with TMA. Overall survival at 3 years was 57%.

Sirolimus clearly has activity in chronic GVHD although it needs to be used in conjunction with other agents. Long-term use of sirolimus mandates careful monitoring of blood lipids to avoid complications of hyperlipidemia.

EXTRACORPOREAL PHOTOIMMUNOTHERAPY

Extracorporeal photoimmunotherapy (ECP) involves extracorporeal exposure of peripheral blood mononuclear cells to photoactivated 8-methoxypsoralen (8-MOP), followed by reinfusion of the treated cells.

The mechanisms of action of ECP in chronic GVHD is not fully understood. It has been proposed that ECP modulates host effector cells, including CD8$^+$ T-lymphocytes, natural killer (NK) cells, and circulating antigen-presenting cells (APC), leading to an attenuation of host antigen-presenting activity, thereby resulting in tolerance [19, 20]. Evidence supporting the role of intact host dendritic cells in GVHD has been derived from studies by Shlomchik and colleagues [21]. ECP induces apoptosis in all leukocyte subsets within 24 to 48 hours. Circulating apoptotic cells are phagocytosed by APCs, a process that is mediated by a highly conserved receptor system of apoptotic cell-associated membrane proteins (ACAMP) and ACAMP receptors on APCs. Other potential mechanisms of ECP-induced immune tolerance include decreased stimulation or depletion of effector T cells, increased production of anti-inflammatory (such as IL-10, IL-4, IL-1 receptor antagonist) or decreased production of proinflammatory cytokines (such as interferon-γ and IL-2), and generation of Tregs [22].

Greinix and colleagues treated 15 patients with extensive chronic GVHD failing steroids and observed responses in 12 of 15 patients with skin involvement, 7 of 10 with liver, and all 11 with oral mucosa [23]. Of the 15 patients, 14 survived with > 90% Karnofsky scores. In addition, a steroid-sparing effect was observed in responding patients with no increase in infectious complications. A larger study of ECP treatment for chronic GVHD in Vienna enrolled 47 patients with a median time of diagnosis at 8 months after HSCT [24]. CR rates were 68% for skin, 81% for mouth, 68% for liver, 28% for ocular, and 11% for joint manifestations. Of the 47 patients, 42 (89%) are currently alive, including 22 patients without GVHD and 18 without immunosuppression.

Complete responses of cutaneous chronic GVHD have been reported in heterogeneous studies (Table 13.3, [23–38]) in up to 80% of steroid-refractory patients with improvement even in sclerodermatous skin [24, 25, 28–30, 32–37]. Improvement in visceral chronic GVHD has been less consistent. Reports of high complete response (CR) rates in liver and gut GVHD [23, 24, 25, 31–33] have not been consistently observed [27–29]. A number of retrospective studies demonstrated efficacy of ECP for patients with chronic GVHD irrespective of the type of transplant (matched unrelated donor vs. matched related donor), duration of chronic GVHD, or Akpek risk stratification. There appears to be no association between dose intensity (number of ECP treatments per month) and clinical response [28, 29]. In view of the variety of ECP schedules investigated in different studies, however, the impact of dose intensity and length of treatment cannot currently be assessed for certain. Importantly, responses to ECP appear to be more frequent in patients treated earlier (<9 months) after diagnosis of chronic GVHD [26]. In line with this suggestion, Couriel and colleagues observed a trend toward higher response rates in de novo chronic GVHD [31].

Several investigators reported a steroid-sparing effect of ECP [23, 28, 29, 31, 32] and the ability to discontinue other immunosuppressive medication in ECP-responders [23, 25, 29]. Foss and colleagues observed a steroid-sparing effect of ECP or discontinuation of immunosuppressants in 80% of patients [29]. Furthermore, a significantly longer survival of patients responding to ECP compared to those failing treatment has been reported [26]. Messina and colleagues observed a 5-year overall survival rate of 96% in ECP-responders compared to 58% in nonresponders ($p = 0.04$, 26). Couriel and colleagues found response to ECP and platelet count at initiation of therapy as strongest predictors of nonrelapse mortality [29]. As surrogate marker for quality of life aspects, an improvement of Karnofsky performance scores from 50 or 60% before ECP to at least 90% after ECP has been reported [23, 26].

In general, ECP was very well tolerated with few major complications reported. These were usually related to the long-term indwelling central venous apheresis catheters such as catheter line infection or venous thrombosis at the catheter site. Mild side effects included transient hypotension during the procedure and intermittent drop of blood cell counts.

In a recent multicenter, prospective, randomized phase II study of ECP in steroid-intolerant, steroid-dependent, or steroid-refractory chronic GVHD, patients were randomized to either conventional treatment with prednisone plus CSP or tacrolimus (n = 47) or conventional treatment plus ECP (n = 48) for 24 weeks [39]. The primary objective was to assess improvement in skin GVHD by use of a validated skin scoring tool [40] by a blinded assessor. Secondary objectives were the assessment of total steroid use, changes in quality of life, the effect of treatment on other organ manifestations of GVHD, and the safety of ECP. Ninety-four percent of patients in both study arms had extensive chronic GVHD. Whereas median percent improvement in total skin score (TSS) per se was not significantly different between the study arms (14.5% in the ECP and 10.4% in the non-ECP arm, $p = 0.510$), a significant steroid-sparing effect defined as at least 50% reduction of steroid dose together with an at least 25% reduction in the TSS were observed in the ECP arm ($p = 0.04$). In addition, 24% of patients in the ECP arm compared to only 7% in the control arm had at least a 50% reduction of the steroid dose and a final steroid dose below 10 mg/day at the end of therapy ($p = 0.027$). Assessment of skin response by the clinical investigators revealed significantly more complete and partial resolution rates in the ECP arm compared to the control arm (40% vs. 10%, $p = 0.0024$).

In summary, ECP has objective activity in the treatment of chronic refractory GVHD and is well tolerated. ECP has the advantage of little in the way of systemic toxicity, and it does not heighten the risk of skin cancers that is observed in topical phototherapy. Further evaluation of the efficacy of ECP in well-designed, prospective, controlled studies with homogeneous patient groups, however, is warranted.

THALIDOMIDE

Thalidomide probably exerts its anti-inflammatory and immunomodulatory properties by inhibiting the production of tumor necrosis factor-α (TNF-α) [41] or by cytokine regulation in T cells [42]. Thalidomide has been investigated in a number of retrospective and phase II studies with significant variability in the reported response rates across studies [43–52] Vogelsang and colleagues evaluated thalidomide in 23 patients with chronic GVHD refractory to conventional immunosuppressants at an initial dose of 800 mg/day in adults and 12 mg/kg/day in children given in 4 divided doses leading to a plasma level of 5 mg/ml 2 hours after the drug administration [44]. Complete resolution was observed in 7 (30%) and partial resolution (PR) in 11 (48%) patients with a survival rate of 76% at 4 years. The median duration of therapy was 240 (range, 2–700) days and the most common adverse effects were sedation (91%) or constipation. Similar response rates have been reported in small series of pediatric and adult patients [46, 48]. Rovelli and colleagues treated 14 children

Table 13.3: Extracorporeal Photoimmunotherapy in Chronic Refractory GVHD

Author	No. pts Involvement	Skin			Liver			Oral			ORR (%)	Med. ECP Cycles	ECP Schedule*	Survival
		No	CR	PR	No	CR	PR	No	CR	PR				
Greinix [23]	15	15	12	3	10	7	2	11	11	1	8 CR, 6 PR (93)	18	2 d/2 w for 3 mo,2 d/4 w	14/15 (93%) at 15 mo
Smith [24]	18	10	5	2	13	2	1	7	1	1	3 CR, 3 PR (33)	20.5	2 d/3 w, 2–3/w	7/18 (39%) at 2 y
Salvaneschi [25]	14	12		5	9	3	3	12	7	1	4 CR, 5 PR (64)		2 d/2 w for 3mo,2 d/3 w	11/14 (79%) at 3 y
Messina [26]	44	36		20	20	8	4				15 CR, 10 PR (68)		2 d/w for 1 mo, every 2 w for 2 mo, monthly for 3 mo	34/44 (77%)
Seaton [27]	28	21	1	9	25		8	14		3	10 PR (36)		2 d/2 w for 4 mo 2 d/mo	24/28 (86%)
Apisarnthanarax [28]	32	32	32	8	11	17					7 CR, 11 PR (56)	36		19/32 (59%)
Foss [29]	25	25	14	16	6	5		13	6		16 PR (64)		2 d/2 w or weekly	15/25 (60)
Rubegni [30]	32	27		8	22		12	25	16	7	9 CR, 13 PR (69)		2–4/w then 1/w, then 2/2 w	
Couriel [31]	71	58		33	21		15	9		7	14 CR, 29 PR (61)		2 d/2 w, 2 d/ 4 w	13/71 (18%) at 5 y
Greinix [32]	47	44	30	11	25	17	4	42	34	6	23 CR, 16 PR (83)		2 d/w for 3w, 2 d/2 w 2d/mo until 6 mo	42/47 (89%)
Perseghin [33]	25	25	25			6			9		11CR, 9 PR (80)	19		19/25 (76%) at 2 y

ECP, Extracorporeal photoimmunotherapy; CR, complete resolution; PR, partial resolution; d, day; med, median; mo, month; No, number; ORR, overall response rate; PR, partial resolution; pts, patients; w, week; y, years.

* Description of the various ECP schedules.
Greinix [23]: 2 consecutive days every 2 weeks for 3 months, then 2 consecutive days every 4 weeks until resolution of GVHD.
Smith [24]: initially patients were treated on 2 days every 3 weeks, then the schedule was changed for other patients to 2 to 3 days per week until maximum response.
Salvaneschi [25]: 2 days every 2 weeks for 3 months, then 2 days every 3 weeks for 3 months.
Messina [26]: 2 days per week for 1 month, then 2 days every 2 weeks for 2 months, then 2 days monthly for 3 months.
Seaton [27]: 2 days every 2 weeks for 4 months, then 2 days every month.
Apisarnthanarax [28]: various schedules.
Foss [29]: 2 days every 2 weeks in the first patients, in later patients 2 days weekly until best response.
Couriel [31]: 2 to 4 days per week until partial response, then 1 day per week, maintenance with 2 days every 2 weeks.
Greinix [32]: 2 consecutive days every 2 weeks until response, then 2 days every 4 weeks until maximum response.
Perseghin [33]: 2 days per week for 3 weeks, then 2 days every 2 weeks for 2 times, then 2 days per month until the 6th month.

Table 13.4: Mycophenolate Mofetil in Chronic Refractory GVHD

Author	Design	No. pts	CR (%)	PR (%)	ORR (%)	Comments
Mookerjee [53]	with T + P	26	2 (8)	10 (38)	12/26 (46)	19% GI toxicity
Busca [54]	with other IS	15 ext	2 (13)	7 (47)	9/15 (60)	only children with progression under CSP + P, 40% GI tox, 33% infections, best responses in GI, oral mucosa and nonsclerodermatous skin, steroid-sparing
Basara [55]	with CSP + P	12			7/12 (58)	response only in limited, 37% 5- year OS
Baudard [56]	with other IS	13			9/13 (69)	increased infection rate
Busca [57]	with other IS	18	5 (28)	8 (44)	13/18 (72)	33% GI tox, 8 serious infections, 71% 2-year OS
Kim [58]	with P +/-CSP	13	1 (8)	9 (69)	10/13 (77)	27% GI tox, 23% infections 54% 2-year OS
Lopez [59]	with CSP/T/P	24	5 (21)	13 (54)	18/24 (75)	83% OS at 2 years
Krejci [60]	with CSP + P	11	3 (27)	4 (36)	7/11 (64)	67% infections, 29% hem. tox

CR, complete resolution; CSP, cyclosporine; ext, extensive chronic GVHD; GI, gastrointestinal; GVHD, graft versus host disease; hem, hematological; IS, immunosuppressants; No, number; nonsclerod., nonsclerodermatous; ORR, overall response rate; OS, overall survival; P, prednisone; pts, eligible patients; PR, partial resolution; T, Tacrolimus; tox, toxicity.

with chronic GVHD (2 limited, 12 extensive) not responding to CSP, steroids, and azathioprine (AZA) with thalidomide at a median dose of 5.5 mg/kg/day (minimum 3, maximum 9.5) achieving 6 (43%) CR and 4 (29%) PR [46]. Treatment duration ranged from 1.3 to 102 months. The best responders had predominantly mucocutaneous involvement of chronic GVHD and quiescent onset. Sedation was the major side effect and 2 patients developed peripheral neuropathy.

In larger series more modest responses to thalidomide have been observed. Parker et al. reported the results of the, so far, largest phase II study of salvage thalidomide treatment of refractory chronic GVHD in 80 patients who had failed to respond to prednisone or prednisone and CSP [45]. Thalidomide was given at 800 to 1200 mg/day in four divided doses in combination with CSP and steroids. Overall 16 patients (20%) showed a sustained response including 9 CR and 7 PR after a median therapy duration of 16 months (range, 0.3–4.5 years). Most of the responses were observed in patients with isolated oral mucosa, liver, and skin involvement without severe sclerodermatous manifestations. Of the 16 patients who responded, 13 (81%) patients were alive with a median follow-up of 2.8 years compared with 30 of 64 (47%) who did not respond. Twenty-nine patients (36%) had thalidomide discontinued because of side effects, which included sedation (n = 7), constipation (n = 3), neuropathy (n = 3), skin rash (n = 6), and neutropenia (n = 10). Kulkarni and colleagues administered thalidomide in addition to CSP and corticosteroids in 59 patients [50]. Thirty-four patients received azathioprine concomitantly. Thirteen patients (22%) had CR, 8 (14%) PR and response rates were comparable for limited (39%) and extensive (33%) chronic GVHD.

In summary, thalidomide has modest activity in chronic GVHD in combination with other immunosuppressive agents but is poorly tolerated. It should be used primarily for lichenoid GVHD, especially oral lichen planus, and it should be used at the lowest dose that maintains a response.

MYCOPHENOLATE MOFETIL

Mycophenolate mofetil (MMF) is an antimetabolite that results in noncompetitive reversible inhibition of inosine monophosphate dehydrogenase. This leads to selective inhibition of lymphocyte purine synthesis and proliferation. Interestingly, it appears to spare Treg, a characteristic that may prove to be beneficial [8]. Experience with MMF in chronic refractory GVHD is limited (Table 13.4). Mookerjee et al. reported the results from 26 patients who had progressive disease on a regimen containing at least steroids and CSP or tacrolimus and were given MMF at a dose of 1 g orally twice a day in association with tacrolimus [53]. The later was initially started at a dose of 1 mg orally twice a day and subsequent doses adjusted to maintain a blood level of 5 to 10 ng/ml. The overall response rate was 46%. Of the responders, 2 patients had complete resolution (8%) and were successfully taken off immunosuppressants, while 10 patients (38.5%) had significant improvement. The number of organs involved did not correlate with response, as about half the patients with either skin alone or multiple organ involvement demonstrated improvement with this regimen that was well tolerated. The most common side effects were gastrointestinal disturbances in 19% and hematotoxicity in 4%. In 7 other studies with small patient numbers, response rates were reported in 58% to 77% of patients refractory to various immunosuppressants including steroids [54–60]. While gut, oral, liver, and nonsclerodermatous skin manifestations were reported to be more responsive to MMF [54, 57], this was not observed by others [56]. Higher serum trough levels of the MMF active metabolite, mycophenolic acid, were associated with an improved response rate (2.48 compared with 1.58 mg/l, $p = 0.058$) in a series of 13 patients reported by Baudard et al [56].

Thus, MMF in combination with other immunosuppressants may be beneficial in patients with chronic GVHD.

However, GI toxicity and serious infections reported previously are of concern. MMF appears to have little long-term toxicity, certainly much less than corticosteroids. A reasonable strategy to avoid the debilitating effects of Cushing syndrome is to get chronic GVHD under control by adding MMF to corticosteroids and/or other agents. The corticosteroids can be tapered first to the lowest dose that maintains the response. This can be followed by tapering of the MMF as tolerated.

TOTAL-LYMPHOID IRRADIATION

Total-lymphoid irradiation (TLI) has been used as an immunosuppressive treatment in autoimmune diseases and in solid organ transplantation [61, 62]. Mechanisms involved in TLI-induced tolerance are not fully understood, but TLI in animal model decreases cytotoxic T-lymphocyte counts, associated with modifications of the Th2/Th1 and CD4/CD8 ratio [63, 64]. TLI has been reported to be effective in a limited number of patients with refractory chronic GVHD [65–67]. Low-dose (1 Gy) thoracoabdominal irradiation (TAI), which irradiates all lymph node areas without requiring extensive organ shielding, has been used in 41 patients with refractory extensive chronic GVHD, predominantly cutaneous, or musculoskeletal involvement, by Robin and colleagues [67]. Before undergoing TAI, 41% of patients had experienced at least five episodes of chronic GVHD, defined as the number of successive and distinct treatment lines. Eighty-two percent of patients achieved a clinical response at a median of 34 days after TAI (range, 15–180 days). Complete resolution was obtained in 11 patients by 2 years post TAI. Best overall responses (CR and partial response [PR]) by 6 months after TAI were observed in fasciitis (79%), oral mucosa (73%), skin (67%), and ocular mucosa (67%). Fifty-seven percent of patients had at least a 50% reduction of their steroid daily dose by 6 months after TAI. Probability of steroid discontinuation was 38% by 2 years post TAI (95% CI, 23%–56%). Ten-year survival from TAI was 57% (95% CI, 42%–78%). Patients with lymphocytes $> 1.0 \times 10^9/l$, and platelets $> 200 \times 10^9/l$ had a better outcome (10-year estimated overall survival [OS], 72% vs. 38%). Hematotoxicity of TAI was low. Fifteen infections were observed during the first year after TAI, giving a 1-year infection incidence of 37% (95% CI, 20%–51%). Secondary malignancies occurred in 4 patients (osteosarcoma, n = 1; head and neck carcinomas, n = 3), giving an estimated 10-year incidence of 8.2% (95% CI, 0%–30%).

TOPICAL PHOTOTHERAPY

Nonionizing radiation has the capacity to profoundly modify immunity and immunogenicity both systemically and locally in the skin. Rejection of transplanted ultraviolet (UV)-induced skin tumors, contact hypersensitivity, delayed-type hypersensitivity, and antigen-presenting-cell functions are all suppressed by UV radiation, whereas other immune reactions, including antibody presentation, CTL induction, macrophage activity, and graft rejection, are not [68]. The effect of UV radiation on Langerhans cells is critical to immunosuppression, resulting in a shift from immunogenic (Th1) to tolerogeneic (Th2) response [68]. This shift may be mediated by cytokine release and expression of costimulatory molecules [32].

UV radiation is divided into two major regions, UVB (290–320 nm) and UVA (320–400 nm). UVA irradiation combined with oral 8-methoxypsoralen (PUVA) has been used as alternative for cutaneous steroid-refractory chronic GVHD manifestations resulting in responses in lichenoid disease in studies with small patient numbers [69–74]. Vogelsang et al. reported the largest series on 40 patients given oral PUVA 4 times per week achieving 78% improvement including 50% CR of skin disease [69]. Poor responses in sclerodermatous skin manifestations and no effect on extracutaneous chronic GVHD were seen. Intraoral PUVA [75, 76] after failure of multiple systemic immunosuppressive therapies resulted in complete resolution in 4 of 7 patients and partial resolution in another 2 of 7 as reported by Wolff et al. [75] Oral application of 8-methoxypsoralen may result in systemic side effects such as nausea, vomiting, cataract formation, and severe accidental phototoxic reactions seen as blistering and marked erythema of the skin [77]. PUVA bath therapy as an alternative reportedly achieved CR in 3 of 6 patients including sclerodermatous manifestations after a median of 14.5 treatments given 3 to 4 times per week and allowed reduction in concomitant immunosuppression [78]. As an important long-term side effect of PUVA, the development of basal cell carcinoma has to be kept in mind [79, 80].

Long-wavelength UVA (340–400 nm, UVA$_1$) phototherapy has been reported to be efficacious in chronic cutaneous GVHD [81–84]. Wetzig and colleagues treated patients 3 to 5 times per week with a median of 30 (range, 13–91) UVA$_1$ therapies with a median total dose of 1330 J/cm² (range, 590–3500) [84]. Six (60%) patients had a CR, 3 (30%) a PR, and 1 patient showed improvement of sclerotic skin lesions and joint mobility. Of the 7 patients with lichenoid skin manifestations, 6 had CR whereas all 3 with sclerodermatous disease had PR. UVA$_1$ has significant advantages over PUVA as nausea, emesis, long-lasting skin photosensitivity, and the need for eye protection are avoided. However, optimal dosing and schedule of UVA$_1$ treatment remain to be determined and long-term results are currently not available. UVA$_1$ appears to be a promising new therapeutic option for chronic cutaneous GVHD as an adjunct to other immunosuppressive therapies. In further detailed studies on the effects of UVA$_1$ phototherapy for chronic GVHD low-, medium-, and high-dose UVA$_1$ therapy should be compared to allow sparing of radiation dose.

Shorter wave UVB radiation (280–320 nm) does not entail prior administration of a photosensitizer and can therefore be given safely to patients who do not tolerate psoralen. Use of UVB phototherapy in the management of chronic GVHD has been limited [85, 86]. Enk et al. reported complete resolution in 1 patient with lichenoid manifestations and no response in 2 patients with sclerodermatous lesions [85].

In summary, phototherapy of skin lesions of chronic GVHD with either UVB or UVA light following oral administration

Table 13.5: CD20 Antagonists in Chronic Steroid-Refractory GVHD

Author	No. pts	Outcome
Ratanatharathorn [87]	8 ext.	4/8 improved (50%), tapered IS, 8/8 alive up to 99 mo
Canninga-van Dijk [88]	6 ext.	5/6 responded (83%) with marked clinical, biochemical, and histologic improvement,
Cutler [89]	21	2 CR (10%), ORR 14/20 (70%), responses in cutaneous and musculoskeletal disease, steroid-sparing
Zaja [90]	38	65% ORR, 63% RR in skin, 48% mouth, 43% eyes, 25% liver, 37% lung, 76% 2-year survival

CR, complete resolution; ext, extensive chronic GVHD; GVHD, graft versus host disease; IS, immunosuppression; mo, months; No, number; ORR, overall response rate; pts, patients; RR, response rate.

of psoralen has been shown to be effective in lichenoid skin changes in addition to systemic immunosuppressive therapies. Anecdotal reports of improvement of oral GVHD with PUVA have also been made. No significant effect is reported in other organs. Thus, for a systemic immunomodulatory effect of phototherapy, ECP should be administered. Whether sclerodermatous chronic GVHD responds better to UVA_1 than PUVA has to be evaluated in larger patient numbers. However, since the risk of skin cancers is already high in chronic GVHD, it seems reasonable to favor ECP over topical therapy when possible.

CD20 ANTAGONISTS (RITUXIMAB)

There is increasing evidence that B-cell dysregulation contributes to the pathogenesis of chronic GVHD prompting several groups to investigate the efficacy of rituximab in the management of patients with chronic refractory GVHD (Table 13.5, [87–90]). Rituximab was administered at a dose of 375 mg/m^2 every week for 4 weeks, with retreatment planned within 8 to 12 weeks in case of incomplete response. Ratanatharathorn et al. reported sustained responses in 4 of 8 patients, even with recovery of B cells in three of these [87]. In addition, disappearance of cold agglutinin titers and resolution of the Raynaud phenomenon (n = 1), decline in urinary protein excretion due to membranous glomerulonephritis (n = 1), and improvement of sclerodermatous changes of the thoracic cage with a marked improvement in the pulmonary spirogram (n = 1) were observed.

Canninga-van Dijk and colleagues treated 6 patients with refractory extensive chronic GVHD with anti-CD20 monoclonal antibody [88]. Of the 6 patients, 5 responded to treatment with marked clinical, biochemical, and histologic improvement.

Cutler and colleagues performed a phase I/II study of rituximab therapy in steroid-refractory chronic GVHD in 21 patients given 38 cycles of rituximab [89]. Seventy percent responded, including 2 patients with CR. Responses were limited to patients with cutaneous and musculoskeletal manifestations of chronic GVHD and were durable through 1 year after therapy. In addition, 68% of patients had a dose reduction of at least 50% in corticosteroid doses and the median prednisone

dose fell from 40 mg/day at trial initiation to 10 mg/day 1 year after rituximab therapy ($p < 0.001$). A chronic GVHD symptom score improved in approximately 50% of treated patients.

Recently, Zaja et al. reported on 38 patients with refractory chronic GVHD given rituximab after a median of 3 (range, 1 to > 6) failed treatment lines [90]. Overall response rate was 65% with best responses in skin (63%), mouth (48%), eyes (43%) and lungs (37.5%). The actuarial 2-year survival in this cohort was 76%.

The specificity of anti-CD20 therapy with rituximab strongly supports the concept that there is a B-cell component in the pathobiology of chronic GVHD. While the response data are encouraging, for the most part anti-CD20 is a useful adjunct to therapy rather than a definitive answer. These data do suggest that specific therapy directed at avoiding the B-cell response may be needed as part of an overall chronic GVHD prevention strategy.

OTHER AGENTS WITH POSSIBLE ACTIVITY

Several additional drugs have been reported to have objective responses in patients with chronic GVHD; however, none of these agents has been studied in well-controlled trials and proven to be useful. Clofazimine is an antimycobacterial drug that has been used in chronic autoimmune skin disorders, such as discoid systemic lupus erythematosus (SLE). Lee and colleagues treated 22 patients with clofazimine for chronic GVHD starting at 300 mg orally in a single daily dose for 90 days [91]. Then, the dose was lowered to 100 mg orally daily and the medication continued indefinitely as tolerated. The drug tends to crystallize in tissues resulting in skin pigmentation and gastrointestinal toxicity; however, by reducing the dose promptly it is generally well tolerated. Responses were observed in 50% of patients with skin involvement, flexion contractures, or oral manifestations including some complete response and 7 of 22 patients were able to reduce other immunosuppressive medications. However, this initial report has not been followed up with further studies.

Retinoids were proposed by the Johns Hopkins group [92] based on reports of activity of etretinate in scleroderma. They treated 32 patients who had a median of 30 months of refractory sclerodermatous chronic GVHD. Although 20 of 27 patients showed some improvement, 6 patients had ulcerations requiring discontinuation of therapy.

Another agent that has been reported to have activity is hydroxychloroquine. Gilman and colleagues studied this drug because of its known activity in autoimmune disorders [93]. It is an antimalarial that interferes with antigen processing and presentation, cytokine production, and cytotoxicity. A phase II trial of hydroxychloroquine (12 mg/kg/day) in 40 patients with steroid-resistant or steroid-dependent chronic GVHD resulted in 3 complete responses and 14 partial responses. The responders were able to undertake a > 50% reduction in their corticosteroid dose while receiving therapy.

Pentostatin is a potent inhibitor of adenosine deaminase, an enzyme that is intrinsic to T-lymphocyte function. It is highly immunosuppressive and induces lymphocyte apoptosis. It was shown by Boleanos-Meade and colleagues to be useful in acute GVHD [94] and has been used in a small number of children with chronic GVHD, with suggestive early results [51]. However, it must be used with caution because of the risk of cytopenias and opportunistic infections.

Anticytokine therapy has been used only minimally in chronic GVHD. There are small series using TNF-α antagonists (etanercept) [95, 96], IL-2 receptor α antagonists (daclizumab) [97, 98], or the combination of infliximab and daclizumab [50]. However, the data are very limited and these drugs and combinations cannot be recommended outside of a clinical trial.

Finally, investigators have considered treating chronic GVHD with an autologous transplantation [52], or by doing a second allogeneic transplantation from a different donor. This idea has a reasonable theoretical basis, but it is unlikely to become a generally useful management approach.

CONCLUSIONS

Typically in medicine, prevention or primary therapy is more effective than secondary therapy, and chronic GVHD is no exception. Optimally, we would be able to prevent all chronic GVHD while maintaining an effective graft-versus-leukemia response. Until we understand the biology of chronic GVHD well enough to adopt effective prophylactic strategies, the need to develop effective primary and secondary therapy will be compelling. The critical features of effective salvage therapy for chronic GVHD are (1) to treat early before irreversible organ injury supervenes, (2) to treat with effective agents with nonoverlapping toxicities, and (3) to treat until chronic GVHD has fully stabilized or resolved to prevent a recurring pattern of remission and exacerbations, while being sensitive to the possibility that there may be organ injury that will not respond to immunosuppression.

REFERENCES

1. Koc S, Leisenring W, Flowers ME, et al Therapy for chronic graft-versus-host disease: a randomized trial comparing cyclosporine plus prednisone versus prednisone alone. *Blood*. 2002;100:48–51.

2. Sullivan KM, Witherspoon RP, Storb R, et al Alternating-day cyclosporine and prednisone for treatment of high-risk chronic graft-vs-host disease. *Blood*. 1988;72:555–561.

3. Sullivan KM, Shulman HM, Storb R, et al. Chronic graft-versus-host disease in 52 patients: adverse natural course and successful treatment with combination immunosuppression. *Blood*. 1981;57:267–276.

4. Sullivan KM, Witherspoon RP, Storb R, et al. Prednisone and azathioprine compared with prednisone and placebo for treatment of chronic graft-vs-host disease: prognostic influence of prolonged thrombocytopenia after allogeneic marrow transplantation. *Blood*. 1988;72:546–554.

5. Deeg HJ, Socie G, Schoch G, et al Malignancies after marrow transplantation for aplastic anemia and Fanconi anemia: a joint Seattle and Paris analysis of results in 700 patients. *Blood*. 1996;87:386–392.

6. Goto T, Kino T, Hatanaka H, et al. FK506: historical perspectives. *Transplant Proc*. 1991;23:2713–2717.

7. Crum A, Woude V, Bierer E. Immunosuppression and immunophilin ligands: cyclosporine A, FK-506 and rapamycin. In: Ferrara JLM, Deeg JH, Burakoff SJ, eds. Graft-versus-host disease. Marcel Dekker, New York, 1996:111–149.

8. Zeiser R, Nguyen VH, Beilhack A, et al Inhibition of CD4+CD25+ regulatory T-cell function by calcineurin-dependent interleukin-2 production. *Blood*. 2006;108:390–399.

9. Baan CC, van der Mast BJ, Klepper M, et al. Differential effect of calcineurin inhibitors, anti-CD25 antibodies and rapamycin on the induction of FOXP3 in human T cells. *Transplantation*. 2005;80:110–117.

10. Tzakis AG, Abu-Elmagd K, Fung JJ, et al FK506 rescue in chronic graft-versus-host disease after bone marrow transplantation. *Transplant Proc*. 1991;23:3225–3227.

11. Kanamaru A, Takemoto Y, Kakishita E, et al FK506 treatment of graft-versus-host disease developing or exacerbating during prophylaxis and therapy with cyclosporine and/or other immunosuppressants. *Bone Marrow Transplant*. 1995;15:885–889.

12. Carnevale-Schianca F, Martin P, Sullivan K, et al Changing from cyclosporine to tacrolimus as salvage therapy for chronic graft-versus-host disease. *Biol Blood Marrow Transplant*. 2000;6:613–620.

13. Nagler A, Menachem Y, Ilan Y. Amelioration of steroid-resistant chronic graft-versus-host-mediated liver disease via tacrolimus treatment. *J Hematother Stem Cell Res*. 2001;10:411–417.

14. Couriel DR, Saliba R, Escalon MP, et al Sirolimus in combination with tacrolimus and corticosteroids for the treatment of resistant chronic graft-versus-host disease. *Brit J Haematol*. 2005; 130:409–417.

15. Johnston LJ, Brown J, Shizuru JA, et al Rapamycin (sirolimus) for treatment of chronic graft-versus-host disease. *Biol Blood Marrow Transplant*. 2005;11:47–55.

16. Jurado M, Vallejo C, Perez-Simon JA, et al Sirolimus as part of immunosuppressive therapy for refractory chronic graft-versus-host disease. *Biol Blood Marrow Transplant*. 2007; 13:701–706.

17. Antin JH, Kim HT, Cutler C, et al Sirolimus, tacrolimus, and low-dose methotrexate for graft-versus-host disease prophylaxis in mismatched related donor or unrelated donor transplantation. *Blood*. 2003;102:1601–1605.

18. Cutler C, Kim HT, Hochberg E, et al. Sirolimus and tacrolimus without methotrexate as graft-versus-host disease prophylaxis

after matched related donor peripheral blood stem cell transplantation. *Biol Blood Marrow Transplant.* 2004;10:328–336.

19. Alcindor T, Gorgun G, Miller KB, et al. Immunomodulatory effects of extracorporeal photochemotherapy in patients with extensive chronic graft-versus-host disease. *Blood.* 2001;98:1622–1625.

20. Gorgun G, Miller KB, Foss FM. Immunologic mechanisms of extracorporeal photochemotherapy in chronic graft-versus-host disease. *Blood.* 2002;100:941–947.

21. Shlomchik WD, Couzens MS, Tang CB, et al. Prevention of graft-versus-host disease by inactivation of host antigen-presenting cells. *Science.* 1999;285:412–415.

22. Peritt D. Potential mechanisms of photopheresis in hematopoietic stem cell transplantation. *Biol Blood Marrow Transplant.* 2006;12:7–12.

23. Greinix HT, Volc-Platzer B, Rabitsch W, et al. Successful use of extracorporeal photochemotherapy in the treatment of severe acute and chronic graft-versus-host disease. *Blood.* 1998; 92:3098–3104.

24. Smith EP, Sniecinski I, Dagis AC, et al. Extracorporeal photochemotherapy for treatment of drug-resistant graft-vs-host disease. *Biol Blood Marrow Transplant.* 1998;4:27–37.

25. Salvaneschi L, Perotti C, Zecca M, et al. Extracorporeal photochemotherapy for treatment of acute and chronic GVHD in childhood. *Transfusion.* 2001;41:1299–1305.

26. Messina C, Locatelli F, Lanino E, et al. Extracorporeal photochemotherapy for paediatric patients with graft-versus-host disease after haematopoietic stem cell transplantation. *Brit J Haematol.* 2003;122:118–127.

27. Seaton ED, Szydlo RM, Kanfer E, et al. Influence of extracorporeal photopheresis on clinical and laboratory parameters in chronic graft-versus-host disease and analysis of predictors of response. *Blood.* 2003;102:1217–1223.

28. Apisarnthanarax N, Donato M, Körbling M, et al. Extracorporeal photopheresis therapy in the management of steroid-refractory or steroid-dependent cutaneous graft-versus-host disease after allogeneic stem cell transplantation: feasibility and results. *Bone Marrow Transplant.* 2003;31:459–465.

29. Foss FM, DiVenuti GM, Chin K, et al. Prospective study of extracorporeal photopheresis in steroid-refractory or steroid-resistant extensive chronic graft-versus-host disease: analysis of response and survival incorporating prognostic factors. *Bone Marrow Transplant.* 2005;35:1187–1193.

30. Rubegni P, Cuccia A, Sbano P, et al. Role of extracorporeal photochemotherapy in patients with refractory chronic graft-versus-host disease. *Brit J Haematol.* 2005;130:271–275.

31. Couriel D, Hosing C, Saliba R, et al. Extracorporeal photochemotherapy for the treatment of steroid-resistant chronic GVHD. *Blood.* 2006;107:3074–3080.

32. Greinix HT, Socie G, Bacigalupo A, et al. Assessing the potential role of photopheresis in hematopoietic stem cell transplant. *Bone Marrow Transplant.* 2006;38:265–273.

33. Perseghin P, Galimberti S, Balduzzi A, et al. Extracorporeal photochemotherapy for the treatment of chronic graft-versus-host disease: Trend for a possible dose-related effect? *Ther Apher Dial.* 2007;11:85–93.

34. Owsianowski M, Gollnick H, Siegert W, et al. Successful treatment of chronic graft-versus-host disease with extracorporeal photopheresis. *Bone Marrow Transplant.* 1994;14:845–848.

35. Rossetti F, Zulian F, Dall'Amico R, et al. Extracorporeal photochemotherapy as single therapy for extensive, cutaneous chronic graft-versus-host disease. *Transplant.* 1995;59:149–151.

36. Dall'Amico R, Rossetti F, Zulian F, et al. Photopheresis in paediatric patients with drug-resistant chronic graft-versus-host disease. *Brit J Haematol.* 1997;97:848–854.

37. Abhyankar S, Godder K, Chiang K, et al. Extracorporeal photopheresis with UVADEX for the treatment of chronic graft-versus-host disease. *Exp Hematol.* 1998;26:32.

38. Child FJ, Ratnavel R, Watkins P, et al. Extracorporeal photopheresis (ECP) in the treatment of chronic graft-versus-host disease (GVHD). *Bone Marrow Transplant.* 1999;23:881–887.

39. Flowers MED, Van Besien, K, Apperley J, et al. A randomized single-blind study of extracorporeal photopheresis with UVADEX plus conventional therapy (CT) compared to CT alone in chronic GVHD. *Blood.* 2006;108:758 (abstract).

40. Greinix HT, Pohlreich D, Maalouf J, et al. A single-center pilot validation study of a new chronic GVHD skin scoring system. *Biol Blood Marrow Transplant.* 2007;13: 715–723.

41. Moriera AL, Sampaio EP, Znuidzinas A, et al. Thalidomide exerts its inhibitory action on tumor necrosis factor alpha by enhancing mRNA degradation. *J Exp Med.* 1993;177:1675–1680.

42. McHugh SM, Rifkin IR, Deighton J, et al. The immunosuppressive drug thalidomide induces T helper cell Type 1 (Th2) and concomitantly inhibits Th1 cytokine production in mitogen-and antigen-stimulated human peripheral blood mononuclear cell cultures. *Clin Exp Immunol.* 1995;99:160–167.

43. Heney D, Norfolk DR, Wheeldon J, et al. Thalidomide treatment for chronic graft-versus-host disease. *Brit J Haematol.* 1991;78:23–27.

44. Vogelsang GB, Farmer ER, Hess AD, et al. Thalidomide for the treatment of chronic graft-versus-host disease. *N Engl J Med.* 1992;326:1055–1058.

45. Parker PM, Chao N, Nademanee A, et al. Thalidomide as salvage therapy for chronic graft-versus-host disease. *Blood.* 1995;86:3604–3609.

46. Rovelli A, Arrigo C, Nesi F, et al. The role of thalidomide in the treatment of refractory chronic graft-versus-host disease following bone marrow transplantation in children. *Bone Marrow Transplant.* 1998;21:577–581.

47. Browne PV, Weisdorf DJ, DeFor T, et al. Response to thalidomide therapy in refractory chronic graft-versus-host disease. *Bone Marrow Transplant.* 2000;26:865–869.

48. Van de Poel MHW, Pasman PC, Schouten HC. The use of thalidomide in chronic refractory graft versus host disease. *Neth J Med.* 2001;59:45–49.

49. Kulkarni S, Powles R, Sirohi B, et al. Thalidomide after allogeneic haematopoietic stem cell transplantation: activity in chronic but not in acute graft-versus-host disease. *Bone Marrow Transplant.* 2003;32:165–170.

50. Rodriguez V, Anderson PM, Trotz BA, Arndt CA, Allen JA, Khan SP. Use of infliximab-daclizumab combination for the treatment of acute and chronic graft-versus-host disease of the liver and gut. *Pediatr Blood Cancer.* 2007;49:212–215.

51. Goldberg JD, Jacobsohn DA, Margolis J, et al. Pentostatin for the treatment of chronic graft-versus-host disease in children. *J Pediatr Hematol Oncol.* 2003;25:584–588.

52. Arat M, Ilhan O, Iayan EA, Celebi H, Koc H, Akan H. Treatment of extensive chronic sclerodermatous graft-versus-host disease with high-dose immunosuppressive therapy and CD34+ autologous stem cell rescue. *Blood.* 2001;98:892–893.

53. Mookerjee B, Altomonte V, Vogelsang G. Salvage therapy for refractory chronic graft-versus-host disease with mycophenolate mofetil and tacrolimus. *Bone Marrow Transplant.* 1999;24:517–520.

54. Busca A, Saroglia EM, Lanino E, et al. Mycophenolate mofetil (MMF) as therapy for refractory chronic GVHD (cGVHD) in children receiving bone marrow transplantation. *Bone Marrow Transplant.* 2000;25:1067–1071.

55. Basara N, Kiehl MG, Blau W, et al. Mycophenolate mofetil in the treatment of acute and chronic GVHD in hematopoietic stem cell transplant patients: four years of experience. *Transplant Proc.* 2001;33:2121–2123.

56 Baudard M, Vincent A, Moreau P, et al. Mycophenolate mofetil for the treatment of acute and chronic GVHD is effective and well tolerated but induces a high risk of infectious complications: a series of 21 BM or PBSC transplant patients. *Bone Marrow Transplant.* 2002;30:287–295.

57. Busca A, Locatelli F, Marmont F, et al. Response to mycophenolate mofetil therapy for refractory chronic graft-versus-host disease. *Haemat.* 2003;88:837–838.

58. Kim JG, Sohn SK, Kim DH, et al. Different efficacy of mycophenolate mofetil as salvage treatment for acute and chronic GVHD after allogeneic stem cell transplant. *Eur J Haematol.* 2004;73:56–61.

59. Lopez F, Parker P, Nademanee A, et al. Efficacy of mycophenolate mofetil in the treatment of chronic graft-versus-host disease. *Biol Blood Marrow Transplant.* 2005;11:307–313.

60. Krejci M, Doubek M, Buchler T, et al. Mycophenolate mofetil for the treatment of acute and chronic steroid-refractory graft-versus-host disease. *Ann Hematol.* 2005;84:681–685.

61. Slavin S. Successful treatment of autoimmune disease in (NZB/NZW)F1 female mice by using fractionated total lymphoid irradiation. *Proc Natl Acad Sci U S A.* 1979;76:5274–5276.

62. Valentine VG, Robbins RC, Wehner JH, et al. Total lymphoid irradiation for refractory acute rejection in heart-lung and lung allografts. *Chest.* 1996;109:1184–1189.

63. Field EH, Rouse TM, Gao Q, et al. Association between enhanced Th2/Th1 cytokine profile and donor T-cell chimerism following total lymphoid irradiation. *Hum Immunol.* 1997;52:144–154.

64. Lan F, Zeng D, Higuchi M, et al. Host conditioning with total lymphoid irradiation and antithymocyte globulin prevents graft-versus-host disease: the role of CD1-recative natural killer T cells. *Biol Blood Marrow Transplant.* 2003;9:355–363.

65. Socie G, Devergie A, Cosset JM, et al. Low-dose (one gray) total-lymphoid irradiation for extensive, drug-resistant chronic graft-versus-host disease. *Transplant.* 1990;49:657–658.

66. Bullorsky EO, Shanley CM, Stemmelin GR, et al. Total lymphoid irradiation for treatment of drug resistant chronic GVHD. *Bone Marrow Transplant.* 1993;11:75–76.

67. Robin M, Guardiola P, Girinsky T, et al. Low-dose thoracoabdominal irradiation for the treatment of refractory chronic graft-versus-host disease. *Transplant.* 2005;80:634–642.

68. Ullrich SE. Mechanisms underlying UV-induced immune suppression. *Mutat Res.* 2005;571:185–205.

69. Vogelsang GB, Wolff D, Altomonte V, et al. Treatment of chronic graft-versus-host disease with ultraviolet irradiation and psoralen (PUVA) *Bone Marrow Transplant.* 1996; 17:1061–1067.

70. Aubin F, Brion A, Deconinck E, et al. Phototherapy in the treatment of cutaneous graft-versus-host disease. *Transplant.* 1995;1:151–155.

71. Volc-Platzer B, Hönigsmann H, Hinterberger W, Wolff K. Photochemotherapy improves chronic cutaneous graft-versus-host disease. *J Am Acad Dermatol.* 1990;23:220–228.

72. Eppinger T, Ehninger G, Steinert M, Niethammer D, et al. 8-Methoxypsoralen and ultraviolet A therapy for cutaneous manifestations of graft-versus-host disease. *Transplant.* 1990;50:807–811.

73. Atkinson K, Weller P, Rayman W, Biggs J. PUVA therapy for drug-resistant graft-versus-host disease. *Bone Marrow Transplant.* 1986;1:227–236.

74. Jampel RM, Farmer ER, Vogelsang GB, et al. PUVA therapy for chronic cutaneous graft-versus-host disease. *Arch Dermatol.* 1991;127:1673–1678.

75 Wolff D, Anders V, Corio R, et al. Oral PUVA and topical steroids for treatment of oral manifestations of chronic graft-versus-host disease. *Photoderm Photoimmunol Photomed.* 2004;20:184–190.

76. Redding SW, Callander NS, Haveman CW, Leonard DL. Treatment of oral chronic graft-versus-host disease with PUVA therapy: case report and literature review. *Oral Surg Oral Med Oral Pathol Oral Radiol Endod.* 1998;86:183–187.

77. Kerscher M, Volkenandt M, Meurer M, et al. Treatment of localized scleroderma with PUVA bath photochemotherapy. *Lancet.* 1994;343:1233.

78. Leiter U, Kaskel P, Krähn G, et al. Psoralen plus ultraviolet-A-bath photochemotherapy as an adjunct treatment modality in cutaneous chronic graft-versus-host disease. *Photoderm Photoimmun Photomed.* 2002;18:183–190.

79. Altman JS, Adler SS. Development of multiple cutaneous squamous cell carcinomas during PUVA treatment for chronic graft-versus-host disease. *J Am Acad Dermatol.* 1994;31:505–507.

80. Lindelöf B, Sigurgeirsson B, Tegner E, et al. PUVA and cancer risk: the Swedish follow-up study. *Br J Dermatol.* 1999; 141:108–112.

81. Grundmann-Kollmann M, Behrens S, Gross C, et al. Chronic sclerodermic graft-versus-host disease refractory to immunosuppressive treatment responds to UVA1 phototherapy. *J Am Acad Dermatol.* 2000;42:134–136.

82. Ständer H, Schiller M, Schwarz T. UVA1 therapy for sclerodermic graft-versus-host disease of the skin. *J Am Acad Dermatol.* 2002;46:799–800.

83. Calzavara Pinton P, Porta F, Izzi T, et al. Prospects for ultraviolet A1 phototherapy as a treatment for chronic cutaneous graft-versus-host disease. *Haematologica.* 2003;88:1169–1175.

84. Wetzig T, Sticherling M, Simon JC, et al. Medium dose long-wavelength ultraviolet A (UVA1) phototherapy for the treatment of acute and chronic graft-versus-host disease of the skin. *Bone Marrow Transplant.* 2005;35:515–519.

85. Enk CD, Elad S, Vexler A, et al. Chronic graft-versus-host disease treated with UVB phototherapy. *Bone Marrow Transplant.* 1998;22:1179–1183.

86. Van Dooren-Greebe RJ, Schattenburg A, Koopman RJJ. Chronic cutaneous graft-versus-host disease: successful treatment with UVB. *Br J Derm.* 1991;125:498–499.

87. Ratanatharathorn V, Ayash L, Reynolds C, et al. Treatment of chronic graft-versus-host disease with anti-CD20 chimeric monoclonal antibody. *Biol Blood Marrow Transplant.* 2003;9:505–511.

88. Canninga-van Dijk MR, Van der Straaten HM, Fijnheer R, et al. Anti-CD20 monoclonal antibody treatment in 6 patients with therapy-refractory chronic graft-versus-host disease. *Blood.* 2004;104:2603–2606.

89. Cutler C, Miklos D, Kim HT, et al. Rituximab for steroid-refractory chronic graft-versus-host disease. *Blood.* 2006;108:756–762.

90. Zaja F, Bacigalupo A, Patriarca F, et al. Treatment of refractory chronic GVHD with rituximab: a GITMO study. *Bone Marrow Transplant.* 2007;40:273–277.

91. Lee SJ, Wegner SA, McGarigle CJ, Bierer BE, Antin JH. Treatment of chronic graft-versus-host disease with clofazimine. *Blood*. 1997;89:2298–2302.

92. Marcellus DC, Altomonte VL, Farmer ER, et al. Etretinate therapy for refractory sclerodermatous chronic graft-versus-host disease. *Blood*. 1999;93:66–70.

93. Gilman AL, Chan KW, Mogul A, et al. Hydroxychloroquine for the treatment of chronic graft-versus-host disease. *Biol Blood Marrow Transplant*. 2000;6:327–334.

94. Bolanos-Meade J, Jacobsohn DA, Margolis J, et al. Pentostatin in steroid-refractory acute graft-versus-host disease. *J Clin Oncol*. 2005;23:2661–2668.

95. Busca A, Locatelli F, Marmont F, Ceretto C, Falda M. Recombinant human soluble tumor necrosis factor receptor fusion proteina s treatment for steroid refractory graft-versus-host disease following allogeneic hematopoietic stem cell transplantation. *Am J Hematol*. 2006;82:45–52.

96. Chiang KY, Abhyankar S, Bridges K, Godder K, Henslee-Downey JP. Recombinant human tumor necrosis factor receptor fusion protein as complementary treatment for chronic graft-versus-host disease. *Transplantation*. 2002;73:665–667.

97. Willenbacher W, Basara N, Blau IW, Fauser AA, Kiehl MG. Treatment of steroid refractory acute and chronic graft-versus-host disease with daclizumab. *Br J Haematol*. 2001;112:820–823.

98. Teachey DT, Bickert B, Bunin N. Daclizumab for children with corticosteroid refractory graft-versus-host disease. *Bone Marrow Transplant*. 2006;37:95–99.

14

Evaluating Therapeutic Response in Chronic Graft versus Host Disease

David A. Jacobsohn, Sandra A. Mitchell, and Steven Z. Pavletic

INTRODUCTION

Importance of Chronic GVHD Response Criteria

Chronic graft versus host disease (GVHD) is one of the major barriers to successful outcomes in allogeneic hematopoietic stem cell transplantation (HSCT). Undoubtedly, one of the key problems has been the lack of well-designed prospective clinical trials that test agents in chronic GVHD. Accepted endpoints for chronic GVHD studies are overall survival or permanent discontinuation of immunosuppression [1, 2]. While these endpoints may work for a large phase III trial, they are not acceptable for early phase trials. Moreover, they are endpoints that require one to control for significant confounding variables, thus necessitating larger sample sizes typically only achievable in multisite studies. Patients, investigators, and clinicians need results from smaller early phase studies that may indicate the potential efficacy of a specific agent for treatment of chronic GVHD. Unfortunately, few such early phase trials have been conducted, and the relative absence of clinically meaningful short, intermediate, and longer-term endpoints that can be feasibly and reliably measured may deter investigators from pursuing such drug development trials (Table 14.1).

The imperative to define response criteria that are reliable, valid, and sensitive to clinically important therapeutic change is clear. Chronic GVHD problem is increasing because of the decrease in early transplant-related mortality, more frequent use of donor-lymphocyte infusions, peripheral blood stem cells, increasing age of transplant recipients, and use of more alternative donors. Systemic corticosteroids as primary therapy for chronic GVHD was shown more than 25 years ago to improve survival as compared to no therapy [3]. Patients with extensive cGVHD require prolonged treatment [1, 2]. There is no standard therapy for patients whose cGVHD does not resolve on steroids. Unless there are very obvious clinical changes, it is can be very difficult to decide whether a drug is actually changing the course of a patient's GVHD. Given the potential toxicities and immunosuppressive effects of these drugs, the therapeutic index is narrow. Thus now more than ever it is incumbent upon the transplant community to develop validated response criteria that can be used to systematically test the activity of different compounds in chronic GVHD. The availability of such criteria could greatly improve the efficiency of drug development in chronic GVHD. There is currently no US Food and Drug Administration-approved medication for use in chronic GVHD. The presence of validated short-term response criteria would likely lead to more phase I and II trials in chronic GVHD, and these would yield valuable information that could identify potential phase III candidates. Currently there are few early-stage trials, and those that are in progress or have been performed have had to use definitions of responses that are usually based on subjective assessments of global complete (disappearance of all symptoms) or partial response (50% reduction in symptoms) based on nonreproducible subjective physician assessments. There is a considerable variability in tools used from one study to the next (review by G. Akpek available at: http://www.asbmt.org/GVHDForms.htm). There has been a trend toward introducing "surrogate" measures of benefit in chronic GVHD trials such as the ability to taper steroids. However, this endpoint is controlled by the physician and of uncertain value unless a double-blinded study is employed or the taper is conducted according to a fixed predefined algorithm. Because the yield from these studies is dampened, caution has to be taken before committing resources to a large phase III trial based on these results.

This chapter summarizes the challenges encountered to date in evaluating therapeutic response in chronic GVHD clinical trials, identifies the desirable clinimetric properties of outcome evaluation measures for this patient population, and outlines the National Institutes of Health (NIH) chronic GVHD response criteria [4]. We conclude by outlining the significant challenges that remain in defining therapeutic response in chronic GVHD clinical trials, and suggest some future directions for the further development of chronic GVHD response criteria.

Table 14.1: Measurement Characteristics

Reliability
Measure produces same score on repeated use in the same setting

Validity
Content/Face Validity
Items appear to measure what they are intended to measure
Items are representative of all aspects of the outcome of interest
Convergent/Discriminant Validity
Measure demonstrates convergence with constructs that are theoretically related (convergent validity) or theoretically unrelated (discriminant validity)
Groups known to be different from each other have significantly different scores on a measure
Criterion Validity/Concurrent validity
Measure is highly associated with a gold-standard measure of the construct but which may not be feasible for routine use
Measure predicts an objective, specific, and clinically meaningful future outcome such as disease-free survival
Sensitive/Responsive to Change
Measure is capable of detecting sufficiently small changes in the outcome or discriminating/differentiating clinically important differences in disease state between individuals and within an individual over time

Feasibility
Measure can be reasonably obtained (e.g., readily available, manageable clinician and patient burden) in the setting in which it is to be used

---

DIAGNOSIS, STAGING, AND RESPONSE CRITERIA

It is important to differentiate between response criteria and diagnosis/staging criteria. For any disease, the goals of diagnosis/staging are to determine the presence and gauge the extent and severity of involvement. For chronic GVHD in particular, adequate staging criteria will allow health-care practitioners to grade the degree and extent of organ involvement [5]. This staging should ideally provide some assessment of risk, or prognosis [6, 7] Therefore, a good staging system should guide the decision of whether or not to begin topical or systemic therapy for chronic GVHD, since the decision will be based on extent of organ involvement, severity, and the prognosis of the current status of the patient's disease. A good example is the staging for acute GVHD [8], which serves multiple purposes. First, it allows to easily communicate about the current status of a patient's GVHD so that someone familiar with the scale will have a clear understanding of the severity of the acute GVHD even without seeing the patient. Second, it risk-stratifies patients [9]; and third, it guides the decision about whether or not to begin or intensify immunosuppressive therapy.

Adequate response criteria fill a very different role as compared to staging criteria in chronic GVHD. Most important, response criteria need to be sensitive to change as compared to staging criteria. While staging criteria need to be broad to accommodate the different segments of the disease spectrum, response criteria must be specific, and sensitive to change, to ensure that even small but potentially clinically meaningful changes can be captured on a clinical trial.

CONSIDERATIONS IN SELECTING INDICATORS FOR MEASURING RESPONSE

In designing a clinical trial, decisions must be made not only about the selection of the outcome(s), but also about how they will be measured. Beyond survival and discontinuation or tapering of immunosuppression, most relevant indicators of therapeutic response include changes in target tissues and organs involved with GVHD (e.g., skin, mouth, eyes, liver hematologic system), symptom burden (severity, frequency, distress and interference with usual function), functional performance and capacity, and quality of life. Desirable approaches to measurement of these variables may include objective indicators (such as MRI, laboratory data), clinician assessments (e.g., body surface area [BSA] involvement, range of motion, walk velocity, Karnofsky Performance Status), and patient-reported outcome measures (e.g., SF-36, symptom scales, patient perception of change). Other measures that are relevant to determinations of therapeutic effect beyond solely determining therapeutic response include the burden of treatment (side effects, time lost from work) and direct and indirect costs.

There is increasing appreciation of the value of incorporating the patient's perception into outcome measurement [10–13]. Objective and clinician-based measures of disease manifestations may fail to fully capture the ways that a chronic illness and its treatment affect an individual's perceived health, mood, functioning, and quality of life. Measurement of patient-reported outcomes (PROs) is a particularly valuable technique to gauge dimensions of improvement such as symptom burden or functional performance that may be less visible to clinicians and are not captured by diagnostic testing.

An ideal outcome measurement system has several characteristics. It should be reliable, valid, specific/relevant, responsive to change, discriminate clinically important changes in disease activity, be associated strongly with treatment outcome, and be feasible for widespread use, and have limited redundancy. The importance of each of these characteristics for chronic GVHD response evaluation is further examined below. As we will later illustrate, the selection of the outcome and the approach taken to measuring that outcome can significantly influence the interpretability of clinical trial results. Therefore, considerable thought and consultation should be given when designing this fundamental component of a research study.

DEFINITIONS OF PROPERTIES THAT APPLY TO MEASUREMENT SCALES

In designing a measurement system to evaluate therapeutic response for a disorder that is characterized by diverse manifestations, a variable time course, and a spectrum of disease activity and residual damage, several important clinimetric criteria or properties should be satisfied. Clinimetrics is the science of characterizing the properties of a clinical measurement instrument including the dimensions of reliability, validity, responsiveness to change, and feasibility, when the measure is applied to measure an outcome in a specific patient population.

The essential property of any measure is that it be both valid and reliable. Considerations of reliability will be assessed differently, depending upon whether a measure is scored by a clinician, is an objective indicator, or is a PRO. For clinician-evaluated measures, there are two types of measures of reliability that need to be taken into consideration: intra-rater reliability (an index of intra-observer variability when one person measures the same item twice and their ratings are compared) and inter-rater reliability (an index of variability when comparing two or more persons measuring the same item) [14]. The measurement of the amount of BSA involved with a lichenoid rash provides an example. If an investigator measures the involved BSA at 25%, how close to that value does the same person need to be when he/she examines the identical rash again (intra-rater) and how close does another investigator need to be when examining the same rash (inter-rater)?

Another important property of a measure is that it is *valid*, in other words, that it measures what it purports to measure. Validity refers to the degree to which a measure accurately reflects or assesses the specific concept that the researcher is attempting to measure. While reliability is concerned with the accuracy of the actual measuring instrument or procedure, validity is concerned with the study's success at measuring *what the researchers set out to measure*. Establishing validity means establishing the relationship between the measurement of a concept and the actual presence or amount of the concept itself.

A measure may be highly reliable but not valid as a measure of the outcome of interest. For example, evaluating the diameter of a skin ulcer on the bottom of the foot may be a very reliable measure (i.e., good agreement between raters and good agreement when one rater assesses the same skin ulcer twice), but the diameter of a skin ulcer is not a particularly valid measure of, for example, functional capacity. On the other hand, a measure may be valid but not reliable. A measure like grip strength, for example, may be a very valid test of upper extremity strength, but if it is not obtained in a consistent fashion on each occasion (e.g., if sometimes the measure is taken on the dominant hand and sometimes the nondominant hand, if the hand dynamometer isn't adjusted for hand size) the measurement obtained is neither a reliable nor a valid test of upper extremity strength. On the other hand, grip strength may not be a valid measure if what we are interested in is functional capacity for ambulation, since upper body strength is not directly involved in ambulation.

In supporting an argument that a measure is valid, several different types of validity evidence may be considered [15–17]. There are two principal categories of validity evidence: content validity and construct validity. The simplest type of validity is content validity (sometimes called *face validity*). Content validity refers to the degree to which the items appear to measure what they are intended to measure and that items are representative of all aspects of the outcome that is being tested. Construct validity is concerned with whether an instrument actually measures the construct it purports to measure. For example, a measure may be said to be a measure of the severity of chronic GVHD skin involvement. Evidence that the measure actually gauges the *severity* of chronic GVHD skin manifestations is needed to support construct validity. A number of different approaches are informative when judging the construct validity of a measure, including convergent, discriminant, and criterion validity. Convergent validity is present when the measure of interest shows a correspondence or convergence with a measure of a similar construct, and discriminant validity is present when measures of constructs that theoretically should not be related to each other are in fact observed to be unrelated (i.e., your measure discriminates between dissimilar constructs). This is sometimes established using correlation coefficients, or by using a "known" or contrasted groups approach. The known groups approach is based on the hypothesis that if a measure is valid, the scores on that measure should be significantly different for members of already constituted groups who have differing characteristics. For example, a new measure of disease severity would have evidence of validity if it were able to discriminate persons who clinicians had divided into groups based on mild, moderate, and severe disease manifestations. Construct validity can also be explored by examining agreement between a new measure and a gold-standard approach to the measurement of that same characteristic (concurrent validity). Lastly, a measure has evidence of validity when it is able to predict a specific and objective future outcome. Methods that examine the underlying structure of a measure, such as factor analysis, can also support conclusions about construct validity. Measurement characteristics that should

Table 14.2: Response Criteria Development Strategies: Need for Accepted and Validated Short-Term Endpoints in Chronic GVHD Clinical Trials

Endpoint	Interpretation	Time of Endpoint	Comment
Survival	Universally accepted direct measure of benefit Easily measured	Long (years) Randomized studies needed	Not suitable for early drug development or pilot studies
Objective response (CR/PR)	Surrogate of clinically meaningful benefit	Short (months) Can assess in single arm studies	Few drugs produce high CR/PR rates Validation complexity
Change in the biomarker	Surrogate endpoint intended to substitute for a major clinical endpoint or early predictor of response	Ultra short (days, weeks) Smaller single arm studies	Very attractive for drug development None exist

CR, complete response; GVHD, graft versus host disease; PR, partial response.

be considered when selecting an outcome measure are summarized in Table 14.2.

EVALUATION OF THERAPEUTIC OUTCOMES IN CHRONIC DISEASE

Having examined the characteristics of an ideal outcome measure, some consideration of the directions taken in evaluating therapeutic outcomes in other chronic illnesses may also inform our understanding of therapeutic response evaluation in chronic GVHD. Systems for measuring clinical response and therapeutic outcomes have been described for a number of rheumatologic conditions including rheumatoid arthritis, systemic vasculitis, Sjogren's syndrome, dermatomyositis, and systemic sclerosis [18–25], as well as for multiple sclerosis, and multiple system atrophy [26, 27]. The systems described in the literature typically incorporated specific criteria for clinician evaluation of disease activity together with some kind of objective radiographic or laboratory measure. Many include PRO measures such as symptom burden, self-assessed functional performance, or health-related quality of life. Many of the response evaluation approaches also include instruments to capture patient and clinicians' view of change over time and their respective perceptions of global disease severity. In some instances, performance-based measures of function (walk distance, muscle strength) are also included. Not every system provides specific guidance concerning the degree of change needed to define a response as improvement. Approaches to defining response have included dichotomous definitions (improved/not improved), ordinal definitions (degrees of response scored on an ordinal scale), change in the overall index of disease activity (all measures either summed or weighted to create an index of disease activity), or a continuous definition of improvement (e.g., percentage change in a measure, mean at time of evaluating response divided by baseline mean value, number of measures improved by X%) [28].

Systems used in evaluating juvenile inflammatory conditions and systemic sclerosis have attempted to dissect disease activity from residual damage [20, 29, 30] and have also attempted to optimize the feasibility and reproducibility of response measurements [31]. Some of the measures of disease activity simply pool findings of activity to create a composite score, and others create a single index measure by weighting specific disease manifestations. Many of the systems emerged through a consensus development approach. Those applied in the evaluation of therapeutic response for rheumatologic disorders have undergone the most extensive clinimetric evaluation.

LIMITATIONS OF HISTORICAL APPROACHES USED TO MEASURE RESPONSE IN CHRONIC GVHD

Table 14.3 summarizes the challenges in response evaluation that may have attenuated the information yield of the clinical trials in cGVHD performed to date. To illustrate the dilemmas these challenges pose in interpreting results, it is useful to look back at main therapeutic trials in chronic GVHD. Some of the first therapeutic trials for chronic GVHD were published in 1988; Sullivan et al. reported on alternating-day cyclosporine/prednisone and prednisone/azathioprine comparing it to prednisone alone [32, 33]. Although the authors presented sites of disease, there is no way of gathering in which domains (i.e., skin, mouth, etc.) the actual response occurred. There is also a very significant weight placed on biopsies. A response in these reports constituted "clinically inactive chronic GVHD" but it was partial if biopsies showed continued GVHD activity and complete if biopsies showed no GVHD activity. Many questions are raised from these important works. What is the definition of active versus inactive chronic GVHD? We may assume that a rash was considered active but it is impossible to know whether sclerotic GVHD was considered active or inactive. In some ways the definition of response is quite demanding – if

Table 14.3: Challenges in Response Evaluation Encountered in Chronic GVHD Trials to Date

Differentiating active versus inactive disease manifestations

Dissecting disease activity versus residual damage

Histopathology may aid for establishing the diagnosis, but is not suitable for monitoring of clinical improvement

Whether response is gauged through *qualitative change* in a manifestation in addition to or instead of *change in the extent* of a manifestation varies depending upon organ system (e.g., skin texture vs. liver function tests)

Variable definitions of complete response, partial response, and progression

Selection of endpoints – to date trials have emphasized long term outcomes of mortality, discontinuation of immunosuppression

Characterizing overall response (improvement in some dimensions vs. stability in others)

Trajectory of disease change prior the time of trial entry (progressive vs. stable vs. improving) can affect the assessment of response versus stability after intervention

Defining minimal clinically important difference

Evaluating response is challenging especially at the extremes: With a lower burden of disease, it is difficult to identify clinically important difference and measurement error may obscure change. With a greater burden of disease, it is easier to demonstrate response but is that response clinically sufficiently meaningful?

GVHD, graft versus host disease.

a patient had had a decrease in rash from 80% to 10%, this patient would not have been classified as a responder using that scheme. What about manifestations that we now know persist and do not improve, such as ocular sicca? Were these manifestations considered active or inactive disease? Finally, we may ask what is the role of a biopsy in assessing response? Is a biopsy useful only for diagnostic purposes (and that is at times questionable) or can it tell us something about the degree of response? Even with this scale, the authors were able to show, in both publications, a degree of responsiveness to therapy, as there was an adequate distribution among complete responders, partial responders, and those that failed therapy. Most importantly though, response predicted outcome: mortality increased incrementally from complete responders to partial responders to those that failed treatment. For complete responders, mortality at 9 months was 0% to 20%, for partial responders it was 15% to 31%, and for those that failed therapy it was 54% to 75%. Establishing that response according to their semi-quantitative scale did correlate with survival was groundbreaking and led to a heightened awareness of the need for early implementation of therapy in chronic GVHD.

Vogelsang et al. took a very different approach in looking at response in their study treating with thalidomide refractory or high-risk chronic GVHD patients [34]. They attempted to quantify percent improvement, and used that change in determining whether a patient had a response or not. To obtain a partial response, patients needed to have greater than 50% but less than 100% improvement in all affected areas. For skin they looked at lichenoid rashes, active sclerodermatous changes, and hair distribution. A few points regarding this skin assessment are worth mentioning. First is that they qualified sclerodermatous changes by the word "active." This implies that "inactive" scleroderma may have been counted as no GVHD. It is not clear how the investigators distinguished between active versus inactive scleroderma? Furthermore, if a patient's skin manifestations maintained the same BSA involvement but changed

from doughy moveable scleroderma to the nonmoveable sclerodermatous skin that is tight and bound to the bone (that may never respond to immunosuppression and may thus be termed "inactive" by some), would that have been considered a response or persistence of disease, or perhaps even worsening of disease? Also, do we require a decrease in the BSA involved by scleroderma, or simply a texture change (e.g., softening) in the quality of the skin involved?

Another important challenge is that of defining the magnitude of improvement necessary for partial response, across the full range of disease severity/burden. Two dilemmas contribute to the challenge that arises in defining the magnitude of change that constitutes partial response. First, the magnitude of improvement that constitutes partial response declines in a nonlinear fashion as the burden of disease declines, with the result that discerning partial response is comparatively more difficult when the burden of disease is lower. Contributing to this is the difficulty of reliably measuring small clinical changes. The second dilemma arises in determining whether a partial response when the disease burden is low constitutes a clinically significant improvement. A 50% improvement is often used to define partial response and clinical benefit in systems of therapeutic response evaluation and illustrates the differential functioning of this criterion with lower and higher burden of disease. While the 50% improvement definition may be acceptable when there is a high burden of disease (where it is easier to demonstrate clinical response), a 50% improvement in a person with a lower burden of disease might represent only a clinically trivial change. Moreover, the difficulty of reliably discerning improvement with a lower burden of disease given the measurement error introduced with clinical evaluation across time further complicates response evaluation. In a patient who has a skin rash involving about 80% of the body surface area, improvement to 20% of the body surface area involved with rash is clearly a greater than 50% response, and in this situation, it is easy for an outcome assessor to determine that this is a partial response. A 75% reduction in the extent of body surface area involved is also clinically significant. There is also a large margin of error that can be accepted to arrive at the same answer – for the most part if the initial evaluation was called anywhere between 70 and 90 involvement and the final anywhere between 10 and 30, it would still be termed a partial response. However, even small imprecision in clinical assessment is amplified as we move to a lower burden of disease. If someone begins with 10% skin involvement, then a partial response requires a decrease to 5% of body surface area involved. Obviously the effects of the variation around such a small number are different from the effects of that same variation around a larger number, rendering assessment of response with lower burden of disease comparatively more difficult. The other closely related issue is that of clinical importance of partial response when the burden of disease is low. Is going from a 10% to a 5% lichenoid rash as meaningful as going from a 80% to a 40% lichenoid rash? These would both be called a partial response in the thalidomide trial example we are discussing. Similarly, that trial would have called a total bilirubin moving from 4 to 2 a partial response as well as a bilirubin moving from 20 to 10. While both scenarios represent a 50% decrease from the baseline, they may have vastly different implications for the patient and for the drug under study.

In 1995, Parker et al. published a larger trial utilizing thalidomide [35] in a very similar group of patients as in Vogelsang et al.'s trial. One of the striking differences is that a partial response on the basis of skin required patients to have > 50% improvement in the extent of skin involvement. One interpretation is that the authors of this clinical trial were in fact more conservative than Vogelsang et al. Here a patient with scleroderma would need to have a significant reduction in the total amount of scleroderma, whereas in the prior trial, a change from active to inactive scleroderma may have constituted a response. One of the concerns with the Parker et al. design is that improvement as gauged by softening of the skin but not resolution of the extent may be missed. A drug may be clinically active and lead to skin softening, which may in turn improve the quality of life of the patient; however, this degree of improvement could be missed if we only look at extent of skin involvement. In sum, assessment of therapeutic response in a complex multiorgan chronic disease such as chronic GVHD poses a number of conceptual challenges. The lag time in determining response and relative event rarity make the classic objective endpoints of survival or disease remission unsuitable for drug development trials in chronic GVHD. There is a need for measures that can quantify and capture eventual intervention-induced changes in diverse clinical manifestations, symptoms, and patient's experiences associated with chronic GVHD (Figure 14.1).

NIH CONSENSUS CRITERIA FOR EVALUATING RESPONSE IN CHRONIC GVHD

Developed by national and international experts through a series of consensus meetings in 2005, and published in 2006, the

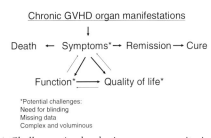

Figure 14.1 Challenges in developing response criteria for chronic GVHD: Lack of accepted outcomes in trials when survival or remission are not adequate endpoints.
GVHD, graft versus host disease.

NIH Criteria for Evaluating Therapeutic Response in Chronic GVHD were developed to overcome the inherent limitations of the current approaches to evaluating response. As shown in Table 14.4 the criteria include core and ancillary measures, and encompass objective indicators, clinician assessed indicators, and patient-reported outcomes. The criteria have also been tailored to the pediatric setting. The measures were developed to be easy to use by transplantation and nontransplantation care providers, using evaluation methods that are feasible for use in busy outpatient settings. The measures focus on the most important and common manifestations of chronic GVHD and emphasize quantitative, continuous level measures. Measurement domains were conceptually defined and measures specifically selected to represent each of those domains, specifically, chronic GVHD-specific signs, symptoms, global ratings, functional status, and quality of life. The selection of measures emphasized those with established measurement properties in other chronically ill patient populations. Initial evaluation at baseline defines irreversible organ damage that is to be excluded from future response assessments, as well as sentinel features to be followed prospectively. The impact of therapy on general aspects of physical and mental health, symptom burden, functional status, and quality of life are followed. Provisional definitions of complete response, partial response, and disease progression for each organ and for overall response have also been proposed. Measures should be made at 3-month intervals and whenever a major change in treatment occurs. An educational program to train investigators in the use of the response criteria has been developed by Mitchell and Pavletic in 2006 and a variety of data collection tools are also available (www.asbmt.org/GVHDForms). Figure 14.2 shows one of the main data collection tools, which captures skin, oral, and ocular manifestations as well as documents gastrointestinal symptoms, hematology, liver, and pulmonary function tests, global ratings, and optional ancillary measures of functional performance. Data collection focuses on quantitative measures of primary organ manifestations. Organ-specific measures are separated from symptoms, function, and therapeutic intention to promote better sensitivity in detecting a therapeutic effect in drug development trials. Functional performance endpoints of grip strength and 2-minute walk distance are optional with the intion to be

Table 14.4: NIH Proposed Response Criteria Measures

Measure	Clinician Assessed	Patient Reported
Core	Organ-specific measures	N/A
Signs	clinician assessed	Patient reported
Symptoms		Lee Symptom Scale
Global rating	7-point change scale	7-point change scale
	Mild–moderate–severe	Mild–moderate–severe
	0–10 severity scale	0–10 severity scale
Ancillary		
Function	Grip strength	HAP
	2-minute walk distance	ASK (children)
Performance status	Karnofsky/Lansky	N/A
Quality of life	N/A	FACT-BMT
		SF-36 v.2
		CHRIs-HSCT (children)

ASK, activities scale for kids; BMT, bone marrow transplantation; CHRI-HSCT, child health ratings inventory-hematopoietic stem cell transplantation module; HAP, human activity profile; N/A, not applicable; SF-36, = Medical Outcomes Study Short Form 36. Source: Based on information from Pavletic et al. *Biol Blood Marrow Transplant.* 2006; 12:252–266.

explored as ancillary supporting endpoints in trials. Measures are collected at baseline and every 3 months until study endpoints are met. Overall determination of response is made by the study coordinating center according to the general guidelines describes in the response criteria documents [4].

It is important to stress the inclusion of symptom severity and bother (both patient-reported and as captured by the health-care team) in the NIH recommendations. Until now, as illustrated in the trials discussed above, response assessment has been solely based on the clinician observing changes in the signs of GVHD – but not the symptoms. The specific patient-reported symptom scale that the GVHD consensus recommends concurrently with clinical assessment is the Lee Symptom Scale [36], which has been validated as a measure of the extent of bother associated with 30 chronic GVHD symptoms in adults. There is currently no analogous scale for children, and it is unclear whether this scale would be useful in that group, particularly in the younger patients. In addition to this scale, patients are asked whether they feel their GVHD is mild, moderate, or severe; they are asked how severe their chronic GVHD symptoms are on a scale of 0 to 10 [37]; and they are asked whether they feel their GVHD is same, better, or worse over the past month, reporting this change on a 7-point scale [38]. The health-care practitioner is asked to fill the same ratings as well with regard to the patient. There is also a short questionnaire for patients to rate their skin, oral, and ocular complaints from a scale of 1 to 10. Here the consensus group took a broad and multifaceted approach. Inclusion of multiple scales and measures may incorporate some redundancy without adding incremental information; however this can be established only in prospective longitudinal studies that explore the clinimetric properties of the response criteria including validity and

sensitivity to change. Investigators in other areas have noted that capturing the patient's view of change offered additional information that was complementary to clinicians' evaluation of change over time [39]. Moreover, such global rating scales can also be used in anchor-based approaches to determine the minimally important clinical difference and patient acceptable symptom state in other outcome measures [18, 40–42].

Another major change to what has been used up to now in evaluating patients with chronic GVHD is the recommendation to more closely assess functional capacity and functional performance. In addition to the GVHD-specific core measures, the NIH Consensus realized that chronic GVHD can greatly affect what a person does on a daily basis (functional performance) and what is their maximum physical capacity. Therefore, a number of tests of function and endurance are recommended, most of which come from the physical therapy and rehabilitation literature. These basic measures of functional capacity, grip strength [43, 44], and the 2-minute walk distance [45], while tested in a number of chronic diseases, have not yet been validated in chronic GVHD. The analysis and interpretation of functional measures in therapeutic trials will also need to control for the presence of comorbidities and consider the degree to which functional impairment may reflect fixed damage [46].

Though development and testing of these measures is ongoing, preliminary studies have contributed initial evidence of the feasibility and inter-rater reliability of the component elements of the response criteria [47]. Across 4 small pilot trials (n = 25 adult and pediatric patients; n = 34 clinician raters), the agreement was modest overall, with median intraclass correlations (ICCs) between novices and experts for movable sclerosis, nonmovable sclerosis, and oral findings began to approach the 0.7 level considered to be acceptable. These

FORM A

Current Patient Weight: _____   Today's Date: _____   MR#Name: _____

CHRONIC GVHD ACTIVITY ASSESSMENT-CLINICIAN

Component	Findings	Scoring (see skin score worksheet)
Skin Front / Back	Erythematous rash of any sort	% BSA (max 100%)
	Moveable sclerosis	% BSA (max 100%)
	Non-moveable sclerosis (hidebound/non-pinchable) or subcutaneous sclerosis/fascitis	% BSA (max 100%)
	Ulcer(s): select the largest ulcerative lesion, and measure its largest dimension in cm and mark location of ulcer	Location: _____ Largest dimension: _____ cm

Eyes Bilateral Schirmer's Tear Test (without anesthesia) in persons 9 years or older	Right Eye: _____ mm of wetting		Left Eye: _____ mm of wetting

Mouth Mouth Hard Palate — Soft Palate Pharynx — Uvula — Tongue	Mucosal change	No evidence of cGVHD		Mild		Moderate		Severe	
	Erythema	None	0	Mild erythema or moderate erythema (<25%)	1	Moderate (≥25%) or Severe erythema (<25%)	2	Severe erythema (≥25%)	3
	Lichenoid	None	0	Hyperkeratotic changes(<25%)	1	Hyperkeratotic changes(25-50%)	2	Hyperkeratotic changes (>50%)	3
	Ulcers	None	0	None	0	Ulcers involving (≤20%)	3	Severe ulcerations (>20%)	6
	Mucoceles*	None	0	1-5 mucoceles	1	6-10 scattered mucoceles	2	Over 10 mucoceles	3
				*Mucoceles scored for lower labial and soft palate only				Total score for all mucosal changes	

Blood Counts	Platelet Count _____ K/uL	ULN _____ K/uL	Total WBC _____ K/uL	ULN _____ K/uL	% Eosinophils _____ %
Liver Function Tests	Total serum bilirubin _____ mg/dL	ULN _____ mg/dL	ALT _____ U/L	ULN _____ U/L	Alkaline Phosphatase _____ U/L	ULN _____ U/L

Gastrointestinal-Upper GI • Early satiely OR • Anorexia OR • Nausea & Vomiting	0=no symptoms 1=mild, occasional symptoms, with little reduction in oral intake _during the past week_ 2=moderate, intermittent symptoms, with some reduction in oral intake _during the past week_ 3=more severe or persistent symptoms throughout the day. with marked reduction in oral intake. on almost every day of the past week
Gastrointestinal-Esophageal • Dysphagia OR • Odynophagia	0=no esophageal symptoms 1=Occasional dysphagia or odynophagia with solid food or pills _during the past week_ 2=Intermittent dysphagia or odynophagia with solid foods or pills, but not for liquids or soft foods, _during the past week_ 3=Dysphagia or odynophagia for almost all oral intake, _on almost every day of the past week_
Gastrointestinal-Lower GI • Diarrhea	0=no loose or liquid stools during the past week 1=occasional loose or liquid stools, on some days _during the past week_ 2=intermittent loose or liquid stools throughout the day, _on almost every day of the past week_ without requiring intervention to prevent or correct volume depletion 3=voluminous diarrhea on almost every day of the past week, requiring intervention to prevent or correct volume depletion
Lungs • Bronchiolitis Obliterans	Pulmonary Function Tests with Diffusing Capacity (attach report for person> 5 yrs old)	FEV-1 _____ % Predicted	Single Breath DLCO (adjusted for hemoglobin) _____ % Predicted

Health Care Provider Global Ratings: In your opinion, do you think that this patient's chronic GVHD is mild, moderate or severe? 0=none 1=mild 2=moderate 2=severe	Where would you rate the severity of this patient's chronic GVHD symptoms on the following scale, where 0 is cGVHD symptoms that are not at all severe and 10 is the most severe cGVHD symptoms possible: 0 1 2 3 4 5 6 7 8 9 10 cGVHD symptoms not at all severe Most severe cGvHD symptoms possible	Over the past <u>month</u> would you say that this patient's cGVHD is +3=Very much better +2=Moderately better +1=A little better 0=About the same −1=A little worse −2=Moderately worse −3=Very much worse
Functional Performance (in persons >4 years old) • Walk Time • Grip Strength	Total Distance Walked in 2 Minutes: Number of laps: _____ (× 50 feet) + final partial lap: _____ feet = _____ feet walked in 2 minutes	Grip Strength (Dominant Hand) Trial #1 _____ psi Trial #2 _____ psi Trial #3 _____ psi	Range of Motion: o Not performed o Physical Therapy Report Attached

Score	Lansky Performance Status Scale Definitions (circel from 0-100) (persons < 16 years old)	Karnofsky Performance Status Scale Definitions (circle from 0-100) (persons 16 years of older)
100	Fully active, normal	Normal no complaints; no evidence of disease
90	Minor restrictions in physically strenuous activity	Able to carry on normal activity; minor signs or symptoms of disease
80	Active, but tires more quickly	Normal acitivity with effort; some signs or symptoms of disease
70	Both greater restriction of and less time spent in play activity	Cares for self: unable to carry on normal activity or to do active work
60	Up and around, but minimal active play; keeps busy with quieter activities	Requires occasional assistance but is able to care for most personal needs
50	Gets dressed but lies around much of the day, no active play but able to participate in all quiet play and activities	Requires considerable assistance and frequent medical care
40	Mostly in bed; participates in quiet activities	Disabled; requires special care and assistance
30	In bed; needs assistances even for quiet play	Severely disabled; hospital admission is indicated although death not imminent
20	Often sleeping; play entirely limited to very passive activities	Very sick; hospital admission necessary; active supportive treatment necessary
10	No play; does not get out of bed	Moribund; fatal processed progressing rapidly
0	Unresponsive	Dead

Figure 14.2 Two Page Data Collection Form for Clinician Assessed Measures – NIH response criteria project. (Based on information from Pavletic et al. *Biol Blood Marrow Transplant.* 2006; 12:252–266.) See Plate 28 in the color plate section.

pilot studies also showed the response measures to be acceptable for clinician implementation. Completion of the patient self-report measures required a median of 16 to 17 minutes, suggesting only a modest respondent burden. Continued evaluation in prospective clinical trials is needed to determine if the various dimensions of the response criteria exhibit high correlation over time, whether they are sensitive to changes in disease manifestations and health status, and to continue to define the signal-to-noise ratio inherent in each measure. It is also important to stress that the proposed NIH criteria are not a final set of mandatory recommendations that must be used in their entirety. These new criteria provide only a set of guidelines and tools that can be selected for use prospectively, most commonly as secondary endpoints, for development in clinical trials. It is ultimately expected that after protracted data collection, validation, and refinements the transplant community would produce a validated set of response measures suitable also for new agent approval trials. The future utility of these response criteria can be perhaps also further enhanced by parallel development and incorporation of new biological markers for evaluation of responses.

FUTURE DIRECTIONS WITH THE NIH RESPONSE CRITERIA

The response criteria that have been set are much more comprehensive than any criteria we have ever seen used in prior clinical trials. However, approaches to evaluating response that have been used in other chronic multisystem diseases suggest that using a number of different tools will lead to important, generalizable knowledge regarding the outcomes of chronic GVHD therapy [18–25]. For example, it is conceivable that on a clinical trial a patient may have measurable decrease in lichenoid skin involvement but may report worse quality of life due to frequent hospitalizations with infection. It is also possible that on therapy with corticosteroids a patient may have less gastrointestinal GVHD symptoms, but owing to the secondary effects of the therapy may have inferior functional performance as measured by 2-minute walk distance and the human activity profile (HAP) questionnaire. Decisions about redundancy will also have to be made thoughtfully, since it is also possible that outcome measures may perform differently at different stages of the disease course such that two measures are strongly correlated prior to commencing treatment, but that their correlation diminishes over time. For example, quality of life and disease severity may be highly correlated prior to the start of treatment; however a therapy may improve disease severity initially while improvements in quality of life and well-being occur as the patient is able to recover from the effects of chronic GVHD and the acute side effects of treatment.

One of the major efforts has been to make the scales as quantitative as possible. The idea is to detract from qualitative assessments of patients on clinical trials and enable assessments that would be sensitive enough to discern the signal of therapeutic effect in a new drug development trial. Clearly this is difficult in GVHD, especially in measuring sclerotic involvement where quantitative methods to measure depth of sclerosis are not available. Therefore the focus is on determining percent body surface area of involvement. One of the limitations that we may see is that (especially because it is hard to assess depth of sclerosis) patients may improve or worsen by having softer or thicker skin, respectively. A measure that only addresses percent skin involvement may be insensitive to these changes. In an effort to overcome these limitations, other groups proposed other skin assessment scales that also incorporate qualitative skin texture assessments [48, 49]. All these approaches should ideally be validated in parallel in prospective trials, which may ultimately result in defining the most desirable tools for skin assessments in trials.

Furthermore, for a quantitative scale such as this one to work in clinical trials, it must be both feasible and reproducible. In other words, the whole tool needs to be able be completed in a reasonable amount of time as this may be occurring in a busy clinic. As important, there must be a certain degree of reproducibility. What this means is that what one observer "sees" needs to be reasonably close to the second observer. For example, if we focus on skin, can two observers agree that the majority of the skin GVHD in a patient is moveable as opposed to nonmoveable sclerosis? And how close to each other, in grading the percent BSA involved, are the two observers? How much variability in reproducibility is too much? Clearly a measure that performs with minimal measurement error is desired; however the extent of variability cannot exceed what is considered a clinically meaningful change – otherwise one could miss detection of a clinically meaningful change by having different observers over time. Moreover, the amount of variability in a measure relative to its absolute values (the signal-to-noise ratio) strongly affects sample size, with measures with a larger signal-to-noise ratio requiring larger samples. In our pilot trials in adults and children, we examined the inter-rater agreement of two evaluators in grading the extent of skin and soft tissue manifestations of chronic GVHD. Clinicians who received a 2-hour instruction in grading chronic GVHD response evaluated a series of patients with chronic GVHD, and their BSA scoring was compared with the scoring of dermatologists. In calculating agreement rates, we took the absolute value of the difference between the clinician and expert score, and if that absolute value was 15 or less, the two clinicians were considered to be within a 15% BSA threshold of agreement. Using this definition, we found that experts and clinicians were in agreement 69% of the time when rating erythema, 80% of the time when rating superficial/movable sclerosis, and 75% of the time when rating deep/nonmoveable sclerosis. Future studies are needed to determine whether inter-rater reliabilities can be improved through opportunities for more intensive training that includes feedback on performance. The evaluation of cGVHD therapeutic response is also an area that might benefit from efforts to automate and digitize assessments through improved instrumentation, imaging methods, biomarkers, and computer-based applications, thus improving reliability by limiting potential sources of measurement error.

In addition to these short-term efforts at assessing reliability and feasibility, it will be very important to determine how these assessment tools perform over time. Are these measures sensitive to change? To what extent can they capture response to therapy? Do the tools measure different aspects of chronic GVHD manifestations, or is there unacceptable overlap? For each measure, what is the minimally clinically important difference metric and are aspects of the response criteria predictive of survival or nonrelapse mortality? There is currently an ongoing large prospective multicenter cohort observational chronic GVHD study that is designed to address many of these questions. Patients will be followed longitudinally, and the NIH response measures, in addition to other measures, will be used to assess participants every 6 months regardless of how they are treated. This study will serve as comprehensive validation of the NIH response criteria, and may provide to define a disease activity index. In the meantime, as new chronic GVHD clinical trials and projects are proposed, the new NIH response criteria should also be incorporated in parallel into the trial design. The experience of using the criteria in prospective trials will provide data that can be applied to further refining the response criteria, and can be used for companion studies to explore validity, reliability, and sensitivity to change.

REFERENCES

1. Koc S, Leisenring W, Flowers ME, et al. Therapy for chronic graft-versus-host disease: a randomized trial comparing cyclosporine plus prednisone versus prednisone alone. *Blood.* 2002; 100:48–51.

2. Stewart BL, Storer B, Storek J, et al. Duration of immunosuppressive treatment for chronic graft-versus-host disease. *Blood.* 2004;104:3501–3506.

3. Sullivan KM, Shulman HM, Storb R, et al. Chronic graft-versus-host disease in 52 patients: adverse natural course and successful treatment with combination immunosuppression. *Blood.* 1981;57:267–276.

4. Pavletic S, Martin P, Lee SJ, et al. Measuring therapeutic response in chronic graft versus host disease. *Biol Blood Marrow Transplant.* 2006;12(3): 252–266.

5. Filipovich AH, Weisdorf D, Pavletic S, et al. National Institutes of Health consensus development project on criteria for clinical trials in chronic graft-versus-host disease: I. Diagnosis and staging working group report. *Biol Blood Marrow Transplant.* 2005;11:945–956.

6. Akpek G, Zahurak ML, Piantadosi S, et al. Development of a prognostic model for grading chronic graft-versus-host disease. *Blood.* 2001;97:1219–1226.

7. Lee SJ, Klein JP, Barrett AJ, et al. Severity of chronic graft-versus-host disease: association with treatment-related mortality and relapse. *Blood.* 2002;100:406–414.

8. Przepiorka D, Weisdorf D, Martin P, et al. 1994 Consensus Conference on Acute GVHD Grading. *Bone Marrow Transplant.* 1995;15:825–828.

9. Cahn JY, Klein JP, Lee SJ, et al. Prospective evaluation of 2 acute graft-versus-host (GVHD) grading systems: a joint Societe Francaise de Greffe de Moelle et Therapie Cellulaire (SFGM-TC), Dana Farber Cancer Institute (DFCI), and International Bone Marrow Transplant Registry (IBMTR) prospective study. *Blood.* 2005;106:1495–1500.

10. Guidance for industry: patient-reported outcome measures: use in medical product development to support labeling claims: draft guidance. *Health Qual Life Outcomes* 2006;4:79.

11. Garcia SF, Cella D, Clauser SB, et al. Standardizing patient-reported outcomes assessment in cancer clinical trials: a patient-reported outcomes measurement information system initiative. *J Clin Oncol.* 2007;25:5106–5112.

12. Sloan JA, Halyard MY, Frost MH, et al. The Mayo Clinic manuscript series relative to the discussion, dissemination, and operationalization of the Food and Drug Administration guidance on patient-reported outcomes. *Value Health.* 2007;10 (Suppl 2):S59-S63.

13. Willke RJ, Burke LB, Erickson P. Measuring treatment impact: a review of patient-reported outcomes and other efficacy endpoints in approved product labels. *Control Clin Trials.* 2004;25:535–552.

14. Shoukri, MM. *Measures of interobserver agreement.* 2004. Boca Raton: Chapman & Hall/CRC.

15. Sechrest L. Validity of measures is no simple matter. *Health Serv Res.* 2005;40:1584–1604.

16. Kelly PA, O'Malley KJ, Kallen MA, Ford ME. Integrating validity theory with use of measurement instruments in clinical settings. *Health Serv Res.* 2005;40:1605–1619.

17. Downing SM. Validity: on meaningful interpretation of assessment data. *Med Educ.* 2003;37:830–837.

18. Ruperto N, Ravelli A, Pistorio A, et al. The provisional Paediatric Rheumatology International Trials Organisation/American College of Rheumatology/European League Against Rheumatism Disease activity core set for the evaluation of response to therapy in juvenile dermatomyositis: A prospective validation study. *Arthritis Rheum.* 2008;59:4–13.

19. Bowman SJ, Sutcliffe N, Isenberg DA, et al. Sjogren's Systemic Clinical Activity Index (SCAI)–a systemic disease activity measure for use in clinical trials in primary Sjogren's syndrome. *Rheumatology.* (Oxford) 2007;46:1845–1851.

20. Ringold S, Wallace CA. Measuring clinical response and remission in juvenile idiopathic arthritis. *Curr Opin Rheumatol.* 2007;19:471–476.

21. Lequesne M. Indices of severity and disease activity for osteoarthritis. *Semin Arthritis Rheum.* 1991;20:48–54.

22. Stucki G, Sangha O, Stucki S, et al. Comparison of the WOMAC (Western Ontario and McMaster Universities) osteoarthritis index and a self-report format of the self-administered Lequesne-Algofunctional index in patients with knee and hip osteoarthritis. *Osteoarthritis Cartilage.* 1998;6:79–86.

23. Gladman DD, Mease PJ, Healy P, et al. Outcome measures in psoriatic arthritis. *J Rheumatol.* 2007;34:1159–1166.

24. Hellmich B, Flossmann O, Gross WL, et al. EULAR recommendations for conducting clinical studies and/or clinical trials in systemic vasculitis: focus on anti-neutrophil cytoplasm antibody-associated vasculitis. *Ann Rheum Dis.* 2007;66:605–617.

25. Furst D, Khanna D, Matucci-Cerinic M, et al. Systemic sclerosis – continuing progress in developing clinical measures of response. *J Rheumatol.* 2007;34:1194–1200.

26. May S, Gilman S, Sowell BB, et al. Potential outcome measures and trial design issues for multiple system atrophy. *Mov Disord.* 2007;22:2371–2377.

27. Rudick RA, Cutter G, Reingold S. The multiple sclerosis functional composite: a new clinical outcome measure for multiple sclerosis trials. *Mult Scler.* 2002;8:359–365.

28. A proposed revision to the ACR20: the hybrid measure of American College of Rheumatology response. *Arthritis Rheum.* 2007;57:193–202.

29. Hudson M, Steele R, Baron M. Update on indices of disease activity in systemic sclerosis. *Semin Arthritis Rheum.* 2007;37:93–98.

30. Miller FW, Rider LG, Chung YL, et al. Proposed preliminary core set measures for disease outcome assessment in adult and juvenile idiopathic inflammatory myopathies. *Rheumatology.* (*Oxford*) 2001;40:1262–1273.

31. Maksymowych WP, Mallon C, Richardson R, et al. Development and validation of the Edmonton Ankylosing Spondylitis Metrology Index. *Arthritis Rheum.* 2006;55:575–582.

32. Sullivan KM, Witherspoon RP, Storb R, et al. Prednisone and azathioprine compared with prednisone and placebo for treatment of chronic graft-v-host disease: prognostic influence of prolonged thrombocytopenia after allogeneic marrow transplantation. *Blood.* 1988;72:546–554.

33. Sullivan KM, Witherspoon RP, Storb R, et al. Alternating-day cyclosporine and prednisone for treatment of high-risk chronic graft-v-host disease. *Blood.* 1988;72:555–561.

34. Vogelsang GB, Farmer ER, Hess AD, et al. Thalidomide for the treatment of chronic graft-versus-host disease. *N Engl J Med.* 1992;326:1055–1058.

35. Parker PM, Chao N, Nademanee A, et al. Thalidomide as salvage therapy for chronic graft-versus-host disease. *Blood.* 1995;86:3604–3609.

36. Lee S, Cook EF, Soiffer R, Antin JH. Development and validation of a scale to measure symptoms of chronic graft-versus-host disease. *Biol Blood Marrow Transplant.* 2002;8:444–452.

37. Cleeland CS, Mendoza TR, Wang XS, et al. Assessing symptom distress in cancer patients: the M.D. Anderson Symptom Inventory. *Cancer.* 2000;89:1634–1646.

38. Osoba D, Rodrigues G, Myles J, Zee B, Pater J. Interpreting the significance of changes in health-related quality-of-life scores. *J Clin Oncol.* 1998;16:139–144.

39. Fischer D, Stewart AL, Bloch DA, et al. Capturing the patient's view of change as a clinical outcome measure. *JAMA.* 1999;282:1157–1162.

40. Revicki D, Hays RD, Cella D, Sloan J. Recommended methods for determining responsiveness and minimally important differences for patient-reported outcomes. *J Clin Epidemiol.* 2008;61:102–109.

41. Ward MM. Response criteria and criteria for clinically important improvement: separate and equal? *Arthritis Rheum.* 2001;44:1728–1729.

42. Kvien TK, Heiberg T, Hagen KB. Minimal clinically important improvement/difference (MCII/MCID) and patient acceptable symptom state (PASS): what do these concepts mean? *Ann Rheum Dis.* 2007;66 (Suppl 3):iii40-iii41.

43. Mathiowetz V, Kashman N, Volland G, et al. Grip and pinch strength: normative data for adults. *Arch Phys Med Rehabil.* 1985;66:69–74.

44. Mathiowetz V, Wiemer DM, Federman SM. Grip and pinch strength: norms for 6- to 19-year-olds. *Am J Occup Ther.* 1986;40:705–711.

45. Waters RL, Lunsford BR, Perry J, Byrd R. Energy-speed relationship of walking: standard tables. *J Orthop Res.* 1988;6:215–222.

46. Ward MM. Interpreting measurements of physical function in clinical trials. *Ann Rheum Dis.* 2007;66 (Suppl 3):iii32-iii34.

47. Mitchell S, Reeve B, and Cowen E. Feasibility and reproducibility of the new NIH consensus criteria to evaluate response in chronic GVHD – a pilot study. [abstract]. *Blood.* 2005;106 (Suppl 1):873a.

48. Jacobsohn DA, Chen AR, Zahurak M, et al. Phase II study of pentostatin in patients with corticosteroid-refractory chronic graft-versus-host disease. *J Clin Oncol.* 2007;25:4255–4261.

49. Greinix HT, Pohlreich D, Maalouf J, et al. A single-center pilot validation study of a new chronic GVHD skin scoring system. *Biol Blood Marrow Transplant.* 2007;13:715–723.

General Principles of Ancillary and Supportive Care

Paul A. Carpenter and Daniel R. Couriel

Chronic graft versus host disease (GVHD) is characterized by polymorphic clinical manifestations with varying severity and clinical course. Prolonged systemic immunosuppressive therapy including glucocorticoids is necessary to control disease severity and nonrelapse mortality. Treatment, combined with delayed immunologic reconstitution associated with chronic GVHD, increases the risk of infections and other complications. Because the clinical manifestations of chronic GVHD can persist for prolonged periods, the complete spectrum of complications may cause significant and sometimes irreversible morbidity. It follows that ancillary therapy and supportive care are central components in the long-term management of chronic GVHD after allogeneic hematopoietic cell transplantation (HCT).

Guidelines for ancillary and supportive care have recently been established by the Ancillary Therapy and Supportive Care Working Group of the National Institutes of Health (NIH) Consensus Development Project on Criteria for Clinical Trials in Chronic GVHD [1]. The committee's recommendations include therapy for organ-specific symptoms, patient education, appropriate follow-up and preventive measures, and guidelines for the prevention and management of infections and other common complications.

The recommendations are organized according to an evidence-based system that reflects the strength of recommendations and the quality of evidence supporting them (Table 15.1). Currently, 44% of the recommendations are supported by higher quality evidence, designated level I or level II, on the basis of data gathered from published phase III or phase II clinical trials respectively. The rating is further designated by lower case "a" if the evidence was derived from a chronic GVHD study (level Ia or IIa) or lower case "b" if the evidence was derived in an analogous disease setting (level Ib or IIb). The remainder of recommendations are rated level III, on the basis of expert consensus opinion (Figure 15.1), highlighting the need for areas of supportive care with the greatest need for clinical research.

The term *ancillary therapy* embraces any frequently prescribed immunosuppressive or anti-inflammatory interventions

that have topical intent like corticosteroid or tacrolimus skin emollients, cyclosporine eye drops, and any other interventions directed at organ-specific control of symptoms, for example, artificial tears or orally administered sialogogue therapy to help relieve sicca symptoms. The term *supportive care* also includes interventions that are directed at organ-specific control of complications resulting from GVHD and its therapy. Examples of the latter include regular use of antibiotics to prevent the development of infections caused by *Pneumocystis jirovecii* and encapsulated bacteria; the use of bisphosphonates to treat glucocorticoid-induced osteoporosis; management of toxicities like hypertension, hyperlipidemia, and renal dysfunction due to other medications; and problems not directly related to chronic GVHD, like iron overload and psychosocial adaptation. Included in this definition are educational, preventive, and psychosocial interventions with this same objective.

In general, close serial monitoring of all organ systems is recommended to promote early detection and intervention directed toward reversing or preventing the progression of chronic GVHD manifestations and preventing infection, secondary malignancy, and treatment-associated toxicities (Table 15.2).

All organ systems potentially affected by chronic GVHD or its treatment should be monitored serially in individuals at risk at least annually for 5 years after HCT [2]. The scope and frequency of monitoring should be individualized as clinically indicated. More frequent monitoring is strongly advised for those with active GVHD, especially during high-risk periods – for example, treatment taper or escalation – and for those who are participating in clinical trials.

Ancillary and supportive care interventions include a preventive focus that is especially relevant for patients with newly diagnosed chronic GVHD (Table 15.3) but also cover the range of organ-specific interventions commonly employed in addition to systemic GVHD treatment (Table 15.4). It is noteworthy that the use of organ-specific ancillary treatment interventions may, in some cases, circumvent the need for systemic treatment or allow doses of systemic agents to be decreased.

Table 15.1: Evidence-Based Rating System for Ancillary Therapy and Supportive Care in Chronic GVHD

Category		Definition
Strength of the recommendation		
	A	Should always be offered
	B	Should generally be offered
	C	Evidence for efficacy is insufficient to support a recommendation for or against, or evidence for efficacy might not outweigh adverse consequences, or cost of the approach. Optional
	D	Moderate evidence for lack of efficacy or for adverse outcome supports a recommendation against use. Should generally not be offered
	E	Good evidence for lack of efficacy or for adverse outcome supports a recommendation against use. Should never be offered
Quality of evidence supporting the recommendation		
	I	Evidence from ≥1 properly randomized, controlled trial
	II	Evidence for ≥1 well-designed clinical trial without randomization, from cohort or case-controlled analytic studies (preferable from > 1 center), or from multiple time series or dramatic results from uncontrolled experiments
	III	Evidence from opinions of respected authorities based on clinical experience; descriptive
Qualifier for categories I and II		
	a	Evidence derived directly from study(s) in graft versus host disease
	b	Evidence derived indirectly from study(s) in analogous or other pertinent disease

From: Couriel D, Carpenter PA, Cutler C, et al. *Biol Blood Marrow Transplant.* 2006;12:375–396

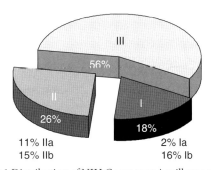

Figure 15.1 Distribution of NIH Consensus Ancillary and Supportive Care Recommendations based on quality of evidence.
From: Couriel D, Carpenter PA, Cutler C, et al. *Biol Blood Marrow Transplant.* 2006;12:375–396 with permission from Elsevier. See Plate 29 in the color plate section.

Just as it is most reliable to make the diagnosis of chronic GVHD by way of a carefully directed history and physical examination that considers multiple organ involvement, comprehensive ancillary and supportive care management should follow the same approach. The list of organs most commonly involved with chronic GVHD after peripheral blood transplantation, in descending order of frequency, includes skin, mouth, liver, eyes, gastrointestinal tract, vagina, esophagus, joints, lungs, and muscles. The distribution of organ involvement is similar after marrow transplantation with the exceptions that skin and vaginal tract involvement occur less frequently [3]. Organ-specific interventions for the skin and its appendages focus on the management of pruritis, rash, pain, dyspigmentation, and limited range of motion. In the oral cavity the focus is on alleviating pain, dryness, taste impairment, odynophagia, and reduced range of motion. Ancillary eye care focuses on the relief of keratoconjunctivitis sicca, more simply termed *the dry eye syndrome*. Interventions for vulvovaginal tissues focus on the relief of dysuria, dryness, and dyspareunia. Gastrointestinal symptoms often pose diagnostic dilemmas, sorting out whether the complaint is exclusively or partly due to GVHD or exclusively or partly due to other etiologies that require a range of interventions to address problems like medication toxicity, esophageal web, reflux esophagitis, or malabsorption due to pancreatic insufficiency. Abnormal liver function tests or weight loss can similarly have a range of etiologies that need to be delineated so that appropriate interventions may be prescribed.

The remainder of this chapter illustrates how these guidelines are typically incorporated into comprehensive management plans for patients with chronic GVHD. The following

Table 15.2: Summary of Monitoring Recommendations

Category	Specific Assessment	Frequency (months)
Interval history	Symptoms	1–12
	Medication review	
Physical examination	General	1–12
	Weight	1–6
	Height	3*–12
	Tanner score*	6–12
	Nutrition	1–12
	Developmental*	1–12
Laboratory	General blood work	1–6
	CBC and differential	
	Creatinine	
	Magnesium serum level	
	Liver function tests	
	Therapeutic drug levels	
	IgG level†	
	Lipid profile	6–12
	Iron indices	6–12
	Pulmonary function tests	3–12
	Bone health:	12
	DEXA densitometry	
	Serum calcium	
	25-OH Vitamin D	
	Thyroid function tests	12
Specialist evaluations	Ophthalmology:	3–12
	Schirmer test	
	Glaucoma test	
	Dental/oral medicine	6–12
	Soft/hard palate examination	As needed
	Culture lesions	,,
	Biopsy lesions	,,
	Photograph lesions	,,
	Radiographs	6–12
	Dermatology	As needed
	Extent and type of lesion	
	Gynecology	As needed
	Vulvovaginal examination	
	Physical therapy	3–12
	Range of motion if sclerosis is present	
	Neuropsychological	As needed

* Applicable to children who have not yet reached final adult height.
† Regular measurement of serum IgG applies during the first 12 months after transplant until the patient is independent of replacement therapy (IgG > 400 mg/dL).
Table modified from Couriel D, Carpenter PA, Cutler C, et al. *Biol Blood Marrow Transplant.* 2006;12:375–396.

case histories describe actual patients who were referred to chronic GVHD clinics at the authors' institutions. The purpose of each case is not to review or justify details about the systemic immunosuppressive therapy that the patient received. Instead, the focus is on the individual ancillary and supportive recommendations that are listed after each case presentation and

the evidence-based rating to support the recommendation (if available).

CASE 1

A 33-year-old woman is seen in clinic for long-term follow-up at 18 months after myeloablative conditioning and peripheral blood

Table 15.3: Summary of Preventive Interventions

Organ System	Interventions			
	Routine Prophylaxis Antibiotics	Routine Surveillance		Organ-Specific
		Malignancy	Infection	
Skin and appendages	No	Yes	No*	Photoprotection
Mouth and oral cavity	No†	Yes	Yes[v,b,y]	Maintain good oral/dental hygiene
				Consider routine dental cleaning
Eyes	No	No	Yes	Photoprotection
				Cataract surveillance
				Glaucoma surveillance
Vulva and vagina	No	Yes	Yes[v,b,y]	Early gynecology consultation
				Estrogen deficiency surveillance
Gastrointestinal (GI) tract and liver	No	Yes††	Yes[v,f]	GI endoscopy
				Excess alcohol avoidance
Lungs	Yes[v,b,p]	No	Yes[v,b,y,f]	Immunizations for prevention of respiratory infections
				Smoking avoidance
Metabolic	–	–	–	Hyperlipidemia screening
				Hypertension screening
				Chronic renal failure screening
				Iron overload screening
Neurologic	–	–	–	Calcineurin inhibitor drug levels
				Seizure prophylaxis: blood pressure control, electrolyte replacement, anticonvulsants
Immunologic and infectious disease	Yes[v,b,p]	–	Yes	Immunizations
				Consider immunoglobulin replacement based on levels and recurrent infections
Musculoskeletal	–	–	–	Range of joint motion surveillance
				Bone density surveillance (DEXA)
				Calcium and 25-OH vitamin D levels
				Physical therapy
				Calcium, vitamin D supplementation
				Bisphosphonate therapy

f, fungal; v, viral; b, bacterial; y, yeast; p, *Pneumocystis jirovecii* pneumonia.
* Erosive or ulcerative skin lesions are exceptions that may warrant routine microbiological cultures.
† Exception is endocarditis prophylaxis with teeth cleaning.
†† Routine at age 50 or earlier for positive family history or bowel cancer.

transplant for myelodysplastic syndrome (MDS)/refractory anemia (RA). When last seen 6 months ago she continued tacrolimus and tapered prednisone therapy for an earlier diagnosis of mild chronic GVHD of the skin and mouth. Since she stopped prednisone 3 months ago her *chief complaint* is dry eyes and mouth. In the *review of systems* she reports mild oral sensitivities and uses artificial tears every 1 to 2 hours. No dysphagia or odynophagia. She endorses postnasal drip and reports occasional sinus headaches. No fevers. She has had a cough, which began not long after stopping prednisone. No dyspnea, chest pain, or palpitations. No weight loss in the past 2 months. No gastrointestinal symptoms. She reports a loss of libido that she relates to dyspareunia. She has ovarian failure secondary to conditioning with busulfan and cyclophosphamide and has not received hormone replacement since her transplant. On *physical examination* her vital signs are satisfactory. Minimal nail dystrophy is present. No rash or palpable deep sclerosis. The corneas appear moist. The conjunctivae are mildly injected. Schirmer's test reveals 5 mm wetting bilaterally. Chest auscultation shows bilateral reduced air entry and occasional wheeze. Range of joint motion is full. The total oral cavity surface shows 25% minimal erythema and 25% to 50% mild lichenoid changes. Gynecological examination shows vulvovaginal atrophy, lichenoid mucosal changes, and vaginal stenosis.

Table 15.4: Summary of Treatment Interventions

Organ System	Organ-Specific Intervention
Skin and appendages	For intact skin: topical emollients, glucocorticoids, antipruritics, psoralen and UVA, calcineurin inhibitors
	For erosions/ulcerations: topical antimicrobials, protective films or other dressings, debridement, hyperbaric oxygen, wound care consultation
Mouth and oral cavity	Topical high- and ultra-high-potency glucocorticoids and analgesics
	Therapy for xerostomia
Eyes	Artificial tears, ocular ointments, topical glucocorticoids, or cyclosporine
	Punctual occlusions, humidified environment, occlusive eyewear, moisture chamber eyeglasses, cevimeline, pilocarpine, tarsorraphy, gas-permeable scleral contact lens, autologous serum
	Topical antimicrobials, doxycycline
Vulva and vagina	Water-based lubricants, topical estrogens, topical corticosteroids or calcineurin inhibitors, dilators, surgery for extensive synechae or obliteration
GI tract and liver	Eliminate other etiologies (infection, malabsorption unrelated to GVHD, hemochromatosis, etc.).
	Dietary modification, enzyme supplementation for malabsorption, gastroesophageal reflux management, esophageal dilatation, ursodeoxycholic acid
Lungs	Eliminate other etiologies (e.g., infection, gastroesophageal reflux)
	Inhaled glucocorticoids, bronchodilators, supplementary oxygen, pulmonary rehabilitation
	Consider lung transplantation for appropriate candidates
Hematopoietic	Eliminate other etiologies (e.g., drug toxicity, infection)
	Hematopoietic growth factors, immunoglobulin for immune cytopenias
Metabolic	Lipid-lowering therapy if appropriate
	Antihypertensive medication if appropriate
	Substitute less nephrotoxic medications if there is significant renal dysfunction
	Regular phlebotomy for iron overload
Neurologic	Occupational and physical therapies
	Treatment of neuropathic syndromes with tricyclic antidepressants, selective serotonin re-uptake inhibitors, or anticonvulsants
Immunologic and infectious disease	Organism-specific antimicrobial agents
	Empiric parenteral broad-spectrum antibacterial coverage for fever
Musculoskeletal	Physical therapy, bisphosphonates for osteopenia and osteoporosis

UVA, ultraviolet A.

Relevant Investigations (Case 1)

Complete blood count:	WBC 6.2, ANC 4.2, eosinophils 0.01, hematocrit 37%, MCV 85, reticulocytes 0.9%, platelets 155,000			
Liver function tests:	Bilirubin 0.3 mg/dL, AST 15 IU, ALT 16 IU, alkaline phosphatase 110 IU, albumin 3.7 mg/dL			
Creatinine/electrolytes:	0.8 mg/dL, magnesium 1.9 mg/dL, calcium 9.4 mg/dL			
Tacrolimus level:	8 ng/mL			
DEXA scan T-scores:	Lumbar spine		Left femoral neck	
Posttransplant				
3 months:	−0.8		−0.9	
18 months:	**−1.8**		**−2.1**	
Fasting lipid panel:	Cholesterol 115 mg/dL, HDL **33**, LDL 60, triglycerides 119 mg/dL			

High-resolution chest CT:	Evidence of air trapping with expiration				
PFTs (% predicted):	FEV1	FVC	FEV1/FVC	RV	Comments
Baseline (pretransplant):	108	118	99	62	Corrected diffusing capacity 104%
Posttransplant					
3 months:	98	108	93	83	
12 months:	81	85	80	110	
18 months:	**69**	**85**	**63**	**160**	FEV1 + 12% after bronchodilator

ALT, alanine aminotransferase activity; ANC, absolute neutrophil count; AST, serum transaminase; FEV1, forced expiratory volume in one second; FVC, forced vital capacity; HDL, high-density lipoprotein; LDL, low-density lipoprotein; MCV, mean corpuscular volume; PFT, pulmonary function test; RV, residual volume; wbc, white blood cells.

Discussion: This patient developed insidious bronchiolitis obliterans almost certainly on the basis of chronic GVHD, which has also progressed in the eyes, mouth, and vagina after stopping prednisone. She developed moderately severe osteopenia while on prednisone and without estrogen replacement therapy. The case illustrates failure to consider the broader history and the omission of timely ancillary and supportive care recommendations. Although spirometry values were normal at 3 and 12 months after transplant, the 10% to 25% drop in forced expiratory volume in one second (FEV1) and serial increase in residual volumes calibrated to the patient's pretransplant baseline values should have prompted closer monitoring. Although her baseline DEXA scan indicated satisfactory bone mineral density, she was at risk for bone loss, as indicated by the history of hypogonadism secondary to busulfan, failure to resume hormone replacement after transplant, and the addition of chronic prednisone therapy. At this visit she was advised to continue tacrolimus and to resume prednisone at a dose of 0.5 mg/kg every other day. Sirolimus was added as a steroid-sparing agent and the following ancillary and supportive care was advised.

Ancillary GVHD Care

1. Inhaled fluticasone and salmeterol (250/50 mg) twice daily with spacer device **(level CIb)**
2. Betamethasone diprorionate gel and vaginal dilator therapy with gynecological follow-up **(level BIII)**
3. Topical estrogen therapy and vaginal dilatation alternating with steroid applications **(level BIII)**
4. Trial of lower punctual plugs **(Level BIb)** or Lacriserts **(Level CIb)** for ocular sicca

Supportive Care

1. Continue daily trimethoprim (TMP)/sulfamethoxazole (SMX) as prophylaxis for encapsulated organisms **(level BIIb)** and PCP **(level AIb)**.
2. Continue *Varicella zoster virus* (VZV) prophylaxis with acyclovir twice daily **(level CIa)**.
3. Administer influenza vaccine if not already given for the current flu season **(level BIII)**.
4. Confirm immunization against Pneumococcus and *Haemophillus influenzae* Type B **(level BIIb)**.
5. Start alendronate to be taken on an empty stomach; erect posture to avoid esophagitis **(level AIIb)**.
6. Supplement to provide daily intakes of 1500 mg calcium and 400 IU vitamin D **(level AIb)**.
7. Gynecological practitioner prescribed topical patch for estrogen replacement therapy.

Monitoring

1. Do serial monthly pulmonary function for at least 3 months to determine trend on therapy.
2. Monitor levels of tacrolimus and sirolimus weekly until the levels are stable and within desired range.
3. Measure serum fasting lipids monthly initially while on sirolimus to determine the need for intervention.
4. Repeat DEXA scan in 12 months to determine progress on estrogen and bisphosphonate therapy.

CASE 2

A 49-year-old man is seen in a chronic GVHD clinic 18 months after peripheral blood transplantation from his human leukocyte antigen (HLA)-matched sister for acute lymphoblastic leukemia (ALL). Prednisone and tacrolimus were discontinued 8 months earlier after resolution of progressive onset chronic GVHD of the skin. Six months ago he started complaining of pruritus but his ***chief complaint*** is progressive skin tightening over the hands, feet, arms, thighs, upper chest, and waist. In the ***review of systems*** he denies fatigue, dyspnea, chest pain, or palpitations. No gastrointestinal or genitourinary complaints. Over the last 2 months he reports numbness and tingling in both hands. ***Family history*** is notable for diabetes and heart disease. One brother had a myocardial infarction at age 40. ***Physical examination*** is notable for severe superficial sclerotic changes in four extremities and around the waist. He has difficulty buttoning his shirt and range of motion is severely limited at wrists, ankles, and, to a lesser extent, at elbows and knees. There is generalized skin dyspigmentation and mild nail dystrophy. Twenty-five percent of the oral cavity surface is covered by mild lichenoid changes. Blood pressure 125/78 mmHg. Remaining physical examination is normal.

Relevant Investigations

Complete blood count:	WBC 8.1, ANC 3.1, eosinophils **0.9 (11%)**,Hematocrit 39%, MCV 90,
Liver function tests:	Bilirubin 0.4 mg/dL, AST 35 IU, ALT 26 IU, alkaline phosphatase **199 IU**, albumin 3.4 mg/dL
Creatinine/electrolytes:	1.2 mg/dL, magnesium 2.0 mg/dL. Fasting blood glucose 98 mg/dL

Management

He begins extracorporeal photopheresis (ECP) and therapy with tacrolimus and tapered prednisone, which began at a dose of 1 mg/kg daily. Six weeks later he reports improved range of joint motion but complains of fatigue and spends half the day lying down. He reports difficulty climbing stairs and standing from a sitting position. He is concerned about high blood glucose levels and dislikes the insulin shots. Formal studies show a 30% to 35% improvement in range of motion at wrists, ankles, and elbows. Blood pressure is 130/82 mmHg. The prednisone dose is at 1 mg/kg alternating with 0.5 mg/kg every other day, and tacrolimus blood levels are within desired range. He was referred to physical therapy and endocrinology. Twelve weeks later, he feels substantially better and can perform his usual activities with little effort. He has been exercising 3 times a week with physical therapy. Formal studies show a 50% to 60% improvement in joint motion compared with the first visit. The skin is now clearly softened at all previously affected sites. His prednisone dose is now 0.75 mg/kg every other day and he has not required insulin therapy for the past 2 weeks. Per the endocrinology report his lipid panel and bone density evaluation were within normal limits.

Discussion: The patient has severe chronic GVHD, diagnosed on the basis of the extent of sclerosis and functional impairment. ECP therapy combined with a standard 2-drug immunosuppressive regimen achieved modest short-term improvement in range of motion but high-dose prednisone caused significant treatment-related toxicity. Addition of physical therapy and attention to diabetes management led to improved outcomes. Ideally, the following ancillary and supportive care should have begun or been discussed at the onset of systemic immunosuppression.

Ancillary GVHD Care

1. Refer to physical therapy for quantitative range of motion measurements, deep tissue massage, and stretching to release joint contractures and to monitor progress (level AIII).

Supportive Care

1. Start antibiotic prophylaxis for encapsulated organisms (level BIIb).
2. Start antibiotic prophylaxis for PCP (level AIb).
3. Add VZV prophylaxis with acyclovir twice daily (level CIa).
4. Advise influenza vaccine if not already given for the current flu season (level BIII).
5. Immunize against Pneumococcus and *H. influenzae* Type B if not already done after transplant (level BIIb).
6. Start alendronate to be taken on an empty stomach; erect posture to avoid esophagitis (level AIIb).
7. Supplement to provide daily intakes of 1500 mg calcium and 400 IU vitamin D (level AIb).

Monitoring

1. Measure serum fasting lipids and blood glucose periodically.
2. Repeat DEXA scan in 12 months and consider stopping bisphosphonate therapy if prednisone is stopped and bone mineral density is normal.
3. Repeat formal range of joint motion studies in 6 months or sooner if clinically indicated.

CASE 3

A 23-year-old man is referred to the clinic and with a new diagnosis of progressive scleurodermatous chronic GVHD 22 months after he received a CY/12 GyTBI conditioning and a peripheral blood transplant for acute myelogenous leukemia (AML). He has an earlier history of moderately severe oral chronic GVHD that was treated with prednisone and cyclosporine. His *chief complaint* is tightness in the arms and flanks that began 2 months ago and that he has to use tricky maneuvers to dress and undress. In the *review of systems* he denies mouth discomfort or ocular sicca but reports excessive tearing. He reports 12 lb. of weight loss since stopping prednisone. No anorexia or vomiting, occasional nausea, and no diarrhea. There is a 5-month history of nonproductive cough and mild exertional dyspnea but he can walk up six flights of stairs without stopping. No chest pain or palpitations. No fevers. No postnasal drip. No sinusitis

or headaches. *Physical examination* is notable for asthenia; weight 62 kg. Pulse 84, respiratory rate 16, blood pressure 112/70. Mild nail dystrophy is present. No erythematous or lichenoid skin changes. No morphea or superficial sclerosis. Postural deformity is noted to be caused by severe contractures at shoulders, elbows, wrists, and small joints of hands, and deep sclerosis of the trunk, arms, and neck. Deltoid muscle wasting is marked. Range of joint motion is full at the ankles, knees, and hips. The vermillion border of the lips is mottled. The total oral cavity surface shows 25% moderate erythema, patchy gingival and lateral glossal erythema, and 25% to 50% lichenoid changes. A hyperkeratotic mucosal plaque is noted to be ~3 to 4 cm long × 1.5 cm in maximal width. Remainder of physical examination is normal.

Relevant Investigations

Complete blood count:	WBC 6.9, ANC 3.1, eosinophils **19%**, Hematocrit **34%, MCV 102, r**eticulocytes **4.9%**, platelets 355,000				
Liver function tests:	Bilirubin 0.4 mg/dL, AST 35 IU, ALT 26 IU, alkaline phosphatase **230 IU**, albumin 3.4 mg/dL				
Creatinine/ electrolytes:	0.7 mg/dL, magnesium 2.0 mg/dL, calcium 9.6 mg/dL				
Cyclosporine level:	244 ng/mL				
DEXA scan T-scores:	**−2.37** (lumbar spine), **−1.47** (left femoral neck)				
Fasting lipid panel:	Cholesterol 145 mg/dL, HDL 69, LDL 60, triglycerides 79 mg/dL.				
High-resolution chest CT:	No evidence of air trapping with expiration				
PFTs (% predicted):	FEV1	FVC	FEV1/ FVC	RV	Comments
Baseline (pretransplant):	78	96	**58**	152	Ex-smoker, FEV1 + 10% with bronchodilator
Posttransplant					
3 months:	**70**	**98**	**59**	143	
12 months:	74	**85**	**72**	**202**	
20 months:	**51**	77	**55**	238	Corrected diffusing capacity 69%
22 months:	**45**	**55**	**67**	228	FEV1 + 8% after bronchodilator

Discussion: The patient has severe chronic GVHD, diagnosed on the basis of the degree of functional limitation in joints and lung. Pulmonary function tests indicate a mixed obstructive and, more recently superimposed, restrictive pattern reflecting chest wall sclerosis. An aggressive therapeutic approach was advised to try to recover or preserve joint motion. In addition to discontinuing cyclosporine and starting systemic therapy with prednisone, sirolimus, and extracorporeal photopheresis, the following ancillary and supportive care recommendations were made.

Ancillary GVHD Care

1. Referral to physical therapy for quantitative range of motion measurements, deep tissue massage for the thorax and stretching (or serial splinting) to release joint contractures at the shoulder girdle, elbows, wrists, and fingers, and to monitor progress **(level AIII)**
2. Clobetasol gel (0.05%) to treat buccal mucosal hyperkeratotic plaque **(level AIIb)**

Supportive Care

1. Start antibiotic prophylaxis for encapsulated organisms **(level BIIb)**.
2. If not allergic to TMP/SMX change PCP prophylaxis **(level AIb)** from dapsone to TMP/SMX because laboratory tests are consistent with a possible dapsone-induced hemolysis.
3. Add VZV prophylaxis with acyclovir twice daily **(level CIa)**.
4. Influenza vaccine if not already given for the current flu season **(level BIII)**.
5. Immunize against Pneumococcus, *H. influenzae* Type B if not already done after transplant **(level BIIb)**.
6. Start alendronate to be taken on an empty stomach; erect posture to avoid esophagitis **(level AIIb)**.
7. Supplement to provide daily intakes of 1500 mg calcium and 400 IU vitamin D **(level AIb)**.

Monitoring

1. Measure serum fasting lipids monthly initially while on sirolimus to determine the need for intervention.
2. Repeat DEXA scan in 12 months.
3. Follow-up of erosive hyperkeratotic plaque with oral medicine in 6 months.
4. Repeat pulmonary function testing in 2 to 3 months and follow-up with pulmonology.
5. Repeat formal range of joint motion studies in 6 months or sooner if clinically indicated.

CASE 4

A 36-year-old man is seen in follow-up for chronic GVHD that is now of 2.5 years duration and which began de novo, at 5 months after myeloablative conditioning and peripheral blood cell transplant for chronic myelogenous leukemia (CML) in chronic phase. Three months ago, he began therapy with prednisone, low-dose beclomethasone six times daily; cyclosporine was changed to tacrolimus because of progressive dysphagia and odynophagia that was attributed to diffuse esophageal ulcerations, webs, and gastric erythema and edema observed endoscopically and confirmed histologically to be due to GVHD. An interim *chief complaint* was major mood disturbance that was affecting his marriage and relationships at work. Prednisone was subsequently tapered more rapidly than intended from 50 mg every other day to 20 mg every other day and he now reports arthralgias and fatigue on the off-prednisone days. On *review of systems* he denied recurrent swallowing difficulties, rash, pruritus, and nail or hair changes. He intermittently and infrequently uses artificial tears for dry eye. He is working full time as a senior administrator. The *physical examination* is normal apart from minimal ridging of the nails, mild patchy atrophy, and very minimal erythema of the oral mucosa. Schirmer's test: 5 mm (L), 10 mm (R).

Relevant Investigations

Complete blood count:	WBC 5.76, ANC 3.22, eosinophils 0.06, Hematocrit 49%, MCV 91, reticulocytes 1.4%, platelets 177,000
Liver function tests:	Bilirubin 0.9 mg/dL, AST 28 IU, ALT 44 IU, alkaline phosphatase 67 IU, GGT 91, albumin 3.5 mg/dL
Creatinine/ electrolytes:	1.1 mg/dL, magnesium 2.1 mg/dL, calcium 9.8 mg/dL
Cyclosporine level:	3 ng/mL
DEXA scan T-scores:	**-1.8** (lumbar spine), **-1.9** (left femoral neck)
Fasting lipid panel:	Cholesterol **210** mg/dL, HDL **31**, LDL **149**, triglycerides **215** mg/dL
Fasting glucose:	84 mg/dL

PFTs (% predicted):	FEV1	FEV1/ FVC	TLC	RV	Comments
	98	**70**	123	148	Stable, corrected diffusing capacity **69%**

Repeat endoscopy:	Esophageal biopsies show no epithelial disturbance but the superficial lamina propria contained a small mixed, predominantly lymphocytic infiltrate. Gastric biopsies were consistent with active GVHD.

GGT, gamma-glutamyltranspeptidase.

Discussion: The marked improvement in esophageal symptoms was attributed to the systemic immunosuppressive therapy and ancillary therapy with oral beclomethasone. The accelerated prednisone taper led to greatly improved mood and behavior but arthralgias, myalgias, and fatigue could relate to either prednisone withdrawal syndrome or adrenal insufficiency (**see Chapter 26**). The patient remained adamant to discontinue prednisone. Therefore, in addition to continuing the prednisone taper by 2.5 mg each week, the following supportive care recommendations were made.

Ancillary GVHD Care

1. Decrease beclomethasone from 0.5 mg six times daily to 1 mg four times daily.
2. Continue preservative-free artificial tears for dry eyes **(level AIb)**.

Supportive Care

1. Because esophageal endoscopy showed inflammation it might be helpful to increase the omperazole dose from once daily to twice daily. Sleep with the head on the bed elevated by 4 inches.

2. Continue Penicillin VK as encapsulated organism prophylaxis **(level BIIb)**.
3. PCP prophylaxis with TMP/SMX **(level AIb)**.
4. Acyclovir prophylaxis is not necessary because he was VZV seronegative pretransplant **(level CIa)**.
5. Complete immunizations by giving shots for diphtheria, tetanus, and *H. influenzae* type b (HIB) **(level BIIb)**.
6. Influezae vaccination as soon as this becomes available in the Fall **(level BIII)**
7. Give a dose of zoledronic acid 4 mg IV for moderately severe osteopenia **(level AIIb)**.
8. Supplement to provide daily intakes of 1500 mg calcium and 400 IU vitamin D **(level AIb)**.
9. Add atorvostatin 10 mg daily and increase to 20 mg daily if no side effects and liver function tests remain satisfactory to address what have become chronic derangements of in his lipid panel.
10. If adrenal insufficiency is confirmed (see monitoring), begin hydrocortisone replacement with 15 mg 8 AM, 5 mg at 6 PM on off-prednisone days. When the prednisone taper reaches a dose of 5 mg every other day, simply replace the prednisone with split dose hydrocortisone given daily instead of every other day.

Monitoring

1. Rule out adrenal insufficiency by measuring early morning (0800 hours) baseline and adrenocorticotropic hormone (ACTH)–stimulated serum cortisol levels when his prednisone dose approximates 10 to 15 mg every other day (testing 4 weeks later when he reported worsening fatigue did confirm adrenal insufficiency with cortisol levels of 5.8 μg/mL at 0800h, 7.6 μg/mL at 30 minutes, and 8.2 μg/mL at 60 minutes after ACTH stimulation).
2. Repeat DEXA scan in 2 months because the last scan was 10 months ago.
3. Continue tacrolimus to maintain levels between 5 and 10 ng/mL and acceptable serum creatinine.
4. Repeat endoscopy and GVHD evaluation in 6 months with a goal to taper tacrolimus if appropriate.
5. Continue to monitor bcr/abl by polymerase chain reaction (PCR) in blood annually.

Key Points

- Ancillary and supportive care embraces the most frequent interventions that have topical intent, and any other intervention directed at organ-specific control of symptoms or complications resulting from GVHD and its therapy.
- Ancillary and supportive care is central to the management of chronic GVHD because clinical manifestations are polymorphic, may be prolonged and cause significant morbidity, or may even be irreversible.
- Forty-four percent of ancillary and supportive care guidelines are based on quality level I or II evidence.
- The recent evidence-based grading of ancillary and supportive care designated 56% of recommendations as being currently based on expert consensus opinion (level III), therefore highlighting several areas with the greatest need for clinical research.
- Ancillary and supportive care may enhance the effects of systemic therapy and prevent significant morbidity from chronic GVHD as well as treatment-related complications.
- The role of ancillary and supportive care as a steroid-sparing strategy needs to be systematically evaluated.

REFERENCES

1. Couriel D, Carpenter PA, Cutler C, et al. Ancillary and supportive care of chronic graft versus host disease: National Institutes of Health consensus development project on criteria for clinical trials in chronic graft versus host disease: V. Ancillary and supportive care working group report. *Biol Blood Marrow Transplant.* 2006;12:375–396.
2. Filipovich AH, Weisdorf D, Pavletic S, et al. National Institutes of Health consensus development project on criteria for clinical trials in chronic graft versus host disease: I. Diagnosis and staging working group report. *Biol Blood Marrow Transplant.* 2005;11:945–956.
3. Flowers ME, Parker PM, Johnston LJ, et al. Comparison of chronic graft versus host disease after transplantation of peripheral bloodstem cells versus bone marrow in allogeneic recipients: long-term follow-up of a randomized trial. *Blood.* 2002;100:415–419.

PART III: ORGAN SITE OR SYSTEM-SPECIFIC MANIFESTATIONS

16

CUTANEOUS MANIFESTATIONS OF CHRONIC GRAFT VERSUS HOST DISEASE

Edward W. Cowen and Sharon R. Hymes

INCIDENCE

Although advances in conditioning regimens, cell delivery, and graft versus host disease (GVHD) prophylaxis have improved the prognosis of patients following allogeneic stem cell transplantation (SCT), chronic GVHD (cGVHD) of the skin continues to be a significant source of long-term patient morbidity in SCT recipients. The skin is the most common target of cGVHD and is remarkably variable in its presentations, resulting in potential cosmetic, functional, and even life-threatening sequelae [1–3].

PRESENTATION

Cutaneous cGVHD may overlap with acute disease, occur *de novo,* or develop after a disease-free interval following acute GVHD [3]. Traditionally, the onset of cGVHD was classified as greater than 100 days after hematopoietic stem cell transplantation (HSCT) and heralded by the appearance of lichen planus-like lesions or sclerodermoid (scleroderma-like) changes. Newer HSCT regimens, as well as the delivery of donor lymphocyte infusions, have altered the timing of this "classic" presentation. Accurate estimation of the true incidence of cutaneous cGVHD is further hindered by the diversity of its clinical presentation (Table 16.1).

An effort to create a systematic classification of the cutaneous manifestations of cGVHD were undertaken as part of the 2005 National Institute of Health (NIH) Consensus Development Project [3]. The proposed criteria for the diagnosis of cutaneous cGVHD include (1) distinction from acute GVHD; (2) at least one diagnostic clinical sign of cGVHD or one distinctive manifestation confirmed by biopsy or relevant testing; (3) exclusion of other possible diagnoses [3]. The third criterion is particularly relevant, as drug eruptions and nonspecific symptoms such as pruritus are common posttransplantation. Other prevalent skin diseases such as eczema and psoriasis occurring in the posttransplant setting may also be confused with cGVHD. In addition, early skin lesions of cGVHD are often subtle and disease progression may be insidious. For example, xerosis (dry skin) and follicular-centered papules may require histopathology and clinical correlation to distinguish follicular eczema and keratosis pilaris from cGVHD.

Diagnostic skin changes of cutaneous cGVHD include poikiloderma (dyspigmentation, atrophy, and telangiectasia), lichen planus-like features, and sclerotic changes (Table 16.2). "Lichenoid" is a term that is better reserved as a histological description of the band-like inflammatory cell infiltrate at the dermal–epidermal junction and vacuolar alteration of the basal cell layer. This histologic pattern frequently results in long-term postinflammatory hyper- and hypopigmentation, especially in darker skin individuals. Sclerotic skin changes may be deep (extending through the dermis and/or subcutaneous tissue), morphea-like (superficial sclerosis with localized patchy areas of moveable skin, often with overlying dyspigmentation), or lichen sclerosus-like (discrete to coalescent atrophic plaques with underlying dermal sclerosis). cGVHD-related sclerosis often starts at sites of skin friction or pressure, such as the waistband, and may be complicated by pain, bullae formation [5], the appearance of benign angiomatous papules and nodules [6], or erosions and ulcerations. Deeper sclerosis may involve the subcutaneous fat, producing a rippled texture to the skin resembling cellulite.

cGVHD-related fasciitis may present in a particularly insidious manner, with the gradual onset of limited range of motion of affected joints. The overlying skin is variably affected and may appear relatively normal. Dorsiflexion of the wrist is often impaired with an inability to bring the palms together ("prayer sign"). Occasionally, there is visible induration or a groove demarcating fascial bundles or following the path of a superficial vessel. Magnetic resonance imaging may be of value in demonstrating evidence of fascial involvement [7].

"Distinctive" features of cutaneous cGVHD include skin depigmentation and nail, hair, and scalp changes [3]. The NIH Consensus Development Project IV includes the term "erythematous rash of any sort" as a broad umbrella term for the many skin eruptions associated with cutaneous cGVHD that affect the epidermis [8].

Table 16.1: Manifestations of Cutaneous cGVHD

cGVHD with Predominantly Epidermal Manifestations	Description
Xerotic/asteatotic/ ichthyosiform (Figure 16.1)	Dry skin, frequently generalized; "dry dandruff" on scalp or fishlike scale as in ichthyosis
Keratosis pilaris-like (Figure 16.2)	Perifollicular erythema or hyperpigmentation with papules or follicular keratotic, spiny protrusions
Lichen planus-like (Figure 16.3)	Purplish to markedly hyperpigmented, polygonal papules with varying configurations: annular, reticulated, or confluent; distribution may be follicular, linear, dermatomal, or lupus-like; may be vesiculobullous
Papulosquamous/psoriasiform/ eczematous (Figure 16.4)	Discrete guttate, annular or confluent erythematous scaly patches and plaques with micaceous scale that may involve any part of the body including scalp, face, hands and feet
Poikiloderma (Figure 16.5)	Variegated colors: erythema, hypo- and hyperpigmentation with cigarette-paper epidermis; suggestive of lupus when present on the face
Dyspigmentation (Figure 16.6)	May be punctate or confetti-like; generally considered to be a postinflammatory phenomenon; may be associated with dermal fibrosis of varying depths and appear "leopard-like"; spontaneous depigmentation suggestive of vitiligo may be prominent
Reactive erythema (Figure 16.7)	Urticarial or annular plaques with variable scale resembling erythema annulare centrifugum or lupus erythematosus
Erythroderma (Figure 16.8)	Diffuse to generalized erythema over ≥80% of the body accompanied by scaling, localized bullae, or superficial erosions
Acral erythema (Figure 16.9)	Diffuse or patchy erythema, edema, and pain of distal fingers, toes, palms, and soles; may appear targetoid or erythema multiforme-like with variable hyperkeratosis and erosions; early cases may resemble hand or foot eczema

cGVHD with Sclerotic Manifestations	Description
Lichen sclerosus-like (Figure 16.10)	May be indistinguishable from the idiopathic variety with purple or gray-white smooth papules and plaques, plugged follicles, and sclerosis of the papillary dermis; at times associated with fibrosis of deeper layers of the dermis or prominent atrophy
Dermal fibrosis, superficial (Figure 16.11)	Superficial and middermal sclerosis resulting in indurated plaques with variable pigmentation; epidermis may be normal, atrophic, or bullous and skin can be moved over underlying structures; resembles morphea clinically
Dermal fibrosis, full thickness/ scleroderma-like (Figure 16.12)	Sclerosis involves all layers of the skin with loss of subcutaneous tissue, making it fixed to underlying bone; early on may be preceded by edema/lymphedema resulting in a peau d'orange appearance, bullae, and occasionally vascular tumors; pipestem fibrosis of the extremities is frequently associated with neuropathy and painful ulcers
Rippled or cellulite-like subcutaneous fibrosis (Figure 16.13)	Skin appears to be rippled in areas rich in adipose tissue-volar arms, abdomen, and lateral thighs; caused by fibrosis of septae of subcutaneous fat
Fasciitis (Figure 16.14)	Prominent grooving may be visible along fascial bundles or in path of superficial vessels; joint contractures; overlying skin may appear normal or minimally affected Superficial skin may have varying degrees of fibrosis or may not be fibrotic at all; prominent grooves are seen along the course of tendons; causes marked reduction of range of motion at joints; "prayer sign" is positive

cGVHD Nail and Scalp Manifestations	Description
Nail dystrophy (Figure 16.15)	Nails are generally thin with vertical ridging and vertical pigment bands; pterygia may be seen and entire nail may be lost; variable periungual telangiectasia
Alopecia (Figure 16.16)	Patchy or moth-eaten scarring alopecia with variable epidermal and pigmentary changes and scarring

Source: Adapted from Hymes et al. [4]

Table 16.2: Diagnostic Features of cGVHD of the Skin, Hair, and Nails

Diagnostic*
Poikiloderma
Lichen planus-like features
Lichen sclerosus-like features
Morphea-like sclerosis
Scleroderma-like sclerosis
Eosinophilic fasciitis-like features

Distinctive†
Depigmentation
New onset scarring or nonscarring scalp alopecia
Scaling, papulosquamous scalp lesions
Nail dystrophy
  Longitudinal ridging, splitting, brittleness
  Onycholysis
  Pterygium unguis
  Anonychia

Other features
Ichthyosis
Hypohidrosis
Keratosis pilaris
Hypopigmentation
Hyperpigmentation
Premature gray hair
Edema
Erythema††
Maculopapular eruption††
Pruritus††

* Sufficient to establish a diagnosis of cutaneous cGVHD in the
  appropriate clinical setting.
† Feature of cGVHD, but insufficient alone to establish a diagnosis
  of cGVHD.
†† Also seen in the setting of acute GVHD.

Source: Adapted from Filipovich *et al.* [3]

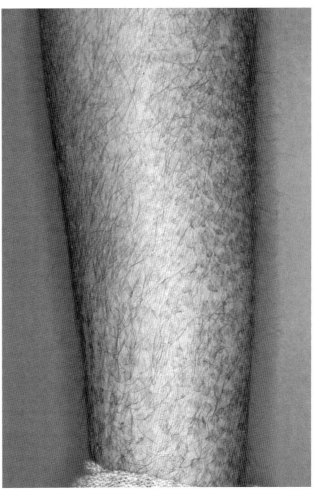

Figure 16.1 Ichthyosiform cGVHD (fish-scale-like changes). See Plate 30 in the color plate section.

Table 16.2 and the accompanying figures show many of the skin manifestations associated with cGVHD. Not infrequently, an individual patient will demonstrate more than one disease pattern or changing morphologies over time. Overlapping involvement of erythematous cGVHD and sclerotic cGVHD is common. In addition, patients may develop features of both acute and chronic GVHD following donor lymphocyte infusion or taper of immunosuppressive medications.

Postinflammatory hyper- and hypopigmentation is a significant concern of many patients and is difficult to reverse. Involvement of the hair follicles of the scalp produces hair loss that may be irreversible, especially when associated with fibrosis. Lichen planus-like GVHD often impacts the nail matrix, producing pterygium and severe nail dystrophy or permanent nail loss. Dermal sclerosis produces a multitude of problems including poor wound healing confounded by infection in the setting of global immune impairment. Fasciitis often results in permanent restriction in joint mobility. Without treatment, the course of cutaneous cGVHD is unpredictable, but usually progressive.

PROGNOSIS AND CLINICAL COURSE

Although many patients with cutaneous cGVHD develop mild symptoms such as xerosis or ichthyosis (dry skin with fish-scale-like changes), which are easily controlled with topical therapy, others develop chronic symptoms relating to cGVHD, which have a lasting impact on quality of life.

DIAGNOSIS

When a classic manifestation of cutaneous cGVHD develops in the appropriate clinical setting (e.g., skin thickening several months following SCT), the diagnosis can usually be made by dermatologic examination alone and histologic confirmation may not be necessary. However, cutaneous cGVHD, in

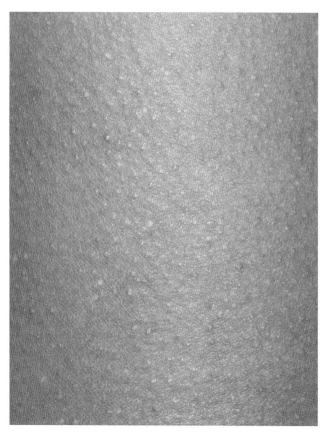

Figure 16.2 Folliculocentric papules resembling keratosis pilaris. See Plate 31 in the color plate section.

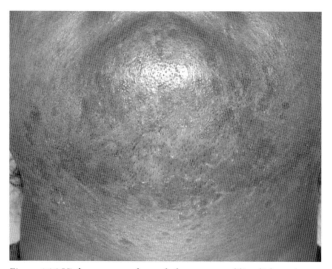

Figure 16.3 Violaceous papules and plaques resembling lichen planus. See Plate 32 in the color plate section.

its protean manifestations, may simulate a variety of dermatological conditions (Table 16.3), or may present in a nonspecific manner, potentially leading to inappropriate therapy or delay in evaluation for other organ involvement.

Table 16.3: Dermatological Conditions Resembling cGVHD

Drug exanthem
Eosinophilic fasciitis
Ichthyosis vulgaris
Keratosis pilaris
Lichen planus
Lichen sclerosus
Lupus erythematosus
Morphea
Phototoxicity
Systemic sclerosis
Toxic epidermal necrolysis
Xerosis

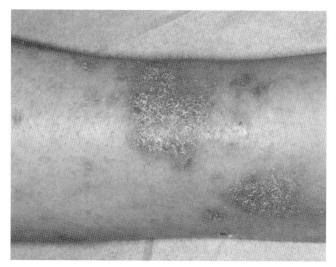

Figure 16.4 Psoriasiform cGVHD. See Plate 33 in the color plate section.

Given the breadth of cutaneous manifestations associated with cGVHD, it is tempting to attribute any new skin problem in the post–allo-SCT setting to cutaneous GVHD. However, as discussed earlier, the NIH Consensus Project has published criteria that distinguish diagnostic and distinctive cGVHD features of the skin, hair, and nails (Table 16.1) [3]. Nonspecific signs and symptoms of cGVHD, such as erythema, scaling, and pruritus, may be attributed to a variety of causes in the post–allo-SCT setting, including drug hypersensitivity and viral exanthem. Infections including *Cytomegalovirus*, *Herpes simplex* and *Varicella zoster*, and, most recently, *humanPapillomavirus* have been associated with flares of cutaneous cGVHD [9]. Generally speaking, the less distinct the clinical features of the eruption, the more likely histological confirmation will be required.

The histology of erythematous papular lesions of cGVHD resembles that of lichen planus, an inflammatory skin condition

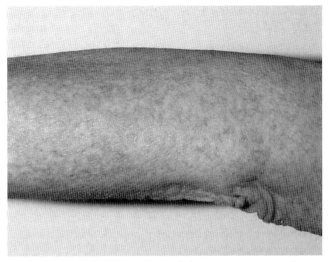

Figure 16.5 Erythema, hypo- and hyperpigmentation due to poikilodermic cGVHD. See Plate 34 in the color plate section.

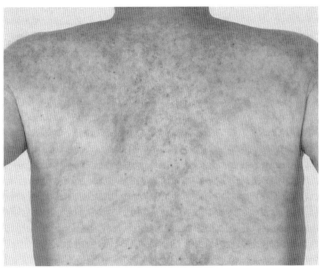

Figure 16.6 Residual hyperpigmentation following resolution of cutaneous cGVHD. See Plate 35 in the color plate section.

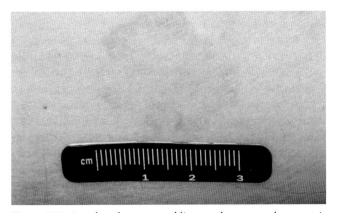

Figure 16.7 Annular plaque resembling erythema annulare centrifugum. See Plate 36 in the color plate section.

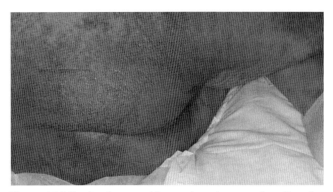

Figure 16.8 Erythroderma; widespread erythema and scaling. See Plate 37 in the color plate section.

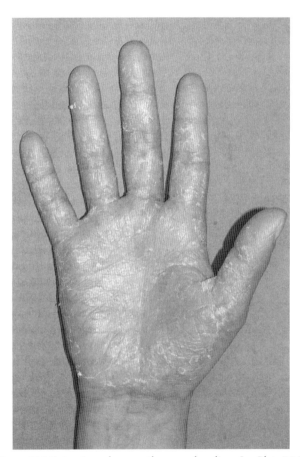

Figure 16.9 Extensive palmar erythema and scaling. See Plate 38 in the color plate section

characterized by basal keratinocyte vacuolar changes, but typically contains a less dense dermal infiltrate than that which is observed in lichen planus [10]. The infiltrate of the papillary and upper reticular dermis contains primarily lymphocytes, mononuclear cells, and melanophages [10]. Scattered shrunken eosinophilic apoptotic keratinocytes with or without pyknotic nuclei are visible within all levels of the epidermis but are usually present in greater numbers in the basal layer. In patients

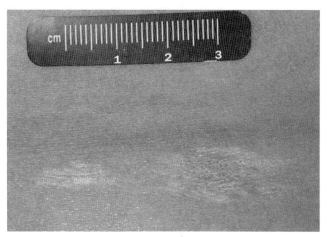

Figure 16.10 Localized atrophic plaques with superficial sclerosis. See Plate 39 in the color plate section.

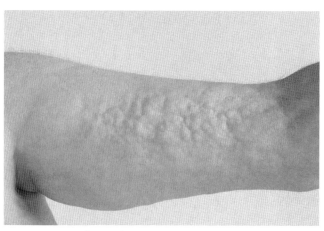

Figure 16.13 Rippling and nodularity of the subcutaneous tissue. See Plate 42 in the color plate section.

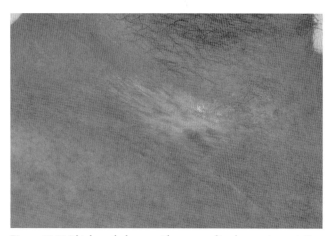

Figure 16.11 Thickened plaque with surrounding hyperpigmentation resembling morphea. See Plate 40 in the color plate section.

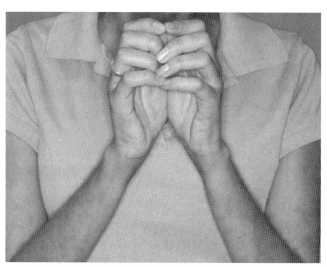

Figure 16.14 cGVHD-related fasciitis, with limited wrist dorsiflexion (positive "prayer sign"). See Plate 43 in the color plate section.

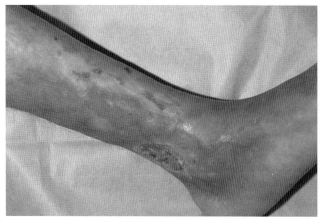

Figure 16.12 Hidebound (nonmoveable) fibrosis of the leg with ulcer formation. See Plate 41 in the color plate section.

with follicular involvement, localization to the hair follicles reminiscent of lichen planopilaris is observed [10].

The epidermis in the sclerotic forms of cGVHD may demonstrate overlying cGVHD changes similar to those described previously or may appear unaffected. The dermal findings in sclerotic cGVHD resemble morphea and scleroderma with replacement of the normal collagen pattern of the papillary and reticular dermis with bundles with thickened collagen and loss of periadnexal fat, and eventually loss of adnexal structures as well. Perivascular and periadnexal lymphocytic inflammation is a variable finding, and in contrast to morphea, inflammation at the dermal–subcutaneous fat border is uncommon [11]. A histologic diagnosis of GVHD-related fasciitis may require an incisional biopsy and demonstrates thickening and edema of subcutaneous and fascial tissue with

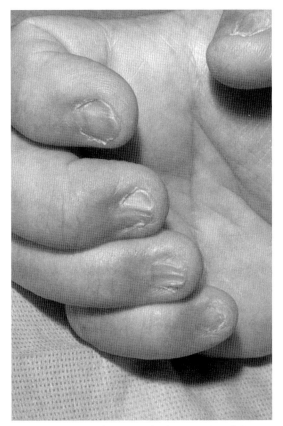

Figure 16.15 Nail dystrophy, vertical ridging, and nail thinning. See Plate 44 in the color plate section.

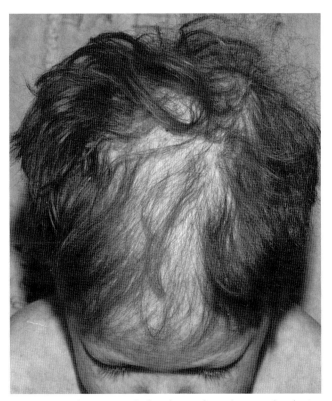

Figure 16.16 Alopecia, patchy hair loss with erythema and scale. See Plate 45 in the color plate section.

Table 16.4: Drugs Commonly Associated with Cutaneous Adverse Reactions in the Setting of cGVHD

Azithromycin (P)
Cephalosporins
Fluoroquinolones (P)
Hydrochlorthiazide (P)
Penicillins
Trimethoprim/sulfamethoxazole (P)
Voriconazole (P)

P, frequently associated with photosensitivity.

lymphocytic infiltration. Diagnosis is usually made on clinical criteria.

Differentiation of GVHD from drug reaction on histopathological grounds may be difficult in some cases. The presence of eosinophils in the inflammatory infiltrate, a frequent finding in drug reactions, does not reliably distinguish between GVHD and drug reaction, as they can be found in both settings [12]. A history of exposure to a medication commonly associated with drug eruptions may provide helpful clinical correlation to the dermatopathologist, who is considering a diagnosis of drug reaction (Table 16.4), whereas the administration of additional donor stem cells, tapering of cGVHD therapy, or recent infections are more suggestive of GVHD.

TREATMENT

The decision to prescribe a topically directed or systemic treatment for cutaneous cGVHD depends on a number of factors, including the extent and rate of progression of skin involvement, the impact of the skin disease on the patient, and its potential for long-term morbidity. Close communication between the dermatologist and transplant physician ensures that other systemic factors are also considered, including the presence of high-risk features such as thrombocytopenia, the rate of overall cGVHD progression, concurrent medical issues, and the status of the underlying disease or malignancy. For patients with isolated skin involvement, the benefit of systemic immunosuppressive therapy must be weighed against the risk of serious adverse affects, including infection, as well as possible interference with graft-versus-leukemia/tumor effect. As infection is a leading cause of death in patients with cGVHD, ideally topically directed therapy is preferable to systemic immunosuppressive therapy for patients with cGVHD limited to the skin. Unfortunately, few topically directed therapies produce a durable remission in skin symptoms, particularly for patients with extensive involvement. Furthermore, an evidence-based approach to skin-targeted therapies is hampered by lack of standardized diagnostic criteria and efficacy endpoints; for instance, "lichenoid" and "sclerodermoid" cGVHD are sometimes reported together without the use of response criteria specific for the different morphologies [13]. Further studies are urgently needed to determine the optimal treatment modality for different clinical presentations of skin involvement.

Topical corticosteroids and immunomodulaters are appropriate first-line therapy for patients with limited cutaneous disease. Erythema and scaling characteristic of the nonsclerotic types of cGVHD respond to midpotency (triamcinolone 0.1%) to ultrahigh potency topical steroid (clobetasol 0.05%) cream or ointment [14], but care should be taken with prolonged use, particularly on the face and intertriginous areas of the body, as skin atrophy may result and systemic absorption may be an issue in pediatric patients. Patients treated with topical steroids should be monitored regularly to ensure that the steroid preparations are being used in the appropriate quantity at the proper anatomic location(s) and that no cutaneous side effects have developed.

The topical immunomodulators tacrolimus ointment (Protopic®) and pimecrolimus cream (Elidel®) are potentially attractive alternatives to topical steroid therapy, because they exert an anti-inflammatory effect similar to that of midpotency topical steroids but do not induce skin atrophy that is associated with long-term topical steroid use. Topical tacrolimus is available in 0.1% and 0.03% ointment concentrations. Topical pimecrolimus is available in 1% cream only. These drugs are currently Food and Drug Administration (FDA) approved as second-line agents for atopic dermatitis for ages 2 years and older (tacrolimus 0.1% is not approved for children aged 2–15). Both may induce localized pruritus or burning, particular when administered to nonintact (eroded) skin.

The topical immunomodulators are most appropriate in areas at high risk of topical steroid-induced skin atrophy, such as the face and intertriginous surfaces. However, the duration of benefit of the topical immunomodulators is often short-lived and the risk of extended use of the agents in the setting of cGVHD is unknown. Choi and Nghiem [15] reported improvement in pruritus and erythema in 18 cGVHD patients treated with tacrolimus 0.1% ointment. However, all patients eventually required systemic therapy or phototherapy to control their skin disease. Subsequent reports have also confirmed a modest benefit from tacrolimus ointment 0.1% and 0.03% as well as pimecrolimus cream [16, 17]. Systemic toxicity is also a potential concern with these agents. Markedly elevated serum tacrolimus levels have been reported in patients on concurrent systemic tacrolimus therapy following the use of tacrolimus 0.1% ointment for acute cutaneous GVHD and for chronic oral GVHD [18, 19]. Systemic toxicity after three applications of topical tacrolimus has also been reported in a pediatric patient with acute skin GVHD who was not on systemic tacrolimus therapy [20]. The product labeling for both topical immunomodulators carries a black box warning regarding a possible association with malignancy, specifically lymphoma

risk, with extended use, although a definite causal relationship has not been established.

Pruritus is a variable finding in cutaneous cGVHD, but in some patients may be severe. Petrolatum-based emollients such as Aquaphor® may provide relief, particularly in patients with xerotic skin. Colloidal oatmeal powder bathtub soaks and topical antipruritic lotions containing camphor and menthol also provide short-term relief for intractable itching. The judicial use of oral sedating antihistamines may be beneficial, but care should be taken as these agents may exacerbate oral and ocular sicca symptoms.

Residual postinflammatory pigmentation often persists for months after resolution of active cutaneous cGVHD, and can be a significant cosmetic concern for patients, particularly darkly pigmented individuals. However, there is little data to support a benefit of topical bleaching agents or fade creams containing hydroquinone with or without retinoids or corticosteroid-containing compounds [14].

Treatment of skin erosions and ulcerations in the setting of cGVHD is challenging, particularly in patients with severe skin sclerosis, and in those with poor general health. Aggressive wound management utilizing protective films, dressings, and wound healing products such as becalpermin may be beneficial [14]. Referral to a dedicated wound care clinic will maximize the likelihood of achieving wound healing. As immunosuppression is common in this population, it is important to remain vigilant for the potential of skin infection and perform appropriate cultures if there is a concern of wound infection. Similarly, areas of skin breakdown that are atypical in appearance or do not respond to aggressive wound management should prompt a search for other causes of skin ulceration, including vasculitis, bullous drug reaction, neuropathy, primary cutaneous malignancy, or metastatic disease.

Patients with sclerotic involvement of the skin, subcutaneous tissue, or fascia may experience an insidious decline in function, resulting in joint range of motion limitations and joint contractures. In some cases, patients may falsely attribute their functional restrictions to deconditioning or may not have noticed the rippled texture of their skin indicative of underlying deep fibrosis. Vigilance by the physician and patient for new areas of sclerotic involvement or progression of joint limitations will allow for early intervention with appropriate medical and/or rehabilitative treatment to limit further functional decline.

Phototherapy

Following allo-HSCT, patients are routinely counseled to avoid ultraviolet (UV) radiation. Paradoxically, UV phototherapy is useful for the treatment of certain forms of cutaneous cGVHD. UV-induced immunosuppression via downregulation of local immune responses has made light therapy a useful modality for a number of nontransplant related inflammatory dermatoses [21, 22]. The mechanism of action is complex and multifactorial; UV radiation inhibits contact sensitivity and proliferative responses of lymphoid cells to mitogens and alloantigens by inactivation of T lymphocytes and antigen-presenting cells. Langerhans cells are depleted and morphologically altered, changing their capacity to present antigens [23], and keratinocytes produce and release immunosuppressive cytokines [24–29].

Phototherapy has demonstrated efficacy in both acute and chronic cutaneous GVHD. It is a particularly attractive option for patients with widespread skin involvement, and patients for whom systemic immunosuppression poses a high risk of infection or might interfere with a graft-versus-leukemia/tumor response. Currently, several different methods of light therapy are available: PUVA (oral psoralen and UVA light [320–400 nm]), broadband UVB (290–320 nm), narrowband UVB (311 nm), and UVA1 (340–400 nm).

PUVA is the only form of phototherapy that requires ingestion of a photosensitizing agent (psoralen) before exposure to UV light, although topically applied psoralens can be used (topi-PUVA, bath-PUVA). The benefit of PUVA for the treatment of lichen planus-like GVHD was first reported in 1985 [30, 31]. PUVA-bath therapy resulted in improvement in both lichenoid and sclerotic cGVHD in a small series of patients [32]. Broadband UVB (290–320 nm), and the more selective narrowband UVB (311 nm), has also demonstrated some benefit in small case reports [28, 33].

In general, sclerotic cGVHD manifestations are less responsive to phototherapy with UVB or PUVA than nonsclerotic cGVHD. As a rule, the longer the wavelength of light, the deeper the skin absorption; UVB is primarily absorbed in the epidermis, whereas UVA penetrates more deeply into the dermis than either broad or narrowband UVB. UVA1, a new phototherapy technique that utilizes a narrower range of UVA wavelength exposure (340–400 nm) without an oral photosensitizer, has been reported to benefit patients with a number of sclerotic skin conditions resembling sclerotic forms of cGVHD, including localized scleroderma (morphea), extragenital lichen sclerosus, and acral sclerosis associated with systemic sclerosis [34]. The efficacy of UVA1 has been described in several patients with lichenoid and sclerotic forms of cGVHD [35–37]; however, relapse after discontinuing therapy has also been reported [38, 39]. In addition, this form of phototherapy is not yet widely available in the United States.

The optimal exposure frequency and UV dosage of phototherapy for cGVHD have not been standardized. Typically, two to five visits/week to a physician's office for treatment are required to maintain a benefit. Certain patients, particularly those with skin sclerosis, may not tolerate PUVA treatment due to nausea, pruritus, skin irritation, or phototoxicity [40, 41] In addition, long-term PUVA treatment for psoriasis is associated with an increased risk of basal cell carcinoma, squamous cell carcinoma, and melanoma [42–43]. Although there is no epidemiologic cutaneous malignancy risk data for phototherapy in the post-HSCT setting, multiple squamous cell carcinomas have been reported following PUVA treatment for cGVHD [44]. Furthermore, melanoma risk is significantly elevated in patients following HSCT [45]. Therefore, the potential for the development of cutaneous malignancy should be made known to patients before initiating phototherapy and routine skin cancer surveillance is warranted. Before initiating phototherapy, testing for antinuclear and Sjogren's syndrome antibodies (SS-A/B, anti-Ro/La) is recommended, as these may be markers of potential phototoxicity. Photosensitizing medications should be avoided, if possible, and the UV dose may need to be adjusted when these medications are added (Table 16.4). Before exposing the whole body to phototherapy, a small area on the back is often tested to determine the minimal dose of light that produces erythema. However, patients may have extensive erythematous involvement that precludes such testing.

Extracorporeal Photopheresis

ECP is a specialized form of phototherapy approved by the U.S. FDA for the treatment of cutaneous T-cell lymphoma. The patient undergoes leukopheresis and the mononuclear cell sample is then mixed *ex vivo* with 8-methoxypsoralen and exposed to a UVA light source before reinfusion into the patient. This treatment has demonstrated efficacy for acute and chronic cutaneous GVHD. Greinix *et al.* [46] reported a 65% complete response rate for acute skin GVHD following 3 months of treatment. Messina *et al.* [47] reported a 76% response for acute skin involvement in a pediatric series. In a large review of 71 patients treated with ECP for chronic cGVHD, 59% of patients with cutaneous involvement responded to therapy, including 67% of those patients categorized as "scleroderma" [48]. ECP has been used successfully in the treatment of cGVHD-related fasciitis [49] as well as eosinophilic fasciitis, a rare disease process characterized by deep soft tissue fibrosis that clinically resembles GVHD-related fasciitis [50].

ECP requires placement of a large, double-lumen pheresis catheter and is not available at all medical centers. In addition, very small children are currently not able to undergo this procedure because of the fluid volume extracted for the procedure. However, modifications in the pheresis process may soon allow this therapy utilizing smaller fluid volumes. The optimal frequency and duration of treatment is unclear, as is the precise mechanism by which ECP is effective against cGVHD. ECP causes an increase in the plasmacytoid DC2 dendritic cell population and a corresponding decrease in the monocytoid DC1 population, which may result in a shift from a primarily Th1 to a Th2 cytokine profile [51]. Increased production of interleukin (IL)-10, in particular, may play an important role in the mitigation of the GVHD response through inhibition of antigen presentation and promotion of regulatory T-cell differentiation [52, 53].

Table 16.5: Preventive Skin Care/Surveillance Recommendations

Dry skin/pruritus

Moisturizing nonscented soaps

Frequent emollients: thick petrolatum-based ointments (Aquaphor®) produce more durable hydration than creams (Eucerin®); water-based lotions are least effective

Patient education

Sun exposure may induce a flare of skin disease

Avoid outdoor activities during peak hours of UV radiation (10 AM–4 PM)

Liberal use of broad spectrum UVA/B sunblock (SPF 30 or higher; note SPF refers only to UVB protection) on photoexposed surfaces

Use broad-brimmed hat, long-sleeves or UV protective clothing, and/or use of laundry additive to increase UV protective factor of clothing (Sun Guard™)

Elevated risk of skin cancer in the setting of iatrogenic/GVHD-associated immunosuppression and with phototherapy treatment

Advise patients on signs of sclerotic forms of cGvHD (skin thickening, rippling, decreasing joint range of motion, joint contractures)

Skin screening at office visits

Evaluate for areas of skin breakdown, potential cutaneous infection

Evaluate for potential skin malignancy; treatment of premalignant lesions (e.g., actinic keratoses)

Review of new photosensitizing medications (e.g., sulfamethoxasole/trimethoprim, voriconazole)

Reinforcement of importance of self-skin examination, skin cancer education, sun protection

Monitor for signs of skin/subcutaneous tissue sclerosis, including rippling, joint range of motion limitations, joint contractures

Systemic Retinoids

There is limited data on the efficacy of systemic retinoids for the treatment of cutaneous cGVHD. In a study by Marcellus *et al.* [54] 20/27 evaluable patients with treatment-refractory sclerotic GVHD had a subjective response to etretinate. Six patients could not tolerate the medication due to scaling and/or skin breakdown. Etretinate is no longer available in the United States, but two oral retinoids, isotretinoin (Accutane®) and acitretin (Soriatane®), are currently FDA approved for nodular acne and psoriasis, respectively. Further prospective studies with these agents are needed to determine if either have a role in the treatment of cutaneous cGVHD. All systemic retinoids are teratogenic and should be used in caution in women of child-bearing potential. In addition, xerosis is the most common side effect of systemic retinoid therapy and may exacerbate symptoms in some patients with cGVHD.

PREVENTION

Systemic infections, excessive sun exposure, and drug eruptions all may induce flares in cutaneous cGVHD symptoms. Preventive strategies include sun avoidance, and the use of sunblock and protective clothing to decrease the risk of excessive UV-induced flares of cGVHD (Table 16.5). This is of particular importance for patients on photosensitizing medications, such as trimethoprim/sulfamethosazole or voriconazole, in whom a phototoxic reaction may be mistaken for a flare of cGVHD skin disease, or which may induce a flare of cutaneous cGVHD (Table 16.4). Careful skin hygiene and monitoring for infection are important in patients with skin erosions/ulcerations to decrease the risk of secondary wound infection. Surveillance at regular intervals for cutaneous malignancy should also be performed.

FUTURE

As our appreciation of the clinical heterogeneity of cutaneous cGVHD continues to evolve, so must the principles of management also change to keep pace with new discoveries and new possibilities of better therapy. Nonmyeloablative conditioning regimens and the use of donor lymphocyte infusions (DLI) that delay the onset of "acute" skin GVHD until greater than 100 days following transplantation have blurred the temporal distinction between "acute" and "chronic" GVHD [55]. Therefore, careful categorization of GVHD skin involvement should be performed whenever skin disease is used as an outcome in therapeutic trials, and validation of cutaneous disease measures is needed to better discern the efficacy of both topical and systemic interventions.

A great need remains for new approaches to the treatment of cutaneous cGVHD. The addition of targeted cancer treatment such as the use of tyrosine kinase inhibitors has added an important new approach to cancer therapy. Similarly, advances in our understanding of chronic cGVHD may soon allow for the identification of more targeted approaches to cutaneous cGVHD therapy. One such approach is the use of agents that target skin fibrosis but do not interfere with the graft-versus-leukemia/tumor response and do not carry the attendant risks associated with conventional immunosuppressive therapy. Platelet-derived growth factor (PDGF) may play a key role in the increased proliferative capacity of fibroblasts, an effect that is enhanced by the presence of transforming growth factor-β (TGF-β) [56]. Increased gene expression of PDGF has been detected in the skin in the murine sclerodermatous GVHD model [57]. Recently, Baroni *et al.* [58] reported stimulatory autoantibodies to the PDGF receptor (PDGFR) in a group of 46 patients with systemic sclerosis. Similar autoantibodies to PDGFR were subsequently reported in a cohort of patients with extensive cGVHD [59]. In these studies, production of reactive oxygen species (ROS) and tyrosine phosphorylation was reversed with the use of PDGFR tyrosine kinase inhibitors, suggesting that agents such as imatinib with activity against the PDGFR may have the potential to inhibit fibrosis associated with the sclerotic forms of cGVHD. If fact, bronchiolitis obliterans, a fibrosing pulmonary complication of cGVHD, has also been associated with PDGF expression [60] and has been reported to respond to treatment with imatinib [61].

Chronic cutaneous GVHD remains a challenging problem for both the patient and the clinician post-HSCT. Multidisciplinary efforts have facilitated the recognition of early disease, but it is still not known why individual patients develop particular skin manifestations. Recent efforts to develop a consensus of characteristic phenotypic skin changes are not only of diagnostic importance but will also help facilitate multiinstitutional communication, leading to a better understanding of the immunology, clinical course, and treatment options.

REFERENCES

1. Wingard JR, Vogelsang GB, Deeg HJ. Stem cell transplantation: supportive care and long-term complications. Hematology/the Education Program of the American Society of Hematology American Society of Hematology 2002:422–444.
2. Goerner M, Gooley T, Flowers ME, et al. Morbidity and mortality of chronic GVHD after hematopoietic stem cell transplantation from HLA-identical siblings for patients with aplastic or refractory anemias. *Biol Blood Marrow Transplant.* 2002;8(1):47–56.
3. Filipovich AH, Weisdorf D, Pavletic S, et al. National Institutes of Health consensus development project on criteria for clinical trials in chronic graft-versus-host disease: I. Diagnosis and staging working group report. *Biol Blood Marrow Transplant.* 2005;11(12):945–956.
4. Hymes SR, Turner ML, Champlin RE, Couriel DR. Cutaneous manifestations of chronic graft-versus-host disease. *Biol Blood Marrow Transplant.* 2006;12(11):1101–1103.
5. Patel AR, Turner ML, Pavletic SZ, Cowen EW. The isomorphic response in morphealike graft-versus-host disease *Arch Dermatol.* 2008;144:1229–31.
6. Adamski H, Le Gall F, Cartron L, et al. Eruptive angiomatous lesions associated with graft–versus-host disease. *Br J Dermatol.* 2003;149(3):667–668.
7. Clark J, Yao L, Turner M, Cowen E. Magnetic resonance imaging for the diagnosis of subcutaneous involvement in patients with chronic graft-versus-host disease. *J Am Acad Dermatol.* 2008;58(2):AB85.
8. Pavletic SZ, Martin P, Lee SJ, et al. Measuring therapeutic response in chronic graft-versus-host disease: National Institutes of Health Consensus Development Project on Criteria for Clinical Trials in Chronic Graft-versus-Host Disease: IV. Response Criteria Working Group report. *Biol Blood Marrow Transplant.* 2006;12(3):252–266.
9. Kunishige JH, Hymes SR, Madkan V, et al. Epidermodysplasia verruciformis in the setting of graft-versus-host disease. *J Am Acad Dermatol.*2007;57(5 Suppl):S78–S80.
10. Weedon D, Strutton G. Skin pathology. 2nd ed. London, New York: Churchill Livingstone; 2002:46–47.
11. Hood A, Farmer ER. Interface dermatitis. In: Farmer ER, Hood AF, eds. *Pathology of the skin.* 2nd ed. New York: McGraw-Hill, Health Professions Division; 2000:201–205.
12. Marra DE, McKee PH, Nghiem P. Tissue eosinophils and the perils of using skin biopsy specimens to distinguish between drug hypersensitivity and cutaneous graft-versus-host disease. *J Am Acad Dermatol.*2004;51(4):543–546.
13. Greinix HT, Volc-Platzer B, Knobler R. Criteria for assessing chronic GVHD. *Bone Marrow Transplant* 2000;25(5):575.
14. Couriel D, Carpenter PA, Cutler C, et al. Ancillary therapy and supportive care of chronic graft-versus-host disease: National Institutes of Health consensus development project on criteria for clinical trials in chronic Graft-versus-host disease: V. Ancillary Therapy and Supportive Care Working Group Report. *Biol Blood Marrow Transplant.* 2006;12(4):375–396.
15. Choi CJ, Nghiem P. Tacrolimus ointment in the treatment of chronic cutaneous graft-vs-host disease: a case series of 18 patients. *Arch Dermatol.* 2001;137(9):1202–1206.
16. Elad S, Or R, Resnick I, Shapira MY. Topical tacrolimus-a novel treatment alternative for cutaneous chronic graft-versus-host disease. *Transpl Int.* 2003;16(9):665–670.
17. Schmook T, Kraft J, Benninghoff B, et al. Treatment of cutaneous chronic graft-versus-host disease with topical pimecrolimus. *Bone Marrow Transplant.* 2005;36(1):87–88.
18. Prot-Labarthe S, Therrien R, Champagne MA, Duval M, Joubert C. Toxic serum levels of tacrolimus after topical administration in an infant with severe cutaneous graft-versus-host disease. *Bone Marrow Transplant.* 2007;40(3):295–296.
19. Conrotto D, Carrozzo M, Ubertalli AV, et al. Dramatic increase of tacrolimus plasma concentration during topical treatment for oral graft-versus-host disease. *Transplantation.* 2006;82(8):1113–1115.
20. Neuman DL, Farrar JE, Moresi JM, Vogelsang GB, Higman MA. Toxic absorption of tacrolimus [corrected] in a patient with severe acute graft-versus-host disease. *Bone Marrow Transplant.* 2005;36(10):919–920.
21. Ozawa M, Ferenczi K, Kikuchi T, et al. 312-nanometer ultraviolet B light (narrow-band UVB) induces apoptosis of T cells within psoriatic lesions. *J Exp Med.* 1999;189(4):711–718.
22. Kripke ML, Morison WL, Parrish JA. Systemic suppression of contact hypersensitivity in mice by psoralen plus UVA radiation (PUVA). *J Invest Dermatol.* 1983;81(2):87–92.
23. Kripke ML. Ultraviolet radiation and immunology: something new under the sun-presidential address. *Cancer Res.* 1994;54(23):6102–6105.
24. Ashworth J, Kahan MC, Breathnach SM. PUVA therapy decreases HLA-DR+ CDIa+ Langerhans cells and epidermal cell antigen-presenting capacity in human skin, but flow cytometrically-sorted residual HLA-DR+ CDIa+ Langerhans cells

exhibit normal alloantigen-presenting function. *Br J Dermatol.* 1989;120(3):329–339.

25. Kim TY, Kripke ML, Ullrich SE. Immunosuppression by factors released from UV-irradiated epidermal cells: selective effects on the generation of contact and delayed hypersensitivity after exposure to UVA or UVB radiation. *J Invest Dermatol.* 1990;94(1):26–32.

26. Kang K, Hammerberg C, Meunier L, Cooper KD. CD11b+ macrophages that infiltrate human epidermis after in vivo ultraviolet exposure potently produce IL-10 and represent the major secretory source of epidermal IL-10 protein. *J Immunol.* 1994;153(11):5256–5264.

27. Krueger JG, Wolfe JT, Nabeya RT, et al. Successful ultraviolet B treatment of psoriasis is accompanied by a reversal of keratinocyte pathology and by selective depletion of intraepidermal T cells. *J Exp Med.* 1995;182(6):2057–2068.

28. Grundmann-Kollmann M, Martin H, Ludwig R, et al. Narrowband UV-B phototherapy in the treatment of cutaneous graft versus host disease. *Transplantation.* 2002;74(11):1631–1634.

29. Cooper KD. Cell-mediated immunosuppressive mechanisms induced by UV radiation. *Pharmacol Physicians.* 1996;63(4):400–406.

30. Hymes SR, Morison WL, Farmer ER, Walters LL, Tutschka PJ, Santos GW. Methoxsalen and ultraviolet A radiation in treatment of chronic cutaneous graft-versus-host reaction. *J Am Acad Dermatol.* 1985;12(1 Pt 1):30–37.

31. Jampel RM, Farmer ER, Vogelsang GB, Wingard J, Santos GW, Morison WL. PUVA therapy for chronic cutaneous graft-vs-host disease. *Arch Dermatol.* 1991;127(11):1673–1678.

32. Leiter U, Kaskel P, Krahn G, et al. Psoralen plus ultraviolet-A-bath photochemotherapy as an adjunct treatment modality in cutaneous chronic graft versus host disease. *Photodermatol Photoimmunol Photomed.* 2002;18(4):183–190.

33. Enk CD, Elad S, Vexler A, Kapelushnik J, Gorodetsky R, Kirschbaum M. Chronic graft-versus-host disease treated with UVB phototherapy. *Bone Marrow Transplant.* 1998;22(12):1179–1183.

34. Breuckmann F, Gambichler T, Altmeyer P, Kreuter A. UVA/UVA1 phototherapy and PUVA photochemotherapy in connective tissue diseases and related disorders: a research based review. *BMC dermatology.* 2004;4(1):11.

35. Ziemer M, Thiele JJ, Gruhn B, Elsner P. Chronic cutaneous graft-versus-host disease in two children responds to UVA1 therapy: improvement of skin lesions, joint mobility, and quality of life. *J Am Acad Dermatol.* 2004;51(2):318–319.

36. Grundmann-Kollmann M, Behrens S, Gruss C, Gottlober P, Peter RU, Kerscher M. Chronic sclerodermic graft-versus-host disease refractory to immunosuppressive treatment responds to UVA1 phototherapy. *J Am Acad Dermatol.* 2000;42(1 Pt 1):134–136.

37. Stander H, Schiller M, Schwarz T. UVA1 therapy for sclerodermic graft-versus-host disease of the skin. *J Am Acad Dermatol.* 2002;46(5):799–800.

38. Calzavara Pinton P, Porta F, Izzi T, et al. Prospects for ultraviolet A1 phototherapy as a treatment for chronic cutaneous graft-versus-host disease. *Haematologica.* 2003;88(10):1169–1175.

39. Wetzig T, Sticherling M, Simon JC, Hegenbart U, Niederwieser D, Al-Ali HK. Medium dose long-wavelength ultraviolet A (UVA1) phototherapy for the treatment of acute and chronic

graft-versus-host disease of the skin. *Bone Marrow Transplant.* 2005;35(5):515–519.

40. Vogelsang GB, Wolff D, Altomonte V, et al. Treatment of chronic graft-versus-host disease with ultraviolet irradiation and psoralen (PUVA). *Bone Marrow Transplant.* 1996;17(6):1061–1067.

41. Stern RS. The risk of melanoma in association with long-term exposure to PUVA. *J Am Acad Dermatol.* 2001;44(5):755–761.

42. Stern RS, Liebman EJ, Vakeva L. Oral psoralen and ultraviolet-A light (PUVA) treatment of psoriasis and persistent risk of nonmelanoma skin cancer. PUVA Follow-up Study. *J Natl Cancer Inst.* 1998;90(17):1278–1284.

43. Stern RS, Lunder EJ. Risk of squamous cell carcinoma and methoxsalen (psoralen) and UV-A radiation (PUVA). A meta-analysis. *Arch Dermatol.* 1998;134(12):1582–1585.

44. Altman JS, Adler SS. Development of multiple cutaneous squamous cell carcinomas during PUVA treatment for chronic graft-versus-host disease. . *J Am Acad Dermatol.* 1994;31(3 Pt 1):505–507.

45. Curtis RE, Rowlings PA, Deeg HJ, et al. Solid cancers after bone marrow transplantation. *N Engl J Med.* 1997;336(13):897–904.

46. Greinix HT, Volc-Platzer B, Kalhs P, et al. Extracorporeal photochemotherapy in the treatment of severe steroid-refractory acute graft-versus-host disease: a pilot study. *Blood.* 2000;96(7):2426–2431.

47. Messina C, Locatelli F, Lanino E, et al. Extracorporeal photochemotherapy for paediatric patients with graft-versus-host disease after haematopoietic stem cell transplantation. *Br J Haematol.* 2003;122(1):118–127.

48. Couriel DR, Hosing C, Saliba R, et al. Extracorporeal photochemotherapy for the treatment of steroid-resistant chronic GVHD. *Blood.* 2006;107(8):3074–3080.

49. Sbano P, Rubegni P, De Aloe GB, Guidi S, Fimiani M. Extracorporeal photochemotherapy for treatment of fasciitis in chronic graft-versus-host disease. *Bone Marrow Transplant.* 2004;33(8):869–870.

50. Romano C, Rubegni P, De Aloe G, et al. Extracorporeal photochemotherapy in the treatment of eosinophilic fasciitis. *J Eur Acad Dermatol Venereol.* 2003;17(1):10–13.

51. Gorgun G, Miller KB, Foss FM. Immunologic mechanisms of extracorporeal photochemotherapy in chronic graft-versus-host disease. *Blood.* 2002;100(3):941–947.

52. Craciun LI, Stordeur P, Schandene L, et al. Increased production of interleukin-10 and interleukin-1 receptor antagonist after extracorporeal photochemotherapy in chronic graft-versus-host disease. *Transplantation.* 2002;74(7):995–1000.

53. Fimiani M, Di Renzo M, Rubegni P. Mechanism of action of extracorporeal photochemotherapy in chronic graft-versus-host disease. *Br J Dermatol.* 2004;150(6):1055–1060.

54. Marcellus DC, Altomonte VL, Farmer ER, et al. Etretinate therapy for refractory sclerodermatous chronic graft-versus-host disease. *Blood.* 1999;93(1):66–70.

55. Couriel DR, Saliba RM, Giralt S, et al. Acute and chronic graft-versus-host disease after ablative and nonmyeloablative conditioning for allogeneic hematopoietic transplantation. *Biol Blood Marrow Transplant.* 2004;10(3):178–185.

56. Bonner JC. Regulation of PDGF and its receptors in fibrotic diseases. *Cytokine Growth Factor Rev.* 2004;15(4):255–273.

57. Zhou L, Askew D, Wu C, Gilliam AC. Cutaneous gene expression by DNA microarray in murine sclerodermatous graft-versus-

host disease, a model for human scleroderma. *J Investigative Dermatol.* 2007;127(2):281–292.

58. Baroni SS, Santillo M, Bevilacqua F, et al. Stimulatory autoantibodies to the PDGF receptor in systemic sclerosis. *N Engl J Med.* 2006;354(25):2667–2676.

59. Svegliati S, Olivieri A, Campelli N, et al. Stimulatory autoantibodies to PDGF receptor in patients with extensive chronic graft-versus-host disease. *Blood.* 2007;110(1):237–241.

60. Hertz MI, Henke CA, Nakhleh RE, et al. Obliterative bronchiolitis after lung transplantation: a fibroproliferative disorder associated with platelet-derived growth factor. *Proc Natl Acad Sci U S A.* 1992;89(21):10385–10389.

61. Majhail NS, Schiffer CA, Weisdorf DJ. Improvement of pulmonary function with imatinib mesylate in bronchiolitis obliterans following allogeneic hematopoietic cell transplantation. *Biol Blood Marrow Transplant.* 2006;12(7):789–791.

17

Oral Chronic Graft versus Host Disease

Nathaniel S. Treister, Mark M. Schubert, and Jane M. Fall-Dickson

INTRODUCTION

The oral cavity is a frequent target of chronic graft versus host disease (cGVHD) with changes observed in the lips, muscles, mucosa, salivary glands, dentition, and also in the facial skin. When severe, oral cGVHD is functionally debilitating; however, even mild involvement can have a significant impact on the conduct of daily activities and overall quality of life (QOL). Early recognition and diagnosis of oral changes, provision of appropriate and effective therapies, and vigilant long-term follow-up are critical to minimize complications and to improve both short- and long-term outcomes.

INCIDENCE

Oral cGVHD is a frequent and, often, very prominent complication following allogeneic hematopoietic cell transplantation (HCT). Almost 80% of patients diagnosed with cGVHD demonstrate some degree of oral involvement, making this one of the most common clinical manifestations [1–3]. In fact, the prevalence of oral and skin cGVHD is nearly equivalent, making these the two most commonly affected tissues [2]. Although a number of risk factors for the development of cGVHD have been characterized, none specific for the oral cavity have been identified. Standard GVHD prophylaxis regimens are the only specific measures that can prevent or minimize the risk of developing oral cGVHD.

Although oral findings may be the initial and in some cases only indication of cGVHD development, this is highly variable and oral changes may occur at any point along the course of evolution of cGVHD. Also, oral cGVHD may first present clinically as other areas (e.g., skin) are resolving. Although it is more common to observe oral complications emerge in the context of tapering immunosuppression, they may develop regardless of increases or reductions in systemic immunomodulatory therapies. Further complicating matters is the increasing utilization of alternate protocols such as reduced-intensity conditioning regimens, umbilical-cord stem cell transplantation, and donor lymphocyte infusions, which may significantly

alter the relationship between acute and chronic GVHD with respect to timing, course, and intensity (e.g., delayed onset or "overlap" syndrome) [4].

Compared with adults, pediatric patients overall have a significantly lower risk of developing cGVHD, although this difference diminishes with increasing age (i.e., late teens). The incidence appears to be increasing with greater utilization of peripheral blood HCT protocols in children [5, 6]. Of those children who develop cGVHD, the oral cavity is affected at approximately the same frequency as adults [7–11]. Although individual cases can be quite severe even in very young children, clinical involvement of the oral cavity is generally less extensive as compared with older patients [11]. Preverbal and younger children may not be able to effectively express their symptoms to their doctor, and therefore obtaining a detailed history from the parent/guardian and conducting a thorough oral examination are essential.

PRESENTATION

Oral cGVHD presents with a spectrum of signs and symptoms that are in large part proportional to the degree, extent, location, and severity of clinical involvement (Table 17.1). Both the oral mucosa and salivary glands (major and minor) are targets of alloreactive donor lymphocytes, and although both organs are often affected concurrently, disease may be restricted to one tissue type. Although salivary gland involvement may be as or more severe than mucosal disease, resulting in significant clinical complications and morbidity, the term "oral cGVHD" is often used to refer specifically to mucosal changes. Of note, one or both systems can be involved at any given time and treatment may be organ-targeted; therefore each organ should be evaluated separately.

Oral Mucosal cGVHD

The classic signs of oral mucosal cGVHD clinically mimic oral lichen planus, and include white hyperkeratotic changes including striations or lacey reticulations and plaques; erythema,

Table 17.1: Presenting Signs and Symptoms of Oral cGVHD

Oral Mucosal cGVHD		Salivary Gland cGVHD	
Signs	Symptoms	Signs	Symptoms
White reticulations and plaques	Sensitivity to foods/drinks	Thickened, sticky, ropey or foamy saliva	Xerostomia
Erythema	– spicy/seasoned foods	Lack of saliva/absence of floor of mouth pooling	Sensitivity to foods/drinks
Ulcerations with pseudomembranes	– acidic foods (citrus, salad dressing, carbonated drinks)	Atrophic mucosa	Difficulty speaking
Atrophic glossitis	– alcoholic beverages and alcohol containing mouth rinses	Dental caries (interproximal and at the cervical margins)	Difficulty chewing
Superficial mucoceles	– salty foods	Oral candidiasis	Difficulty swallowing/throat constriction
Blisters on palate after meals	– hard/crunchy/crusty foods	Frequent water sipping	Waking at night due to severe dryness
	– warm (temperature) foods/drinks	Tongue "clicking" while speaking	Taste changes
	Sensitivity to mint-flavored toothpaste/brushing	Food debris inside the mouth	
	Taste changes	Inability to eat dry foods without fluids	

A number of findings are common to both mucosal and salivary gland involvement.

also accompanied with mucosal thinning or atrophy, presenting as distinct areas of redness; and ulcerations, or pseudomembranes, appearing as well-defined yellowish-white lesions that are often distinctly painful [11–15] (Figure 17.1A–G). Reticulation and erythema are the most common clinical findings, with ulcerations observed less frequently [12, 15, 16]. Patients often present with a combination of reticulation, erythema, and ulcerations, with specific findings that are remarkably variable, even in the same patient at different points in time.

Ulcerations are considered the most severe and generally the most painful manifestation. However, there is a tremendous range in reported symptoms as seen in patients who have only reticular lesions experiencing significant oral sensitivity and resulting in reduced oral intake, while some patients with ulcerations do not report significant pain or disability. The buccal mucosa, labial mucosa, and tongue are the most frequently affected mucosal sites, although, any intraoral location may be involved [12, 15, 16]. Of particular note, the soft palate and posterior oropharynx are infrequently affected, and esophageal involvement is rare. Symptoms of throat discomfort are invariably related to salivary gland changes or pharyngeal candidiasis [15, 16]. Secondary oral infections with candidiasis, *Herpes simplex virus*, and *Cytomegalovirus* may lead to unusual clinical presentations in patients with oral cGVHD and often require culture and/or biopsy for definitive diagnosis [17]. Laboratory studies to rule out these infections are needed in conjunction with expert clinical observations as part of the diagnostic, as well as, disease monitoring process.

Many patients with oral cGVHD involvement will report no symptoms. However, when present, the symptoms of oral mucosal cGVHD can range from mildly annoying to completely debilitating, leading to weight loss, malnutrition, poor oral hygiene, and significantly compromised QOL. Commonly reported symptoms include mouth pain; mouth sensitivity (e.g., intolerance to normally tolerated spicy, acidic, salty, carbonated, and strongly flavored foods, drinks, and oral healthcare products); inability to tolerate hard, crunchy, and crusty foods; mouth tightness with opening; restricted oral intake; altered or diminished taste; and a sensation of "roughness" on the inside of the mouth [11–15]. Such findings, in large part, can be attributed to the degree and extent of mucosal changes, with the location and distribution of lesions having a significant impact on symptoms and functional limitations [15]. Although, the extent to which weight loss and malnutrition are directly correlated with oral cGVHD activity is unclear, patients suffering from profound oral sensitivity can have tremendous difficulty maintaining adequate nutritional and caloric intake even when limited to an exclusively soft, bland diet [3, 18].

The histopathological and molecular features of oral mucosal cGVHD have been well-characterized. Histopathological findings include hyperkeratosis, epithelial atrophy, an interface submucosal lymphocytic infiltrate, and basal-cell apoptosis and degeneration, with specific findings dependent on the location and clinical characteristics of the biopsy site (e.g., hyperkeratosis observed in reticular but not ulcerative lesions, Figure 17.2) [10, 12, 17, 19–23]. The inflammatory infiltrate is composed primarily of CD4+ and CD8+ T lymphocytes, with most studies reporting a predominance of CD8+ cells, and CD68+ macrophages and Langerhans cells, with B cells infrequently detected [20–26]. However, it is unclear to what extent these histopathologic features and molecular mechanisms correlate with actual clinical disease activity and related symptoms, or importantly, how these parameters may be influenced by various systemic and local therapies.

Salivary Gland cGVHD

Saliva plays a critical role in maintaining oral health and function, and when compromised, can result in tremendous

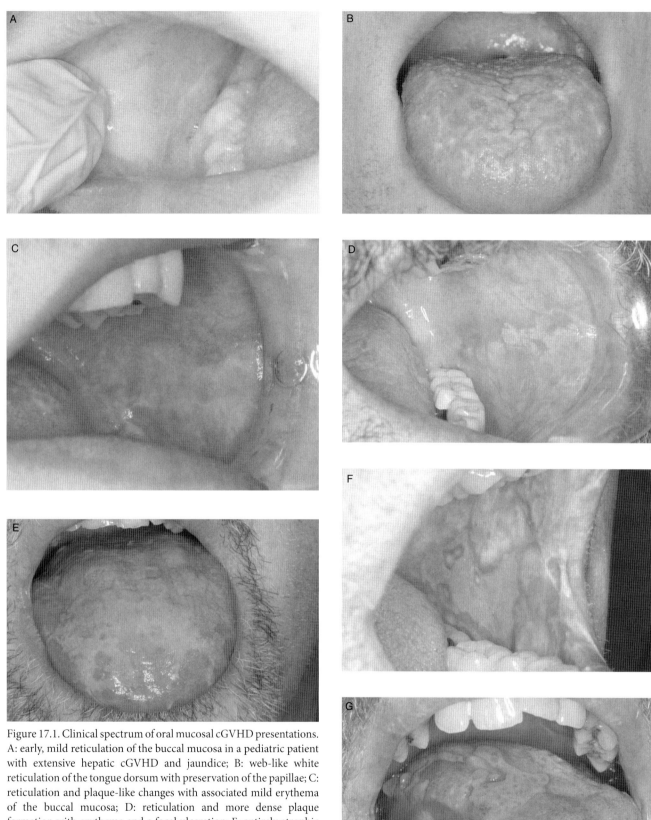

Figure 17.1. Clinical spectrum of oral mucosal cGVHD presentations. A: early, mild reticulation of the buccal mucosa in a pediatric patient with extensive hepatic cGVHD and jaundice; B: web-like white reticulation of the tongue dorsum with preservation of the papillae; C: reticulation and plaque-like changes with associated mild erythema of the buccal mucosa; D: reticulation and more dense plaque formation with erythema and a focal ulceration; E: entirely atrophic tongue dorsum with extensive atypical plaque-like changes; F: heavy reticulation with intense erythema and a very large area of ulceration; G: extensive ulceration of the tongue with areas of atrophic glossitis adjacent to areas with entire preservation of the papillae. See Plate 46 in the color plate section.

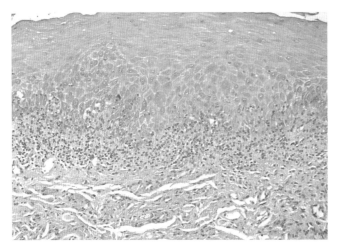

Figure 17.2 Oral mucosal cGVHD histopathology. Oral squamous mucosa with a band-like infiltrate of T lymphocytes at the interface between the connective tissue and basement membrane with basal-cell degeneration, acanthosis, and hyperkeratosis. This specimen corresponds to a white reticular lesion clinically. See Plate 47 in the color plate section.

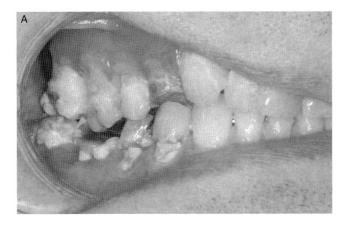

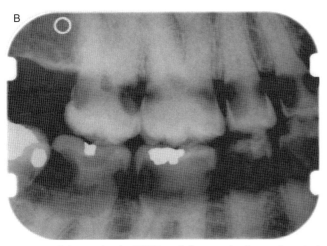

Figure 17.3 Salivary gland cGVHD oral changes. A: advanced cervical decay in a patient 1 year after HCT due to both salivary gland and mucosal cGVHD; B: intraoral periapical radiograph of same patient showing extent of interproximal decay. See Plate 48 in the color plate section.

morbidity due to dysfunction and hard- and soft-tissue infections [27–29]. Signs of salivary gland cGVHD include dry and atrophic appearing mucosa, hyposalivation (e.g., lack of floor of mouth pooling), thick, viscous and ropey saliva, rampant dental caries (in particular cervical, interproximal, and at the margins of preexisting restorations), and recurrent oral candidiasis [13, 14, 30, 31] (Figure 17.3A, B). Salivary gland cGVHD results in both quantitative (i.e., decreased output or hyposalivation), and qualitative alterations (e.g., increased levels of sodium, magnesium, epidermal growth factor, total protein, albumin, and IgG, and decreased levels of IgA) in saliva flow and composition [7, 10, 12, 22, 23, 32–45]. The degree of salivary gland hypofunction has been found to correlate with overall cGVHD severity, with flow rates decreased up to 70% compared to those without cGVHD [46]. Of note, conditioning regimens that include total-body irradiation have not been found to be associated with significant long-term salivary gland hypofunction [46–48].

Clinical signs and symptoms of salivary gland cGVHD include thickened saliva, lack of saliva, mouth and throat dryness (xerostomia), difficulty chewing, difficulty swallowing, sensation of throat constriction, increased sensitivity to food and drinks, altered or diminished taste, difficulty speaking, and frequent waking at night due to severe oral dryness [14, 49]. Clinicians may note that the degree of symptoms appears to be out of proportion to the observed clinical signs of hyposalivation; this is most likely explained by qualitative rather than quantitative changes. Over time, patients may develop tolerance to long-standing xerostomia, further complicating the ability to evaluate salivary gland disease activity, treatment responses, and risks for developing secondary complications [31].

Superficial mucoceles are small (<0.5 cm) mucous filled vesicles that are commonly seen on the soft palate and less frequently on the buccal and labial mucosa and tongue (Figure 17.4A, B) [10, 12, 50]. Inflammation of the minor salivary glands, due to direct targeting or secondary to mucosal cGVHD, results in ductal damage and vesicle formation. These often develop abruptly during meals and are typically described more as an annoyance than actually painful, and may subside within hours of forming only to be replaced by new lesions at the next meal. Occasionally, deeper and more symptomatic mucoceles develop that do not resolve without surgical intervention (Figure 17.5A–D).

Owing to their high concentration and accessibility within the oral labial mucosa, lower labial minor salivary gland biopsies (often collected with the labial mucosa intact using a 4.0-mm skin punch) can be easily performed to support a diagnosis of cGVHD and are collected at some centers at standardized time points for routine staging purposes following HCT [32]. Detailed histopathological scoring guidelines for both salivary glands and mucosa have been recently published [17]. Histopathological analysis of minor salivary gland biopsies demonstrates lymphocyte exocytosis into intralobular ducts and acini, infiltration and accumulation of intralobular, periductal lymphocytes, and periductal fibrosis [12, 19, 22, 23, 31]. The lymphocytic infiltrate is characterized predominantly by CD8+ T cells and few B

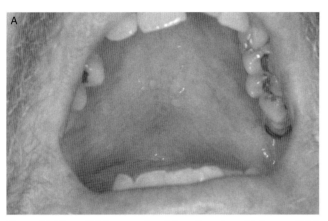
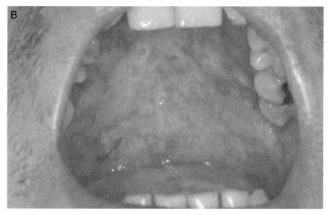

Figure 17.4 Superficial mucoceles of the palate. A: multiple superficial mucoceles both intact and burst with several areas of secondary ulceration; B: numerous superficial mucoceles in the context of severe mucosal cGVHD. See Plate 49 in the color plate section.

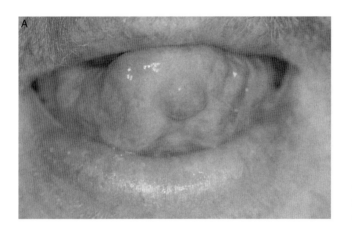
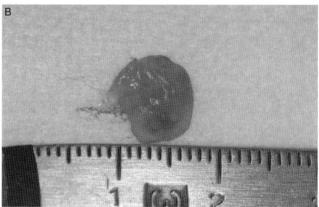
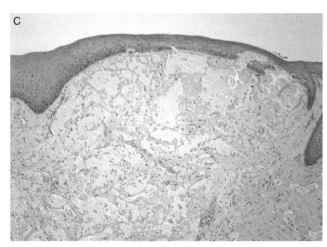
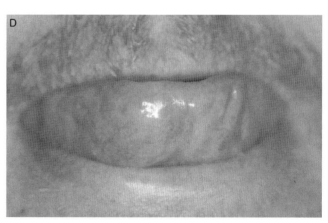

Figure17.5 Symptomatic deep mucocele. A: large 1.0 cm well-defined dome-shaped mucocele in the anterior ventral tongue; B: gross pathology following excision; C: histopathology demonstrating extensive mucous collection in the connective tissue with normal appearing surface mucosa; D: excision site 1 week later showing complete healing. See Plate 50 in the color plate section.

cells with associated cytokine dysregulation [21, 30, 51, 52]. The intensity of cellular and molecular changes has been found to correlate with the clinical degree of salivary gland hypofunction, supporting a strong relationship with this hypofunction and the infiltrating alloreactive lymphocytes [21, 51].

While not routinely performed, salivary gland scintigraphy has been utilized to evaluate glandular function following allogeneic HCT [46, 53]. Comparative studies before and up to 100 days postallogeneic HCT did not demonstrate significant changes in flow despite subjective reports of xerostomia [46,

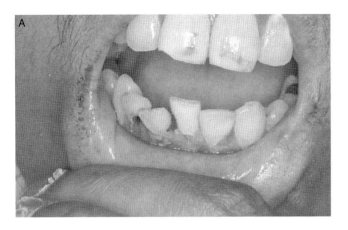
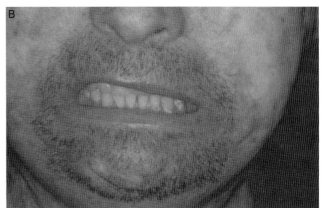
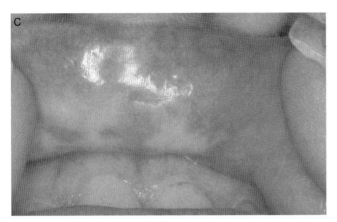
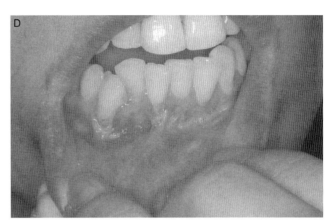

Figure 17.6 Sclerotic oral cGVHD. A: advanced sclerosis of the facial skin resulting in limited maximum opening, inability to maintain oral hygiene resulting in gingival bleeding, and subsequent rampant dental caries; B: extensive sclerotic changes resulting in painful myospasm and dystonia; C: severe penetrating skin sclerosis replacing normal mucosa with dense fibrous tissue; D: sclerotic changes of the mucosa resulting in loss of the labial vestibule and localized areas of advanced recession due to pulling away of the gingival tissues. See Plate 51 in the color plate section.

53]. However, reduced uptake, accumulation, and excretion were observed in patients with cGVHD compared to those that did not develop cGVHD[46].

Sclerotic Oral cGVHD

Although an exceedingly rare complication that tends to develop late in the course of cGVHD, sclerosis of the oral and perioral structures can lead to severe limitations in an individual's ability to eat, speak, maintain oral hygiene, and receive dental treatment (Figure 17.6A–D) [49]. More commonly, complaints of "tightness" are due to lichenoid changes affecting the buccal mucosa; this sensation often resolves following topical therapy. Orofacial sclerosis, most commonly, develops secondary to involvement of the facial skin associated with extensive sclerotic skin cGVHD, resulting in progressive trismus (limited opening) and infrequently, painful myospasm. In rare cases, the mucosa may be directly affected as a primary sclerotic process or due to scarring in areas of long-standing chronic ulcerative mucosal disease (i.e., "band" formation that when palpated feels like a tightened rubber band). The end result is "tightening" of the affected structures, which may

result in functional deficits and localized soft tissue and periodontal defects. Independent of salivary gland involvement, patients with sclerotic changes and trismus are at high risk for dental disease due to challenges in maintaining adequate oral hygiene.

DIAGNOSIS

In the majority of cases, oral cGVHD can be diagnosed by history, context, and clinical examination alone. The National Institutes of Health (NIH) Consensus Development Project on Criteria for Clinical Trials in Chronic Graft-versus-Host Disease has recently introduced standardized criteria for oral cGVHD diagnosis, clinical and histopathological scoring, and measuring treatment response [17, 54–57]. The intent of these instruments is to facilitate standardized criteria for research in oral cGVHD to allow meaningful comparisons to be made across studies and between institutions [58]. Diagnostic features sufficient to establish a clinical diagnosis of oral cGVHD include lichenoid or reticular lesions and hyperkeratotic plaques; erythematous and ulcerative changes (in the absence of lichenoid reticulations)

Table 17.2: The NIH Consensus Development Project on Criteria for Clinical Trials in Chronic Graft versus Host Disease Staging Score

Score 0	Score 1	Score 2	Score 3
No symptoms	Mild symptoms with disease signs but *not* limiting oral intake significantly	Moderate symptoms with disease signs with *partial* limitation of oral intake	Severe symptoms with disease signs with *major* limitation of oral intake

are considered "distinctive" but not diagnostic [55]. The clinical scoring system, which is meant to be used for baseline and cross-sectional evaluations at any given point in time, measures the severity of involvement according to a 4-point scale, based on a combination of oral signs and the degree of functional impact (Table 17.2). Histopathological criteria grade-specific findings and features on a 4-point scale based on the likelihood of supporting a diagnosis of cGVHD [17].

For repeated observations, for example in the context of a cGVHD clinical trial, more detailed objective and subjective measures are evaluated [56]. The clinician-assessed instrument takes into account: (1) extent of reticulation/lichenoid changes; (2) severity and extent of erythema; (3) extent of ulcerations; and (4) the number of superficial mucoceles, and generates a score from 0 to 15 (Figure 17.7). Patient reported most severe pain, sensitivity, and dryness are collected using an 11-point scale (0–10) from "not present" to "as bad as you can imagine."

Diagnostic Biopsy

When indicated, obtaining a tissue biopsy of the oral mucosa or minor salivary glands is a simple and safe outpatient procedure. Confirmation by histopathological diagnosis can be useful when clinical presentation is equivocal or when definitive diagnosis is absolutely essential. Non-ulcerated mucosal lesions should be selected to ensure inclusion of the epithelium. In most cases the biopsy should be performed with a 4.0-mm skin punch biopsy and must include the full thickness of epithelium and underlying connective tissue. For minor salivary gland biopsies, a small incision or ellipse is made in the lower labial mucosa and five to six minor salivary gland lobules are removed with tissue forceps and scissors. The biopsy site is closed with resorbable chromic gut sutures, heals within a few days and rarely scar. Biopsy specimens should be submitted to general or oral pathologists who are experienced in the interpretation and diagnosis of cGVHD (Figure 17.2).

Clinical trials for cGVHD require consistently applied and interpreted criteria for pathologic diagnosis [17]. Validation of these criteria should be carried out through multi-institutional studies with biopsies correlated with clinically observed disease [17]. There are several factors that may result in a false-negative histopathologic assessment of cGVHD: (1)

biopsy may be performed immediately after the onset of symptoms and signs of presumptive cGVHD; (2) suboptimal tissue sampling that samples an oral ulcer and not the adjacent intact mucosa; (3) oral labial biopsies may not include enough glandular lobules to differentiate between active disease and previously damaged tissue; and (4) suboptimal processed and sectioned samples [17].

SIGNIFICANCE FOR PROGNOSIS AND CLINICAL COURSE

The oral cavity is a readily visualized, easily accessible site from which to make the clinicopathologic assessment of the presence and severity of oral cGVHD [59]. Although oral lesions are most common in patients with extensive cGVHD, patients may also present with limited disease involving only the oral cavity. While there is some evidence that subclinical cGVHD diagnosed through skin or buccal mucosal biopsy may serve as a predictor of subsequent development of cGVHD [60], there is no way to predict overall incidence, extent, or progression of systemic cGVHD on the basis of the timing or severity of oral findings. Similarly, for those affected there are no reliable signs or indicators that predict the long-term course or duration of oral involvement.

It has long been recognized that oral sensitivity is one of the symptoms strongly associated with cGVHD and may be the first indication of cGVHD onset or flare [12]. Intensity of oral cGVHD-related sensitivity has been described as severe [61], and this pain may increase patient distress in already difficult clinical situations. However, this oral pain does not have a one-to-one correlation with observed severity of oral cGVHD, is not limited to patients with ulcerative lesions [12, 15], and may be accompanied by complaints of burning, irritation, and dryness. This oropharyngeal pain may alter the ability to swallow both liquids, and solid foods contributing to weight loss and malnutrition, which are serious clinical problems in this population [18, 62].

Randomized and observational studies have shown decreased QOL and impaired functional status in the setting of cGVHD [63, 64]. The constellation of symptoms experienced with oral cGVHD may be a key component in the decreased QOL in these patients. Furthermore, systemic immunosuppressive therapy with corticosteroids and steroid-sparing

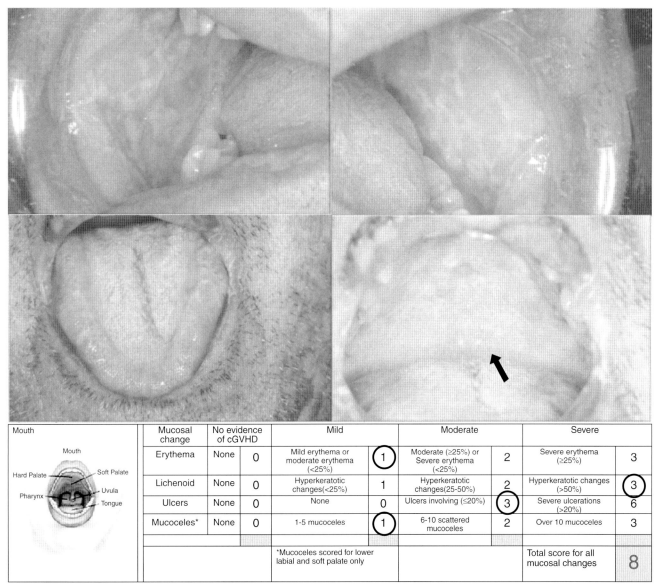

Mouth	Mucosal change	No evidence of cGVHD		Mild		Moderate		Severe	
	Erythema	None	0	Mild erythema or moderate erythema (<25%)	(1)	Moderate (≥25%) or Severe erythema (<25%)	2	Severe erythema (≥25%)	3
	Lichenoid	None	0	Hyperkeratotic changes(<25%)	1	Hyperkeratotic changes(25-50%)	2	Hyperkeratotic changes (>50%)	(3)
	Ulcers	None	0	None	0	Ulcers involving (≤20%)	(3)	Severe ulcerations (>20%)	6
	Mucoceles*	None	0	1-5 mucoceles	(1)	6-10 scattered mucoceles	2	Over 10 mucoceles	3
				*Mucoceles scored for lower labial and soft palate only				Total score for all mucosal changes	8

Figure 17.7 Use of the NIH Oral cGVHD clinical scoring instrument. In this example, all affected areas are shown, and those not shown can be assumed to be uninvolved. When estimating percentages, the entire mucosal surface area of all anatomic sites, both affected and unaffected, must be considered. The areas of *erythema* are primarily perilesional surrounding ulcerations and are not severe (the deep red areas on the lips are bleeding from the ulcers). All sites show extensive *lichenoid* changes accounting for greater than 50% of the overall surface areas. There are multiple *ulcers* of the lips, tongue, palate, and buccal mucosa; however, when considered as a percentage of all of these sites, these do not account for more than 20% of the entire surface areas. The *mucoceles* are highlighted by the black arrow. See Plate 52 in the color plate section.

immunomodulatory agents is often needed even for isolated oral involvement, leading to long-term consequences of immunosuppression [65, 66].

MANAGEMENT

The primary objective in managing oral cGVHD is to reduce or minimize symptoms, with the intent of improving oral function and overall QOL. Oral symptoms do not necessarily correlate with the extent or severity of clinical findings; therefore when considering the need for treatment, greater

emphasis should be placed on patient-reported outcomes rather than purely clinical signs. Patient education is vital to provide an understanding of the nature of their condition, what to expect, specific management instructions, and potential long-term complications; a patient information sheet is available for download from the American Academy of Oral Medicine website (http://www.aaom.com). During the early stages of involvement, patients may benefit tremendously from consultation with an oral health care specialist experienced in the diagnosis and management of oral cGVHD, its short- and long-term sequelae, and its overall impact on oral and systemic health. Regularly scheduled

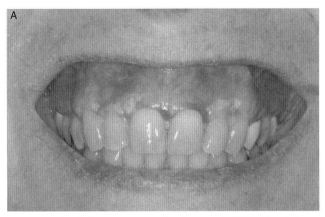
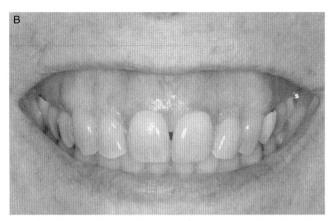

Figure 17.8 Topical management of oral mucosal cGVHD involving attached gingiva. A: extensive painful mucosal involvement with reticulation, severe erythema, and focal ulceration of the maxillary anterior attached gingiva extending onto unattached gingival mucosa; B: less than one month later following intensive treatment with topical corticosteroids and tacrolimus with no changes in systemic medications. See Plate 53 in the color plate section.

oral and dental evaluations are critical for patients with oral cGVHD because they are at greater risk for dental caries, as well as second malignancies. When oral intake is sufficiently compromised, consultation with a nutritionist or dietician should be coordinated [62, 67, 68].

Oral Health Care

Basic oral health care and preventive measures (e.g., routine dental cleanings, home fluoride therapy), while not specific treatments for oral cGVHD, are critical elements of overall management strategies [49]. Patients with gingival involvement may avoid brushing due to pain, which then leads to dental plaque accumulation that further exacerbates the inflammation and puts them at high risk for developing cervical caries (Figure 17.3A). Patients with salivary gland involvement are at especially high risk for developing new and recurrent dental caries. All patients should brush their teeth with a soft-bristled toothbrush (manual or electric) and fluoride-containing toothpaste three times-a-day (in particular, after meals) and floss daily to prevent plaque and calculus formation. Patients often have difficulty or avoid brushing altogether due to oral sensitivity to toothpaste flavoring agents and detergents. A children's or mild adult toothpaste (e.g., Biotene, Rancho Dominguez, CA) are generally well-tolerated in such cases. Running hot water over the toothbrush before brushing softens the bristles, also helping to reduce gingival sensitivity. In more severe cases, rinsing with 2% viscous lidocaine just before brushing may be necessary to minimize discomfort. Alcohol containing mouth rinses should be avoided as these tend to be quite painful and may exacerbate oral cGVHD.

In most cases, patients should return to their dentist 6 months after HCT for a comprehensive examination including bitewing radiographs [49]. In patients with significant oral cGVHD, intraoral manipulation during dental work may induce

a localized flare; therefore needs should be prioritized and treatment delivered only when considered urgent (e.g., symptomatic dental pain or extensive clinical/radiographic caries). There is no consensus on the indication(s) or need for antibiotic prophylaxis before invasive procedures (e.g., deep scaling, dental extractions); however, some centers recommend this practice due to long-term immunosuppression following the American Heart Association/American Dental Association prescribing guidelines [49, 69].

Management of Oral Mucosal cGVHD

The majority of patients with oral cGVHD will already be managed with a combination of systemic immunomodulatory medications [70, 71]. Owing to the lack of oral cGVHD specific endpoints and inconsistent methods of evaluation in published studies, oral response to these agents is poorly characterized; however, it is clear that oral cGVHD often persists and remains problematic despite aggressive systemic therapy [72]. Localized and topical ancillary care measures can provide critical supportive care for symptomatic management of oral cGVHD and its complications [49]. Following treatment, symptomatic relief may be more readily achieved than actual resolution of lesions (e.g., complete healing of ulcerations, Figure 17.8A, B). Therefore, special emphasis should be placed on assessing changes in patient-reported outcomes [13].

Topical treatment of oral mucosal cGVHD has not been systematically evaluated and there is little evidence-based data to support the use of any given therapy; however, expert consensus and the literature refer to topical steroids with high and ultra-high potency agents as standard treatment [14, 49, 72–74]. Many of the strategies for treating skin cGVHD, as well as comparable intraoral conditions, such as oral lichen planus, have been adapted and applied for the management of oral cGVHD [72, 75]. The highest potency topical corticosteroids are generally recommended, however, within a specific category (e.g., ultrapotent) there is no evidence-based data to support the use of one agent versus another [73, 74]. Selection is typically determined by commercially available formulations (which vary geographically), patient acceptance, and provider preference [76–78]. Steroid gels are easily applied to distinct areas and, due to their hydrophyllic properties, are generally better absorbed than creams or ointments.

When application is difficult and retention compromised due to the location of lesions (e.g., ventral tongue, soft palate) and the presence of saliva, addition of a bioadhesive methylcellulose base, either by the patient mixing in an over-the-counter product (e.g., Orabase, Colgate-Palmolive, New York, NY) or prepared by a compounding pharmacist, permits greater mucosal adherence and contact time. Alternatively, and especially when lesions are widespread (e.g., bilateral buccal and tongue lesions), rinsing with a steroid elixir (e.g., dexamethasone) for approximately 5 minutes is easier, well-tolerated, and often more effective than localized gel applications. Rinses can significantly improve both compliance and efficacy in pediatric patients although very young children must be closely monitored to ensure that the medication is not swallowed. Specific dispensing guidelines and instructions are provided in Table 17.3.

A small subset of patients is at risk for developing secondary oral candidiasis during topical steroid therapy. Patients may report a change or increase in the quality of oral symptoms, typically 3 to 7 days following the start of topical therapy. Classic signs include diffuse patchy white mucosal lesions, often described as "cottage cheese" like in appearance that in most cases can be easily removed with gauze, revealing a raw and erythematous underlying mucosa (Figure 17.9) [73, 79]. Candidiasis may also present as purely erythematous lesions with atrophic changes, especially evident on the tongue dorsum. Angular cheilitis, another candidal infection characterized by painful crusted and cracked erythematous lesions at the corners of the mouth, is often associated with intraoral fungal infection. Antifungal therapy is effective for both treatment and preventing recurrence, permitting the continuation of topical steroid therapy. Hyperkeratotic cGVHD changes must not be mistaken for candidiasis and will not improve with antifungal therapy.

A number of reports have demonstrated the efficacy of topical tacrolimus therapy for the management of oral mucosal cGVHD [80–82]. Despite only being commercially available in ointment form (Protopic 0.1% and 0.03% ointment, Astellas Pharma US, Deerfield, IL), localized application either directly, via gauze, or mixed with a bioadhesive base may result in significant clinical and symptomatic improvement. The majority of published reports have evaluated the 0.1% ointment, which should be prescribed over the 0.03% formulation for maximum benefit, due to poor absorption and limited contact time with a hydrophobic petroleum base in the oral environment. Detectable tacrolimus serum levels have been observed following topical oral therapy, presumably via transmucosal systemic absorption (rather than by swallowing) and although these are typically well below clinically therapeutic levels, routine measurements may be considered in young children and in patients already taking tacrolimus orally [82, 83].

Alternative treatments that have been proposed, including topical azathioprine, topical cyclosporine, CO_2 laser, low-level laser, and phototherapy (including PUVA, broad-band and narrow-band UVB), have been reported only in individual cases or small series with variable results [76, 77, 80, 81, 84–93]. In most of these studies inclusion/exclusion criteria and concomitant medications were poorly-defined, and there was no standard approach for defining and evaluating oral mucosal lesions, symptoms, or improvement, making comparisons between various studies and overall assessment of efficacy (and toxicity) difficult, if not impossible. While the safety and efficacy of these therapies is unclear, their use may be considered in refractory cases when delivered by experienced clinicians with appropriate training.

Regardless of specific treatments, pain control is a critical component of overall management strategies. Topical anesthetics such as viscous lidocaine may be especially effective in reducing sensitivity before eating, oral hygiene, or applying topical therapies [49]. Use of systemic analgesics, including opioids, should be considered in patients with significant oral pain.

Management of Salivary Gland cGVHD

Management of salivary gland cGVHD focuses on decreasing symptoms, improving salivary flow, and preventing infections (Table 17.3). Response to therapy is evaluated by measuring changes in symptoms over time. While sialometric evaluation of salivary gland function can be performed [30, 94, 95], this requires specialized equipment, is time consuming, and may not reflect the extent of symptoms. Basic oral/dental measures include hydration with sugar-free beverages, limiting caffeine and alcohol intake (due to their dehydrating effects), restricting consumption of refined carbohydrates (to reduce caries risk), brushing after all meals, flossing regularly, and nightly application of topical prescription-strength fluoride to the teeth [49]. Stimulation of the salivary glands with sugar-free or xylitol-sweetened gum or candies can be very effective in reducing symptoms of xerostomia. Use of over-the-counter oral wetting agents can also be an important component of management, with the choice of specific products dependent on patient preference.

Sialogogue therapy is safe and often very effective in improving salivary flow and reducing symptoms, although no agent has been evaluated in large randomized trials for cGVHD specifically [41, 94–97] (Table 17.3). These agents stimulate muscarinic cholinergic receptors (M1 and M3) on the salivary glands and have been shown to not only improve flow and subjective complaints of xerostomia, but to also normalize sialochemical

Table 17.3: Treatment Guidelines for Management of Oral cGVHD

Mucosal Disease

Category	Agent	Dispensing Instructions	Precautions	Level of Evidence
Corticosteroids	*Topical Gels*			
	Clobetasol propionate 0.05% gel (Class 1, super high potency)	60 g tube	Do not swallow.	AIIb
	Betamethasone diproprionate 0.05% gel (Class 1, super high potency)	Dry affected area with gauze, apply with finger 2–4 times/day, do not eat or drink for 15–20 minutes after application. Wash hands afterwards	Do not use long-term (>1–2 weeks) on lips due to risk of permanent atrophy. This is *not* a concern on the mucosa	AIIb
	Fluocinonide 0.05% gel (Class 2, high potency)	May help to mix 1:1 with an over-the-counter mucoadhesive base (e.g., Orabase {Colgate-Palmolive, New York, NY}), or can be compounded for improved retention. Can also apply to gauze and hold over lesion. Good for distinct, limited, easy to reach lesions	Secondary oral candidiasis in small subset of susceptible patients; antifungal prophylaxis with fluconazole 100 mg 1–3 times/week is generally effective, *or* daily treatment with clotrimazole troches 5 times/day. Fungal culture generally not useful in determining susceptibility	AIIb
	Topical Rinses			
	Dexamethasone 0.5 mg/5 mL	500 mL bottle. Rinse with 5.0 mL for 5 minutes, 2–6 times/day, then spit out. Do not eat or drink for 15–20 minutes afterwards	Do not swallow.	AIIIa
	Prednisolone 15 mg/5 mL	Good for more widespread or difficult to reach lesions. Other corticosteroids, such as clobetasol proprionate, may be compounded into a rinse and *may* have greater efficacy than those listed; however, no such comparative data exists	Secondary oral candidiasis (see previous text)	BIII
	Inhalers			
	Beclomethasone Fluticasone Betamethasone Triamcinolone	Apply 1–2 puffs in mouth to affected areas 2–4 times/day, hold in mouth, then spit out. Good for distinct, difficult to reach areas	Do not inhale / Do not swallow / Secondary oral candidiasis (see previous text)	BIII
	Intralesional			
	Triamcinolone acetonide 40 mg/mL (Bristol-Myers Squibb, New York, NY)	For refractory and/or large painful ulcerations. 0.3–0.4 mL for 1.0 cm² lesion. Draw into 1.0 mL tuberculin syringe, inject below ulceration. Inject multiple locations for large ulcerations	May require multiple consecutive weekly injections	BIII
Nonsteroidal Immunomodulatory Agents	Tacrolimus 0.1% ointment (Astellas Pharma US, Inc., Deerfield, IL)	60 g tube. Dry affected area with gauze, apply with finger 2–4 times/day, do not eat or drink for 15–20 minutes after application. Wash hands afterwards	May cause transient burning upon application. Consider monitoring plasma levels especially in young children. FDA black box warning	BIIa

Salivary Gland Disease

		Especially useful for treating the lips; can be used safely long-term		
		May help to mix 1:1 with a mucoadhesive base (e.g., Orabase) for improved mucosal retention. Can also apply to gauze and hold over lesion		
		Tacrolimus may be compounded into a rinse for improved topical dosing; however, there is no published data on this treatment approach		
Caries Prevention	Neutral sodium fluoride 5,000 ppm gel	Apply with toothbrush at night before bed *following* routine oral hygiene, do not rinse with water Consider having dentist fabricate soft custom trays; apply in trays for 30 minutes or leave overnight	Do not swallow, especially in young children Dispense one tube	AIb
Salivary Stimulants	Sugar-free hard candies and gum	Use as needed for xerostomia relief	May not be effective in patients with minimal residual gland function Must be sugar-free to prevent caries Xylitol containing products may be preferred due to sweetness without cariogenic potential	AIII
Oral Wetting Agents	Many over-the-counter products available. Biotene Oral Balance products (Laclede, Rancho Dominguez, CA) generally well tolerated	Follow manufacturer's instructions and use as needed throughout the day For patients with nighttime dryness, use before bed and keep at bedside	Generally safe to swallow but read manufacturer's insert before using	AIIb
Sialogogues	Pilocarpine hydrochloride	5 mg 3 times/day; before meals Can be increased to 10 mg 3 times/day; however, the likelihood of adverse events increases Counsel patient regarding possible adverse events	Side effects include sweating and gastrointestinal discomfort. Excessive sweating infrequently encountered in patients with cGVHD Contraindicated in patients with narrow-angle glaucoma Use with caution in patients with chronic obstructive pulmonary disease and asthma	BIb/IIa
	Cevimeline hydrochloride	30 mg 3 times/day; before meals	Same as pilocarpine; may be less due to higher selectivity for M3 receptors	BIb/III
	Bethanechol	10–50 mg 3 times/day	Similar to pilocarpine and cevimeline	CIb/III

Only commonly used therapies that are supported by published evidence (in oral cGVHD or closely related conditions such as oral lichen planus and Sjögren syndrome) or expert consensus opinion are included. Many other treatments that have been reported only in very small, uncontrolled studies and that are not widely used or regularly available (e.g., phototherapy) are not included and cannot be recommended at this time.

Level of evidence definitions. Strength of the recommendation: A, should always be offered; B, should generally be offered; C, evidence for efficacy insufficient to support a recommendation for or against. Quality of evidence supporting the recommendation: I, ≥1 randomized, controlled clinical trial; II, >1 well-designed clinical trial without randomization, from cohort or case-controlled analytic studies (preferable from >1 center), or from multiple time series or dramatic results from uncontrolled experiments; III, opinions of respected authorities on the basis of clinical experience, descriptive, Qualifiers for categories I and II: a, evidence derived directly from study(s) in cGVHD; b, evidence derived indirectly from study(s) in analogous or other pertinent diseases.

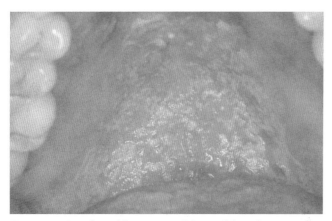

Figure 17.9. Pseudomembranous candidiasis of the palate secondary to topical steroid rinses. Note the numerous superficial mucoceles and fainter more macular areas of reticular cGVHD changes. Once weekly fluconazole therapy with ongoing topical therapy was effective in treating and preventing recurrence. See Plate 54 in the color plate section.

changes [41, 96]. While excessive sweating is common following treatment in patients with Sjögren syndrome and radiation xerostomia [98, 99], the authors note that this is rarely experienced in patients with cGVHD. Sialogogues, however, are contraindicated in patients with narrow-angle glaucoma and should be prescribed with caution in those with chronic obstructive pulmonary disease (e.g., brochiolitis obliterans with organizing pneumonitis, pulmonary cGVHD), asthma, and certain cardiac conditions. While an initial response can be immediate, benefits may not be noticeable for several weeks; therefore at least 6 to 8 weeks of therapy should be prescribed before determining that an individual is a nonresponder [94]. For those who do benefit, response does not diminish over time and there are no known long-term safety concerns.

Superficial mucoceles generally do not require treatment, and even when symptomatic, do not tend to respond to topical therapies. Rarely, deeper symptomatic lesions must be excised surgically.

Management of Sclerotic Oral cGVHD

In most cases, primary management of sclerotic changes is appropriate systemic immunomodulatory therapy. Early intervention is critical for effective long-term management and can often prevent significant deterioration of function. Daily passive stretching exercises may be beneficial in maintaining or increasing mouth opening in patients with trismus secondary to skin sclerosis or mucosal band formation [49, 100]. This can be accomplished by relaxing the jaw muscles and opening "passively" using two hands (placing the thumbs against the incisal edges of the front teeth), stacked tongue depressors, or a physical therapy device (e.g., Therabite, Atos Medical Inc., West Allis, WI); the jaw is opened to the point of resistance and held for several seconds then repeated 5 to 10 times, then repeated several times throughout the day. In the case of

secondary myospasm, muscle relaxants, systemic and topical nonsteroidal anti-inflammatory agents, trigger point injections (e.g., with local anesthetics or corticosteroids), and botulinum toxin injections may be considered [101].

Surveillance for Second Cancers

Second malignancies have long been recognized as a significant complication for long-term survivors of allogeneic HCT [102–104]. Oral squamous cell carcinoma is one of the most common solid malignancies in both adult and pediatric long-term survivors [105]. As oral cGVHD can present in many different ways and associated mucosal changes may persist indefinitely even when asymptomatic and clinically quiescent, only biopsy can discriminate between cGVHD, dysplasia, and malignancy. Patients should be carefully evaluated annually by an experienced oral health care specialist, and should routinely monitor their own oral tissue and report any suspicious changes immediately to their health care providers.

FUTURE

No standard treatment exists for oral cGVHD that fails to respond to initial therapy or becomes refractory [106]. Therefore there is a critical need to develop nontoxic adjuvant therapies that are both efficacious and avoid the long-term consequences of systemic corticosteroid therapies [107]. The majority of management strategies for oral cGHVD have not been evidence based, resulting in modest advances in treatment. Clinical trials are needed to test novel agents as proposed by the NIH cGVHD Consensus Development Project. Consistency of assessment of oral cGVHD across clinical trials and in clinical practice settings is a key component of the clinical research efforts targeted at elucidating the pathogenesis of this disease and the effect of investigational and routinely used agents.

REFERENCES

1. Ratanatharathorn V, Ayash L, Lazarus HM, Fu J, Uberti JP. Chronic graft-versus-host disease: clinical manifestation and therapy. *Bone Marrow Transplant.* Jul 2001;28(2):121–129.
2. Flowers ME, Parker PM, Johnston LJ, et al. Comparison of chronic graft-versus-host disease after transplantation of peripheral blood stem cells versus bone marrow in allogeneic recipients: long-term follow-up of a randomized trial. *Blood.* Jul 15 2002;100(2):415–419.
3. Lee SJ, Klein JP, Barrett AJ, et al. Severity of chronic graft-versus-host disease: association with treatment-related mortality and relapse. *Blood.* Jul 15 2002;100(2):406–414.
4. Subramaniam DS, Fowler DH, Pavletic SZ. Chronic graft-versus-host disease in the era of reduced-intensity conditioning. *Leukemia.* May 2007;21(5):853–859.

5. Zecca M, Prete A, Rondelli R, et al. Chronic graft-versus-host disease in children: incidence, risk factors, and impact on outcome. *Blood*. Aug 15 2002;100(4):1192–1200.

6. Diaz MA, Vicent MG, Gonzalez ME, et al. Risk assessment and outcome of chronic graft-versus-host disease after allogeneic peripheral blood progenitor cell transplantation in pediatric patients. *Bone Marrow Transplant*. Sep 2004;34(5):433–438.

7. Berkowitz RJ, Strandjord S, Jones P, et al. Stomatologic complications of bone marrow transplantation in a pediatric population. *Pediatr Dent*. Jun 1987;9(2):105–110.

8. Dahllof G, Heimdahl A, Modeer T, Twetman S, Bolme P, Ringden O. Oral mucous membrane lesions in children treated with bone marrow transplantation. *Scand J Dent Res*. Jun 1989;97(3):268–277.

9. Majorana A, Schubert MM, Porta F, Ugazio AG, Sapelli PL. Oral complications of pediatric hematopoietic cell transplantation: diagnosis and management. *Support Care Cancer*. Sep 2000;8(5):353–365.

10. Nicolatou-Galitis O, Kitra V, Van Vliet-Constantinidou C, et al. The oral manifestations of chronic graft-versus-host disease (cGVHD) in paediatric allogeneic bone marrow transplant recipients. *J Oral Pathol Med*. Mar 2001;30(3):148–153.

11. Treister NS, Woo SB, O'Holleran EW, Lehmann LE, Parsons SK, Guinan EC. Oral chronic graft-versus-host disease in pediatric patients after hematopoietic stem cell transplantation. *Biol Blood Marrow Transplant*. Sep 2005;11(9):721–731.

12. Schubert MM, Sullivan KM, Morton TH, et al. Oral manifestations of chronic graft-v-host disease. *Arch Intern Med*. Aug 1984;144(8):1591–1595.

13. Schubert MM, Sullivan KM. Recognition, incidence, and management of oral graft-versus-host disease. *NCI Monogr*. 1990(9):135–143.

14. Woo SB, Lee SJ, Schubert MM. Graft-vs.-host disease. *Crit Rev Oral Biol Med*. 1997;8(2):201–216.

15. Treister N, Cook EF, Antin JA, Lee S, Soiffer R, Woo S. Clinical evaluation of oral chronic graft-versus-host disease. *Biol Blood Marrow Transplant*. 2008;14:110–115.

16. Busca A, Locatelli F, Vai S, Dall'Omo AM, Gargiulo A, Falda M. Clinical grading of oral chronic graft-versus-host disease in 104 consecutive adult patients. *Haematologica*. Apr 2005;90(4):567–569.

17. Shulman HM, Kleiner D, Lee SJ, et al. Histopathologic diagnosis of chronic graft-versus-host disease: National Institutes of Health Consensus Development Project on Criteria for Clinical Trials in Chronic Graft-versus-Host Disease: II. Pathology Working Group Report. *Biol Blood Marrow Transplant*. Jan 2006;12(1):31–47.

18. Jacobsohn DA, Margolis J, Doherty J, Anders V, Vogelsang GB. Weight loss and malnutrition in patients with chronic graft-versus-host disease. *Bone Marrow Transplant*. Feb 2002;29(3):231–236.

19. Nakhleh RE, Miller W, Snover DC. Significance of mucosal vs salivary gland changes in lip biopsies in the diagnosis of chronic graft-vs-host disease. *Arch Pathol Lab Med*. Aug 1989;113(8):932–934.

20. Mattsson T, Sundqvist KG, Heimdahl A, Dahllof G, Ljungman P, Ringden O. A comparative immunological analysis of the oral mucosa in chronic graft-versus-host disease and oral lichen planus. *Arch Oral Biol*. 1992;37(7):539–547.

21. Hiroki A, Nakamura S, Shinohara M, Oka M. Significance of oral examination in chronic graft-versus-host disease. *J Oral Pathol Med*. May 1994;23(5):209–215.

22. Nakamura S, Hiroki A, Shinohara M, et al. Oral involvement in chronic graft-versus-host disease after allogeneic bone marrow transplantation. *Oral Surg Oral Med Oral Pathol Oral Radiol Endod*. Nov 1996;82(5):556–563.

23. Soares AB, Faria PR, Magna LA, et al. Chronic GVHD in minor salivary glands and oral mucosa: histopathological and immunohistochemical evaluation of 25 patients. *J Oral Pathol Med*. Jul 2005;34(6):368–373.

24. Fujii H, Ohashi M, Nagura H. Immunohistochemical analysis of oral lichen-planus-like eruption in graft-versus-host disease after allogeneic bone marrow transplantation. *Am J Clin Pathol*. Feb 1988;89(2):177–186.

25. Yamada H, Chihara J, Hamada K, et al. Immunohistology of skin and oral biopsies in graft-versus-host disease after bone marrow transplantation and cytokine therapy. *J Allergy Clin Immunol*. Dec 1997;100(6 pt 2):S73-S76.

26. Sato M, Tokuda N, Fukumoto T, Mano T, Sato T, Ueyama Y. Immunohistopathological study of the oral lichenoid lesions of chronic GVHD. *J Oral Pathol Med*. Jan 2006;35(1):33–36.

27. Amerongen AV, Veerman EC. Saliva–the defender of the oral cavity. *Oral Dis*. Jan 2002;8(1):12–22.

28. Porter SR, Scully C, Hegarty AM. An update of the etiology and management of xerostomia. *Oral Surg Oral Med Oral Pathol Oral Radiol Endod*. Jan 2004;97(1):28–46.

29. Atkinson JC, Grisius M, Massey W. Salivary hypofunction and xerostomia: diagnosis and treatment. *Dent Clin North Am*. Apr 2005;49(2):309–326.

30. Nagler RM, Nagler A. Major salivary gland involvement in graft-versus-host disease: considerations related to pathogenesis, the role of cytokines and therapy. *Cytokines Cell Mol Ther*. Dec 1999;5(4):227–232.

31. Alborghetti MR, Correa ME, Adam RL, et al. Late effects of chronic graft-vs.-host disease in minor salivary glands. *J Oral Pathol Med*. Sep 2005;34(8):486–493.

32. Sale GE, Shulman HM, Schubert MM, et al. Oral and ophthalmic pathology of graft versus host disease in man: predictive value of the lip biopsy. *Hum Pathol*. Nov 1981;12(11):1022–1030.

33. Izutsu KT, Sullivan KM, Schubert MM, et al. Disordered salivary immunoglobulin secretion and sodium transport in human chronic graft-versus-host disease. *Transplantation*. May 1983;35(5):441–446.

34. Izutsu KT, Schubert MM, Truelove EL, et al. The predictive value of elevated labial saliva sodium concentration: its relation to labial gland pathology in bone marrow transplant recipients. *Hum Pathol*. Jan 1983;14(1):29–35.

35. Janin-Mercier A, Devergie A, Arrago JP, et al. Systemic evaluation of Sjogren-like syndrome after bone marrow transplantation in man. *Transplantation*. May 1987;43(5):677–679.

36. Lindahl G, Lonnquist B, Hedfors E. Lymphocytic infiltration and HLA-DR expression of salivary glands in bone marrow transplant recipients: a prospective study. *Clin Exp Immunol*. May 1988;72(2):267–273.

37. Mattsson T, Arvidson K, Heimdahl A, Ljungman P, Dahllof G, Ringden O. Alterations in taste acuity associated with allogeneic bone marrow transplantation. *J Oral Pathol Med*. Jan 1992;21(1):33–37.

38. Quiquandon I, Janin A, Noel-Walter MP, et al. Cytomegalovirus expression in minor salivary glands and chronic graft-versus-host disease. *Bone Marrow Transplant*. Jul 1994;14(1):31–35.

39. Mariette X, Cazals-Hatem D, Agbalika F, et al. Absence of cytomegalovirus and Epstein-Barr virus expression in labial salivary glands of patients with chronic graft-versus-host disease. *Bone Marrow Transplant*. Apr 1996;17(4):607–610.

40. Chaushu G, Chaushu S, Slavin S, Or R, Garfunkel AA, Yefenof E. Salivary immunoglobulins in recipients of bone marrow grafts. III. A longitudinal follow-up of CMV specific antibodies. *Bone Marrow Transplant*. Feb 1996;17(2):237–241.

41. Nagler RM, Nagler A. The effect of pilocarpine on salivary constituents in patients with chronic graft-versus-host disease. *Arch Oral Biol*. Aug 2001;46(8):689–695.

42. Nagler RM, Nagler A. Sialometrical and sialochemical analysis of patients with chronic graft-versus-host disease – a prolonged study. *Cancer Invest*. 2003;21(1):34–40.

43. Nagler RM, Nagler A. The molecular basis of salivary gland involvement in graft-vs.-host disease. *J Dent Res*. Feb 2004;83(2):98–103.

44. Chen A, Wai Y, Lee L, Lake S, Woo S. Using the modified Schirmer test to measure mouth dryness: a preliminary study. *J Amer Dent Assoc*. 2005;136:164–170.

45. Imanguli MM, Atkinson JC, Harvey KE, et al. Changes in salivary proteome following allogeneic hematopoietic stem cell transplantation. *Exp Hematol*. Feb 2007;35(2):184–192.

46. Nagler R, Marmary Y, Krausz Y, Chisin R, Markitziu A, Nagler A. Major salivary gland dysfunction in human acute and chronic graft-versus-host disease (GVHD). *Bone Marrow Transplant*. Feb 1996;17(2):219–224.

47. Jones LR, Toth BB, Keene HJ. Effects of total body irradiation on salivary gland function and caries-associated oral microflora in bone marrow transplant patients. *Oral Surg Oral Med Oral Pathol*. Jun 1992;73(6):670–676.

48. Chaushu G, Itzkovitz-Chaushu S, Yefenof E, Slavin S, Or R, Garfunkel AA. A longitudinal follow-up of salivary secretion in bone marrow transplant patients. *Oral Surg Oral Med Oral Pathol Oral Radiol Endod*. Feb 1995;79(2):164–169.

49. Couriel D, Carpenter PA, Cutler C, et al. Ancillary therapy and supportive care of chronic graft-versus-host disease: national institutes of health consensus development project on Criteria for Clinical Trials in Chronic Graft-Versus-Host Disease: V. Ancillary Therapy and Supportive Care Working Group Report. *Biol Blood Marrow Transplant*. Apr 2006;12(4):375–396.

50. Campana F, Sibaud V, Chauvel A, Boiron JM, Taieb A, Fricain JC. Recurrent superficial mucoceles associated with lichenoid disorders. *J Oral Maxillofac Surg*. Dec 2006;64(12):1830–1833.

51. Hiroki A, Nakamura S, Shinohara M, et al. A comparison of glandular involvement between chronic graft-versus-host disease and Sjogren's syndrome. *Int J Oral Maxillofac Surg*. Aug 1996;25(4):298–307.

52. Nagler RM, Nagler A. Salivary gland involvement in graft-versus-host disease: the underlying mechanism and implicated treatment. *Isr Med Assoc J*. Mar 2004;6(3):167–172.

53. Coracin FL, Pizzigatti Correa ME, Camargo EE, et al. Major salivary gland damage in allogeneic hematopoietic progenitor cell transplantation assessed by scintigraphic methods. *Bone Marrow Transplant*. May 2006;37(10):955–959.

54. Pavletic S, Vogelsang G. National Institutes of Health Consensus Development Project on Criteria for Clinical Trials in Chronic Graft-versus-Host Disease: preface to the Series. *Biol Blood Marrow Transplant*. Dec 2005;11(12):943–944.

55. Filipovich AH, Weisdorf D, Pavletic S, et al. National Institutes of Health consensus development project on criteria for clinical trials in chronic graft-versus-host disease: I. Diagnosis and staging working group report. *Biol Blood Marrow Transplant*. Dec 2005;11(12):945–956.

56. Pavletic SZ, Martin P, Lee SJ, et al. Measuring therapeutic response in chronic graft-versus-host disease: National Institutes of Health Consensus Development Project on Criteria for Clinical Trials in Chronic Graft-versus-Host Disease: IV. Response Criteria Working Group report. *Biol Blood Marrow Transplant*. Mar 2006;12(3):252–266.

57. Pavletic SZ, Lee SJ, Socie G, Vogelsang G. Chronic graft-versus-host disease: implications of the National Institutes of Health consensus development project on criteria for clinical trials. *Bone Marrow Transplant*. Nov 2006;38(10):645–651.

58. Shlomchik WD, Lee SJ, Couriel D, Pavletic SZ. Transplantation's greatest challenges: advances in chronic graft-versus-host disease. *Biol Blood Marrow Transplant*. Jan 2007;13(1 Suppl 1):2–10.

59. Demarosi F, Bez C, Sardella A, Lodi G, Carrassi A. Oral involvement in chronic graft-vs-host disease following allogenic bone marrow transplantation. *Arch Dermatol*. Jun 2002;138(6):842–843.

60. Wagner JL, Flowers ME, Longton G, Storb R, Schubert M, Sullivan KM. The development of chronic graft-versus-host disease: an analysis of screening studies and the impact of corticosteroid use at 100 days after transplantation. *Bone Marrow Transplant*. Jul 1998;22(2):139–146.

61. Eggleston TI, Ziccardi VB, Lumerman H. Graft-versus-host disease. Case report and discussion. *Oral Surg Oral Med Oral Pathol Oral Radiol Endod*. Dec 1998;86(6):692–696.

62. Lenssen P, Sherry ME, Cheney CL, et al. Prevalence of nutrition-related problems among long-term survivors of allogeneic marrow transplantation. *J Am Diet Assoc*. Jun 1990;90(6):835–842.

63. Syrjala KL, Chapko MK, Vitaliano PP, Cummings C, Sullivan KM. Recovery after allogeneic marrow transplantation: prospective study of predictors of long-term physical and psychosocial functioning. *Bone Marrow Transplant*. Apr 1993;11(4):319–327.

64. Chiodi S, Spinelli S, Ravera G, et al. Quality of life in 244 recipients of allogeneic bone marrow transplantation. *Br J Haematol*. Sep 2000;110(3):614–619.

65. Vogelsang GB, Hess AD, Santos GW. Acute graft-versus-host disease: clinical characteristics in the cyclosporine era. *Medicine (Baltimore)*. May 1988;67(3):163–174.

66. Vogelsang GB. How I treat chronic graft-versus-host disease. *Blood*. Mar 1 2001;97(5):1196–1201.

67. Roberts S, Thompson J. Graft-vs-host disease: nutrition therapy in a challenging condition. *Nutr Clin Pract*. Aug 2005;20(4):440–450.

68. Doyle C, Kushi LH, Byers T, et al. Nutrition and physical activity during and after cancer treatment: an American Cancer Society guide for informed choices. *CA Cancer J Clin*. Nov-Dec 2006;56(6):323–353.

69. Wilson W, Taubert KA, Gewitz M, et al. Prevention of infective endocarditis: guidelines from the American Heart Association: a guideline from the American Heart Association Rheumatic Fever, Endocarditis, and Kawasaki Disease Committee, Council on Cardiovascular Disease in the Young, and the Council on Clinical Cardiology, Council on Cardiovascular Surgery and Anesthesia, and the Quality of Care and Outcomes Research Interdisciplinary Working Group. *Circulation*. Oct 9 2007;116(15):1736–1754.

70. Stewart BL, Storer B, Storek J, et al. Duration of immunosuppressive treatment for chronic graft-versus-host disease. *Blood*. Dec 1 2004;104(12):3501–3506.

71. Cutler C, Antin JH. Chronic graft-versus-host disease. *Curr Opin Oncol*. Mar 2006;18(2):126–131.

72. Imanguli MM, Pavletic SZ, Guadagnini JP, Brahim JS, Atkinson JC. Chronic graft versus host disease of oral mucosa: review of available therapies. *Oral Surg Oral Med Oral Pathol Oral Radiol Endod*. Feb 2006;101(2):175–183.

73. Gonzalez-Moles MA, Scully C. Vesiculo-erosive oral mucosal disease-management with topical corticosteroids: (2) Protocols, monitoring of effects and adverse reactions, and the future. *J Dent Res*. Apr 2005;84(4):302–308.

74. Gonzalez-Moles MA, Scully C. Vesiculo-erosive oral mucosal disease–management with topical corticosteroids: (1) Fundamental principles and specific agents available. *J Dent Res*. Apr 2005;84(4):294–301.

75. Penas PF, Fernandez-Herrera J, Garcia-Diez A. Dermatologic treatment of cutaneous graft versus host disease. *Am J Clin Dermatol*. 2004;5(6):403–416.

76. Elad S, Or R, Garfunkel AA, Shapira MY. Budesonide: a novel treatment for oral chronic graft versus host disease. *Oral Surg Oral Med Oral Pathol Oral Radiol Endod*. Mar 2003;95(3):308–311.

77. Wolff D, Anders V, Corio R, et al. Oral PUVA and topical steroids for treatment of oral manifestations of chronic graft-vs.-host disease. *Photodermatol Photoimmunol Photomed*. Aug 2004;20(4):184–190.

78. Sari I, Altuntas F, Kocyigit I, et al. The effect of budesonide mouthwash on oral chronic graft versus host disease. *Am J Hematol*. May 2007;82(5):349–356.

79. Glick M, Siegel MA. Viral and fungal infections of the oral cavity in immunocompetent patients. *Infect Dis Clin North Am*. Dec 1999;13(4):817–831, vi.

80. Eckardt A, Starke O, Stadler M, Reuter C, Hertenstein B. Severe oral chronic graft-versus-host disease following allogeneic bone marrow transplantation: highly effective treatment with topical tacrolimus. *Oral Oncol*. Sep 2004;40(8):811–814.

81. Sanchez AR, Sheridan PJ, Rogers RS. Successful treatment of oral lichen planus-like chronic graft-versus-host disease with topical tacrolimus: a case report. *J Periodontol*. Apr 2004;75(4):613–619.

82. Albert MH, Becker B, Schuster FR, et al. Oral graft vs. host disease in children – treatment with topical tacrolimus ointment. *Pediatr Transplant*. May 2007;11(3):306–311.

83. Conrotto D, Carrozzo M, Ubertalli AV, et al. Dramatic increase of tacrolimus plasma concentration during topical treatment for oral graft-versus-host disease. *Transplantation*. Oct 27 2006;82(8):1113–1115.

84. Epstein JB, Reece DE. Topical cyclosporin A for treatment of oral chronic graft-versus-host disease. *Bone Marrow Transplant*. Jan 1994;13(1):81–86.

85. Vogelsang GB, Wolff D, Altomonte V, et al. Treatment of chronic graft-versus-host disease with ultraviolet irradiation and psoralen (PUVA). *Bone Marrow Transplant*. Jun 1996;17(6): 1061–1067.

86. Kuusilehto A, Lehtinen R, Happonen RP, Heikinheimo K, Lehtimaki K, Jansen CT. An open clinical trial of a new mouth-PUVA variant in the treatment of oral lichenoid lesions. *Oral Surg Oral Med Oral Pathol Oral Radiol Endod*. Nov 1997;84(5):502–505.

87. Redding SW, Callander NS, Haveman CW, Leonard DL. Treatment of oral chronic graft-versus-host disease with PUVA therapy: case report and literature review. *Oral Surg Oral Med Oral Pathol Oral Radiol Endod*. Aug 1998;86(2):183–187.

88. Elad S, Garfunkel AA, Enk CD, Galili D, Or R. Ultraviolet B irradiation: a new therapeutic concept for the management of oral manifestations of graft-versus-host disease. *Oral Surg Oral Med Oral Pathol Oral Radiol Endod*. Oct 1999;88(4):444–450.

89. Epstein JB, Nantel S, Sheoltch SM. Topical azathioprine in the combined treatment of chronic oral graft-versus-host disease. *Bone Marrow Transplant*. Mar 2000;25(6):683–687.

90. Epstein JB, Gorsky M, Epstein MS, Nantel S. Topical azathioprine in the treatment of immune-mediated chronic oral inflammatory conditions: a series of cases. *Oral Surg Oral Med Oral Pathol Oral Radiol Endod*. Jan 2001;91(1):56–61.

91. Menillo SA, Goldberg SL, McKiernan P, Pecora AL. Intraoral psoralen ultraviolet A irradiation (PUVA) treatment of refractory oral chronic graft-versus-host disease following allogeneic stem cell transplantation. *Bone Marrow Transplant*. Oct 2001;28(8):807–808.

92. Elad S, Or R, Shapira MY, et al. CO2 laser in oral graft-versus-host disease: a pilot study. *Bone Marrow Transplant*. Nov 2003;32(10):1031–1034.

93. Chor A, de Azevedo AM, Maiolino A, Nucci M. Successful treatment of oral lesions of chronic lichenoid graft-vs.-host disease by the addition of low-level laser therapy to systemic immunosuppression. *Eur J Haematol*. Mar 2004;72(3):222–224.

94. Singhal S, Powles R, Treleaven J, Rattenbury H, Mehta J. Pilocarpine hydrochloride for symptomatic relief of xerostomia due to chronic graft-versus-host disease or total-body irradiation after bone-marrow transplantation for hematologic malignancies. *Leuk Lymphoma*. Feb 1997;24(5–6):539–543.

95. Agha-Hosseini F, Mirzaii-Dizgah I, Ghavamzadeh L, Ghavamzadeh A, Tohidast-Acrad Z. Effect of pilocarpine hydrochloride on unstimulated whole saliva flow rate and composition in patients with chronic graft-versus-host disease (cGVHD). *Bone Marrow Transplant*. Apr 2007;39(7):431–434.

96. Nagler RM, Nagler A. Pilocarpine hydrochloride relieves xerostomia in chronic graft-versus-host disease: a sialometrical study. *Bone Marrow Transplant*. May 1999;23(10):1007–1011.

97. Carpenter PA, Schubert MM, Flowers ME. Cevimeline reduced mouth dryness and increased salivary flow in patients with xerostomia complicating chronic graft-versus-host disease. *Biol Blood Marrow Transplant*. Jul 2006;12(7):792–794.

98. Rieke JW, Hafermann MD, Johnson JT, et al. Oral pilocarpine for radiation-induced xerostomia: integrated efficacy and safety results from two prospective randomized clinical trials. *Int J Radiat Oncol Biol Phys*. Feb 1 1995;31(3):661–669.

99. Vivino FB, Al-Hashimi I, Khan Z, et al. Pilocarpine tablets for the treatment of dry mouth and dry eye symptoms in patients with Sjogren syndrome: a randomized, placebo-controlled, fixed-dose, multicenter trial. P92–01 Study Group. *Arch Intern Med*. Jan 25 1999;159(2):174–181.

100. Vissink A, Burlage FR, Spijkervet FK, Jansma J, Coppes RP. Prevention and treatment of the consequences of head and neck radiotherapy. *Crit Rev Oral Biol Med*. 2003;14(3):213–225.

101. Clark GT. The management of oromandibular motor disorders and facial spasms with injections of botulinum toxin. *Phys Med Rehabil Clin N Am*. Nov 2003;14(4):727–748.

102. Curtis RE, Rowlings PA, Deeg HJ, et al. Solid cancers after bone marrow transplantation. *N Engl J Med*. Mar 27 1997;336(13):897–904.

103. Hasegawa W, Pond GR, Rifkind JT, et al. Long-term follow-up of secondary malignancies in adults after allogeneic bone marrow transplantation. *Bone Marrow Transplant*. Jan 2005;35(1):51–55.

104. Gallagher G, Forrest DL. Second solid cancers after allogeneic hematopoietic stem cell transplantation. *Cancer*. Jan 1 2007;109(1):84–92.

105. Curtis RE, Metayer C, Rizzo JD, et al. Impact of chronic GVHD therapy on the development of squamous-cell cancers after hematopoietic stem-cell transplantation: an international case-control study. *Blood*. May 15 2005;105(10):3802–3811.

106. Lee SJ, Vogelsang G, Gilman A, et al. A survey of diagnosis, management, and grading of chronic GVHD. *Biol Blood Marrow Transplant*. 2002;8(1):32–39.

107. Arora M, Burns LJ, Davies SM, et al. Chronic graft-versus-host disease: a prospective cohort study. *Biol Blood Marrow Transplant*. Jan 2003;9(1):38–45.

18

CHRONIC OCULAR GRAFT VERSUS HOST DISEASE

Stella K. Kim, Janine A. Smith, and James P. Dunn, Jr.

INTRODUCTION

Chronic ocular graft versus host disease is one of the most common manifestations of chronic GVHD (cGVHD). It has been well recognized from the early allogeneic transplantation experience [1–3]. Ocular GVHD affects approximately 60–80% of patients with cGVHD and can cause significant decrease in quality of life with high morbidity [2–4]. The most common form of chronic ocular GVHD is dry eye syndrome (DES) with lacrimal gland dysfunction (reduced aqueous tear production) and keratoconjunctivitis sicca (KCS). Much of the early chronic ocular GVHD literature came from the experience at Johns Hopkins and elsewhere in the early 1980s. Since then, various studies and observations have been made in pathophysiology and in clinical experience in chronic ocular GVHD, in particular in treatment paradigm of organ-specific GVHD in the era of graft versus tumor considerations. National Institute of Health (NIH) Consensus Development Project on Criteria for Clinical Trials in Chronic Graft versus Host Disease published six papers [5–10], of which four papers are relevant to the chronic ocular GVHD [5, 6, 8, 9]. This chapter will describe in detail the clinical manifestations, diagnosis, pathophysiology, and management of chronic ocular GVHD and summarize the relevance of the NIH Consensus to ophthalmology.

CLINICAL MANIFESTATIONS

Dry eye syndrome/KCS is the hallmark of chronic ocular GVHD [3, 11–13]. An earlier study noted that over 80% of patients with cGVHD experienced KCS [14]. A later, multi-center retrospective study showed that 69% of patients who experienced KCS posttransplantation had cGVHD [15]. KCS in this study was more frequently observed in women and in older patients, which is also true for Sjogren's syndrome [15]. Prospective studies also demonstrated high incidence of chronic ocular GVHD with KCS [3, 16, 17]. Most recent study of 44 patients reported that 50% of patients developed KCS, with worse symptoms and clinical signs in patients with meibomian gland dysfunction and chronic systemic GVHD [13].

Symptoms of chronic ocular GVHD include dry eye, irritation, itchiness, epiphora (paradoxical), photophobia, burning, pain, redness (though "redness" qualifies as a clinical sign rather than a symptom, patients often report this as their sentinel symptom), and transient blurred vision [18]. A classic picture of chronic ocular GVHD is a patient who is constantly squinting due to debilitating ocular symptoms (Figure 18.1). Most bothersome symptom for a given patient should be considered the "sentinel symptom" for the patient, and it can be used to track his disease or response to any treatment [8]. Sentinel symptoms can be evaluated with a 0 to 10 scale, and symptoms may often be out of proportion to the clinical findings on the examinations. There is no specific symptom that is pathognomonic for chronic ocular GVHD, though "dry eye" is common. Myriad of nonspecific ocular symptoms of chronic ocular GVHD (blurred vision, for example) may represent ocular toxicities from preparative regimen or other medications, steroid-induced cataract [19] or even serious ocular infections. As such, prompt ophthalmic evaluation in symptomatic cGVHD patients should be considered.

Symptomatic patients may exhibit an obvious conjunctival injection ("red eye") but may also have relatively unimpressive external ocular appearance. Slit lamp examination is required to appreciate keratitis with changes on the ocular surface and uptake of various dyes used during an ophthalmic examination (fluorescein, Rose Bengal stain, and Lissamine Green). While chronic ocular GVHD can affect the lid, meibomian glands, anterior chamber, sclera, vitreous, choroids [13, 20–25], and theoretically every layer of the eye [25], it is typically considered a disease of the lacrimal gland and the conjunctiva [3, 12].

Conjunctival disease has been described in a clinical staging by Jabs et al.: Stage I conjunctival hyperemia; Stage II hyperemia with chemosis and/or serosanguineous exudates; Stage III pseudomembranous conjunctivitis; and Stage IV, pseudomembranous conjunctivitis with corneal epithelial sloughing [12] (Figure 18.2). Unlike the stages of acute GVHD for skin, GI, and liver, conjunctival staging does not impact the overall GVHD grade of a patient in the acute setting. Clinically, however, having multiple organ involvement may influence the clinician to

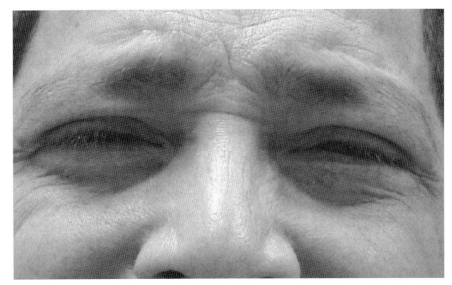

Figure 18.1 Classic appearance of a patient with chronic ocular GVHD with keratoconjunctivitis sicca. See Plate 55 in the color plate section.

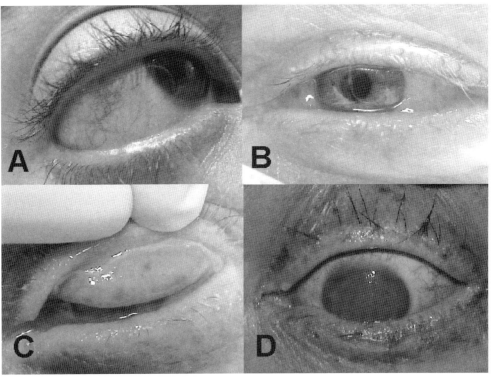

Figure 18.2 Conjunctival staging typically seen in acute GVHD settings. A: Stage I. hyperemia; B: Stage II. hyperemia with chemosis; C: Stage III. pseudomembranous conjunctivitis. Fluoresceine dye uptake at the palpebral conjunctiva D: Stage IV. pseudomembranous conjunctivitis with corneal epithelial sloughing. The corneal defect is also visible by the fluorsceine dye. See Plate 56 in the color plate section.

treat GVHD more aggressively. The conjunctival staging is useful in its description of severity, but the presence of these clinical manifestations may not always represent GVHD. For example, patients who may be retaining fluids (due to systemic steroid treatment or due to electrolyte imbalance) may show impressive conjunctival chemosis without other evidence of ocular GVHD. Also, severe viral infection can cause pseudomembranous keratoconjunctivitis and corneal epithelial defect. Moreover, pseudomembranous pattern with and without corneal epithelial sloughing is typically considered an acute pattern of chronic ocular GVHD. Conjunctival disease in bone marrow transplantation (BMT) patients, therefore, should be considered in the context of the patient's medical history, clinical course, and systemic GVHD status.

Bulbar conjunctival hyperemia ("red eye") may be chronically present when chronic ocular GVHD is not well controlled. Other forms of conjunctival disease in chronic ocular GVHD can be seen in the palpebral conjunctiva. Cicatricial changes on the palpebral conjunctiva may be observed after episodes of pseudomembranous keratoconjunctivis, with resulting fibrovascular scarring (Figure 18.3). Robinson et al. proposed the grading scale of cicatricial changes in order to better assess the palpebral conjunctival disease in chronic ocular GVHD [26–28]. Other forms of conjunctival disease include superior limbic keratoconjunctivitis, and episcleritis [28]. In fact, the spectrum of ocular GVHD may encompass clinical features of ocular inflammatory diseases associated with other autoimmune/collagen vascular diseases. The most common form of chronic ocular GVHD, however, is keratoconjunctivitis sicca [15, 29, 30].

Sicca syndrome (decreased aqueous tear production by the lacrimal gland) can be measured by Schirmer's test. Schirmer's test (Type I), which serves as a surrogate for lacrimal gland function, is crucial in the evaluation and diagnosis of GVHD patients [5]. A thin filter-paper strip is placed at the lateral canthal region in the patient's eyes, and the soaked regions of the strip is measured after 5 minutes (typically without topical anesthetic) (Figure 18.4). Schirmer's score is considered within normal limits if it is greater or equal to 10 mm of tear production with or without topical anesthetic. Normal level measurement is highly variable, though a value less 5 mm is diagnostic of aqueous tear deficiency, whereas, the result is equivocal if the value is between 5 to 10 mm. Schirmer's Type II (with nasal stimulation) is rarely performed for the evaluation of ocular GVHD patients. Lacrimal gland dysfunction do occur in both acute and chronic settings [2, 3], and Schirmer's test can be diagnostic in ocular GVHD in both settings (see Diagnosis) [5]. The result of Schirmer's test, however, may vary depending on a variety of factors, such as medications, history of various chemotherapy agents and/or radiotherapy (such as total-body irradiation), and even the hydration status of the patient. A decrease in the Schirmer's score in the setting of worsening ocular symptoms is suggestive of ocular GVHD, even if the scores are within normal limits. Similar to conjunctival diseases in ocular GVHD, the lacrimal gland dysfunction (i.e., Schirmer's score) must be considered in the context of the overall clinical status of the patient.

In addition to conjunctival and lacrimal gland disease, chronic ocular GVHD includes other clinical manifestation that is thought to be either direct or indirect result of GVHD, such as meibomien gland dysfunction [13, 31]. Meibomian gland dropout from ocular GVHD can decrease the tear break up time (TBUT), causing increased evaporative state, leading to DES with normal Schirmer's score (Figure 18.5). The impact of meibomian gland dysfunction in the severity of chronic ocular GVHD is perhaps underappreciated, and careful evaluation of the lid margins may be helpful in determining the cause of ocular GVHD. Filamentary keratitis can be a recurrent problem in chronic ocular GVHD with significant symptoms of pain and blurred vision. Other ocular abnormalities such as

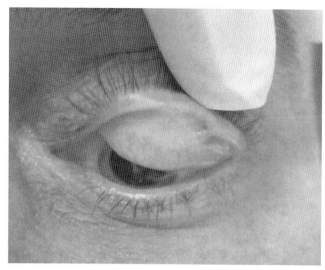

Figure 18.3 Palpebral conjunctiva (everted upper lid): cicatricial scarring from chronic ocular GVHD. See Plate 57 in the color plate section.

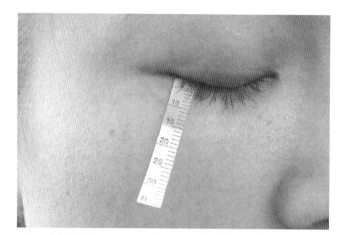

Figure 18.4 Schirmer's test: diagnostic tool for ocular GVHD. See Plate 58 in the color plate section.

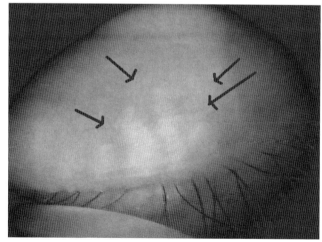

Figure 18.5 Meibomian gland drop outs (see arrows) in chronic ocular GVHD patient. Glands should be linear and extend further toward the fornix of the lid. Decrease in tear break up time (TBUT) is observed in patient with meibomian gland dysfunction. See Plate 59 in the color plate section.

trichiasis, hyperkeratosis, blepharitis, or cicatricial ectropion of the lids from chronic GVHD contribute to the adverse ocular surface environment [12, 30–32].

Posterior pole involvement of ocular GVHD, such as vitritis [24], is exceedingly rare and is a diagnosis of exclusion. Choroidal infiltrations with serous retinal detachments and scleritis are also rare and are typically associated with hyperacute or acute GVHD [21, 22, 33]. Other clinical entities (e.g., steroid-induced cataract, subconjunctival, or retinal hemorrhages, etc.) in allogeneic transplant patients may be associated with the patients medications or with the blood count, and they do not represent chronic ocular GVHD [34, 35].

DIAGNOSIS AND STAGING

Prior to the NIH Consensus Panel for Chronic GVHD, acute and chronic forms of ocular GVHD were categorized by day 100 as the distinguishing point of terminology, irrespective of what pattern of disease patients experienced [36].

In general, however, the acute patterns of ocular GVHD include severe flare of conjunctival inflammation and pseudomebranous keratoconjunctivitis with or without corneal disease, while chronic oGVHD pattern is considered as DES [12, 30, 37].

For the diagnosis of chronic ocular GVHD, Schirmer's test is considered the gold standard. In the presence of one or more organ involvement with cGVHD, Schirmer's score of < 5 mm or Schirmer's score of 6 to 10 mm with a new onset of KCS on the slit lamp exam is diagnostic of chronic ocular GVHD [5]. In pediatric patients, Schirmer's test is typically difficult to perform before age 9 [8]. New onset of symptoms (dry, gritty, painful eyes), cictricial conjuncitivitis, keratoconjunctivitis sicca, or confluent areas of punctate keratopathy individually is insufficient to establish a diagnosis of chronic systemic GVHD [5]. After a full ocular workup and evaluation, including patients' ocular sentinel symptoms, infection history, overall medical and GVHD history, Schirmer's test, specialized corneal staining, viral swabs, all of the information should be used to make the diagnosis of chronic ocular GVHD.

Severity of ocular GVHD may be assessed using the Common Terminology Criteria for Adverse Events, version 3.0 (CTC AE v3.0), in which the grade II and III are delineated by whether the patient's activities of daily living (ADL) are affected and whether the management requires medical versus surgical inventions [38]. While CTC AE v3.0 can be applicable to any type of ocular toxicity of cancer treatment, including transplantation, it is not specific for GVHD. Existing conjunctival staging/grading system [12, 26] may be useful to categorize the severity of the conjunctival disease.

Proposed by the NIH Consensus, the severity of chronic ocular GVHD may be assessed by applying the ocular portion of the comprehensive organ scoring system [5]. The proposed scoring-system divides the signs and symptoms between 0 and 3, in which score 1 is mild symptoms of dry eye, score 2 is moderate symptoms without vision impairment,

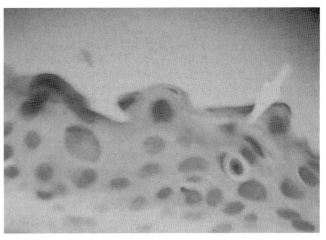

Figure 18.6 Conjunctival biopsy specimen of ocular GVHD: arrow points to an apoptic cell. Attenuated epithelial layer and loss of goblet cells also present. See Plate 60 in the color plate section.

and score 3 is severe symptoms impacting ADL. The organ scoring of cGVHD may be useful for clinical trials (for which the Consensus was developed), and its application in ophthalmology is currently being studied.

Conjunctival biopsy has a role in the evaluation and the diagnosis of ocular GVHD, albeit in a limited capacity [6]. It may be particularly helpful in symptomatic patients with normal Schirmer's score, with no other documented GVHD [39]. Unlike a lacrimal gland biopsy which is relatively invasive, conjunctival biopsy is safe and may be performed in the clinic with topical anesthetic, with minimal risk to the patient. Histologic features of conjunctival GVHD include conjunctival lymphocyte exocytosis, satellitosis, vacuolization of the basal epithelium, and epithelial cell necrosis [12, 25, 39, 40]. These changes of apoptosis are similar to changes that are observed in other organs (Figure 18.6). For select cases, conjunctival specimen may be evaluated for viral inclusions to differentiate the cause of KCS. Other features of conjunctival histopathology include decreased goblet cell density and epithelial attenuation, which are not sufficient for the diagnosis of ocular GVHD [6].

PATHOPHYSIOLOGY

Lacrimal gland has been the focus of many studies to elucidate the pathogenesis of chronic ocular GVHD. Clinically, chronic ocular GVHD shares much similarities with Sjogren's syndrome, both characterized by decreased tear function and chronic inflammation with atrophy of the lacrimal gland. Earlier histopathological study of GVHD patients revealed "lacrimal gland stasis," with distended ductules and obliteration of lumina, similar to bile duct damage seen it liver GVHD [15, 25]. Ogawa et al. have demonstrated by immunohistochemical and ultrastructural studies of lacrimal glands from chronic ocular GVHD patients the presence of excess fibrosis in the extracellular matrix, increased fibroblasts with multilayered basal lamina of the ducts, vessels, and lobules, and have suggested the importance of a subset of fibroblasts in the periductal regions that play a key role in the activation of CD4+ and CD8+ T cells in ocular GVHD [41, 42]. Furthermore, recent study has revealed that a subset of CD34+ fibroblasts in lacrimal gland specimen from chronic ocular GVHD patients are donor derived, suggesting the participation of donor-derived circulating precursor fibroblasts producing excess fibrosis that may lead to KCS in chronic ocular GVHD [43].

A few studies have been conducted on conjunctival tissues from chronic ocular GVHD. Increased CD4/CD8 ratios were observed in the conjunctival stroma of chronic ocular GVHD patients when compared with conjunctival specimen from autologous transplantation patients. This finding may not be unique to chronic ocular GVHD, given that these inflammatory cells were also present in increased numbers in conjunctiva of autologous transplantation specimen when compared to normal specimen, suggesting that these conjunctival changes may be partially due to medications/preparative regimen [44]. It has been shown that there is an increased expression of an inflammatory marker (ICAM-1) in the conjunctiva that is associated with decreased Schirmer's scores and decreased goblet cell density [45]. How increased expression of ICAM-1 impacts decreased goblet cells and decreased in Schirmer's scores (or vice versa) has not been established.

MANAGEMENT

Systemic treatment of cGVHD can improve the signs and symptoms of chronic ocular GVHD. Given the obvious limitations and risks of prolonged systemic immunosuppression, however, the consideration of organ-specific treatment without altering systemic immunosuppression should be the primary approach in managing chronic ocular GVHD. The overview of chronic ocular management is to increase lubrication on the ocular surface, minimize evaporation, prevent drainage of the tear film, and control the inflammation on the ocular surface. Depending on the severity of the symptoms and clinical findings of ocular GVHD, topical and oral medications, surgical intervention, and/or environmental strategies should be explored in each category [9] (Table 18.1).

The use of **lubrication** can alleviate mild symptoms of dry eye syndrome. It is optimal to use preservative-free artificial tears, as they do not cause irritation from topical preservative overexposure. Supplement with preservative-free lubricating ointment before bedtime is also recommended, given that KCS symptoms become worse throughout the day. By coating the ocular surface and decreasing corneal punctuate keratopathy, patient may have a decrease in the sentinel symptoms such as dryness, photophobia, or foreign body sensations, and experience improved quality of vision (up to 30% of clarity of vision is dependant on the natural tear film). For patients requiring artificial tears more than every hour, slow-dissolving hydroxypropyl methylcellulose pellets (Lacriserts) may be inserted into the inferior cul-de-sac for convenience [46]. It may be more convenient than the frequent topical application of tears, but it may not be tolerated due to the constant foreign body sensation. The frequency of tear application may serve as a surrogate for severity of chronic ocular GVHD, and the data can be used to follow the course of ocular GVHD, in particular during a clinical trial.

Oral agents can also be used to increase lubrication by stimulating aqueous tear flow. The selective muscarinic agonists (such as pilocarpine or cevimeline) may be effective in improving sicca symptoms in patients with Sjogren syndrome. The use of these agents, however, has been limited due to their contraindications with heart disease and its possible drug interactions/toxicities in transplant patients [47–50].

Second consideration to management of chronic ocular GVHD is to **control evaporation** of topical lubrication from the ocular surface. Warm compresses and lid care is a simple daily maintenance regimen that should be recommended to all chronic ocular GVHD patients [51]. Lid care may increase the output of the outer oil layer of the tear film from meibomian glands, resulting in decreased aqueous tear evaporation. For patients who have significant meibomitis with chronic ocular GVHD, oral doxycycline should be considered. It has been used to treat meibomian gland dysfunction and blepharitis in rosacea patients [52]. Avoiding sun exposure is important in patients taking oral doxycycline, especially for patients with skin GVHD [9].

Judicious use of bandage contact lens (BCTL) should be explored in patients who have severe chronic ocular GVHD [2, 53]. It has been well recognized that BCTL can be used in select refractory dry eye patients [54]. With BCTL, risks of microbial keratitis in an immunocompromised patient must be weighed against the benefits of alleviating signs and symptoms of refractory chronic ocular GVHD. Prophylactic antibiotic is typically necessary [55]. Those who fail BCTL, scleral lenses may still be beneficial [56]. Unfortunately, they are available in very few centers. In some cases, surgical approach is necessary to decrease exposed ocular surface [57]. Permanent partial tarsorrhphy while beneficial is rarely performed for DES due to cosmesis.

All patients can benefit from environmental strategies to reduce evaporative state, such as using eye protections with moisture chamber goggles [58, 59] and avoiding low humidity, direct wind, or air-conditioning.

To **decrease drainage** of the tear film from the ocular surface into the nasolacrimal duct apparatus, silicone punctal plugs can be placed into the punctum [60]. Punctal occlusion should be considered for patients with moderate to severe ocular GVHD with Schirmer's score of less than 5 mm. There are various designs of punctal plugs and the type that is placed deep into the canalicular system should be avoided, as they have the potential risk of infections [61, 62]. Often, collared plugs (visible placement) fall out in occlusion-dependent individuals, triggering recurrent symptoms and reactive inflammatory keratoconjunctivitis sicca. With repeated episodes, permanent thermal cautery should be performed. If the puncti reopen, the

Table18.1: Treatment of Chronic Ocular GVHD

Topical treatment	Preservative-free artificial tears
	Preservative-free artificial tears ointment
	Slow-dissolving hydroxypropyl methylcellulose
	Cyclosporine eye drops
	Steroid eye drops/ointment*
Surgical approach	Punctal occlusion (via plugs or thermal cauterization)
	Superficial debridement of filamentary keratitis
	Partial tarsorrhaphy
Oral medications	Pilocarpine
	Cevimeline
	Flaxseed oil
	Doxycycline or tetracycline
Environmental/eye wear strategies	Daily lid care/warm compress
	Occlusive eye wear/goggles/moisture chamber glasses
	Bandage contact lens
Treatment available in limited centers	Scleral lens
	Autologous serum

*Judicious use with careful follow-up needed.
Reprinted from *Biology of Blood and Marrow Transplant*, 12, Couriel D, Carpenter PA, Cutler C, et al. Ancillary therapy and supportive care of chronic graft-versus-host disease: National institutes of health consensus development project on criteria for clinical trials in chronic Graft-versus-host disease: V. Ancillary Therapy and Supportive Care Working Group Report, 375–396, 2006 with permission from Elsevier.

procedure should be repeated, even when the punctal openings appear minimal.

To **decrease ocular surface inflammation** is one of the most important goals of chronic ocular GVHD management [5]. Similar to the management of ocular inflammation in collagen vascular disease/autoimmune diseases, the treatment approach to the ocular disease depends on the status of the systemic disease. Systemic immunosuppression is used to control ocular inflammation of collagen vascular/autoimmune conditions; however, the emphasis for controlling ocular inflammation in GVHD patients is on both ocular and systemic treatment. Therefore, topical treatment (steroid, in particular) is more relevant for the treatment of ocular GVHD when compared to the treatment strategies of ocular inflammation from other systemic autoimmune/collagen vascular diseases [26, 28, 37].

Flares of ocular GVHD with no change in systemic GVHD can be addressed with topical medication alone without altering systemic immunosuppression, even when tapering of systemic medications triggered ocular GVHD [37]. Topical steroids is also beneficial in cicatricial conjunctivitis in ocular GVHD [26]. Prolong use of topical steroid is generally avoided for all types of ocular conditions in ophthalmology. For chronic ocular GVHD, low dose topical steroid and judicious follow-up may be a strategy without altering systemic immunosuppression. Because of the side effects of topical steroid (increased risk of cataract, steroid-induced glaucoma, higher susceptibility to infections), topical steroids for ocular GVHD should be initiated by an ophthalmologist who understands issues of GVHD.

Topical cyclosporine treatment for chronic ocular GVHD has shown to decrease ocular symptoms and clinical findings (symptom-scores, corneal sensitivity, tear evaporation rate,

TBUT, vital staining scores) and to decrease inflammatory cells while increasing goblet cell density and MUC5AC mRNA expression [63–65]. Unlike topical steroids, however, intolerance to topical cyclosporine is relatively common. Autologous serum (AS) may also provide anti-inflammatory effect when applied to the ocular surface. It has been used in chronic ocular GVHD with success [66–68]. Use of AS is limited due to a relatively low number of centers that offer this treatment.

Oral supplement of flaxseed oil may help patients with inflammation associated with KCS in Sjogren's patients [69] and may be helpful in ocular GVHD.

Increasing systemic immunosuppression or delaying its taper may be necessary if the ocular disease is refractory and cannot be managed via eye-specific treatment [5, 70]. It is important for the treating ophthalmologist, to understand the patients' systemic immunosuppression regimen, the tapering schedule, and previous history of GVHD flares, to optimize and individualize the ocular treatment for GVHD.

FUTURE DIRECTION

Better treatment options for chronic ocular GVHD should be explored. Implantable immunosuppression has been studied for ocular GVHD in animals [71]. Phase I human trial for a cyclosporine implant in chronic ocular GVHD (currently closed for new accrual at National Eye Institute) is on going with its follow-up safety data collection.

Studies to predict and/or to prevent chronic ocular GVHD should be the focus of future clinical trials. Recent findings in the NIH Consensus Workshop have outlined the metrics for clinical trials in cGVHD. These findings are relevant to chronic ocular GVHD and should be critically studied and validated to implement these metrics for ophthalmic clinical trials.

SUMMARY

Ocular surface disease with KCS (dry eye syndrome) is a common form of chronic ocular GVHD. By recognizing clinical presentations of chronic ocular GVHD and managing organ-specific treatment strategies, the ophthalmologist's role is to work with BMT service, not only to address the ocular disease, but to participate in optimizing the patients' overall immunosuppression profile. Ophthalmologists who are knowledgeable about ocular GVHD should be involved in the multidisciplinary approach when managing GVHD, to achieve the optimal quality of life while minimizing ocular morbidity in cGVHD patients.

REFERENCES

1. Lawley TJ, et al. Scleroderma, Sjogren-like syndrome, and chronic graft-versus-host disease. *Ann Intern Med*, 1977; 87(6):707–709.
2. Franklin RM, et al. Ocular manifestations of graft-vs-host disease. *Ophthalmology*, 1983;90(1):4–13.
3. Hirst LW, et al. The eye in bone marrow transplantation. I. Clinical study. *Arch Ophthalmol*, 1983;101(4):580–584.
4. Arocker-Mettinger E, et al. Manifestations of graft-versus-host disease following allogenic bone marrow transplantation. *Eur J Ophthalmol*, 1991;1(1):28–32.
5. Filipovich AH, et al. National Institutes of Health consensus development project on criteria for clinical trials in chronic graft-versus-host disease: I. Diagnosis and staging working group report. *Biol Blood Marrow Transplant*, 2005. 11(12):945–956.
6. Shulman HM, et al. Histopathologic diagnosis of chronic graft-versus-host disease: National Institutes of Health Consensus Development Project on Criteria for Clinical Trials in Chronic Graft-versus-Host Disease: II. Pathology Working Group Report. *Biol Blood Marrow Transplant*, 2006;12(1):31–47.
7. Schultz KR, et al. Toward biomarkers for chronic graft-versus-host disease: National Institutes of Health consensus development project on criteria for clinical trials in chronic graft-versus-host disease: III. Biomarker Working Group Report. *Biol Blood Marrow Transplant*, 2006;12(2):126–137.
8. Pavletic SZ, et al. Measuring Therapeutic Response in Chronic Graft-versus-Host Disease: National Institutes of Health Consensus Development Project on Criteria for Clinical Trials in Chronic Graft-versus-Host Disease: IV. Response Criteria Working Group Report. *Biol Blood Marrow Transplant*, 2006;12(3):252–266.
9. Couriel D, et al. Ancillary therapy and supportive care of chronic graft-versus-host disease: national institutes of health consensus development project on criteria for clinical trials in chronic Graft-versus-host disease: V. Ancillary Therapy and Supportive Care Working Group Report. *Biol Blood Marrow Transplant*, 2006;12(4):375–396.

10. Martin PJ, et al. National Institutes of Health Consensus Development Project on Criteria for Clinical Trials in Chronic Graft-versus-Host Disease: VI. Design of Clinical Trials Working Group Report. *Biol Blood Marrow Transplant*, 2006;12(5):491–505.
11. Jack MK, et al. Ocular manifestations of graft-v-host disease. *Arch Ophthalmol*, 1983;101(7):1080–1084.
12. Jabs DA, et al. The eye in bone marrow transplantation. III. Conjunctival graft-vs-host disease. *Arch Ophthalmol*, 1989;107(9):1343–1348.
13. Ogawa Y, et al., Dry eye after haematopoietic stem cell transplantation. *Br J Ophthalmol*, 1999;83(10):1125–1130.
14. Livesey SJ, Holmes JA, Whittaker JA. Ocular complications of bone marrow transplantation. *Eye*, 1989;3(pt 3):271–276.
15. Tichelli A, et al. Late-onset keratoconjunctivitis sicca syndrome after bone marrow transplantation: incidence and risk factors. European Group or Blood and Marrow Transplantation (EBMT) Working Party on Late Effects. *Bone Marrow Transplant*, 1996;17(6):1105–1111.
16. Calissendorff B, el Azazi M, Lonnqvist B. Dry eye syndrome in long-term follow-up of bone marrow transplanted patients. *Bone Marrow Transplant*, 1989;4(6):675–678.
17. Mencucci R, et al. Ophthalmological aspects in allogenic bone marrow transplantation: Sjogren-like syndrome in graft-versus-host disease. *Eur J Ophthalmol*, 1997;7(1):13–18.
18. Kim SK. *Ocular Graft versus Host Disease*, in *Cornea*, J.H. Krachmer, M. J. Mannis, and E. J. Holland, Editors. 2004, Mosby: St. Louis. p. 879–885.
19. Dunn JP, et al. Bone marrow transplantation and cataract development. *Arch Ophthalmol*, 1993;111(10):1367–1373.
20. Cheng LL, et al. Graft-vs-host-disease-associated conjunctival chemosis and central serous chorioretinopathy after bone marrow transplant. *Am J Ophthalmol*, 2002;134(2):293–295.
21. Fawzi AA, Cunningham, Jr., ET. Central serous chorioretinopathy after bone marrow transplantation. *Am J Ophthalmol*, 2001;131(6):804–805.
22. Kim RY, et al. Scleritis as the initial clinical manifestation of graft-versus-host disease after allogenic bone marrow transplantation. *Am J Ophthalmol*, 2002;133(6):843–845.
23. Hettinga YM, et al. Anterior uveitis: a manifestation of graft-versus-host disease. *Ophthalmology*, 2007;114(4):794–797.
24. Sheidow TG, et al. Vitritis as the primary manifestation of graft-versus-host disease: a case report with vitreous cytopathology. *Can J Ophthalmol*, 2004;39(6):667–671.
25. Jabs DA, et al. The eye in bone marrow transplantation. II. Histopathology. *Arch Ophthalmol*, 1983;101(4):585–590.
26. Robinson MR, et al. Topical corticosteroid therapy for cicatricial conjunctivitis associated with chronic graft-versus-host disease. *Bone Marrow Transplant*, 2004;33(10):1031–1035.
27. Karwacka E, et al. Pemphigoid-like ocular lesions in patients with graft-versus-host disease following allogeneic bone marrow transplantation. *Transplant Proc*, 2006;38(1):292–294.
28. Kim SK, et al. Ocular graft vs. host disease experience from MD Anderson Cancer Center: Newly described clinical spectrum and new approach to the management of Stage III and IV ocular GVHD. *Biol Blood Marrow Transplant*, 2006;12(2 (S1)):49.
29. Ogawa Y, Kuwana M. Dry eye as a major complication associated with chronic graft-versus-host disease after hematopoietic stem cell transplantation. *Cornea*, 2003;22(Suppl 7):S19-S27.
30. Johnson DA, Jabs DA. The ocular manifestations of graft-versus-host disease. *Int Ophthalmol Clin*, 1997;37(2):119–133.

31. Balaram M, Rashid S, Dana R. Chronic ocular surface disease after allogeneic bone marrow transplantation. *Ocul Surf,* 2005;3(4):203–211.

32. Kim SK. Ocular graft vs. host disease. *Ocul Surf,* 2005;3 (Suppl 4):S177–S179.

33. Kaiserman I, Or R. Laser photocoagulation for central serous retinopathy associated with graft-versus-host disease. *Ocul Immunol Inflamm,* 2005;13(2–3):249–256.

34. Moon SJ, Mieler WF. Retinal complications of bone marrow and solid organ transplantation. *Curr Opin Ophthalmol,* 2003;14(6):433–442.

35. Coskuncan NM, et al. The eye in bone marrow transplantation. VI. Retinal complications. *Arch Ophthalmol,* 1994; 112(3):372–379.

36. Armitage JO. Bone marrow transplantation. *N Engl J Med,* 1994;330(12):827–838.

37. Kim SK. Update on ocular graft versus host disease. *Curr Opin Ophthalmol,* 2006;17(4):344–348.

38. Trotti A, et al. CTCAE v3.0: development of a comprehensive grading system for the adverse effects of cancer treatment. *Semin Radiat Oncol,* 2003;13(3):176–181.

39. West RH, Szer J, Pedersen JS. Ocular surface and lacrimal disturbances in chronic graft-versus-host disease: the role of conjunctival biopsy. *Aust N Z J Ophthalmol,* 1991;19(3):187–191.

40. Wagner JE, Jr., Vogelsang GB, Beschorner WE. Pathogenesis and pathology of graft-vs.-host disease. *Am J Pediatr Hematol Oncol,* 1989;11(2):196–212.

41. Ogawa Y, et al. A significant role of stromal fibroblasts in rapidly progressive dry eye in patients with chronic GVHD. *Invest Ophthalmol Vis Sci,* 2001;42(1):111–119.

42. Ogawa Y, et al. Periductal area as the primary site for T-cell activation in lacrimal gland chronic graft-versus-host disease. *Invest Ophthalmol Vis Sci,* 2003;44(5):1888–1896.

43. Ogawa Y, et al. Donor fibroblast chimerism in the pathogenic fibrotic lesion of human chronic graft-versus-host disease. *Invest Ophthalmol Vis Sci,* 2005;46(12):4519–4527.

44. Rojas B, et al. Cell populations and adhesion molecules expression in conjunctiva before and after bone marrow transplantation. *Exp Eye Res,* 2005;81(3):313–325.

45. Aronni S, et al. Upregulation of ICAM-1 expression in the conjunctiva of patients with chronic graft-versus-host disease. *Eur J Ophthalmol,* 2006;16(1):17–23.

46. Hill JC. Slow-release artificial tear inserts in the treatment of dry eyes in patients with rheumatoid arthritis. *Br J Ophthalmol,* 1989;73(2):151–154.

47. Papas AS, et al. Oral pilocarpine for symptomatic relief of dry mouth and dry eyes in patients with Sjogrens syndrome. *Adv Exp Med Biol,* 1998;438:973–978.

48. Tsifetaki N, et al. Oral pilocarpine for the treatment of ocular symptoms in patients with Sjogren's syndrome: a randomised 12 week controlled study. *Ann Rheum Dis,* 2003;62(12):1204–1207.

49. Papas AS, et al. Successful Treatment of Dry Mouth and Dry Eye Symptoms in Sjogren's Syndrome Patients With Oral Pilocarpine: A Randomized, Placebo-Controlled, Dose-Adjustment Study. *J Clin Rheumatol,* 2004;10(4):169–177.

50. Ono M, et al. Therapeutic effect of cevimeline on dry eye in patients with Sjogren's syndrome: a randomized, double-blind clinical study. *Am J Ophthalmol,* 2004;138(1):6–17.

51. Olson MC, Korb DR, Greiner JV. Increase in tear film lipid layer thickness following treatment with warm compresses in patients with meibomian gland dysfunction. *Eye Contact Lens,* 2003;29(2):96–99.

52. Frucht-Pery J, et al. Efficacy of doxycycline and tetracycline in ocular rosacea. *Am J Ophthalmol,* 1993;116(1):88–92.

53. Russo PA, Bouchard CS, Galasso JM. Extended-wear silicone hydrogel soft contact lenses in the management of moderate to severe dry eye signs and symptoms secondary to graft-versus-host disease. *Eye Contact Lens,* 2007;33(3):144–147.

54. Levinson A, Weissman BA, Sachs U. Use of the Bausch & Lomb Soflens Plano T contact lens as a bandage. *Am J Optom Physiol Opt,* 1977;54(2):97–103.

55. Hovding G. Hydrophilic contact lenses in corneal disorders. *Acta Ophthalmol (Copenh),* 1984;62(4):566–576.

56. Takahide K, et al. Use of fluid-ventilated, gas-permeable scleral lens for management of severe keratoconjunctivitis sicca secondary to chronic graft-versus-host disease. *Biol Blood Marrow Transplant,* 2007;13(9):1016–1021.

57. Cosar CB, et al. Tarsorrhaphy: clinical experience from a cornea practice. *Cornea,* 2001;20(8):787–791.

58. Gresset J, Simonet P, Gordon D. Combination of a side shield with an ocular moisture chamber. *Am J Optom Physiol Opt,* 1984;61(9):610–612.

59. Hart DE, Simko M, Harris E. How to produce moisture chamber eyeglasses for the dry eye patient. *J Am Optom Assoc,* 1994;65(7):517–522.

60. Murube J, Murube E. Treatment of dry eye by blocking the lacrimal canaliculi. *Surv Ophthalmol,* 1996;40(6):463–480.

61. SmartPlug Study Group. Management of complications after insertion of the SmartPlug punctal plug: a study of 28 patients. *Ophthalmology,* 2006; 113(10):1859 e1–e6.

62. Mazow ML, McCall T, Prager TC. Lodged intracanalicular plugs as a cause of lacrimal obstruction. *Ophthal Plast Reconstr Surg,* 2007;23(2):138–142.

63. Kiang E, et al. The use of topical cyclosporin A in ocular graft-versus-host-disease. *Bone Marrow Transplant,* 1998;22(2): 147–151.

64. Lelli GJ, Jr., et al. Ophthalmic cyclosporine use in ocular GVHD. *Cornea,* 2006;25(6):635–638.

65. Wang Y, et al. Ocular surface and tear functions after topical cyclosporine treatment in dry eye patients with chronic graft-versus-host disease. *Bone Marrow Transplant,* 2008; 41(3):293–302.

66. Rocha EM, et al. GVHD dry eyes treated with autologous serum tears. *Bone Marrow Transplant,* 2000;25(10):1101–1103.

67. Ogawa Y, et al. Autologous serum eye drops for the treatment of severe dry eye in patients with chronic graft-versus-host disease. *Bone Marrow Transplant,* 2003;31(7):579–583.

68. Chiang CC, et al. Allogeneic serum eye drops for the treatment of severe dry eye in patients with chronic graft-versus-host disease. *Cornea,* 2007;26(7):861–863.

69. Pinheiro MN, Jr., et al. [Oral flaxseed oil (Linum usitatissimum) in the treatment for dry-eye Sjogren's syndrome patients]. *Arq Bras Oftalmol,* 2007;70(4):649–655.

70. Ogawa Y, et al. Successful treatment of dry eye in two patients with chronic graft-versus-host disease with systemic administration of FK506 and corticosteroids. *Cornea,* 2001;20(4): 430–434.

71. Kim H, et al. Preclinical evaluation of a novel episcleral cyclosporine implant for ocular graft-versus-host disease. *Invest Ophthalmol Vis Sci,* 2005;46(2):655–662.

19

GYNECOLOGICAL MANIFESTATIONS OF CHRONIC GRAFT VERSUS HOST DISEASE

Maria L. Turner and Pamela Stratton

INTRODUCTION

Chronic graft versus host disease (cGVHD) is a multisystem disorder that occurs in 60% to 70% of long-term survivors [1] of allogeneic hematopoietic stem cell transplantation (HSCT) and has been increasing in incidence because of improved survival of posttransplant recipients. The longer survival and unrelenting progression of cGVHD affect several aspects of health and may result in loss of organ function and impaired quality of life.

Under the leadership of the National Institutes of Health, a multidisciplinary group of investigators studying cGVHD established a consortium to study, assemble, and broadcast information about this disease and its treatment as well as to influence the direction of new research into its pathogenic mechanisms. The group has since published several papers relating to the diagnosis and staging [2] histology, [3], and ancillary care [4] of patients with cGVHD. In these consensus reports, the gynecologic aspects of this disease are barely mentioned.

The report on ancillary care recommends that as most transplant physicians are not in a position to address gynecologic problems, women with complaints of vulvar irritation should be referred to their gynecologists. Unfortunately, most gynecologists know very little about stem cell transplant recipients and cGVHD. It is with the hope of furthering knowledge regarding this heretofore neglected aspect of cGVHD that we contribute our experiences at the National Institutes of Health derived from evaluating and caring for the gynecologic problems of women with cGVHD.

The first mention of vaginal problems related to cGVHD occurred in 1982 with a report of vaginal scarring and narrowing occurring in five women following allogeneic transplantation [5]. The authors recognized the importance of surgery followed by the use of dilators to treat this complication. Surprisingly, there was a hiatus of 17 years until other individual case reports of posttransplant vaginal stenosis

and its surgical treatment were published [6–8]. Thus, vaginal stenosis became recognized as a late manifestation of cGVHD.

A case series by Flowers suggested that there may be other genital tract manifestations, but vulvar and vaginal symptoms were not reported separately [9]. Only in the past 5 years have four case series been published, which distinguished vulvar from vaginal disease [10–13]. These have provided some insights about the clinical course and treatment of cGVHD affecting the female genital tract.

INCIDENCE

The incidence of vulvovaginal cGVHD is not really known because all women have not been examined when they develop symptoms and at regular intervals. For example, our calculated 11% prevalence among women undergoing allogeneic peripheral blood stem cell transplantation (PBSCT) is an underestimate as our cohort consisted of some women referred for vulvar complaints and others seen as part of an evaluation of a natural history protocol of cGVHD [13]. Higher rates are reported by both Spinelli and Zantomio [10, 12]. In Spinelli's retrospective study of a cohort of 213 women [10], all of whom had traditional allogeneic bone marrow transplantation (BMT) for hematologic malignancies, 24.9% had vulvar cGVHD.

In a prospective study, Zantomio [12] showed that with a median period of observation of 24 months, 29 of 61 (48%) women developed genital cGVHD. Despite the fact that these women were enrolled in a prospective, interventional protocol focused on prevention of vulvovaginal cGVHD, the estimated probability of genital tract cGVHD was 36% after 1 year and 49% by 2 years. The nearly doubled prevalence of genital cGVHD noted in Zantomio's study may be related to the differences in study design (prospective vs. retrospective). In addition, this study focused on genital involvement and women were instructed to report any genital tract signs or symptoms. Their increased awareness may have led to a higher incidence and, perhaps, an earlier recognition of the disease.

Acknowledgment: This was funded in part by the intramural programs of the National Cancer Institute, the National Institute of Child Health and Human Development, and the NIH Clinical Center.

RISK FACTORS

The risk factors for genital cGVHD have been difficult to determine. Spinelli [10] did not find a statistically significant correlation between genital cGVHD and parity or presence of lower genital tract infections. Among those who developed genital cGVHD, a greater percentage of patients used topical or systemic estrogen ($p = 0.049$). The relation between estrogen and the development of genital cGVHD is debatable, as many are placed on estrogen for genital tract symptoms that could be ascribed to either hypoestrogenism or genital cGVHD. Thus, estrogen use for treating cGVHD symptoms may be a confounding factor, rather than a causal association. An earlier study from Spinelli's group [14], comparing a 24-month follow-up among a cohort of women taking hormone replacement therapy (HRT) with those not on HRT did not find any difference in genital cGVHD.

Our own observations regarding estrogen use have been the opposite of those found by Spinelli et al. [10] In our series [13], cobweb and arcuate vaginal synechiae representing early vaginal cGVHD resolved with use of a ultra–low-dose estrogen vaginal ring (7.5 mcg/24 hours; Pfizer, NY, NY). In some cases, even though vaginal scarring has completely resolved in the upper vagina where the ring is situated, we have observed new vaginal scarring below it, just inside the introitus. We have noted that both vulvar and vaginal disease have begun or worsened when women suddenly stopped either systemic or local estrogen. Furthermore, we have found that topical estrogen was especially useful in treating genital atrophy and mucosal friability of genital cGVHD which were persistent even after resolution of inflammatory symptoms following the use of topical steroids.

The type of stem cell transplant might also be a factor as some reports suggest that cGVHD is more likely to occur after PBSCT than BMT [15, 16]. Although Flowers [9] did not find a significant difference between the prevalence of cGVHD after PBSCT versus BMT, she nevertheless found that cGVHD was more protracted and more difficult to control after PBSCT. More importantly, she also reported that the skin and female genital tract were more frequently involved as a manifestation of cGVHD in patients undergoing PBSCT in comparison with those receiving BMT.

In Zantomio's study [12], 40 of the 61 women received PBSCT and 21 had BMT. In a multivariate analysis of potential risk factors for developing genital cGVHD, receiving donor peripheral blood stem cells was the only factor with a statistically significant increased risk, having a hazard ratio of 3.07 ($p = 0.017$). In this model, the conditioning regimen, donor source, GVHD prophylaxis, donor sex or age of recipient or donor did not influence the prevalence of genital tract cGVHD.

The possible relationship between PBSCT and genital cGVHD is an observation that will be important to study over time. It is anticipated that use of peripheral blood rather than bone marrow for stem cell transplantation will continue to be more common because of the ease and safety of collecting donor cells, earlier neutrophil and platelet recovery, and suggestions of better graft-versus-leukemia effect.

CLINICAL FEATURES

At the time that they developed genital disease, most patients in the reports cited in this chapter, had coexisting cGVHD in other organs. Most of them were on topical or systemic immunosuppressive agents.

From the three studies [10, 12, 13] with relatively large cohorts of women with genital cGVHD, 73%, 90%, and 100% of them, respectively, had evidence of cGVHD affecting other organs, especially skin and oral mucosa. Stratton and Turner's 29 patients, almost all of whom had undergone allogeneic PBSCT, had cGVHD of the skin, mouth, and eyes 93%, 90%, and 79%, respectively [13]. All these organs, including the genital tract, have epithelial or mucosal surfaces, so that their simultaneous vulnerability might be expected. All patients with genital cGVHD had cGVHD in at least one other organ system. Vaginal synechiae, the most severe expression of genital cGVHD was associated with sclerotic skin involvement, a more severe and recalcitrant manifestation of cutaneous cGVHD.

Although the three studies differed in design, the time to onset of symptoms of genital cGVHD was around 10 months from the time of transplantation [10, 12, 13]. In all of these studies, vaginal scarring only occurred in women who also had vulvar cGVHD. In Stratton and Turner's series [13], the onset of vulvar disease had a median of 10 months with the onset of vaginal disease much later, at 19 months. While only 17% had vaginal synechiae at their first visit, by the end of the observation period, additional patients developed vaginal involvement with about half of the patients (48%) affected. Spiryda [11] also found that many women developed vaginal disease despite aggressively treating their vulvar disease, with 7 of her 11 patients requiring surgery for vaginal disease. This time lag of 9 months offers an opportunity to institute preventive measures and treatments targeted to the vaginal mucosa to prevent the need for surgery. Since women develop vaginal cGVHD after vulvar disease, the presence of the latter identifies an at-risk population for whom interventions may be developed to prevent vaginal cGVHD.

CLINICAL GRADING SYSTEM

Spinelli [10] introduced a system for grading the severity of genital involvement into mild, moderate, and severe. Minimal involvement consisted of vulvar redness, pain on touching the labia, and small areas of vulvar denudation. When vulvar denudation was extensive, genital cGVHD was considered to be moderate. Vaginal adhesions or complete vaginal closure was considered severe. Using his grading system, Spinelli reported that 66% of his patients with genital cGVHD had minimal, 22% had moderate, and 12% had severe involvement. By contrast, using Spinelli's same system, Zantomio [13] reported that his patients were divided evenly among each of the three categories.

Stratton and Turner observed that clitoral hood scarring and other vulvar architectural changes were coincident with

Table 19.1: Severity Scoring for Chronic Genital GVHD

Grade I (Minimal)
Generalized erythema and edema of the vulva
Reticulated leukokeratosis
Erythematous patches on mucosal surfaces of the vulva
Erythema and tenderness on light pressure over opening(s) of Skene's and/orBartholin's ducts

Grade II (Moderate) – Grade I plus
Erosions over any part of the vulva
Fissures in vulvar folds – interlabial sulcus; posterior fourchette

Grade III (Severe)
Agglutination of clitoral hood
Introital stenosis
Vaginal synechiae
Hematocolpos/hematometria or complete vaginal closure
Fasciitis of levator sling

Stratton P, Turner ML, Childs R, et al. Vulvovaginal chronic graft-versus-host disease with allogeneic hematopoietic stem cell transplantation. *Obstet Gynecol.* 2007;110(5):1041–1049.

Table 19.2: Symptoms and Signs of Chronic Genital GVHD

Symptoms
Dryness
Burning – when urine touches the vulva
Dyspareunia – superficial or deep
Loss of libido
Amenorrhea

Signs
Dryness
Erythema – generalized or patchy
Erosions and fissures
Pain on light pressure over openings of Skene's and Bartholin's ducts
Reticulated leukokeratosis
Resorption of labia minora
Clitoral agglutination
Introital stenosis
Vaginal synechiae including cobweb, arcuate, or dense scarring
Vaginal narrowing or shortening

vaginal scarring [13]. Thus, these vulvar changes were considered as evidence of severe genital cGVHD. This modification of Spinelli's grading system can be seen in Table 19.1. Using their modified grading system, Stratton and Turner [13] reported that at initial examination, 31% of their patients presented with mild disease while 41% had moderate and 28% had severe involvement that included those with vaginal scarring, vaginal fasciitis, and clitoral hood agglutination.

SYMPTOMS AND SIGNS

Ascertaining the symptoms and signs of genital cGVHD is an important part of the diagnosis (see summary in Table 19.2). Dryness or lack of lubrication in both the vulva and vagina is often described and would be expected in women following induction and conditioning chemotherapy as these treatments often cause premature ovarian failure. Ovarian failure results in loss of estrogen, which is necessary to maintain genital mucosal integrity. On examination, loss of lubrication, thinning of the mucosal surface, and loss of vaginal rugae are noted.

Vulvar burning is a very common complaint and it should be determined whether this occurs when the woman senses the need to void, when urine touches the vulva, after intercourse or unprovoked, at rest. In these patients, vulvar burning that occurs when urine touches the vulva often is associated with eroded or fissured vulvar mucosa with patches of erythema surrounding and underlying these lesions. Burning may be noted when a woman first presents with genital cGVHD, when cGVHD flares as immunosuppressive therapy is being tapered, or it may be a problem for a few days after intercourse as the fragile mucosa may become damaged and needs several days to

heal. Constant vulvar burning, even while at rest, with nothing touching the vulva, suggests a neuropathic etiology rather than cGVHD. BK virus infection should be considered in those with severe dysuria, urinary retention, and gross hematuria.

Another common complaint is dyspareunia. When this occurs with an attempt at deep penetration, it suggests vaginal scarring or shortening. Superficial or introital dyspareunia, a much more common complaint, occurs in those with mucosal damage from fissures or erosions but is also frequently observed in those with minimal inflammation confined to the openings of the vestibular glands (Bartholin's, Skene's, and minor vestibular glands). Occasionally, introital dyspareunia can be caused by extensive labial fusion. Dyspareunia of either type may sometimes be so severe as to cause patients to avoid intercourse altogether.

Findings on visual inspection include erythema that may be diffuse but is most often patchy. The mucosal surfaces of the vestibule as well as the medial surfaces of the labia minora and majora are most often involved (Figure 19.1). Histology may demonstrate chronic vulvitis.

A significant and nearly constant finding among those presenting with vulvar pain and burning is exquisite tenderness on exerting light pressure with an applicator tip over the ostia of one or more of the paired openings of Skene's and Bartholin's ducts, whether erythema surrounds the openings or not (Figure 19.2). These findings are characteristic of "vulvar vestibulitis syndrome," a chronic vulvar pain syndrome that, by definition, is idiopathic [17]. Among those whose fissures and erosions heal with treatment but have continuing introital dyspareunia, we have often found persistence of tenderness on light pressure over the ostia of vestibular glands.

Fissures with accompanying erythema are most often seen in the interlabial sulci (Figure 19.3) and at the posterior

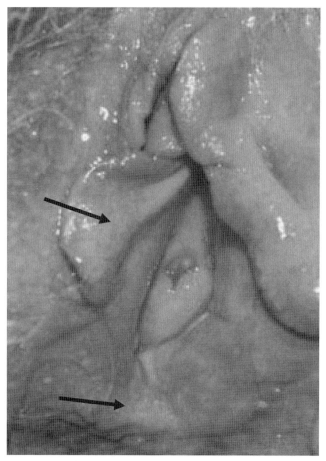

Figure 19.1 Mild genital GVHD: Diffuse erythema and edema of the vulva with reticulated leukokeratosis indicated by arrows of the right labia minora and posterior fourchette. See Plate 61 in the color plate section.

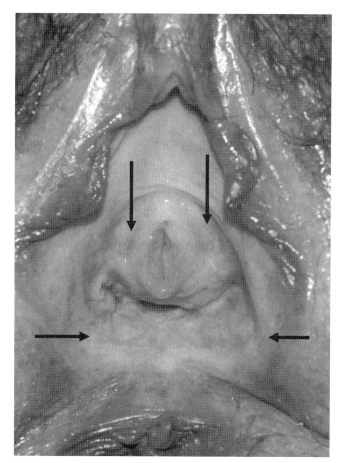

Figure 19.2 Mild genital GVHD: Erythematous patches at the introitus indicated with horizontal arrows. Erythematous areas around the opening of Skene's ducts noted with vertical arrows. These findings are similar to those seen in idiopathic vulvar vestibulitis syndrome. See Plate 62 in the color plate section.

fourchette (Figure 19.4), where the fine fissures may sometimes be hidden by white, macerated desquamated epithelium. A fine retiform or lace-like pattern of leukokeratosis may be seen along the edges of the interlabial fissures or on the skin over the perineal body (Figure 19.1). This very same pattern is seen in lichen planus (an idiopathic inflammatory skin disease that is not related to cGVHD) of the vulva and reflects the lichenoid histology shared by both conditions.

Architectural changes include atrophy and scarring, and characterize severe cGVHD (Figures 19.4 and 19.5). In the vulva, these changes include resorption of the labia minora and agglutination of the clitoral hood and may be attributed to both estrogen deficiency and persistent lichenoid inflammation, the basic histologic finding in cGVHD. Young, menstruating women with lichen planus, a disease that shares a lichenoid histology with cGVHD, also have similar findings of labia minora resorption. Thus, in the patients with genital cGVHD, who also have premature ovarian failure, there may be more than one reason for resorption of the labia minora.

In the clitoral hood region, vulvar mucosal erosions caused by the lichenoid inflammation will cause the free edges of the clitoral hood to stick together in the reparative process, forming

a scar over the clitoris (Figure 19.4). When combined with labial resorption or fusion, this can cause narrowing of the introitus, with labial fusion needing surgical repair [18] (Figure 19.6).

The same erosive and scarring process occurs in the vaginal mucosa leading first to the formation of cobweb-like filaments that eventually become sclerotic, pulling the vaginal walls together with resultant narrowing and shortening of the vaginal canal. The early cobweb-like filaments may be easily lysed during examination. Untreated and unrecognized scarring vaginal cGVHD occurring in either menstruating women or those on cyclic hormonal therapy may lead to the accumulation of menstrual blood proximally causing severe pain and hematometra or hematocolpos, both of which may require surgical intervention.

HISTOLOGY

The classic histology of cGVHD consists of basal vacuolar degeneration with apoptotic keratinocytes in the epidermis or mucosa overlying a superficial perivascular lympho-histiocytic infiltrate [3]. We have found this in some, but not all, biopsies.

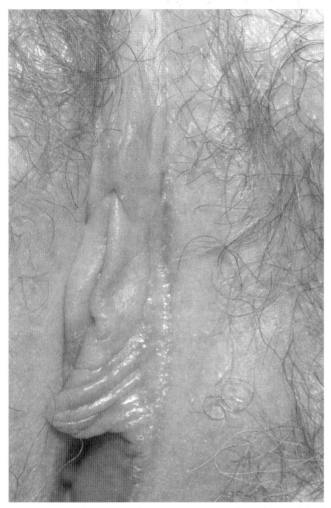

Figure 19.3 Moderate genital GVHD: Fissuring along the interlabial sulcus. This can cause burning on urination. See Plate 63 in the color plate section.

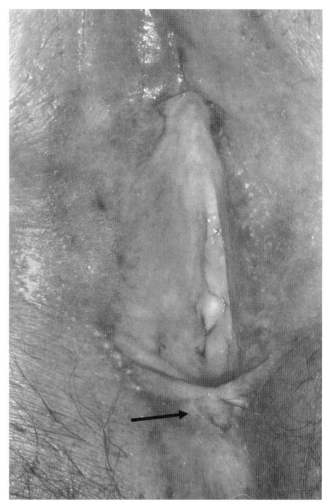

Figure 19.4 Moderate to severe genital GVHD: Marked architectural atrophy and sclerosis of the labia; note tear/fissure at posterior commissure indicated by arrow. See Plate 64 in the color plate section.

At times, biopsies of painful erythematous but noneroded patches are more consistent with nonspecific chronic vulvitis, where the pattern is not lichenoid and the infiltrate is more pleomorphic with a predominance of plasma cells. Apoptotic cells are not always seen. Similar findings have been reported by Spiryda in the seven biopsies in her case series [11].

CLINICAL EVALUATION

After the genital tract symptoms are ascertained, an examination to include the vulva and, if possible, a vaginal examination should be done (Table 19.3). The vulva, perineum, and perianal area should be inspected for the signs of genital GVHD (noted in Table 19.2) and other diseases with attention paid to erythema, fissures, erosions, tender vestibular gland ostia, labial changes, discharge, papules, and changes in pigmentation. The vaginal examination should begin with a gentle digital examination (using water as a lubricant) to evaluate for the different types of synechiae described earlier. During the vulvar and speculum examination, cultures should be obtained for yeast,

Herpes simplex virus (HSV), or other pathogens, if indicated. Cervical cytology should be obtained at least yearly with colposcopy as indicated. Vulvar, vaginal, or cervical biopsy should be done to diagnose squamous intraepithelial lesions or when discrete erythematous or leukokeratotic patches/plaques do not respond to topical therapy.

TREATMENT AND RESPONSE

Many case reports regarding genital cGVHD report the surgical treatment of vaginal stenosis and its complication, hematocolpos. Some advocated lysis of adhesions as the sole intervention [7]. Others recommended postsurgical treatments to prevent or treat vaginal restenosis by using topical corticosteroids, [8 dilators alone, 19], dilators with topical estrogen, [4] dilators with systemic and topical estrogen [20], or dilators with topical cyclosporine [11].

After classifying the genital disease of his patients as mild, moderate, or severe, Spinelli [10] tailored treatment accordingly. Sixty-eight percent of the women with genital cGVHD

Table 19.3: Evaluation

Vulvar examination – inspect cutaneous and mucosal surfaces including the perineum and perianal areas for erythema, fissures, and erosions. Use a q tip to determine whether vestibular gland ostia are tender. Also note papules and changes in pigmentation

Vaginal examination – start with manual examination before doing a speculum examination and use water as the glove lubricant. Determine whether there are adhesions or scars, and check the patency and caliber of the vagina

Cultures, KOH examination – as indicated, especially for yeast, and HSV infection

Pap smear – should be done at least yearly

Colposcopy – as indicated after abnormal cervical cytology

Biopsy – verrucous, acetowhite, mosaic, or punctuated lesions to diagnose squamous intraepithelial lesions including HPV (human papilloma virus) disease, dysplasia, and cancer, or when discrete erythematous or leukokeratotic patches/plaques do not respond to topical therapy

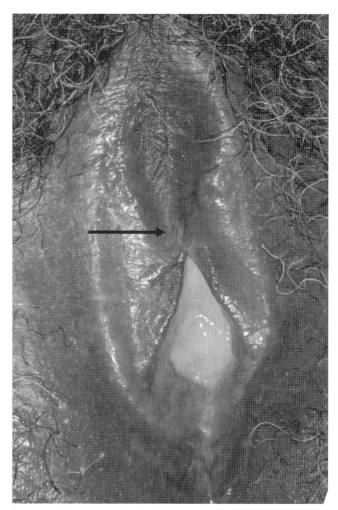

Figure 19.6 Severe genital GVHD: Narrowed introitus from fusion of labia minora as indicated by arrow. See Plate 66 in the color plate section.

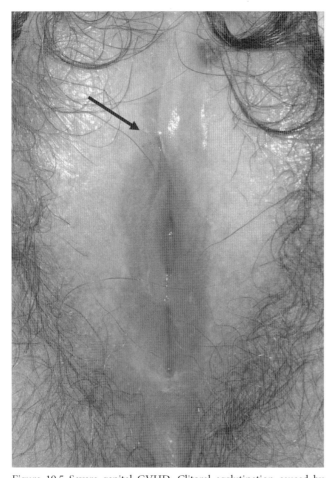

Figure 19.5 Severe genital GVHD: Clitoral agglutination caused by healing of apposing eroded surfaces of the clitoral hood and labia minora designated by arrow. Labial resorption and diffuse erythema are noted as well indicated by arrow. See Plate 65 in the color plate section.

were on systemic hormone therapy. He treated the mild and moderate cases with a combination of topical estrogen and an emollient cream with poor results. He switched nonresponding cases to a medium strength topical steroid (triamcinolone), which proved more effective. He treated the more recalcitrant ones with a superpotent topical steroid, clobetasol propionate cream, or ointment, starting with twice daily applications and tapering to a maintenance dose of 2 to 3 times a week. The most severe cases still needed surgical treatment.

Topical compounded cyclosporine was used by Spiryda's subjects, which was successful in treating vulvar disease but not in preventing vaginal disease [11].

Zantonio [12] recently published a study that included pretransplant education of the participants about the signs and symptoms of genital cGVHD, regular genital self-examination by the patient and scheduled pelvic examinations starting at 3 months posttransplant. Realizing that it was clinically difficult to differentiate mild vulvar or vaginal cGVHD from the genital manifestations of premature ovarian failure associated with chemotherapy and stem cell transplantation, these patients were started on topical and systemic estrogen plus

Table 19.4: Treatment

Topical steroids – for erosions, fissures, erythematous patches

  Superpotent topical steroid ointment* such as clobetasol propionate, applied in a very thin layer to involved areas at bedtime every day until lesions are markedly improved. Applications can be tapered to a maintenance dose of one application 2 to 3 times a week

Estrogen for hormone replacement and to improve skin integrity (assuming no contraindications)

  Estradiol cream or ointment – may start using on the vulva after erosions and fissures are healed. Begin with a layer to involved areas at bedtime every day for 2 weeks and then decrease to one application 2 to 3 times a week

  Estrogen vaginal ring (7.5 mcg/24 hours) for continuous ultralow dose replacement; lasts 90 days

  Consider systemic oral contraceptives or other hormone replacement for women who were not menopausal at time of transplant and who are younger than age 50

Dilators – such as those made by Syracuse Medical Devices (Fayetville, NY) are available in several sizes – extrasmall, small, medium, and large are used for vaginal scarring

  A pea-sized amount of clobetasol and one half inch of estrogen cream is applied to the tip. It is used 2 to 3 times a week until the vaginal scarring is lysed

Cobweb and other newly formed scars – may be lysed by manual manipulation at time of vaginal examination

Thick fibrotic vaginal scars in the setting of hematocolpos or extensive labial fusion may need surgical correction

---

* A pure white petrolatum ointment base without preservatives or alcohol is best tolerated.

progesterone replacement early in the posttransplant period. Ancillary therapies consisted of intravaginal hydrocortisone foam daily for 4 to 6 weeks, topical cyclosporine daily for 4 to 6 weeks in those who did not respond to hydrocortisone foam, and dilators twice a week in those who developed vaginal narrowing despite the other treatments. In this well-designed study, early institution of topical and systemic estrogen replacement did not prevent genital cGVHD in half of the enrolled patients, but no one required surgery for vaginal scarring.

One of this chapter's authors (MLT) had extensive experience with the safety and efficacy of long-term use of superpotent topical steroids for the treatment of erosive, inflammatory mucosal diseases such as lichen sclerosus and erosive lichen planus, while the other (PS) was equally comfortable with the use of topical estrogen for the prevention of scarring and restoration of suppleness of genital mucosa following inflammation. In light of the well-established safety of long-term superpotent topical steroids for treatment of vulvar lichen sclerosus [21], we launched a two-pronged program, starting topical therapy with 0.05% clobetasol propionate ointment applied twice a day in a very thin layer to the vulvar mucosa and accessible vaginal mucosa for 4 to 6 weeks [13] (see summary in Table 19.4). This was tapered to once a day for another 4 to 6 weeks to control inflammation and heal any fissures or erosions. Usually, within 6 to 8 weeks of starting clobetasol ointment, the vulvar erosions and fissures would have healed and vulvar pain was reduced so that an internal examination could be done to determine the extent of vaginal involvement. In the absence of vaginal involvement and if the vulva was healed, clobetasol ointment application was tapered to twice or thrice weekly.

If vaginal synechiae were present such that there was profound vaginal scarring or shortening, the use of vaginal dilators of graduated diameters (Syracuse Medical Devices, Fayetteville, NY) was instituted [13]. The patients were instructed to use dilators two to three times a week with a pea-sized amount of clobetasol ointment and a half inch of estrogen cream applied to the tip. If the vagina only had cobweb or small arcuate synechaie, or as soon as it was lengthened with the use of dilators to approximately 5 cm with a similar width (of 5 cm in diameter), a low dose, slow release estradiol vaginal ring (7.5 mcg/24 hours; Pfizer, NY, NY), was inserted. This ring allowed for direct delivery of estrogen to the genital mucosa without the unwanted side effects of systemic estrogen administration and had the advantage of not needing to be replaced for 3 months. By mechanically keeping the vaginal walls opened, it enabled healing and further dissolution of synechiae.

Only three women in the group were on HRT at the time of their first visit [13]. This low rate of estrogen replacement therapy (ERT) was a response to the recent publication of conflicting reports about the risks and benefits of ERT [22, 23], as well as the tendency for transplanters not to consider use of these agents.

Twenty-one of the twenty-nine women in the group had been sexually active until the onset of genital cGVHD [13]. When first evaluated, these 21 women had severe enough dyspareunia to prevent intercourse. Using the regimen described in the preceding text, most of these women were able to resume sexual activity.

As is true for cGVHD in other organs, genital cGVHD had its remissions and exacerbations requiring adjustments in therapy. We noted exacerbations of cGVHD when women were first tapered off immunosuppressive or hormone therapy, after donor lymphocyte infusion (DLI) or with intercurrent viral infection [13].

Like Zantomio [12], we generally were able to avoid surgery in our patients with only one woman in our cohort needing surgical intervention for hematocolpos. She was regularly menstruating and could not be evaluated frequently [13].

TOPICS FOR FUTURE INVESTIGATION

Quality-of-Life Issues

Now that more women are surviving the major organ complications of cGVHD, consideration should be given to restoration of normal sexual health and function, and other aspects of quality of life. As PBSCT becomes the more commonly practiced method for HSCT, vulvovaginal cGVHD might increase in incidence. In a study regarding the quality of life in bone marrow transplant recipients, Chiodi [24] showed that women had significantly poorer scores in the sexual and psychological domains when compared to men. Syrjala et al. recently published a prospective study which evaluated sexual function through 5 years after myeloablative HSCT compared to controls [25]. Rates of sexual function and activity were lower among both male and female survivors compared to controls and women were more severely affected. Our patients have shared their frustration with their inability to resume a normal sexual life even after erosions, fissures, and scarring have cleared. They speak of a lack of interest, a loss of libido, even as they intellectually crave sexual intimacy. The physical changes wrought by vulvovaginal cGVHD combined with premature ovarian failure as well as psychological factors and their interactions are well discussed by Basson [26] as it pertains to chronic illnesses in general.

Human Papilloma Virus Disease

Squamous cell cancers, which include cervical cancer, are the most common second malignancy after HSCT [27]. There have been preliminary reports of a loss of HPV seroreactivity among transplant recipients [28]. Among the women, who are posttransplant, under care at NHLBI, we have recently noted that 40% developed low- or high-grade genital tract squamous intraepithelial lesions, usually years after transplantation [29]. These abnormal cervical cytology results represent HPV disease that does not appear to be newly acquired HPV infection as many are not having intercourse. It is reasonable to hypothesize that a loss of antibody titers and/or T-cell immunity to HPV can cause a recurrence of HPV disease. These observations point to the necessity of including Pap smears in the evaluation of women after transplantation regardless of whether they have cGVHD or not.

The quadrivalent HPV vaccine (GARDASIL®, Merck & Co.) is a noninfectious recombinant vaccine prepared from the highly purified virus-like particles (VLPs) of the major capsid (L1) protein of HPV types 6, 11, 16, and 18 that was licensed for clinical use in young women 12 to 26 years of age in June 2006. Efficacy was assessed in four placebo-controlled, double-blinded, randomized Phase II and III clinical studies involving 2,942 and 17,599 subjects, respectively [30]. The efficacy of GARDASIL® against HPV 16/18-related disease was 100% for CIN 3, or AIS and 100% for VIN 2/3 or VaIN 2/3 and 100% against HPV 6-, 11-, 16-, and 18-related VIN or VaIN 1. However, the immunogenicity of the vaccine in women at risk for HPV-related disease, who have undergone HSCT is unknown. If quadrivalent HPV vaccine can induce immunity in HSCT recipients, it may potentially prevent HPV-related preneoplastic conditions and squamous cell cancer in these patients and perhaps should be considered as part of the vaccines women receive posttransplant.

REFERENCES

1. Higman MA, Vogelsang GB. Chronic graft versus host disease. *Br J Haematol.* 2004;125(4):435–454.
2. Filipovich AH, Weisdorf D, Pavletic S, et al. National Institutes of Health consensus development project on criteria for clinical trials in chronic graft-versus-host disease: I. Diagnosis and staging working group report. *Biol Blood Marrow Transplant.* 2005;11(12):945–956.
3. Shulman HM, Kleiner D, Lee SJ, et al. Histopathologic diagnosis of chronic graft-versus-host disease: National Institutes of Health Consensus Development Project on Criteria for Clinical Trials in Chronic Graft-versus-Host Disease: II. Pathology Working Group Report. *Biol Blood Marrow Transplant.* 2006; 12(1):31–47.
4. Couriel D, Carpenter PA, Cutler C, et al. Ancillary therapy and supportive care of chronic graft-versus-host disease: National Institutes of Health consensus development project on criteria for clinical trials in chronic Graft-versus-host disease: V. Ancillary Therapy and Supportive Care Working Group Report. *Biol Blood Marrow Transplant.* 2006;12(4):375–396.
5. Corson SL, Sullivan K, Batzer F, August C, Storb R, Thomas ED. Gynecologic manifestations of chronic graft-versus-host disease. *Obstet Gynecol.* 1982;60(4):488–492.
6. DeLord C, Treleaven J, Shepherd J, Saso R, Powles RL. Vaginal stenosis following allogeneic bone marrow transplantation for acute myeloid leukaemia. *Bone Marrow Transplant.* 1999;23(5):523–525.
7. Yanai N, Shufaro Y, Or R, Meirow D. Vaginal outflow tract obstruction by graft-versus-host reaction. *Bone Marrow Transplant.* 1999;24(7):811–812.
8. Louis-Sylvestre C, Haddad B, Paniel BJ. Treatment of vaginal outflow tract obstruction in graft-versus-host reaction. *Am J Obstet Gynecol.* 2003;188(4):943–944.
9. Flowers ME, Parker PM, Johnston LJ, et al. Comparison of chronic graft-versus-host disease after transplantation of peripheral blood stem cells versus bone marrow in allogeneic recipients: long-term follow-up of a randomized trial. *Blood.* 2002;100(2):415–419.
10. Spinelli S, Chiodi S, Costantini S, et al. Female genital tract graft-versus-host disease following allogeneic bone marrow transplantation. *Haematologica.* 2003;88(10):1163–1168.
11. Spiryda LB, Laufer MR, Soiffer RJ, Antin JA. Graft-versus-host disease of the vulva and/or vagina: diagnosis and treatment. *Biol Blood Marrow Transplant.* 2003;9(12):760–765.
12. Zantomio D, Grigg AP, Macgregor L, Panek-Hudson Y, Szer J, Ayton R. Female genital tract graft-versus-host disease: incidence, risk factors and recommendations for management. *Bone Marrow Transplant.* 2006;38(8):567–572.
13. Stratton P, Turner ML, Childs R, et al. Vulvovaginal chronic graft-versus-host disease with allogeneic hematopoietic stem cell transplantation. *Obstet Gynecol.* 2007;110(5):1041–1049.

14. Balleari E, Garre S, Van Lint MT, et al. Hormone replacement therapy and chronic graft-versus-host disease activity in women treated with bone marrow transplantation for hematologic malignancies. *Ann N Y Acad Sci.* 2002;966:187–192.

15. Solano C, Martinez C, Brunet S, et al. Chronic graft-versus-host disease after allogeneic peripheral blood progenitor cell or bone marrow transplantation from matched related donors. A case-control study. Spanish Group of Allo-PBT. *Bone Marrow Transplant.* 1998;22(12):1129–1135.

16. Cutler C, Giri S, Jeyapalan S, Paniagua D, Viswanathan A, Antin JH. Acute and chronic graft-versus-host disease after allogeneic peripheral-blood stem-cell and bone marrow transplantation: a meta-analysis. *J Clin Oncol.* 2001;19(16):3685–3691.

17. Marinoff SC, Turner ML. Vulvar vestibulitis syndrome. *Dermatol Clin.* 1992;10(2):435–444.

18. Norian JM, Stratton P. Labial fusion: a rare complication of chronic graft versus host disease. *Obstet Gynecol.* Aug 2008;112(2):437–439.

19. Hayes EC, Rock JA. Treatment of vaginal agglutination associated with chronic graft-versus-host disease. *Fertil Steril.* 2002;78(5):1125–1126.

20. Anguenot JL, Ibecheole V, Helg C, Piacenza JM, Dumps P, Bonnefoi H. Vaginal stenosis with hematocolpometra, complicating chronic graft versus host disease. *Eur J Obstet Gynecol Reprod Biol.* 2002;103(2):185–187.

21. Cooper SM, Wojnarowska F. Influence of treatment of erosive lichen planus of the vulva on its prognosis. *Arch Dermatol.* 2006;142(3):289–294.

22. Rossouw JE, Anderson GL, Prentice RL, et al. Risks and benefits of estrogen plus progestin in healthy postmenopausal women: principal results From the Women's Health Initiative randomized controlled trial. *JAMA.* 2002;288(3):321–333.

23. Barrett-Connor E, Grady D, Stefanick ML. The rise and fall of menopausal hormone therapy. *Annu Rev Public Health.* 2005;26:115–140.

24. Chiodi S, Spinelli S, Ravera G, et al. Quality of life in 244 recipients of allogeneic bone marrow transplantation. *Br J Haematol.* 2000;110(3):614–619.

25. Syrjala KL, Kurland BF, Abrams JR, Sanders JE, Heiman JR. Sexual function changes over the 5 years after high dose treatment and hematopoietic cell transplantation for malignancy, with case-matched controls at 5 years. *Blood.* Feb 1 2008;111(3):989–996.

26. Basson R, Schultz WW. Sexual sequelae of general medical disorders. *Lancet.* 2007;369(9559):409–424.

27. Leisenring W, Friedman DL, Flowers ME, Schwartz JL, Deeg HJ. Nonmelanoma skin and mucosal cancers after hematopoietic cell transplantation. *J Clin Oncol.* 2006;24(7):1119–1126.

28. Lewensohn-Fuchs I, Ljungman P, Kjerrstrom A, Ringden O, Dalianis T. Loss of seroreactivity against human papillomavirus (HPV) in bone marrow transplant recipients. *Bone Marrow Transplant.* 1996;18(2):333–337.

29. Savani BN, Stratton P, Shenoy A, et al. Increased risk of cervical dysplasia in long term survivors of allogeneic stem cell transplantation––implications for screening and HPV vaccination. *Biol Blood Marrow Transplant.* Sep 2008;14(9):1072–1075.

30. Ault KA. Effect of prophylactic human papillomavirus L1 virus-like-particle vaccine on risk of cervical intraepithelial neoplasia grade 2, grade 3, and adenocarcinoma in situ: a combined analysis of four randomised clinical trials. *Lancet.* 2007;369(9576):1861–1868.

20

Gastrointestinal and Hepatic Manifestations of Chronic Graft versus Host Disease

Miwa Sakai and George B. McDonald

INTRODUCTION

Gastrointestinal and hepatobiliary problems are extremely common in patients with signs and symptoms of chronic GVHD elsewhere in the body, but only esophageal desquamation, webs, and submucosal fibrosis leading to strictures in the upper third of the esophagus are considered diagnostic of cGVHD per se [1]. While a strict definition of what constitutes cGVHD is useful for research purposes, these distinctions are lost on patients whose lives are made miserable by dysphagia, persistent anorexia, nausea, vomiting, diarrhea, abdominal pain, and weight loss. This chapter reviews gastrointestinal and hepatobiliary problems in long-term survivors of allogeneic hematopoietic cell transplant according to causes of these problems (cGVHD-related, infection-related, or related to other disease processes). These categories of causes of symptoms are not mutually exclusive, as transplant survivors with gastrointestinal problems may have multiple disease processes at any one time.

ESOPHAGEAL COMPLICATIONS

Incidence

The incidence of esophageal involvement in patients with cGVHD is not known, as only patients who have esophageal symptoms undergo endoscopy. In the era of before cyclosporine, about 13% of patients with extensive chronic GVHD complained of esophageal symptoms [2, 3]. In some cases, esophageal cGVHD is a disease of medical neglect, or, more accurately, of undertreatment of an ongoing mucosal inflammatory process by physicians unfamiliar with cGVHD.

Acknowledgements: Our research in the field of gastrointestinal and hepatobiliary complications of hematopoietic cell transplant is supported by grants from the U.S. National Institutes of Health, National Cancer Institute (CA 18029, CA 15704). Dr. Sakai is supported by funding from the Bureau of Social Welfare and Public Health of the Tokyo Metropolitan Government and the Japan Clinical Research Support Unit.

Presentation

The most common symptom is dysphagia, particularly for solid food and pills. Some patients present with insidious weight loss, retrosternal pain and aspiration of gastric contents, leading to pulmonary disease that can be mistaken for GVHD-related bronchiolitis obliterans syndromes. Esophageal symptoms may not be obvious, especially in children, in whom a common presentation is weight loss and failure to thrive. Some patients fail to mention dysphagia, believing that mouth pain and poor dentition are responsible for their swallowing difficulty. Poor dentition often leads to inadequately chewed food boluses and severe symptoms if there is esophageal narrowing. In most patients, esophageal involvement occurs in the setting of extensive cGVHD, but in others, oropharyngeal GVHD with isolated esophageal involvement can be seen, without other manifestations. Whether or not they have extensive cGVHD, almost all patients with esophageal cGVHD have oropharyngeal cGVHD.

Esophageal dysfunction may contribute to pulmonary disease in some patients; new-onset air flow obstruction may develop in up to one third of the patients who develop cGVHD [4]. In some patients, aspiration is the primary cause of reactive airway disease. The mechanisms by which esophageal cGVHD may lead to pulmonary problems are aspiration of food and liquid and the reflux of gastric contents because of lack of secondary peristalsis (inability to clear material refluxed into the esophagus) [2]. Myasthenia gravis may also complicate cGVHD, with dysphagia as its presenting complaint, in the absence of esophageal mucosal inflammation [5].

Significance for prognosis

The longer the period of neglect and delay in recognizing esophageal involvement with cGVHD, the worse the submucosal fibrosis in the esophagus and the more difficult the management. The overall prognosis is worse in patients with extensive cGVHD than in those with cGVHD involving only oropharyngeal and esophageal mucosa.

Diagnosis

The diagnosis is made by barium contrast Xray and endoscopy, which should be done with caution, as perforations have been reported [2]. Radiologic findings include bullae, webs, concentric rings, narrowings, strictures, and aperistalsis (Figures 20.1 and 20.2) [3, 6, 7].

The typical desquamation of esophageal epithelium in cGVHD (Figures 20.3A, 3B, and 4B) generally goes undetected at Xray, particularly when the desquamation is a very shallow epithelial peeling.

In other patients, sloughed mucosa hangs in shreds into the lumen, visible to the radiologist as a web or a fibrous shelf at the level of the cricopharyngeus (Figure 20.1) [2, 3, 7]. Upper esophageal rings are also associated with epithelial desquamation; by x-ray, these rings are symmetrical and short. Long, tapering strictures in the proximal and midesophagus are better seen by x-ray than by endoscopy (Figure 20.2). The distal esophagus is generally spared, although some patients have distal esophagitis and esophageal strictures related to acid peptic reflux. Esophagrams are useful for identifying structural abnormalities that might cause problems during endoscopy, such as narrow strictures near the esophageal inlet, a risk factor for perforation.

Endosopic findings include bullae, desquamation of the epithelium (desquamative esophagitis – reddened, friable, and peeled mucosa, very similar to a second degree burn of the skin), upper esophageal webs, ring-like narrowings, and tapering strictures (Figure 20.3) [2]. Histologic findings in endoscopic biopsy specimens include infiltration of the esophageal mucosa with lymphocytes, neutrophils and eosinophils, necrosis of individual squamous cells in the basal layer, and desquamation of the superficial epithelium (Figure 20.4).

These changes are analogous to the findings of cGVHD in skin and oral mucosa. The desquamation, webs, and strictures in human cGVHD are similar to the changes described in the autoimmune diseases pemphigoid and dystrophic epidermolysis bullosa.

There is a wide differential diagnosis of esophageal symptoms in long term survivors (Table 21.1). Sporadic cases of fungal and rarely viral esophagitis may occur in patients with cGVHD who are receiving immunosuppressive or antibiotic therapy. These opportunistic infections of the esophagus are rarely seen in patients receiving continuous prophylaxis against infection caused by fungus or herpesviruses. Infectious causes for esophageal symptoms should be considered when risk factors are present, for example, severe cGVHD, high-dose immunosuppressive treatment, or lack of antimicrobial prophylaxis. Esophageal strictures may also be sequelae of any kind of prior inflammation, for example, earlier herpesvirus infection, severe mucositis involving the esophagus, or chronic reflux of gastric contents. In patients with sicca syndrome due to oral cGVHD, poor saliva production may make swallowing difficult and contribute to esophagitis because of a lack of salivary bicarbonate for acid neutralization. In series of secondary cancers developing late after hematopoietic cell transplant, squamous cell carcinoma of the esophagus has

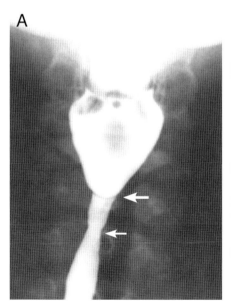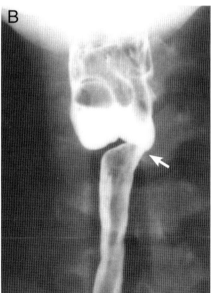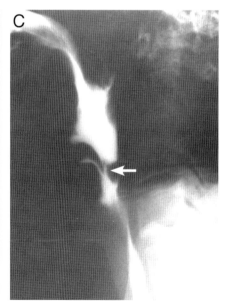

Figure 20.1 Barium contrast x-ray manifestations of chronic GVHD of the esophagus: Webs and rings.
A: x-ray of the upper esophagus, anterior view, showing a thin web (upper arrow) above a ring-like narrowing (lower arrow), from a patient at day 148 after allogeneic transplant. The web was confluent with epithelial desquamation and was easily broken with the passage of the endoscope.
B: x-ray of the hypopharynx and upper esophagus, anterior view, showing a thick, eccentric web distorting the esophageal inlet (arrow), from a patient with extensive cGVHD 770 days after allogeneic transplant.
C: x-ray of the hypopharynx and upper esophagus from the same patient as in Figure 20.1B, two years later. Lateral view, showing that the esophageal inlet had narrowed to a thread-like lumen (arrow).

Table 20.1: Causes of Esophageal Symptoms in Long-Term Transplant Survivors

Chronic GVHD	Infection	Other Causes
Transfer dysphagia (oropharyngeal cGVHD)	Fungal (usually Candida sp.)	Acid-peptic esophagitis
Esophageal webs, concentric rings	Viral (CMV, HSV, rarely VZV)	Strictures (peptic, post-infectious)
Submucosal fibrosis with longitudinal strictures of esophagus		Barrett's columnar lined esophagus with stricture or ulcer
Poor dentition		Pill esophagitis
Xerostomia		Carcinoma (squamous cell > adenocarcinoma)
Esophageal aperistalsis		
Myasthenia gravis		

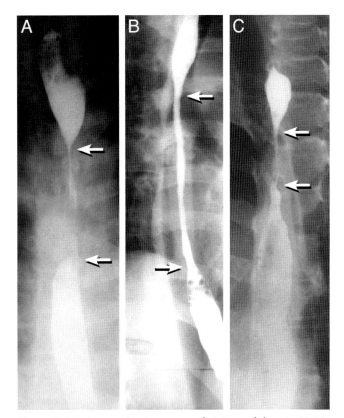

Figure 20.2 Barium contrast x-ray manifestations of chronic GVHD of the esophagus: Strictures.

A: x-ray showing a 5 cm. long, very narrow stricture in the upper to mid esopohagus (arrows), in a patient with extensive cGVHD and severe dysphagia at 383 days after allogeneic transplant.

B: x-ray from the same patient as in 2A, a year later, following immunosuppressive therapy and repeated esophageal dilations. Although the luminal diameter is wider than at baseline, the stricture is now ~10 cm. in length, extending from the upper to the lower third of the esophagus (arrows).

C: x-ray showing a 3 cm. long, very narrow stricture (arrows) limited to the upper third of the esophagus, with a dilated esophageal lumen below the stricture.

been reported, usually in patients with concomitant cGVHD of the oropharynx [8].

Site-Specific Therapy

Patients with extensive cGVHD need systemic immunosuppressive therapy. However, when the inflammatory component is under control, submucosal esophageal fibrosis may lead to abnormal peristalsis, luminal narrowing and persistent symptoms. Esophageal strictures and webs may require endoscopic dilation concomitantly with immunosuppressive therapy to avoid progressive luminal narrowing, but dilations must be done with extreme care, as the perforation risk is higher than with peptic strictures [2]. Diaphanous webs can be easily disrupted by either an endoscope or a dilator, but tight strictures are difficult to dilate safely. Our practice is to dilate with Savary dilators over a fluoroscopically-placed guidewire. Failure to dilate strictures may lead to progressive esophageal narrowing and require a feeding gastrostomy. If extensive submucosal fibrosis persists, rings and tapering strictures may require repeated dilation, in spite of improvement in other organs involved with cGVHD. A fibrotic, stenotic esophagus that cannot be dilated may require esophagectomy and interposition surgery. Therapy with a proton pump inhibitor given twice daily should be considered in patients with esophageal cGVHD, as there is usually uncontrolled acid reflux into an esophagus unprotected by salivary bicarbonate secretion or normal esophageal peristalsis. Night-time oral antacid therapy and head-of-bed elevation (in the reverse Trendelenberg position) are useful additional measures for treating esophagitis, severe retrosternal pain, or recurrent aspiration of gastric contents.

Prevention

It is possible that esophageal involvement can be prevented by prompt treatment of cGVHD at its early stages, but this is an inferential hypothesis, based on the certainty that neglect of

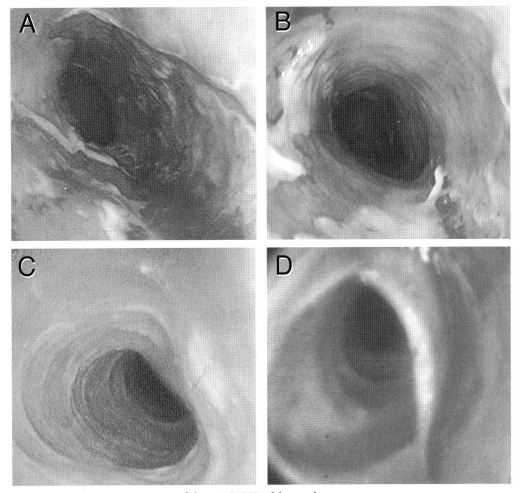

Figure 20.3 Endoscopic appearance of chronic GVHD of the esophagus.

A and B: Upper third of the esophagus, showing exposed submucosa (red areas) adjacent to desquamating squamous epithelium (pale areas). When touched with the biopsy forceps, the epithelial layer peeled away from the underlying submucosa.

C: Middle third of the esophagus, showing multiple ring-like narrowings; epithelium in the upper third of the esophagus, above the rings, was friable.

D: A nearly circumferential web just below the cricopharyngeal inlet to the esophagus, composed of desquamated epithelium. Although some webs in patients with chronic GVHD are wispy and easily broken with the endoscope, this web was thick and firmly attached to the underlying submucosa. See Plate 67 in the color plate section.

cGVHD will lead to intractable esophageal disease. Patients whose esophagus is affected by a submucosal fibrotic process from cGVHD appear to have better outcomes if they undergo serial esophageal dilations as the inflammatory component is brought under control, rather than having to dilate the end-result of esophageal stricturing later.

Future Advances

Topical glucocorticoid therapy is effective for oral [9, 10] and gastrointestinal [11–15] GVHD, and may be effective for esophageal involvement if a formulation can be developed that achieves increased contact time with upper esophageal mucosa. Topical glucocorticoid medications appear to be effective in eosinophilic esophagitis, another inflammatory mucosal process [16].

STOMACH, SMALL INTESTINE, AND COLON DISORDERS

Incidence

The frequency of nausea, anorexia, and diarrhea among patients with typical cGVHD elsewhere is very common, but on closer examination, the endoscopic, histologic, and clinical findings are identical to those of acute GVHD [17, 18]. In some long-term survivors, gastrointestinal symptoms resulting from this type of protracted aGVHD can occur in isolation, without

Table 20.2: Causes of Anorexia, Nausea, or Vomiting in Long-Term Transplant Survivors

Chronic GVHD	Infection	Other Causes
Rare	CMV, HSV, VZV disease *H. pylori* infection Fungal infection (*Candida,* *Zygomyces*) *Giardia, Cryptosporidia* infection	Protracted acute gastrointestinal GVHD Gastrointestinal dysmotility Drug side effect Secondary adrenal insufficiency Inflammatory bowel disease Celiac sprue

Table 20.3: Causes of Diarrhea and in Long-Term Transplant Survivors

Chronic GVHD	Infection	Other Causes
Pancreatic insufficiency	Viral enteritis (CMV, *Rotavirus,* *Norovirus, Adenovirus*) Clostridial colitis (*C.difficile,* *C.septicum*) Giardiasis Cryptosporidia	Protracted gastrointestinal aGVHD Drug effect (MMF colitis, antibiotic associated disease, tacrolimus, metoclopramide, Mg^{++} salts) Disaccharide malabsorption

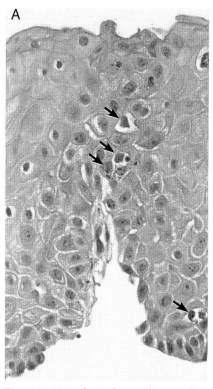
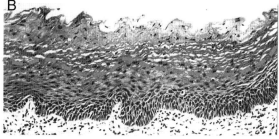

Figure 20.4 Histologic abnormalities in chronic GVHD involving the esophagus.
A: Photomicrograph of esophageal mucosa, showing multiple apoptotic epithelial cells within the basal layer (arrows). (Hematoxylin and eosin; photomicrograph courtesy of KR Loeb)
B: Photomicrograph of esophageal mucosa, showing desquamation of squamous cells (area superior to the dotted line best seen in the color plate). At endoscopy, the esophageal epithelium peeled away when touched with a biopsy forceps. (Hematoxylin and eosin; photomicrograph courtesy of HM Shulman). See Plate 68 in the color plate section.

manifestations of cGVHD, for up to 15 years after allogeneic HCT. Thus, while gastrointestinal GVHD in long-term survivors may not qualify as a typical component of cGVHD, gastrointestinal symptoms of protracted aGVHD are frequently intertwined with those of typical cGVHD [1].

There is one distinctive manifestation of cGVHD involving the intestine that is parallel to esophageal cGVHD, that is, a mucosal inflammatory process in the small intestine and colon that leads to submucosal fibrosis, a form of cGVHD that has become rare. Before the advent of calcineurin inhibitor therapy, and before the natural history of cGVHD was understood, a syndrome of diarrhea, abdominal distention, and severe malabsorption was seen in patients with uncontrolled cGVHD. The histologic appearance of the gastrointestinal tract was that of extensive submucosal and subserosal fibrosis (Figure 20.5) [19].

Severe segmental fibrosis and small intestinal strictures may also be seen in patients with severe aGVHD that has not healed [20].

Presentation

For most long term survivors, gastrointestinal symptoms of satiety, poor appetite, nausea, episodic diarrhea, and weight loss are manifestations of either protracted aGVHD [17, 18, 1] or other gastrointestinal diseases (see Tables 21.2 and 21.3) [21]. Symptoms of protracted aGVHD can be seen as long as 10 to 15 years after transplant. Manifestations of acute gastrointestinal GVHD may present after day 100, particularly after reduced intensity conditioning regimens [22]. There are also patients whose severe aGVHD has not resolved and who remain symptomatic for over 100–200 days [23]; these patients seldom survive long-term because they require continued high-level immunosuppression [24].

Significance for prognosis

For long-term survivors with gastrointestinal symptoms, prognosis depends on a) whether cGVHD is present elsewhere; b) whether GVHD per se is responsible for gastrointestinal symptoms; and c) what doses of immune suppressive drugs are needed to control symptoms. Patients with protracted aGVHD often have less severe symptoms that tend to wax and wane with intensity of immunosuppressive therapy and rarely lead to mucosal necrosis and ulceration.

There is a wide differential diagnosis for anorexia/nausea and diarrhea, such that an inflammatory GVHD process may co-exist with another cause of diarrhea, for example, carbohydrate malabsorption related to down-regulation of small intestinal disaccharidases (lactase, sucrase-isomaltase) or malabsorption of bile salts. If symptoms can be controlled by use of lactase in milk without having to resort to chronic immunosuppressive drugs, the prognosis is usually good. If gastrointestinal symptoms can be controlled only by ongoing immunosuppression, the prognosis is worse. Over-treatment of mild GVHD symptoms may carry a greater risk than the underlying inflammatory

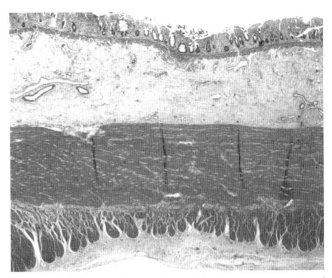

Figure 20.5. **Submucosal and subserosal fibrosis of the intestine of a patient with untreated chronic GVHD.** Full thickness section of colon taken at autopsy from a patient who died of extensive chronic GVHD 458 days after allogeneic marrow transplant during the 1970s. There was extensive submucosal and subserosal fibrosis (pale bluish stain) from the stomach through the colon; symptoms included intractable diarrhea, steatorrhea, and abdominal pain. (Masson trichrome; photomicrograph courtesy of HM Shulman). See Plate 69 in the color plate section.

process. When new gastrointestinal symptoms appear during immunosuppressive therapy, reexamination of the differential diagnosis should be done. The prognosis of patients with severe aGVHD beyond day 100 is very poor.

Diagnosis

Diagnosis of cGVHD with submucosal intestinal fibrosis is rarely made now, as this entity is rare, and full-thickness biopsies may be needed to document the pathology (Figure 20.5) [19]. Histologic findings include submucosal and subserosal fibrosis, significant mucosal architectural crypt distortion, and increased lymphocyte/plasma cell infiltration in the lamina propria.

Endoscopic and histologic findings in patients with protracted aGVHD are identical to those of aGVHD before day 100, that is, mucosal edema and erythema, histologic evidence of epithelial single cell necrosis (apoptosis), and reactive epithelial changes or loss of crypt epithelium [25]. Endoscopic and histologic findings are complementary; the predictive value of negative histology for GVHD is not high, as the pathologist cannot readily see the mucosal edema so apparent to the endoscopist. There are sporadic cases of infections caused by *C. difficile*, Cytomegalovirus, *H. pylori*, and rarely Giardia and Cryptosporidia in long-term survivors. Rarely, chronic intestinal viral infection can be seen in patients who remain on immunosuppressive drugs, for example, Rotavirus, Norovirus, and Adenovirus. Secondary adrenal insufficiency due to glucocorticoid use sometimes causes anorexia, nausea, vomiting and weight loss; this diagnosis should be considered if patient develops upper gastrointestinal symptoms and general fatigue after discontinuation of a glucocorticoid (including oral beclomethasone dipropionate or budesonide). Mycophenolate mofetil may cause gastrointestinal toxicity, usually manifest as diarrhea and colon ulcerations, with apoptotic crypt cells indistinguishable from the histology of aGVHD [26, 27]. In a patient with intestinal symptoms whose immunosppressive drug regimen includes MMF, it may be difficult to make a diagnosis of GVHD until MMF has been discontinued. Another approach is to switch to enteric-coated mycophenolate sodium which has significantly less gut toxicity than MMF [27]. Rare cases of "transmission" of intestinal disease via donor T cells have been reported, for example, inflammatory bowel disease and celiac sprue [28]. In the intestine affected by protracted aGVHD, not all symptoms that result from the inflammatory process are a result of mucosal necrosis or ulceration. For example, mucosal inflammation may lead to the suppression of intestinal disaccharidases and malabsorption of bile salts, leading to osmotic and bile salt diarrhea, respectively.

Site-Specific Therapy

Two randomized trial of oral beclomethasone dipropionate (BDP) have shown that topical glucocorticoid therapy can control the inflammatory activity of aGVHD without prolonged exposure to prednisone, resulting in better outcomes [11, 15]. Long-term use of oral BDP has been reported to be effective in patients with protracted aGVHD [12]. However, topical glucocorticoids such as BDP and enteric-coated budesonide can lead to suppression of the hypothalamic-pituitary-adrenal axis, particularly in children, and the long-term effects of topical glucocorticoid therapy in treating protracted aGVHD are not known. However, oral budesonide has been given at 9 mg/day for 2–3 years without serious adverse events, in a patient population with primary biliary cirrhosis, suggesting a level of safety for this approach [29, 30].

Prevention

Prompt treatment of severe aGVHD will reduce the risk of GVHD-related mucosal necrosis and submucosal fibrosis in the small intestine and colon, now a rarity. We know of no method to prevent protracted aGVHD involving the gastrointestinal tract other than with continuous exposure to immunosuppressive drugs.

Future Advances

Topical glucocorticoid therapy with beclomethasone dipropionate, while effective for acute gastrointestinal GVHD [11, 15] and useful for protracted acute GVHD [12] has never been studied in properly-stratified, dose-finding protocols in long-term survivors with gastrointestinal GVHD. One might also envision protocols that direct oral topical glucocorticoids (beclomethasone dipropionate, budesonide) to the upper gut when symptoms of satiety, nausea, and anorexia dominate, and to the small intestine and colon, when diarrhea is present. Oral topical glucocorticoids hold promise as prednisone-sparing

agents in patients with protracted aGVHD, but optimal doses and formulations remain to be determined.

LIVER DISEASES

Incidence

It is difficult to estimate the incidence of GVHD involving the liver in long-term survivors, as non-specific elevation of serum ALT and alkaline phosphatase is very common and liver biopsies confirming GVHD are not always available. Long-term survivors with histologic evidence of GVHD in the liver usually have features of cGVHD elsewhere in the body. Evidence of cholestasis (elevated alkaline phosphatase (AP) and gamma glutamyl transpeptidase (GGT), usually without pruritus) is present in approximately 80% of patients with extensive cGVHD [31, 32]. Bile duct damage in a transplant survivor is not considered to be diagnostic of cGVHD, but rather a manifestation of protracted aGVHD, similar to protracted aGVHD in the gastrointestinal tract.

Presentation

Patients with cGVHD elsewhere may have three manifestations of liver involvement. 1) Asymptomatic elevation of serum ALT, AP, and GGT as isolated laboratory abnormalities, in the absence of jaundice. 2) Slowly progressive cholestatic jaundice, that is, hyperbilirubinemia often associated with elevated serum AP, a result of damage to small bile ducts. Elevations of AP and GGT usually precede the development of jaundice. 3) Acute hepatocellular injury (hepatitic GVHD), that is, abrupt elevations of serum ALT to over 500 U/L without preceding hepatic dysfunction [33–35]. This presentation tends to occur especially in the setting of tapering immunosuppressive therapy, or donor lymphocyte infusion. Long-term survivors who are infected with hepatitis C virus may also be at risk for liver GVHD, making the attribution of elevations in serum ALT difficult; about a third of HCV-infected transplant survivors will progress to cirrhosis and end-stage liver disease over a 20–35 year time period [36, 37, 38]. There are sporadic case-reports of chronic hepatic GVHD leading to liver failure, but this is an uncommon event.

Significance for Prognosis

Extensive cGVHD carries a poor prognosis, with most deaths resulting from infection, multi-organ failure and recurrent or secondary malignancy. Although patients may become deeply jaundiced, death from hepatic failure is generally rare. Patients with isolated elevations of AP in the absence of jaundice should be followed closely, but may not require extended doses of high-dose immunosuppressive therapy. However, for patients with jaundice secondary to destruction of small bile ducts by GVHD, or those with an acute hepatitic presentation of GVHD, delay in starting immunosuppressive therapy may lead to fatality [33].

Diagnosis

Because of many possible alternative diagnoses, liver biopsy is required to confirm hepatic GVHD in patients with cGVHD elsewhere, particularly if a decision about the intensity and duration of immunosuppressive therapy hinges on proving liver involvement. The decision to biopsy the liver is also dependent on the severity of the liver disease.

1) Patients with asymptomatic elevations of serum ALT, AP, and GGT should be evaluated for other causes of elevated enzymes. If none are apparent, one is left with the questions of whether a biopsy is indicated to identify GVHD as a cause and whether immunosuppressive drug therapy would be given. These questions are moot if a patient has cGVHD elsewhere. While elevated ALT, AP, and GGT may presage destructive damage to small bile ducts and ductules, immunosuppressive therapy (and thus, liver biopsy) are not usually indicated when stable, minor elevation of serum enzymes is the only finding.

2) Patients with jaundice without a proven cause should undergo liver biopsy, as jaundice is a poor prognostic sign whether associated with GVHD or not [39]. In long-term survivors, the differential diagnosis is narrower than it is before day 100, but there is an imperative for immediate treatment according to cause. Early treatment of hepatitic GVHD is important to prevent extensive ductular damage [33]. Histological findings include lymphocytic infiltration in and around small bile ducts, extensive damage to, and loss of, small bile duct epithelial cells, cholestasis, portal fibrosis and piecemeal necrosis [40]. The differential diagnosis of cholestatic jaundice includes biliary obstruction and drug-induced liver injury (DILI). Iron overload has been reported to mimic GVHD [32, 41].

3) Patients who present with an acute hepatitis, that is, steeply rising serum ALT with or without jaundice, present a differential diagnosis of viral infection, DILI, and hepatitic GVHD and thus, require urgent evaluation. Hepatic histology is usually needed to confirm the diagnosis of GVHD and exclude other etiologies. Histological findings of GVHD are lobular hepatitis, portal inflammation, and damage to small bile ducts [33, 40] (Figures 9.1–9.18). A serum autoantibody test for CYP1A2 may prove useful in the diagnosis of hepatic GVHD, as this enzyme appears to be a target antigen in GVHD [42]. Serological testing is also essential to exclude acute viral hepatitis due to a herpesvirus (HSV or VZV) or a hepatitis virus (Hepatitis A-E). Acyclovir should be started pending in case of results of viral tests, and if negative, treatment with a calcineurin inhibitor and prednisone 1–2 mg/kg/day should begun.

The differential diagnosis of liver disease in a transplant survivor includes viral infection, DILI, iron overload, recurrent malignancy, nodular regenerative hyperplasia, focal nodular hyperplasia, and cirrhosis, but these disorders may also co-exist with GVHD. Hepatitis C virus infection in survivors almost always results in chronic hepatitis. In the first 10 years of HCV infection after HCT, there is little liver-related morbidity [32, 43, 44] but there may then be rapid progression of necroinflammatory and fibrotic changes from 10 to 30 years after transplant [36–38]. The prevalence of chronic HBV infection among survivors varies widely depending on the country. The serologic pattern of HBV infection may be atypical in HCT survivors, probably as a consequence of immunosuppression. Clearance of surface antigenemia may be observed and is particularly likely if the donor was anti-HBs positive because of prior HBV infection [45]. Patients who remain HBsAg positive after HCT are at risk of flares of hepatitis activity particularly at times of reduction of immunosuppression, such as during taper of cessation of treatment for cGVHD. Newer agents, such as rituximab and alemtuzumab, have a particularly high risk of reactivation or latent hepatitis B (HBsAg negative, anti-HBc positive) [46–50]. Careful monitoring of HBV DNA levels on therapy and early introduction of an antiviral drug (lamivudine, entecavir) is strongly recommended. DILI may be related to antihypertensive drugs, lipid lowering agents, hypoglycemic agents, nonsteroidal anti-inflammatory drugs, antidepressants, antibiotics, or herbal preparations. Some drug reactions may result in chronic liver disease. Iron overload may be an important co-factor in liver disease in long-term survivors and should be part of a screening panel. Iron overload is particularly severe in thalassemic patients who have undergone HCT [51, 52]. Iron overload is caused by a combination of multiple red cell transfusions and dyserythropoiesis leading to aberrant hepcidin regulation and increased iron transport by the intestine. After HCT, iron accumulation stops and body iron stores fall slowly over time [53]. Clinically significant iron overload is usually only present when serum ferritin levels are over 1000 μg/dL. An elevated serum ferritin level, particularly in patients with cGVHD, chronic viral hepatitis or other causes of liver disease, may not reflect tissue iron stores and thus, it may be important to document the degree of tissue iron overload. In the past, liver biopsy with liver iron determination was required, however increasingly non-invasive methods (e.g. magnetic resonance imaging, Ferriscan®) are being utilized to provide assessments of liver iron concentration and distribution [54]. The consequences of extreme iron overload in HCT survivors are primarily those of cardiac, pituitary, and pancreatic endocrine dysfunction. Mobilization of iron from heavily overloaded patients improves cardiac function, normalizes serum ALT levels, and results in improved liver histology [55, 56]. Iron overload may also be a cause of persistent hepatic dysfunction after HCT that responds to iron mobilization [32, 41, 57–59]. Fungal abscesses can recur after apparently successful antifungal therapy, when high-dose immunosuppressive drugs are started for GVHD. Non-sterile herbal remedies contaminated by molds may lead to liver abscesses in immunosuppressed HCT survivors [60].

Table 20.4: Causes of Hyperbilirubinemia, Elevations of Serum Alt and Alkaline Phosphatase, or Portal Hypertension in Long-Term Transplant Survivors

Chronic GVHD	Infection	Other Causes
Elevation of serum aminotransferase enzymes [64]	Chronic viral hepatitis (HBV, HCV)	Iron overload
Elevation of serum alkaline phosphatase, gamma glutamyl transpeptidase	Fungal abcess	Drug-induced liver injury (DILI)
Cholestatic liver disease	VZV hepatitis	Gallstones, sludge, common duct obstruction
Acute hepatitic presentation of GVHD		Nodular regenerative hyperplasia
		Focal nodular hyperplasia
		Hepatocellular carcinoma
		Cirrhosis

Cirrhosis of the liver related to chronic HCV infection is rising in frequency among patients transplanted before the 1990s. The reasons for more rapid fibrosis progression after HCT are unclear, but may be related to extensive viral replication during immune suppression, concomitant liver involvement with GVHD, and iron overload [36–38]. Clues to the presence of cirrhosis include a switch in the normal ratio of serum aminotransferases so that AST is higher than ALT, thrombocytopenia, and hepatic nodularity and splenomegaly on imaging, although some of these features may not relate to liver disease in HCT survivors. Compared to the general population, patients who survive over 10 years post-HCT have an 8-fold risk of developing a new solid malignancy [61]. Because of the increased rate of chronic viral hepatitis, particularly hepatitis C, among patients transplanted before 1992, the risk of hepatocellular carcinoma is particularly elevated in survivors from this era [62]. Transplant survivors with specific risk factors for hepatocellular carcinoma (HCV or HBV infection, obesity, diabetes, low platelet count) should be screened at yearly intervals [63]. Focal nodular hyperplasia, a common finding on liver imaging in transplant survivors, should not be confused with hepatocellular carcinoma, a less common lesion [64].

Site-Specific Therapy

The addition of ursodeoxycholic acid (UDCA) (12–15 mg/kg/day) to the immunosuppressive regimen results in significant biochemical improvement in patients with cGVHD involving the liver [65]. The long-term use of UDCA is safe and well tolerated and should be considered for long-term transplant survivors with cholestatic liver injury [66, 67]. It is possible that oral beclomethasone dipropionate or budesonide could be used site-specific therapy for hepatic cGVHD, as ~30% of these topical glucocortoids reach the portal circulation [68] and thus, the liver; this approach to other inflammatory liver diseases has been reported to be effective [30]. Liver transplantation, including living-donor transplantation from the original hematopoietic cell donor, has been performed patients with refractory cholestasis due to GVHD [69, 70].

Prevention

The three common manifestations of GVHD involving the liver in patients with cGVHD (Table 4) include one with little clinical import (isolated elevations of serum liver enzymes) and two associated with jaundice, destruction of small bile duct epithelium, and potentially poor outcomes. Pre-emptive therapy of systemic manifestations of cGVHD is likely effective in minimizing the extent of bile duct destruction and hepatic inflammation, but it is especially important to monitor serum ALT and bilirubin levels frequently during tapering and discontinuation of immunosuppressive drug therapy and following DLI, particularly if there has been hepatic involvement with aGVHD. While the differential diagnosis of an acute hepatitis in a long-term transplant survivor includes viral infection and drug-induced liver injury, there should be a sense of urgency in evaluation, as delays in instituting immunosuppressive therapy for hepatitic GVHD may lead to poor outcomes [33].

Future Advances

Considerable hepatology research is focused on the inflammatory and fibrosis processes, fields that are likely to impact liver GVHD. The use of UDCA as prophylaxis of cholestatic liver injury after HCT has had a profound impact on the frequency of clinical jaundice, and should be considered for long-term use in patients with ongoing liver GVHD. Newer, more potent drugs with similar mechanism of action may supplant UDCA.

GALLBLADDER AND BILIARY PROBLEMS

There are no gallbladder manifestations of cGVHD, but long-term survivors appear to have an increased incidence of gallstones and gallstone complications in the years following transplant. The pathogenesis of gallstones in this setting likely relates to the nearly universal formation of calcium bilirubinate microliths (biliary sludge) in the gallbladder in the weeks following myeloablative conditioning therapy [71]. Biliary sludge is found by ultrasound in approximately 70% [72] and

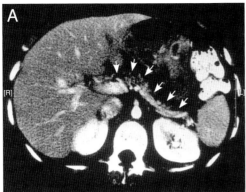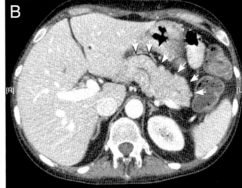

Figure 20.6. Imaging of the abdomen showing pancreatic damage in transplant survivors.
A: Pancreatic atrophy (arrows) in a patient with long-standing extensive chronic GVHD; symptoms of diarrhea and steatorrhea responded to oral pancreatic enzyme supplements.
B: Pancreatic edema (arrows) in a patient with mild protracted acute GVHD involving the gastrointestinal tract, treated with tacrolimus and glucocorticoids. Although serum lipase was elevated, there were no symptoms referable to the pancreas. The cause of pancreatitis was thought to be chronic exposure to tacrolimus.

at autopsy in 100% of HCT patients [71]. These microliths serve as nucleating material for development of gallstones. Cyclosporine has effects on bile composition, decreasing both bile flow and bile salt secretion, which may enhance gallstone formation. Biliary sludge, gall stones, and crystals of calcineurin inhibitor medications may cause cystic duct obstruction, common bile duct obstruction, and acute pancreatitis.

PANCREATIC DISEASES

Incidence

Overt pancreatic disease (either acute pancreatitis or insufficiency) is uncommon in long-term survivors but there is evidence that sub-clinical pancreatic abnormalities are more prevalent. First, there are histologic changes in pancreatic ductular tissue in patients with prolonged GVHD, but it is not clear whether these histologic changes cause either clinical symptoms or pancreatic damage [73, 74]. Second, there is a high frequency of asymptomatic acute pancreatitis that develops during the first 200 days after HCT, related to prolonged GVHD, its treatments (prednisone and calcineurin inhibitors), and possibly to passage of biliary sludge through the ampulla of Vater [75]. Tacrolimus may also cause pancreatitis directly (Figure 20.6B).

Third, the long-term result of persistent pancreatic damage may be fibrosis and atrophy (Figure 20.6A), as pancreatic insufficiency has been noted in a small number of transplant survivors, usually diagnosed because of evidence of fat malabsorption and diarrhea [76–78]. Extreme iron overload may also contribute to pancreatic damage.

Presentation

Pancreatic insufficiency in patients with cGVHD presents with steatorrhea, foul-smelling stools, and weight loss despite adequate caloric intake. Pancreatic enzyme supplement is effective for pancreatic insufficiency but never completely corrects the coefficient of fat absorption.

Significance for Prognosis

Chronic pancreatic atrophy may result from prolonged treatment for GVHD or biliary sludge, but prognosis is more related to the extent and duration of cGVHD.

Diagnosis

Acute pancreatitis is detected by measurement of serum lipase and pancreatic amylase levels, but clinical signs may be absent [75]. Most cases of fat malabsorption caused by pancreatic insufficiency are diagnosed by a finding of excessive fat in stool sample with a qualitative Sudan stain plus a dramatic response to pancreatic replacement therapy. The Sudan stain of a random specimen of stool after adequate fat ingestion is convenient for fecal fat determination. The finding of more than 6 globules per high-power field is considered a positive result. Useful screening tests include measurement of serum trypsinogen (very low levels of serum trypsinogen (<20 ng/mL) are reasonably specific for chronic pancreatitis) and measurement of fecal elastase-1 and chymotrypsin. Pancreatic atrophy is detected by CT or MRI imaging (Figure 20.6A) [78].

Site-Specific Therapy

Oral pancreatic enzymes are the only available treatment for pancreatic insufficiency unless the cause is obstruction of the pancreatic duct in the head of the pancreas. Use of proton pump inhibitor may lessen denaturation of pancreatic lipase in the stomach and thus, increase the effectiveness of oral pancreatic enzymes.

Prevention

Nothing is known about prevention of either acute pancreatitis or pancreatic atrophy in the transplant setting. Detection of subclinical pancreatic damage using serum lipase or imaging tests might be useful in patients who are taking calcineurin inhibitor medication for extended periods of time, as these medications may be a proximate cause of subclinical pancreatic injury (Figure 20.6B).

REFERENCES

1. Filipovich A, Weisdorf D, Pavletic S, et al. National Institutes of health consensus developement project 1on criteria for clinical trials in chronic graft-versus-host disease. I Diagnosis of staging working group report. *Biology of Blood & Marrow Transplantation* 2005;11:945–55.
2. McDonald GB, Sullivan KM, Schuffler MD, Shulman HM, Thomas ED. Esophageal abnormalities in chronic graft-versus-host disease in humans. *Gastroenterology* 1981;80:914–21.
3. McDonald GB, Sullivan KM, Plumley TF. Radiographic features of esophageal involvement in chronic graft-versus-host disease. *Am J Roentgenol* 1984;142:501–6.
4. Chien JW, Martin PJ, Gooley TA, et al. Airflow obstruction after myeloablative allogeneic hematopoietic stem cell transplantation. *American Journal of Respiratory & Critical Care Medicine* 2003;168:208–14.
5. Mackey JR, Desai S, Larratt L, Cwik V, Nabholtz JM. Myasthenia gravis in association with allogeneic bone marrow transplantation: clinical observations, therapeutic implications and review of literature. *Bone Marrow Transplant* 1997;19:939–42.
6. Schima W, Pokieser P, Forstinger C, et al. Videofluoroscopy of the pharynx and esophagus in chronic graft-versus-host disease. *Abdom Imaging* 1994;19:191–4.
7. Minocha A, Mandanas RA, Kida M, Jazzar A. Bullous esophagitis due to chronic graft-versus-host disease. *Am J Gastroenterol* 1997;92:529–30.
8. Shimada K, Yokozawa T, Atsuta Y, et al. Solid tumors after hematopoietic stem cell transplantation in Japan: incidence, risk factors and prognosis. *Bone Marrow Transplantation* 2005;36:115–21.
9. Elad S, Or R, Garfunkel AA, Shapira MY. Budesonide: a novel treatment for oral chronic graft versus host disease. *Oral Surgery Oral Medicine Oral Pathology Oral Radiology & Endodontics* 2003;95:308–11.
10. Sari I, Altuntas F, Kocyigit I, et al. The effect of budesonide mouthwash on oral chronic graft versus host disease. *American Journal of Hematology* 2007;82:349–56.
11. McDonald GB, Bouvier M, Hockenbery DM, et al. Oral beclomethasone dipropionate for treatment of intestinal graft-versus-host disease: a randomized, controlled trial. Gastroenterology 1998;115:28–35.
12. Iyer RV, Hahn T, Roy HN, et al. Long-term use of Oral Beclomethasone Dipropionate for the treatment of gastrointestinal graft-versus-host disease. *Biology of Blood & Marrow Transplantation* 2005;11:587–92.
13. Miura Y, Narimatsu H, Kami M, et al. Oral beclomethasone dipropionate as an initial treatment of gastrointestinal acute graft-versus-host disease after reduced-intensity cord blood transplantation. *Bone Marrow Transplantation* 2006;38:577–9.
14. Castilla C, Perez-Simon JA, Sanchez-Guijo FM, et al. Oral beclomethasone dipropionate for the treatment of gastrointestinal acute graft-versus-host disease (GVHD). *Biology of Blood & Marrow Transplantation* 2006;12:936–41.
15. Hockenbery DM, Cruickshank S, Rodell TC, et al. A randomized, placebo-controlled trial of oral beclomethasone dipropionate as a prenisone-sparing therapy for gastrointestinal graft-versus-host diesease. *Blood* 2007;109:4557–63.
16. Aceves SS, Bastian JF, Newbury RO, Dohil R. Oral viscous budesonide: a potential new therapy for eosinophilic esophagitis in children. *American Journal of Gastroenterology* 2007;102:2271–9.
17. Patey-Mariaud de Serre N, Reijasse D, Verkarre V, et al. Chronic intestinal graft-versus-host disease: clinical, histological and immunohistochemical analysis of 17 children. *Bone Marrow Transplantation* 2002;29:223–30.
18. Akpek G, Chinratanalab W, Lee LA, et al. Gastrointestinal involvement in chronic graft-versus-host disease: a clinicopathologic study. *Biology of Blood & Marrow Transplantation* 2003:46–51.
19. Shulman HM, Sullivan KM, Weiden PL, et al. Chronic graft-versus-host syndrome in man. A long-term clinicopathologic study of 29 Seattle patients. *Am J Med* 1980;69:204–17.
20. Spencer GD, Shulman HM, Myerson D, Thomas ED, McDonald GB. Diffuse intestinal ulceration after marrow transplantation: a clinical-pathological study of 13 patients. *Hum Pathol* 1986;17:621–33.
21. Strasser SI, McDonald GB. Gastrointestinal and hepatic complications. In: Forman SJ, Negrin RS, Blume KG, eds. *Thomas' Hematopoietic Cell Transplantation*. Fourth ed. Oxford, UK, Wiley-Blackwell Publishing, 2009;1434–1455.
22. Mielcarek M, Martin PJ, Leisenring W, et al. Graft-versus-host disease after nonmyeloablative versus conventional hematopoietic stem cell transplantation. *Blood* 2003;102:756–62.
23. Martin PJ, Schoch G, Fisher L, et al. A retrospective analysis of therapy for acute graft-versus-host disease: secondary treatment. *Blood* 1991;77:1821–8.
24. Leisenring W, Martin P, Petersdorf E, et al. An acute graft-versus-host disease activity index to predict survival after hematopoietic cell transplantation with myeloablative conditioning regimens. *Blood* 2006;108:749–55.
25. Ponec RJ, Hackman RC, McDonald GB. Endoscopic and histologic diagnosis of intestinal graft-vs.-host disease after marrow transplantation. *Gastrointest Endosc* 1999;49:612–21.
26. Parfitt JR, Jayakumar S, Driman DK, Mycophenolate mofetil-related gastrointestinal mucosal injury: variable patterns, including graft-versus-host disease-like changes. *Am J Surg Pathol* 2008;32:1367–1372.
27. Hardinger KL, Hebbar S, Bloomer T, Murillo D. Adverse drug reaction driven immunosuppressive drug manipulations: a single-center comparison of enteric-coated mycophenolate sodium vs. mycophenolate mofetil. *Clin Transplant* 2008;22:555–561.
28. Borgaonkar MR, Duggan PR, Adams G. Differing clinical manifestations of celiac disease transmitted by bone marrow transplantation. *Digestive Diseases & Sciences* 2006;51:210–2.
29. Leuschner M, Maier KP, Schlichting J, et al. Oral budesonide and ursodeoxycholic acid for treatment of primary biliary cirrhosis: results of a prospective double-blind trial. *Gastroenterology* 1999;117:918–25.

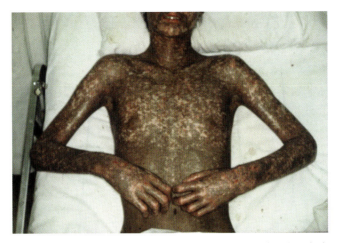

Plate 1. Severe chronic graft versus host disease in one of the first-described patients [22].

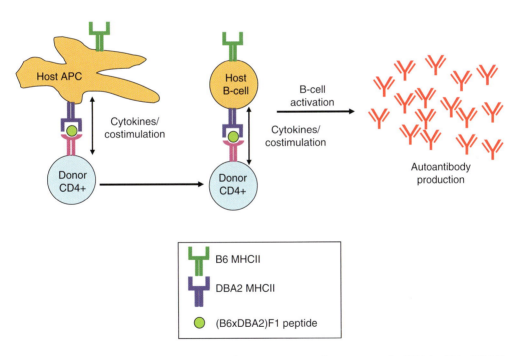

Plate 2. Murine SLE-cGVHD. Illustrated are the events presumed to occur in the DBA2→(B6 × DBA2) F1 model of SLE-cGVHD. Donor DBA2 CD4 T cells are stimulated by host (B6 × DBA2)F1 APCs by interactions with H-2^b allogeneic MHCII molecules bearing B6- or DBA-derived peptides. Activated CD4 T cells in turn stimulate (and likely are stimulated by) host B cells (again bearing H-2^b) to produce autoantibodies.

APC, antigen-presenting cells; GVHD, graft versus host disease; MHCII, major histocompatibility complex II; SLE, systemic lupus erythematosus.

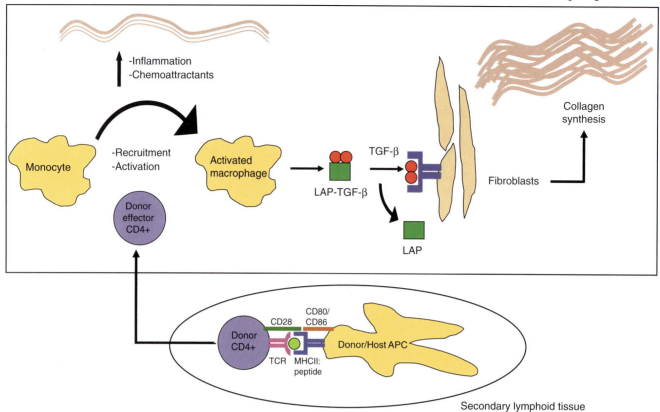

Plate 3. Murine Scl-cGVHD. A potential scenario for generation of fibrotic skin lesions in B10.D2→BALB/c miHA mismatched transplant model. Upon activation by donor and/or host APC, CD4 T cells are recruited into target tissue and signal macrophages to produce TGF-β. TGF-β, in turn, binds to its receptor in fibroblasts resulting in increased collagen synthesis, resulting in fibrosis.

APC, antigen-presenting cells; LAP, latency associated peptide; MHCII, major histocompatibility complex II; TCR, T-cell receptor; TGF-β, tumor growth factor.

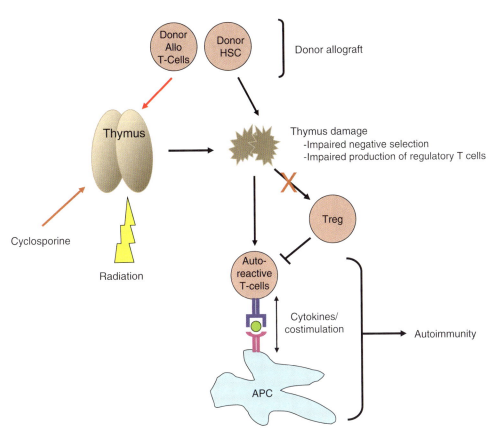

Plate 4. cGVHD resulting from thymus dysfunction. Negative selection could be impaired as a consequence of thymic damage by alloreactive T cells, acting in concert with irradiation. CsA may also interfere with negative selection. As a result, autoreactive T cells that would normally be deleted may escape into the periphery, where they can be activated by antigen-presenting cells. It is also possible that the thymic environment posttransplant does not favor the generation of regulatory T cells.

APC, antigen-presenting cells; HSC, hematopoietic stem cells; Treg, regulatory T cells.

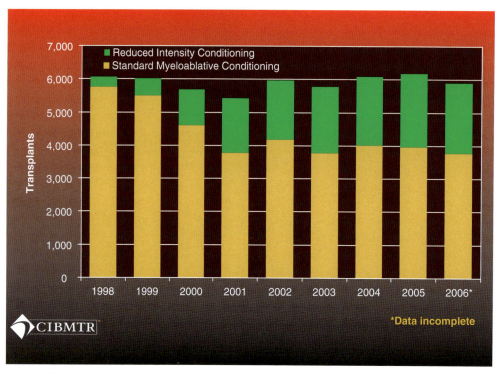

Plate 5. Allogeneic transplantations registered with CIBMTR by conditioning regimen intensity, 1998–2006. Pasquini M. Wang Z., Schneider L. CIBMTR summary slides, 2007. CIBMTR newsletter 2007;13:5–9.

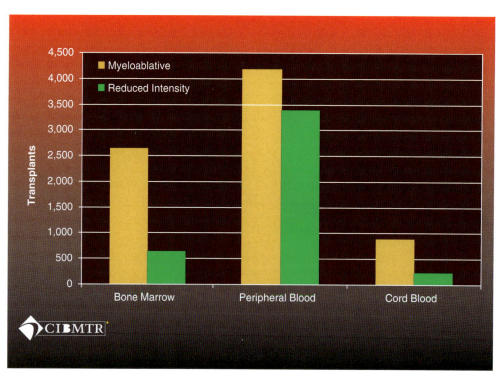

Plate 6. Allogeneic transplantations by graft source and conditioning regimen intensity, registered with CIBMTR, 2005–2006. Data was obtained from CIBMTR [37].

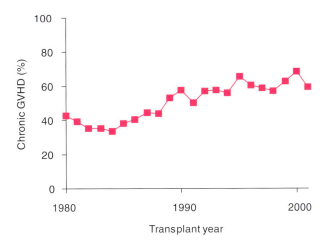

Plate 7. Trend of increasing cGVHD incidence/year over two decades in patients surviving at least 100 days at the Fred Hutchinson Cancer Research Center – all graft sources and regimens. Printed with permission from Elsevier, Ltd. [71]

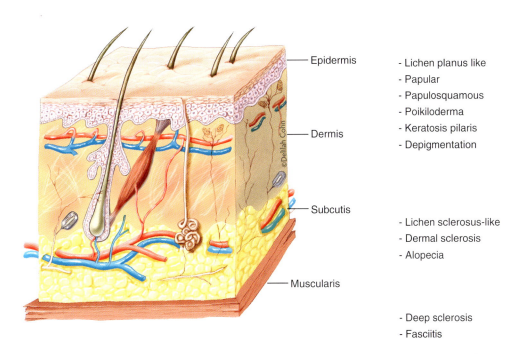

Plate 8. A skin cross section depicting the diverse manifestations of chronic graft versus host disease (cGVHD).

The diverse manifestations of cGVHD are as follows:

Lichen planus-like, Papular, Papulosquamous, Poikiloderma, Keratosis pilaris, Depigmentation, Deep Sclerosis, Fasciitis, Lichen-sclerosus like, Dermal sclerosis, Alopecia

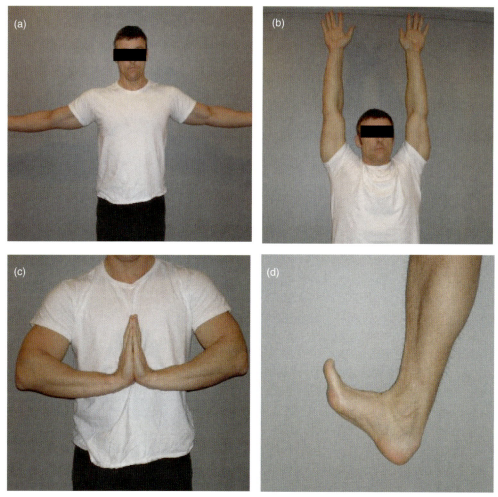

Plate 9. Assessment of limited range of motion (ROM).
A: extension of the arms laterally; B: extension of the arms above the head; C: Flexion of wrists "Buddha hands prayer position" with palms and fingers together; D: extension of ankles.

Lichen planus-like

Lichen sclerosus

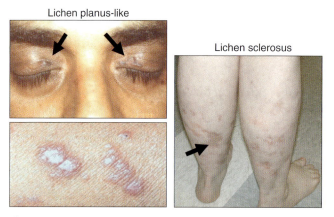

Plate 10. Lichen planus-like and lichen-sclerosus types of cGVHD manifestation.

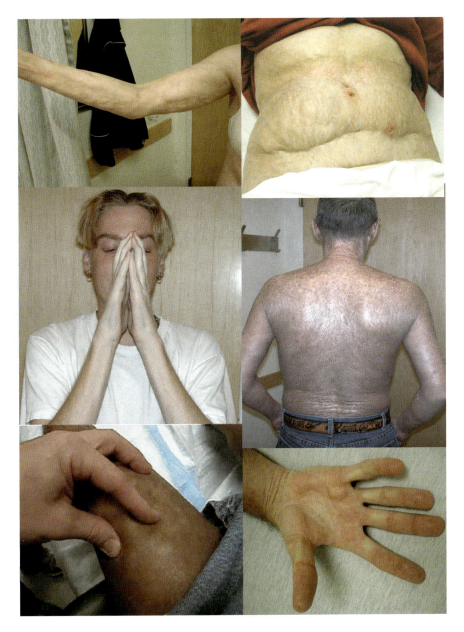

Plate 11. Sclerotic manifestation of cGVHD

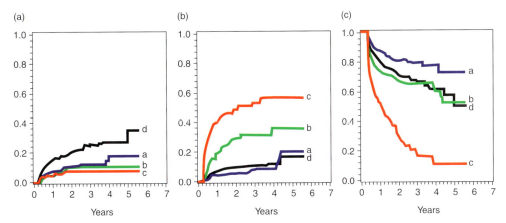

Plate 12. Relapse. B: Treatment-related mortality. C: Disease-free survival. Lines indicate low risk (a); intermediate risk (b); high risk (c); and no cGVHD (d).

Lee SJ, Klein JP, Barrett AJ et al. Severity of chronic graft-versus-host disease :association with trament-related mortality and relapse. *Blood*. 2002;100:406–414.

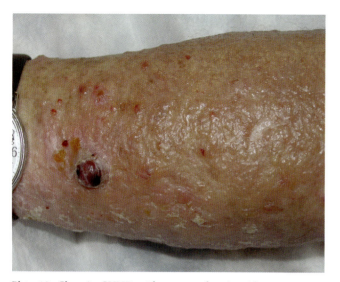

Plate 13. Chronic GVHD with severe sclerosis with angiomatous proliferations. (Courtesy Dr. Daniel Couriel.)

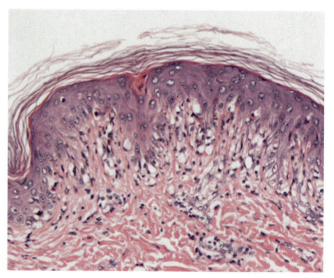

Plate 14. Skin, fatal acute GVHD day 30. The epidermis has an extensive interface dermatitis with continuous vacuolization along the basal, lymphocytic infiltration of the epidermis and superficial perivascular inflammation. The epidermal surface has mild basketweave (loose) hyperkeratosis and is of normal thickness. Along the basal layer of a rete ridge are contiguous keratinocyte apoptotic bodies, clear spaces containing the contracted dense eosinophilic cytoplasm with dark membrane bound nuclear fragments. Lymphocytes partially surround the apoptotic bodies (lymphocytic satellitosis)

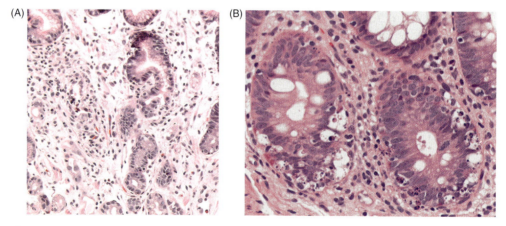

Plate 15. Severe, acute GVHD of gastrointestinal tract day 48. A: in the edematous gastric antrum are loosely scattered lymphocytes and a few eosinophils. The collapsed lumen of a nearly destroyed gland is filled with apoptotic debris. Many of the adjacent glands are infiltrated by lymphocytes and contain multiple contiguous apoptotic bodies in the glandular and neck regions. Apoptosis in the neck region of a gastric gland is particularly characteristic of GVHD. B: colonic biopsy shows adjacent crypts with multiple contiguous apoptotic bodies.

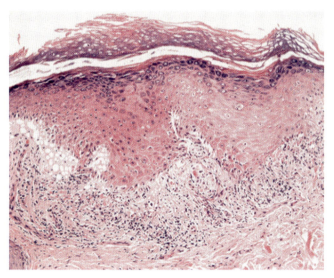

Plate 16. Chronic GVHD of skin with lichen planus-like appearance, day 1,267. The epidermis has compact hyperkeratosis, a thickened granular cell layer and irregular acanthosis (thickening). The rete ridges are blunted with a sawtooth shape. A band-like lymphocytic infiltrate occupies the papillary dermis and focally infiltrates the lower layers of the damaged rete ridges where there are abundant apoptotic bodies.

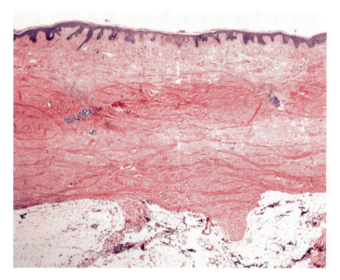

Plate 18. Pan-dermal sclerosis in late chronic GVHD day 1,280. Low power of skin with markedly thickened dermis composed of dense waxy collagen. The entrapped eccrine coils in the center of the dermis indicate the boundary where a normal reticular dermis would end. There was little or no inflammation or apoptotic change in the epidermis to whether the GVHD was still active. This appearance resembles progressive systemic sclerosis; hence the term sclerodermoid to describe the later skin changes of chronic GVHD.

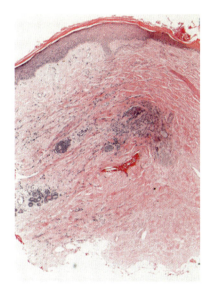

Plate 17. Chronic GVHD of skin developing dermal sclerosis, day 1,069. The collagen in both the papillary (upper) and reticular dermis has developed smudgy dense appearance that has replaced most of the normal collagen bundles. The entrapped dermal appendages, eccrine coils and remnants of a follicle are infiltrated by lymphocytes. The epidermis displays features of chronic GVHD with hyperkeratosis acanthosis, loss of rete ridges with and apoptosis along the straightened the dermal epidermal border.

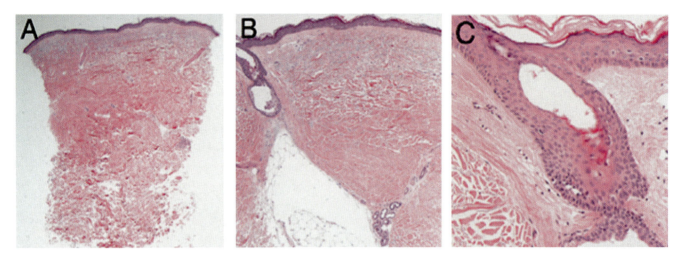

Plate 19. Morpheic variant of chronic GVHD day 2,028. These localized lesions on the back have a nodular focus of dermal fibrosis with dense closely packed collagen without bundles. A: is located in the mid-portion of the reticular dermis B: along the dermal subcutaneous junction shows a nodular focus of smudgy dense collagen containing an entrapped eccrine unit. In contrast, the normal collagen bundles in adjacent uninvolved reticular dermis have a curlicue pattern. C: higher power of B shows a dilated degenerative hair follicle containing a minimal focal lymphocytic infiltrate. The fibrosis appears to track along the perifollicular adventitial dermis and extend up into part of the papillary dermis. Activity is based on progression of fibrosis in serial biopsies, the development of new gross lesions or chronic inflammation. Apoptosis of the epidermis or appendages is often minimal and sometimes absent in morpheic lesions.

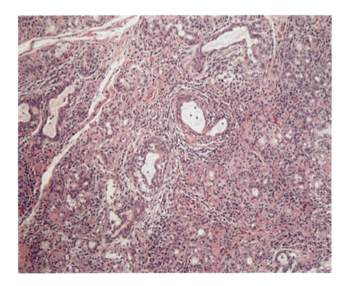

Plate 20. Oral GVHD early changes day 150. Extensive chronic inflammation in the corresponding minor salivary glands has resulted in subtotal destruction of the acinar tissue. The dilated and extensively infiltrated intralobular ducts display prominent vacuolization, apoptosis and segmental loss of nuclei.

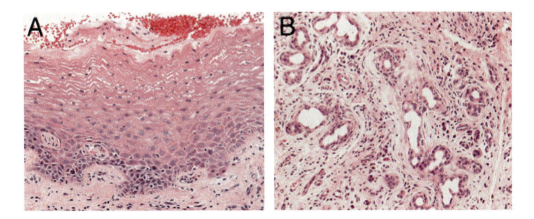

Plate 21. Late stage oral chronic GVHD. A: the mucosa resembles the lichenoid lesion in Figure 9.7 with sawtoothing of the rete ridges and a band-like infiltrate beneath the nonkeratinized squamous mucosa. Apoptosis is present along the basal layer though generally less marked than in cutaneous chronic GVHD. B: the destroyed glandular acinii have been completely replaced by loose fibroblastic stroma containing loosely scatted lymphocytes and plasma cells. The GVHD remains active with lymphocytic infiltration and apoptosis in the atypical proliferated ducts. The denser fibrosis in the interstitium represents more distant damage.

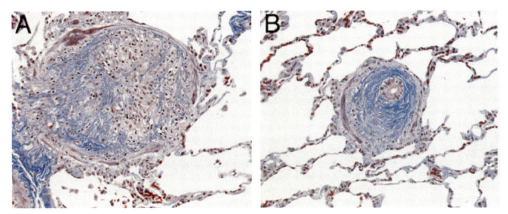

Plate 22. Pulmonary GVHD with obliterative bronchiolitis, day 1,822. Patient with progressive shortness of breath, worsening oxygen requirements, pulmonary function testing profile of airflow obstruction unimproved with bronchodilators, and diffuse ground glass changes on the CT scan of the lungs. Trichrome stains shows over expanded alveoli without any inflammation or consolidation. A: shows a bronchiole whose obstructed lumen contains a mixture of wispy collagen, chronic inflammatory cells and disordered respiratory epithelial cells, that is, obstructive bronchiolitis. B: is a small bronchiole with dense concentrically arranged collagen in the widened subepithelial zone surrounding the small lumen. Other small bronchioles had complete fibrous obliteration of their lumina more accurately termed *constrictive bronchiolitis*.

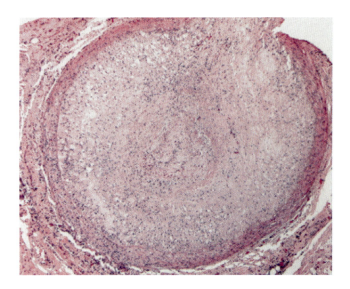

Plate 23. Coronary arteritis from GVHD day 615. Teenager developed severe substernal chest pain for 1 month and reduced cardiac function tests before she died suddenly with myocardial infarction. Coronary arteries were diffusely narrowed from 50% to 100%. The histology resembles the "transplant atherosclerosis" found in chronically rejected cardiac allografts. The wall and lumen of this large artery are nearly obliterated by an arteritis of chronic inflammatory cells admixed with loose extracellular matrix.

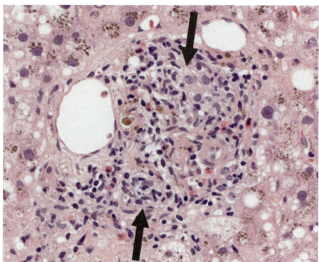

Plate 25. Hepatic GVHD day 454. Arrows in portal space point to damaged bile ducts that consist of a collapsed syncytium of variable sized irregularly arranged nuclei. There are segments where the nuclei are missing. Despite the marked lymphocytic ductitis with cytoplasmic vacuolization, apoptosis of bile duct epithelium is uncommon with hepatic GVHD.

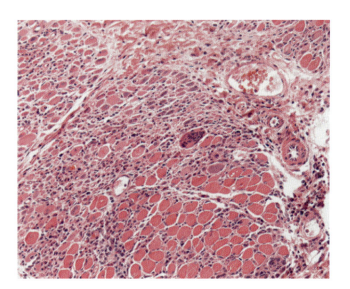

Plate 24. Polymyositis day 1,129. This patient's chronic GVHD, was quiescent after a complete response to treatment for histologically florid lichen-planus like skin lesions. After a hiatus, muscle tenderness with marked elevation of muscle related serum enzymes developed. This muscle biopsy from the deltoid shows a florid polymyositis. The interstitial infiltrate of macrophages, plasma cells and lymphocytes surrounds clusters of small regenerative basophilic fibers with large central nuclei. There are occasional large multinucleated fibers as well as areas of active necrosis with acute interstitial inflammation. The patient made a complete recovery and as of 2007 is status 32 years post-HCT.

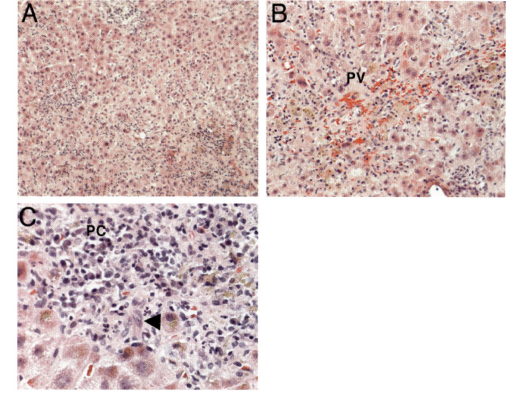

Plate 26. Acute hepatitic onset of liver GVHD day 757 with rapidly rising liver tests AST 1,200, ALT 2,200, bilirubin 6.5. Cultures and serologies for viruses were negative. A; low power shows a lobular and portal hepatitis. B: perivenular area (PV) shows an extensive necroinflammatory infiltrate of lymphocytes and plasma cells, hepatocyte dropout with many acidophilic bodies, and spotty hemorrhage. Endothelialitis, lymphocytic infiltration and adhesion to the venular endothelial is much less common in GVHD than orthotopic liver rejection. C: high power view shows an interface hepatitis (piecemeal necrosis) along the limiting plate of enlarged portal space. The cellular infiltrate has a prominent plasmacytic (PC) component The proliferated ductules (arrowhead) along the limiting plate appear damaged. Early in the acute hepatitic onset of GVHD the portal and lobular inflammation are the predominant features while later histologic features show more definitive bile duct injury and hepatocellular cholestasis.

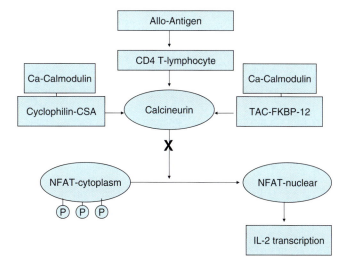

Plate 27. CSA and TAC inhibit calcineurin catalyzed de phosphorylation of NFAT and it's subsequent translocation into the nucleus. Net effect is inhibition of lymphokine (IL-2) transcription. CSA, cyclosporine A; IL, interleukin; NFAT, nuclear factor of activated T cells; TAC, tacrolimus.

FORM A

Current Patient Weight: _____   Today's Date: _____   MR#Name: _____

CHRONIC GVHD ACTIVITY ASSESSMENT-CLINICIAN

Component	Findings	Scoring (see skin score worksheet)
Skin	Erythematous rash of any sort	% BSA (max 100%)
	Moveable sclerosis	% BSA (max 100%)
	Non-moveable sclerosis (hidebound/non-pinchable) or subcutaneous sclerosis/fascitis	% BSA (max 100%)
	Ulcer(s): select the largest ulcerative lesion, and measure its largest dimension in cm and mark location of ulcer	Location: _____ Largest dimension: _____ cm

Eyes Bilateral Schirmer's Tear Test (without anesthesia) in persons 9 years or older	Right Eys: mm of wetting	Left Eys: mm of wetting

Mouth

Mucosal change	No evidence of cGVHD		Mild		Moderate		Severe	
Erythema	None	0	Mild erythema or moderate erythema (<25%)	1	Moderate (≥25%) or Severe erythema (<25%)	2	Severe erythema (≥25%)	3
Lichenoid	None	0	Hyperkeratotic changes(<25%)	1	Hyperkeratotic changes(25-50%)	2	Hyperkeratotic changes (>50%)	3
Ulcers	None	0	None	0	Ulcers involving (≤20%)	3	Severe ulcerations (>20%)	6
Mucoceles*	None	0	1-5 mucoceles	1	6-10 scattered mucoceles	2	Over 10 mucoceles	3
			*Mucoceles scored for lower labial and soft palate only				Total score for all mucosal changes	

Blood Counts	Platelet Count k/uL	ULN k/uL	Total WBC k/uL	ULN k/uL	% Eosinophils	%
Liver Function Tests	Total serum bilirubin mg/dL	ULN mg/dL	ALT U/L	ULN U/L	Alkaline Phosphatase U/L	ULN U/L

Gastrointestinal-Upper GI • Early satiely OR • Anorexia OR • Nausea & Vomiting	0=no symptoms 1=mild, occasional symptoms, with little reduction in oral intake _during the past week_ 2=moderate, intermittent symptoms, with some reduction in oral intake _during the past week_ 3=more severe or persistent symptoms throughout the day. with marked reduction in oral intake. on almost every day of the past week
Gastrointestinal-Esophageal • Dysphagia OR • Odynophagia	0=no esophageal symptoms 1=Occasional dysphagia or odynophagia with solid food or pills _during the past week_ 2=Intermittent dysphagia or odynophagia with solid foods or pills, but not for liquids or soft foods, _during the past week_ 3=Dysphagia or odynophagia for almost all oral intake, _on almost every day of the past week_
Gastrointestinal-Lower GI • Diarrhea	0=no loose or liquid stools during the past week 1=occasional loose or liquid stools, on some days _during the past week_ 2=intermittent loose or liquid stools throughout the day, _on almost every day of the past week_ without requiring intervention to prevent or correct volume depletion 3=voluminous diarrhea on almost every day of the past week, requiring intervention to prevent or correct volume depletion
Lungs • Bronchiolitis Obliterans	Pulmonary Function Tests with Diffusing Capacity (attach report for person> 5 yrs old) FEV-1 % Predicted Single Breath DLCO (adjusted for hemoglobin) % Predicted

Health Care Provider Global Ratings: In your opinion, do you think that this patient's chronic GVHD is mild, moderate or severe? 0=none 1=mild 2=moderate 2=severe	Where would you rate the severity of this patient's chronic GVHD symptoms on the following scale, where 0 is cGVHD symptoms that are not at all severe and 10 is the most severe cGVHD symptoms possible: 0 1 2 3 4 5 6 7 8 9 10 cGvHD symptoms Most severe cGvHD not at all severe symptoms possible	Over the past _month_ would you say that this patient's cGVHD is +3=Very much better +2=Moderately better +1=A little better 0=About the same −1=A little worse −2=Moderately worse −3=Very much worse

Functional Performance (in persons >4 years old) • Walk Time • Grip Strength	Total Distance Walked in 2 Minutes: Number of laps: (× 50 feet) + final partial lap: feet = feet walked in 2 minutes	Grip Strength (Dominant Hand) Trial #1 Trial #2 Trial #3 psi psi psi	Range of Motion: ○ Not performed ○ Physical Therapy Report Attached

Score	Lansky Performance Status Scale Definitions (circel from 0-100) (persons < 16 years old)	Karnofsky Performance Status Scale Definitions(circle from 0-100) (persons 16 years of older)
100	Fully active, normal	Normal no complaints; no evidence of disease
90	Minor restrictions in physically strenuous activity	Able to carry on normal activity, minor signs or symptoms of disease
80	Active, but tires more quickly	Normal acitivity with effort; some signs or symptoms of disease
70	Both greater restriction of and less time spent in play activity	Cares for self: unable to carry on normal activity or to do active work
60	Up and around, but minimal active play; keeps busy with quieter activities	Requires occasional assistance but is able to care for most personal needs
50	Gets dressed but lies around much of the day, no active play but able to participate in all quiet play and activities	Requires considerable assistance and frequent medical care
40	Mostly in beat participates in quiet activities	Disabled; requires special care and assistance
30	In bed, needs assistances even for quiet play	Severely disabled; hospital admission is indicated although death not imminent
20	Often sleeping; play entirely limited to very passive activities	Very sick; hospital admission necessary; active supportive treatment necessary
10	No play; does not get out of bed	Moribund; fatal processed progressing rapidly
0	Unresponsive	Dead

Plate 28. Two Page Data Collection Form for Clinician Assessed Measures – NIH response criteria project. (Based on information from Pavletic et al. _Biol Blood Marrow Transplant._ 2006; 12:252–266.)

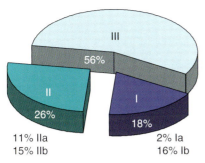

Plate 29. Distribution of NIH Consensus Ancillary and Supportive Care Recommendations based on quality of evidence. From: Couriel D, Carpenter PA, Cutler C, et al. *Biol Blood Marrow Transplant.* 2006;12:375–396 with permission from Elsevier.

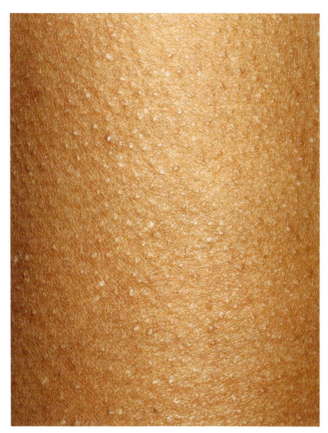

Plate 31. Folliculocentric papules resembling keratosis pilaris.

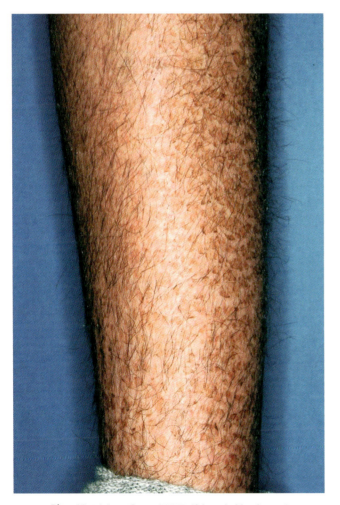

Plate 30. Ichthyosiform cGVHD (fish-scale-like changes).

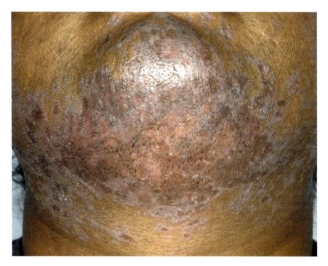

Plate 32. Violaceous papules and plaques resembling lichen planus.

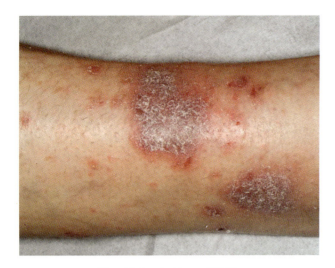

Plate 33. Psoriasiform cGVHD.

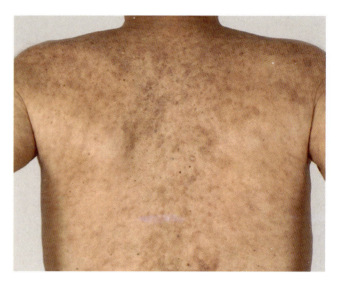

Plate 35. Residual hyperpigmentation following resolution of cutaneous cGVHD.

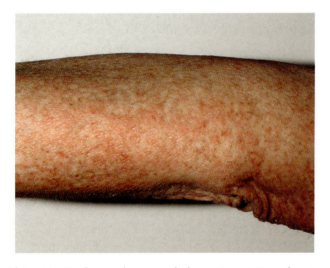

Plate 34. Erythema, hypo- and hyperpigmentation due to poikilodermic cGVHD.

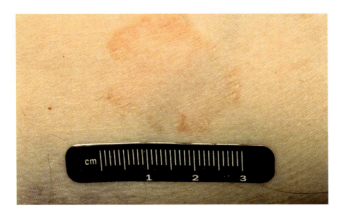

Plate 36. Annular plaque resembling erythema annulare centrifugum.

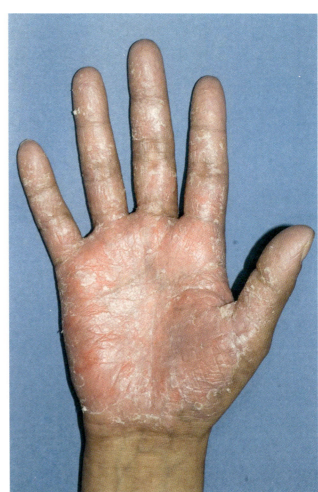

Plate 38. Extensive palmar erythema and scaling.

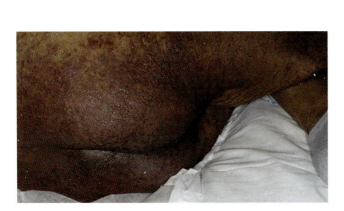

Plate 37. Erythroderma; widespread erythema and scaling.

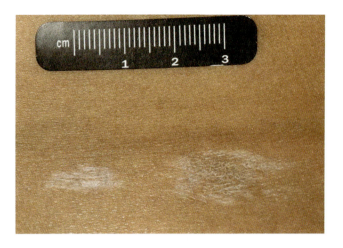

Plate 39. Localized atrophic plaques with superficial sclerosis.

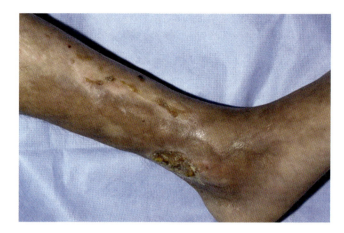

Plate 41. Hidebound (nonmoveable) fibrosis of the leg with ulcer formation.

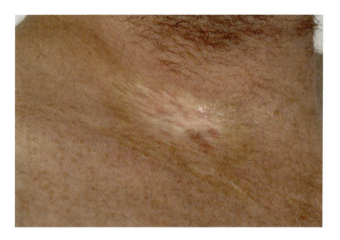

Plate 40. Thickened plaque with surrounding hyperpigmentation resembling morphea.

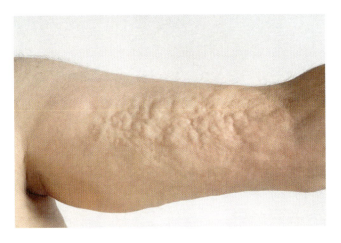

Plate 42. Rippling and nodularity of the subcutaneous tissue.

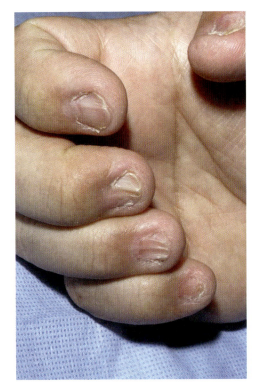

Plate 44. Nail dystrophy, vertical ridging, and nail thinning.

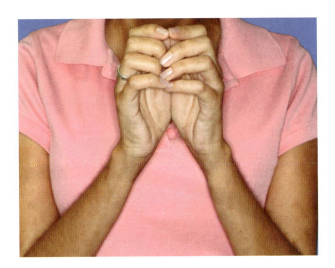

Plate 43. cGVHD-related fasciitis, with limited wrist dorsiflexion (positive "prayer sign").

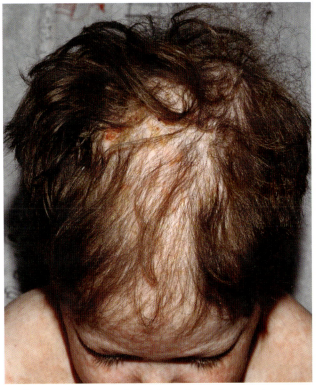

Plate 45. Alopecia, patchy hair loss with erythema and scale.

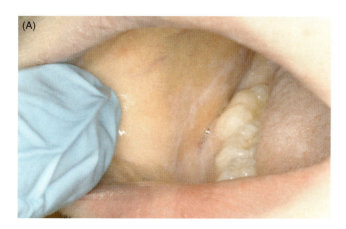

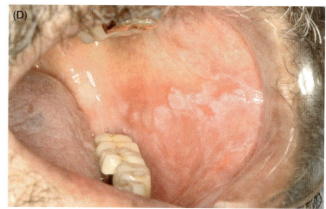

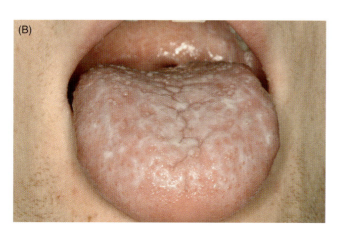

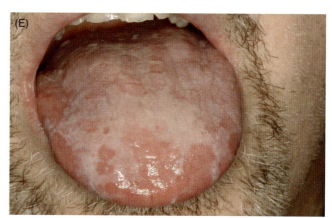

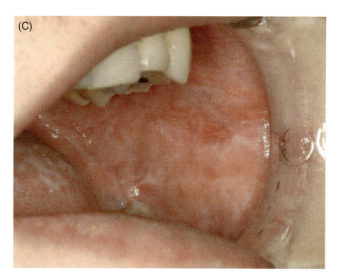

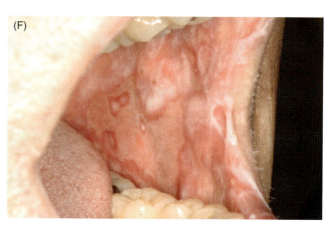

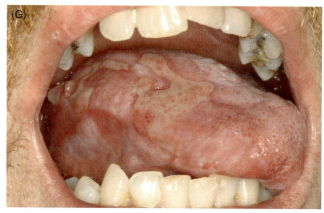

Plate 46. Clinical spectrum of oral mucosal cGVHD presentations. A: early, mild reticulation of the buccal mucosa in a pediatric patient with extensive hepatic cGVHD and jaundice; B: web-like white reticulation of the tongue dorsum with preservation of the papillae; C: reticulation and plaque-like changes with associated mild erythema of the buccal mucosa; D: reticulation and more dense plaque formation with erythema and a focal ulceration; E: entirely atrophic tongue dorsum with extensive atypical plaque-like changes; F: heavy reticulation with intense erythema and a very large area of ulceration; G: extensive ulceration of the tongue with areas of atrophic glossitis adjacent to areas with entire preservation of the papillae.

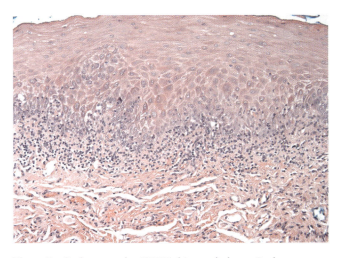

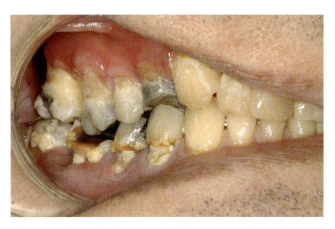

Plate 47. Oral mucosal cGVHD histopathology. Oral squamous mucosa with a band-like infiltrate of T lymphocytes at the interface between the connective tissue and basement membrane with basal-cell degeneration, acanthosis, and hyperkeratosis. This specimen corresponds to a white reticular lesion clinically.

Plate 48. Salivary gland cGVHD oral changes. A: advanced cervical decay in a patient 1 year after HCT due to both salivary gland and mucosal cGVHD; B: intraoral periapical radiograph of same patient showing extent of interproximal decay.

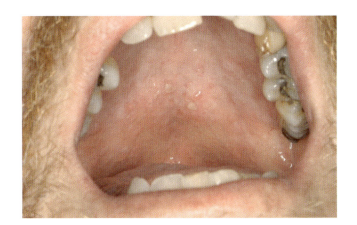

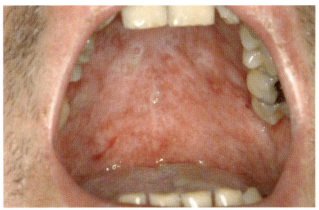

Plate 49. Superficial mucoceles of the palate. A: multiple superficial mucoceles both intact and burst with several areas of secondary ulceration; B: numerous superficial mucoceles in the context of severe mucosal cGVHD.

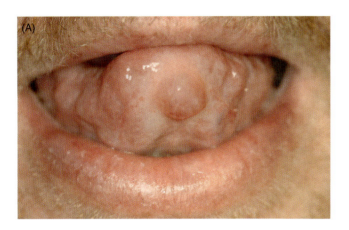

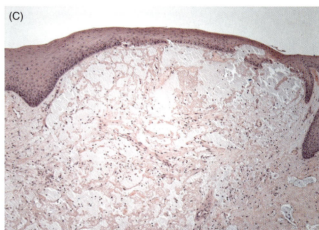

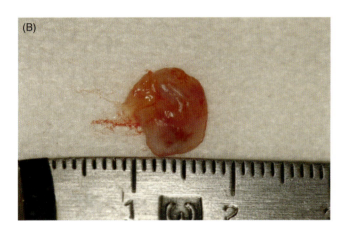

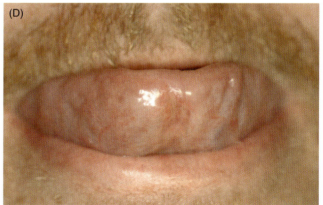

Plate 50. Symptomatic deep mucocele. A: large 1.0 cm well-defined dome-shaped mucocele in the anterior ventral tongue; B: gross pathology following excision; C: histopathology demonstrating extensive mucous collection in the connective tissue with normal appearing surface mucosa; D: excision site 1 week later showing complete healing.

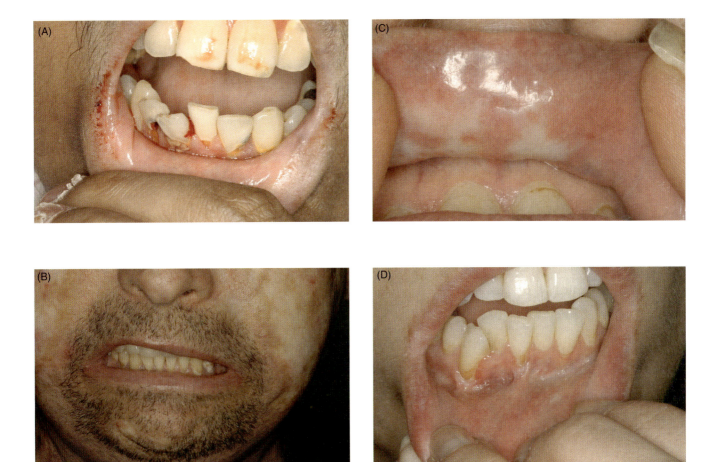

Plate 51. Sclerotic oral cGVHD. A: advanced sclerosis of the facial skin resulting in limited maximum opening, inability to maintain oral hygiene resulting in gingival bleeding, and subsequent rampant dental caries; B: extensive sclerotic changes resulting in painful myospasm and dystonia; C: severe penetrating skin sclerosis replacing normal mucosa with dense fibrous tissue; D: sclerotic changes of the mucosa resulting in loss of the labial vestibule and localized areas of advanced recession due to pulling away of the gingival tissues.

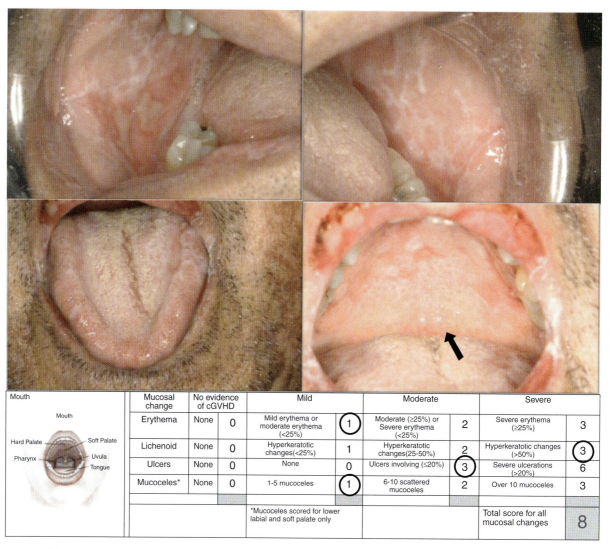

Mouth									
Mucosal change	**No evidence of cGVHD**		**Mild**		**Moderate**		**Severe**	
Erythema	None	0	Mild erythema or moderate erythema (<25%)	①	Moderate (≥25%) or Severe erythema (<25%)	2	Severe erythema (≥25%)	3
Lichenoid	None	0	Hyperkeratotic changes(<25%)	1	Hyperkeratotic changes(25-50%)	2	Hyperkeratotic changes (>50%)	③
Ulcers	None	0	None	0	Ulcers involving (≤20%)	③	Severe ulcerations (>20%)	6
Mucoceles*	None	0	1-5 mucoceles	①	6-10 scattered mucoceles	2	Over 10 mucoceles	3
			*Mucoceles scored for lower labial and soft palate only				Total score for all mucosal changes	8

Mouth — Hard Palate, Mouth, Soft Palate, Pharynx, Uvula, Tongue

Plate 52. Use of the NIH Oral cGVHD clinical scoring instrument. In this example, all affected areas are shown, and those not shown can be assumed to be uninvolved. When estimating percentages, the entire mucosal surface area of all anatomic sites, both affected and unaffected, must be considered. The areas of *erythema* are primarily perilesional surrounding ulcerations and are not severe (the deep red areas on the lips are bleeding from the ulcers). All sites show extensive *lichenoid* changes accounting for greater than 50% of the overall surface areas. There are multiple *ulcers* of the lips, tongue, palate, and buccal mucosa; however, when considered as a percentage of all of these sites, these do not account for more than 20% of the entire surface areas. The *mucoceles* are highlighted by the black arrow.

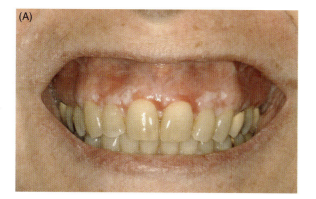
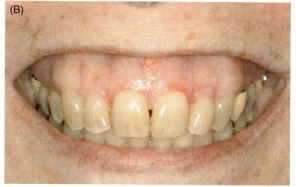

(A) (B)

Plate 53. Topical management of oral mucosal cGVHD involving attached gingiva. A: extensive painful mucosal involvement with reticulation, severe erythema, and focal ulceration of the maxillary anterior attached gingiva extending onto unattached gingival mucosa; B: less than 1 month later following intensive treatment with topical corticosteroids and tacrolimus with no changes in systemic medications.

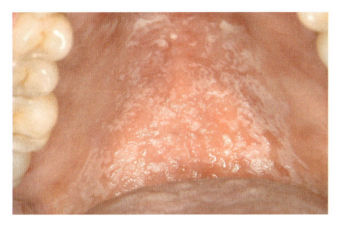

Plate 54. Pseudomembranous candidiasis of the palate secondary to topical steroid rinses. Note the numerous superficial mucoceles and fainter more macular areas of reticular cGVHD changes. Once weekly fluconazole therapy with ongoing topical therapy was effective in treating and preventing recurrence.

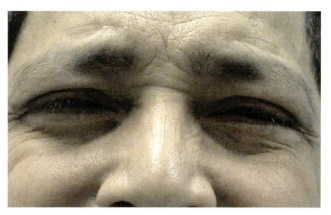

Plate 55. Classic appearance of a patient with chronic ocular GVHD with keratoconjunctivitis sicca.

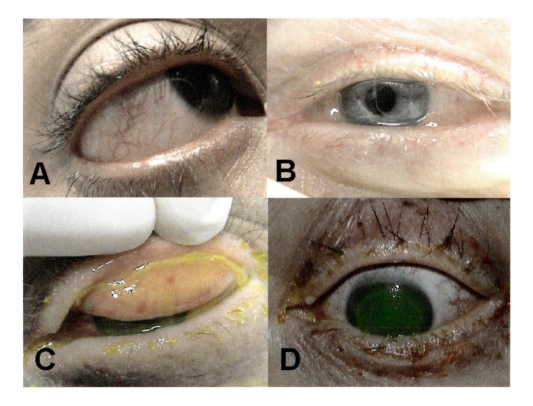

Plate 56. Conjunctival staging (typically seen in acute GVHD settings). (A) Stage I. hyperemia; (B) Stage II. hyperemia with chemosis; (C) Stage III. pseudomembranous conjunctivitis. Fluoresce dye uptake at the palpebral conjunctiva (D) Stage IV. pseudomembranous conjunctivitis with corneal epithelial sloughing. The corneal defect is also visible by the fluorscene dye.

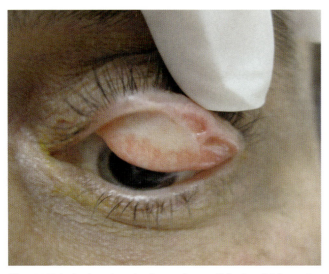

Plate 57. Palpebral conjunctiva (everted upper lid): cicatricial scarring from chronic ocular GVHD.

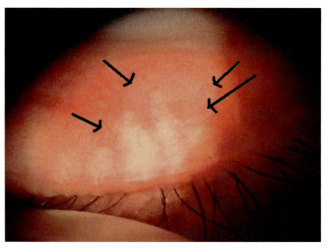

Plate 59. Meibomian gland drop outs (see arrows) in chronic ocular GVHD patient. Glands should be linear and extend further toward the fornix of the lid. Decrease in tear break up time (TBUT) is observed in patient with meibomian gland dysfunction.

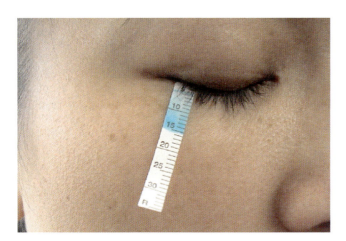

Plate 58. Schirmer's test: diagnostic tool for ocular GVHD.

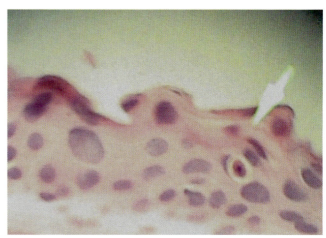

Plate 60. Conjunctival biopsy specimen of ocular GVHD: arrow points to an apoptic cell. Attenuated epithelial layer and loss of goblet cells also present.

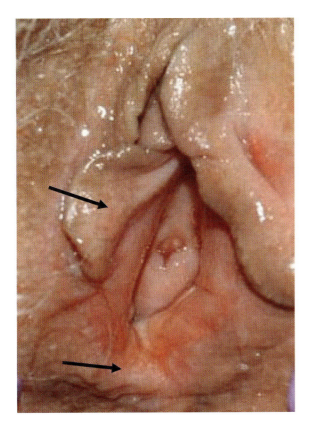

Plate 61. Mild genital GVHD: Diffuse erythema and edema of the vulva with reticulated leukokeratosis of the right labia minora and posterior forchette.

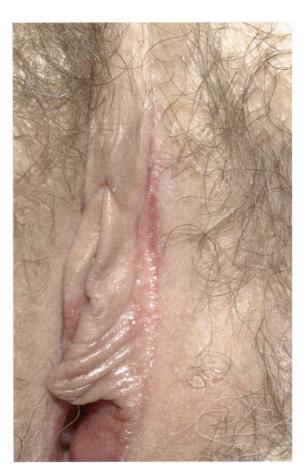

Plate 63. Moderate genital GVHD: Fissuring along the interlabial sulcus. This can cause burning on urination.

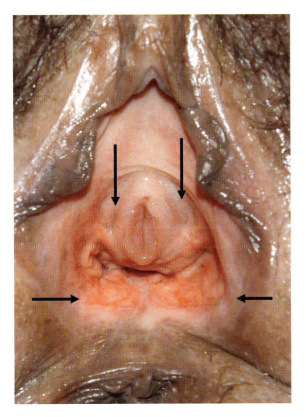

Plate 62. Mild genital GVHD: Erythematous patches at the introitus indicated with horizontal arrows. Erythematous areas around the opening of Skene's ducts noted with vertical arrows. These findings are similar to those seen in idiopathic vulvar vestibulitis syndrome.

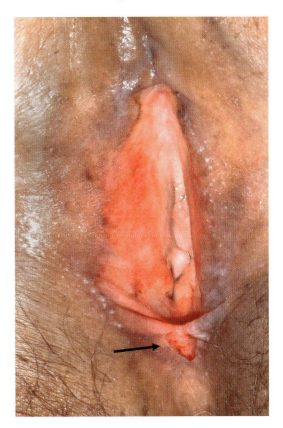

Plate 64. Moderate to severe genital GVHD: Marked architectural atrophy and sclerosis of the labia; note tear/fissure at posterior commissure.

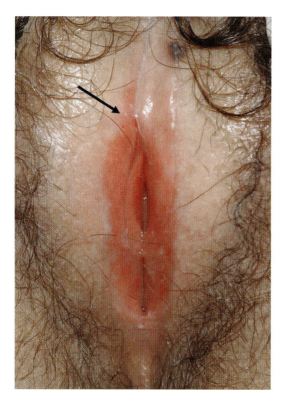

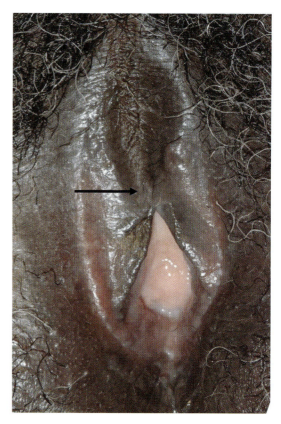

Plate 65. Severe genital GVHD: Clitoral agglutination caused by healing of apposing eroded surfaces of the clitoral hood and labia minora designated by arrow. Labial resorption and diffuse erythema are noted as well.

Plate 66. Severe genital GVHD: Narrowed introitus from fusion of labia minora.

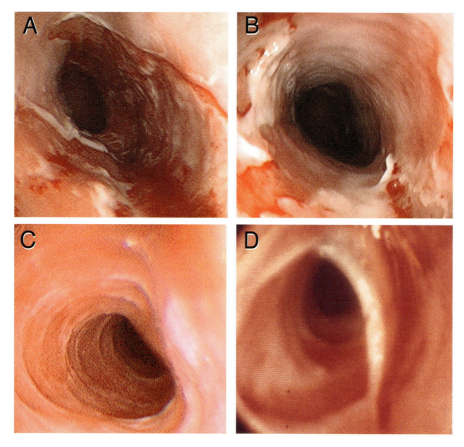

Plate 67. Endoscopic appearance of chronic GVHD of the esophagus. A and B. Upper third of the esophagus, showing exposed submucosa (red areas) adjacent to desquamating squamous epithelium (pale areas). When touched with the biopsy forceps, the epithelial layer peeled away from the underlying submucosa. C. Middle third of the esophagus, showing multiple ring-like narrowings; epithelium in the upper third of the esophagus, above the rings, was friable. D. A nearly circumferential web just below the cricopharyngeal inlet to the esophagus, composed of desquamated epithelium. Although some webs in patients with chronic GVHD are wispy and easily broken with the endoscope, this web was thick and firmly attached to the underlying submucosa.

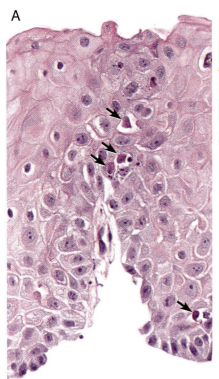

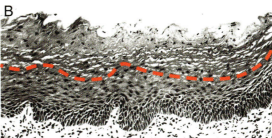

Plate 68. Histologic abnormalities in chronic GVHD involving the esophagus. Photomicrograph of esophageal mucosa, showing multiple apoptotic epithelial cells within the basal layer (arrows). (Hematoxylin and eosin; photomicrograph courtesy of KR Loeb) Photomicrograph of esophageal mucosa, showing desquamation of squamous cells (area superior to the dotted line). At endoscopy, the esophageal epithelium peeled away when touched with a biopsy forceps. (Hematoxylin and eosin; photomicrograph courtesy of HM Shulman)

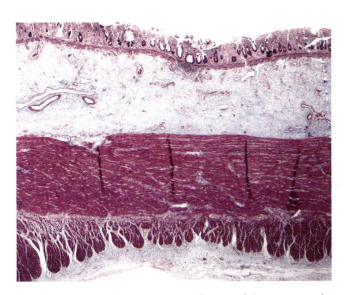

Plate 69. **Submucosal and subserosal fibrosis of the intestine of a patient with untreated chronic GVHD.** Full thickness section of colon taken at autopsy from a patient who died of extensive chronic GVHD 458 days after allogeneic marrow transplant during the 1970s. There was extensive submucosal and subserosal fibrosis (pale bluish stain) from the stomach through the colon; symptoms included intractable diarrhea, steatorrhea, and abdominal pain. (Masson trichrome; photomicrograph courtesy of HM Shulman).

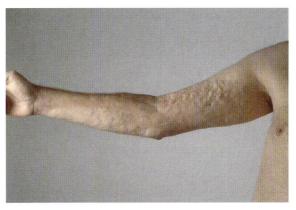

Plate 70. cGVHD-associated Fasciitis.

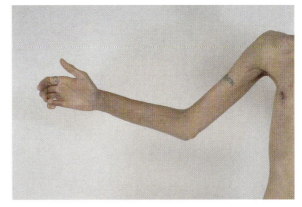

Plate 71. cGVHD-associated contractures. Image reprinted with permission from eMedicine.com, 2008. Available at: http://www.emedicine.com/Med/topic2924.htm.

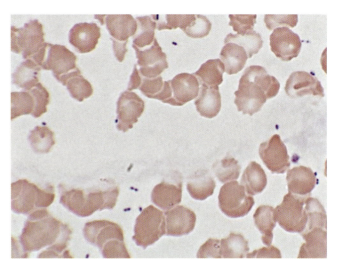

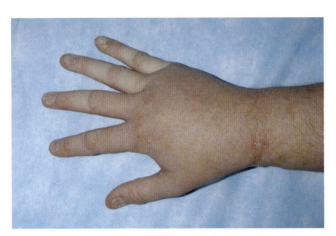

Plate 72. cGVHD-associated edema.

Plate 73. Pneumococcal pneumonia and overwhelming sepsis in cGVHD. A 59-year-old man with chronic GVHD presented with a history of 36 hours of shortness of breath and fever. On admission he was on florid septic shock. The chest radiograph showed left upper lobe pneumonia (A). His peripheral blood smear showed intracellular and extracellular diplococci. (B: Giemsa stain). The blood cultures grew *Streptococcus pneumoniae*, partially susceptible to penicillin. The patient suffered cardiorespiratory arrest and resuscitation was ineffective.

The patient had received a reduced-intensity matched-sibling allo-HCT for CLL 5 years earlier, and was in complete remission. He had suffered chronic extensive GVHD involving skin, eyes, mouth, and liver, but at the time of the event he was not on any systemic immunosuppressive therapy. He had received the pneumococcal vaccine (23-valent). He had been on penicillin VK, but more than a year had passed since the last time he had refilled his prescription.

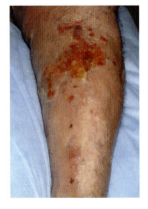 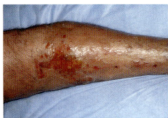 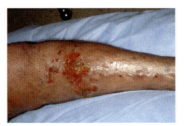

Plate 74. Secodarily infected skin ulcers in a patient with chronic extensive GVHD.

A

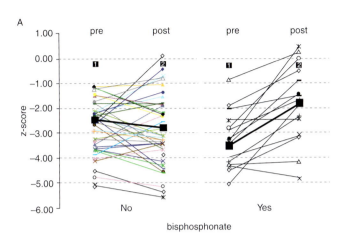

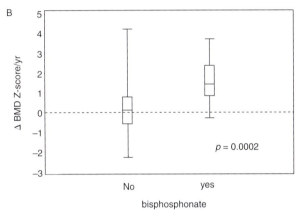

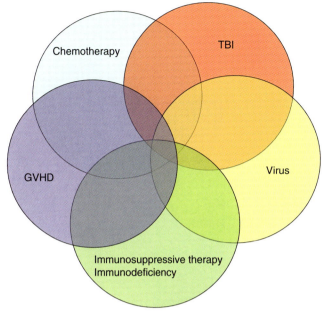

Plate 76. Multifactorial etiology of posttransplantation late effects. GVHD, graft versus host disease; TBI, total body irradiation.

Plate 75. Annualized bone mineral density at baseline and after follow-up. Shown for the patients treated without ($n = 48$) and with ($n = 18$) bisphosphonate are as follows: A: the BMD z-scores for each patient, together with the median z-score (■), at baseline (pre) and at follow-up (post), and B: the median, 25th and 75th percentiles (box), and range of the rates of change of z-scores (whiskers). Reproduced with permission from Elsevier (2007) Carpenter et al. *Biology of Blood and Marrow Transplantation*, 13:683–690 BMD,

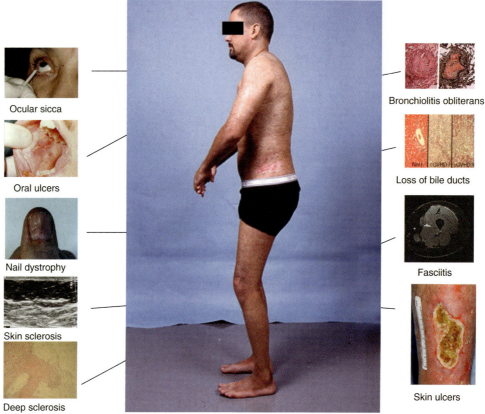

Ocular sicca

Oral ulcers

Nail dystrophy

Skin sclerosis

Deep sclerosis

Bronchiolitis obliterans

Loss of bile ducts

Fasciitis

Skin ulcers

- Infections
- Pulmonary decline (SOB, dyspnea, hypoxemia)
- Endocrinopathies
- Metabolic abnormalities
- Arthralgias/myalgias/fasciitis/contractures
- Oral/dental complications
- Nutritional compromise
- Side effects of chronic immunosuppression (second malignancies, bone density, end-organ toxicity)
- Functional disability- physical, emotional, role, social, sexual
- Distressing symptoms including fatigue, odynophagia, dysphagia, pruritis, ocular pain and dryness
- Body image changes
- Psychosocial distress and adjustment difficulties characteristic of chronic illness

Plate 77. Clinical manifestations of cGVHD and its effects on health status, symptoms, functional status and quality of life.

30. Rautiainen H, Karkkainen P, Karvonen AL, et al. Budesonide combined with UDCA to improve liver histology in primary biliary cirrhosis: a three-year randomized trial. *Hepatology* 2005;41:747–52.

31. Sullivan KM, Shulman HM, Storb R, et al. Chronic graft-versus-host disease in 52 patients: adverse natural course and successful treatment with combination immunosuppression. *Blood* 1981;57:267–76.

32. Tomas JF, Pinilla I, Garcia-Buey ML, et al. Long-term liver dysfunction after allogeneic bone marrow transplantation: Clinical features and course in 61 patients. *Bone Marrow Transplantation* 2000;26:649–55.

33. Strasser SI, Shulman HM, Flowers ME, et al. Chronic graft-vs-host disease of the liver: presentation as an acute hepatitis. *Hepatology* 2000;32:1265–71.

34. Malik AH, Collins JRH, Saboorian MH, Lee WM. Chronic graft versus host disease (GVHD) following hematopoietic cell transplantation (HCT) presenting as an acute hepatitis. *American Journal of Gastroenterology* 2001;96:588–90.

35. Akpek G, Boitnott JK, Lee LA, et al. Hepatitic variant of graft-versus-host disease after donor lymphocyte infusion. *Blood* 2002;100:3903–7.

36. Strasser SI, Sullivan KM, Myerson D, et al. Cirrhosis of the liver in long-term marrow transplant survivors. *Blood* 1999;93:3259–66.

37. Peffault de Latour R, Levy V, Asselah T, et al. Long-term outcome of hepatitis C infection after bone marrow transplantation. *Blood* 2004;103:1618–24.

38. Pergam S, Strasser SI, Flowers ME, Sullivan KM, McDonald GB. Chronic hepatitis C, cirrhosis, and end-stage liver disease in 30-year survivors of bone marrow transplantation. *Biology of Blood & Marrow Transplantation* 2008; 14 (Suppl 2): 31.

39. Gooley TA, Rajvanshi P, Schoch HG, McDonald GB. Serum bilirubin levels and mortality after myeloablative allogeneic hematopoietic cell transplantation. *Hepatology* 2005;41:345–52.

40. Shulman HM, Sharma P, Amos D, Fenster LF, McDonald GB. A coded histologic study of hepatic graft-versus-host disease after human marrow transplantation. *Hepatology* 1988;8:463–70.

41. Kamble R, Selby G, Mims M, Kharfan-Dabaja M, Ozer H, George J. Iron Overload manifesting as apparent exacerbation of hepatic graft-versus-host disease after allogeneic hematopoietic stem cell transplantation. *Biology of Blood & Marrow Transplantation* 2006;12:506–10.

42. Mullighan CG, Bogdanos DP, Vergani D, Bardy PG. Cytochrome P450 1A2 is a target antigen in hepatitic graft-versus-host disease. *Bone Marrow Transplantation* 2006;38:703–5.

43. Strasser SI, Myerson D, Spurgeon CL, et al. Hepatitis C virus infection after bone marrow transplantation: A cohort study with 10 year follow-up. *Hepatology* 1999;29:1893–9.

44. Ljungman P, Johansson N, Aschan J, et al. Long-term effects of hepatitis C virus infection in allogeneic bone marrow transplant recipients. *Blood* 1995;86:1614–8.

45. Lau GKK, Strasser SI, McDonald GB. Hepatitis virus infections in patients with cancer. In: Wingard JR, Bowden RA, eds. Management of Infection in Oncology Patients. London,UK: Martin Dunitz; 2003:321–42.

46. Hui C-K, Cheung WWW, Zhang H-Y, et al. Kinetics and risk of de novo hepatitis B infection in HBsAg-negative patients undergoing cytotoxic chemotherapy. *Gastroenterology* 2006;131:1363. *Gastroenterology* 2006;131:59–68.

47. Dai M-S, Chao T-Y, Kao W-Y, Shyu R-Y, Liu T-M. Delayed hepatitis B virus reactivation after cessation of preemptive lamivudine in lymphoma patients treated with rituximab plus CHOP. *Annals of Hematology* 2004;83:769–74.

48. Iannitto E, Minardi V, Calvaruso G, et al. Hepatitis B virus reactivation and alemtuzumab therapy. *European Journal of Haematology* 2005;74:254–8.

49. Thursky KA, Worth LJ, Seymour JF, Miles Prince H, Slavin MA. Spectrum of infection, risk and recommendations for prophylaxis and screening among patients with lymphoproliferative disorders treated with alemtuzumab. *British Journal of Haematology* 2006;132:3–12.

50. Yeo W, Johnson PJ. Diagnosis, prevention and management of hepatitis B virus reactivation during anticancer therapy. *Hepatology* 2006;43:209–20.

51. Angelucci E, Brittenham GM, McLaren CE, et al. Hepatic iron concentration and total body iron stores in thalassemia major. *New England Journal of Medicine* 2000;343:327–31.

52. Angelucci E, Muretto P, Nicolucci A, et al. Effects of iron overload and hepatitis C virus positivity in determining progression of liver fibrosis in thalassemia following bone marrow transplantation. *Blood* 2002;100:17–21.

53. Lucarelli G, Angelucci E, Giardini C, et al. Fate of iron stores in thalassaemia after bone-marrow transplantation. *Lancet* 1993;342:1388–91.

54. St Pierre TG, Clark PR, Chua-anusorn W, et al. Noninvasive measurement and imaging of liver iron concentrations using proton magnetic resonance. *Blood* 2005;105:855–61.

55. Mariotti E, Angelucci E, Agostini A, Baronciani D, Sgarbi E, Lucarelli G. Evaluation of cardiac status in iron-loaded thalassaemia patients following bone marrow transplantation: improvement in cardiac function during reduction in body iron burden. *British Journal of Haematology* 1998;103:916–21.

56. Angelucci E, Muretto P, Lucarelli G, et al. Phlebotomy to reduce iron overload in patients cured of thalassemia by bone marrow transplantation. Italian Cooperative Group for Phlebotomy Treatment of Transplanted Thalassemia Patients. *Blood* 1997;90:994–8.

57. Mahendra P, Hood IM, Bass G, Patterson P, Marcus RE. Severe hemosiderosis post allogeneic bone marrow transplantation. *Hematol Oncol* 1996;14:33–5.

58. Harrison P, Neilson JR, Marwah SS, Madden L, Bareford D, Milligan DW. Role of non-transferrin bound iron in iron overload and liver dysfunction in long term survivors of acute leukaemia and bone marrow transplantation. *J Clin Pathol* 1996;49:853–6.

59. Kamble R, Mims M. Iron-overload in long-term survivors of hematopoietic transplantation. *Bone Marrow Transplantation* 2006;37:805–6.

60. Oliver MR, Van Voorhis WC, Boeckh M, Mattson D, Bowden RA. Hepatic mucormycosis in a bone marrow transplant recipient who ingested naturopathic medicine. *Clin Infect Dis* 1996;22:521–4.

61. Curtis RE, Rowlings PA, Deeg HJ, et al. Solid cancers after bone marrow transplantation. *N Engl J Med* 1997;336:897–904.

62. Bhatia S, Louie AD, Bhatia R, et al. Solid cancers after bone marrow transplantation. *Journal of Clinical Oncology* 2001;19:464–71.

63. Ioannou GN, Splan MF, Weiss NS, McDonald GB, Beretta L, Lee SP. Incidence and predictors of hepatocellular carcinoma in

patients with cirrhosis. *Clinical Gastroenterology & Hepatology* 2007;5:938–45.

64. Sudour H, Mainard L, Bauman C, Clement L, Salmon A, Bordigoni P. Focal nodular hyperplasia of the liver following hematopoietic SCT. *Bone Marrow Transplant* 2009;43:127–132.

65. Fried RH, Murakami CS, Fisher LD, Willson RA, Sullivan KM, McDonald GB. Ursodeoxycholic acid treatment of refractory chronic graft-versus-host disease of the liver. *Ann Intern Med* 1992;116:624–9.

66. Ruutu T, Eriksson B, Remes K, et al. Ursodeoxycholic acid for the prevention of hepatic complications in allogeneic stem cell transplantation. *Blood* 2002;100:1977–83.

67. Arat M, Idilman R, Soydan EA, et al. Ursodeoxycholic acid treatment in isolated chronic graft-vs.-host disease of the liver. *Clinical Transplantation* 2005;19:798–803.

68. Daley-Yates PT, Price AC, Sisson JR, Pereira A, Dallow N. Beclomethasone dipropionate: absolute bioavailability, pharmacokinetics and metabolism following intravenous, oral, intranasal and inhaled administration in man. *British Journal of Clinical Pharmacology* 2001;51:400–9.

69. Shimizu T, Kasahara M, Tanaka K. Living-donor liver transplantation for chronic hepatic graft-versus-host disease. *New England Journal of Medicine* 2006;354:1536–7.

70. Orlando G, Ferrant A, Schots R, et al. Liver transplantation for chronic graft-versus-host disease: case report with 10-year follow-up. *Transplant International* 2005;18:125–9.

71. Ko CW, Murakami C, Sekijima JH, Kim MH, McDonald GB, Lee SP. Chemical composition of gallbladder sludge in patients after marrow transplantation. *Am J Gastroenterol* 1996;91:1207–10.

72. Teefey SA, Hollister MS, Lee SP, et al. Gallbladder sludge formation after bone marrow transplant: sonographic observations. *Abdom Imaging* 1994;19:57–60.

73. Foulis AK, Farquharson MA, Sale GE. The pancreas in acute graft-versus-host disease in man. *Histopathology* 1989;14:121–128.

74. Washington K, Gossage DL, Gottfried MR. Pathology of the pancreas in severe combined immunodeficiency and DiGeorge syndrome: acute graft-versus-host disease and unusual viral infections. *Hum Pathol* 1994;25:908–14.

75. Ko CW, Gooley T, Schoch HG, et al. Acute pancreatitis in marrow transplant patients: prevalence at autopsy and risk factor analysis. *Bone Marrow Transplant* 1997;20:1081–6.

76. Akpek G, Valladares JL, Lee L, Margolis J, Vogelsang GB. Pancreatic insufficiency in patients with chronic graft-versus-host disease. *Bone Marrow Transplantation* 2001;27:163–6.

77. Maringhini A, Gertz MA, DiMagno EP. Exocrine pancreatic insufficiency after allogeneic bone marrow transplantation. *International Journal of Pancreatology* 1995;17:243–7.

78. Radu B, Allez M, Gornet JM, et al. Chronic diarrhoea after allogenic bone marrow transplantation. *Gut* 2005;54:161–174.

21

Chronic Graft versus Host Disease and the Lung

Javier Bolaños-Meade and Jason W. Chien

INTRODUCTION

Many patients undergoing allogeneic blood and bone marrow transplantation are expected to survive decades after the procedure [1], many of whom will develop chronic graft versus host disease (GVHD) and respiratory complications. Contrary to acute GVHD of the Lung where the syndrome is not common or universally recognized, cryptogenic organizing pneumonia (COP, also known as with bronchiolitis obliterans organizing pneumonia or BOOP) and bronchiolitis obliterans syndrome (BOS) are well-recognized complications that are associated with chronic GVHD [2–4]. BOS and COP can become extremely disabling disorders, resulting in high morbidity and mortality. Therefore, the clinician caring for transplant patients should be familiar with these syndromes.

Recently, the National Institutes of Health Consensus Conference on chronic GVHD published a set of comprehensive recommendations for supportive care of patients with chronic GVHD [5]. These guidelines included recommendations for patients with COP and BOS. The purpose of this chapter is to provide additional details regarding the clinical features, diagnostic approach, and management of these complicated syndromes.

CLINICAL CASE

A 49-year-old female with chronic myelogenous leukemia underwent a human leukocyte antigen (HLA)-matched bone marrow transplant from a sibling after failure to respond to imatinib. Her GVHD prophylaxis consisted of methotrexate and cyclosporine, but cyclosporine was switched to tacrolimus due to severe nausea. She did not develop acute GVHD but 7 months posttransplant presented with chronic GVHD (overlap acute-chronic according to the National Institute of Health [NIH] classification) involving the skin, which was treated with oral corticosteroids and tacrolimus. Her skin condition improved. However, she complained of shortness of breath during the steroid taper. She underwent a bronchoscopy and was diagnosed with *Pseudomonas* pneumonia, which was

treated with broad spectrum antibiotics. A couple of months later, her pulmonary function testing showed a decline with a forced expiratory volume (FEV$_1$) of 56% of predicted. Her thoracic scans showed bilateral patchy infiltrates. She was started on high doses of steroids given the potential diagnosis of COP. As her condition did not improve, she underwent an open lung biopsy that showed mixed lung injury patterns with obliterative bronchiolitis and acute and chronic bronchitis and bronchiolitis with areas of COP associated with giant cells.

APPROACH TO DIAGNOSIS

In general, there are four main components in the diagnostic approach for assessment of respiratory symptoms occurring among long-term survivors of transplantation: clinical assessment, pulmonary function testing, chest imaging, and diagnostic procedures. Due to the potential need for immunosuppressive therapy and the often immunosuppressed state of the transplantation patient, the priority for all of these components is to determine whether the respiratory symptoms may have an infectious etiology.

Clinical Assessment

Clinical assessment should not only inquire about potential lower respiratory tract causes but also address potential upper respiratory tract causes of lower respiratory tract symptoms (e.g., postnasal drip, sinus congestion, or sinus drainage), which can cause intermittent airflow obstruction. Once it is determined that the pulmonary syndrome is unlikely to be caused by an infectious agent, the focus should turn to determining whether there is an intrathoracic versus extrathoracic cause of the respiratory symptoms. The most common noninfectious extrathoracic cause of respiratory symptoms among long-term survivors of transplantation are sclerotic changes of the skin around the chest wall or abdomen, severe kyphosis, and respiratory muscle weakness secondary to deconditioning or long-term corticosteroid use. The most common noninfectious intrathoracic causes include large pleural effusions, pulmonary fibrosis due to previous chest irradiation, complicated infection, chronic interstitial lung disease, large pleural effusions, COP, and BOS. Unfortunately, clinical symptoms for both extrathoracic and intrathoracic causes are generally nonspecific. Both causes may result in shortness of breath, dyspnea on exertion, and a dry cough. However, a sense of inability to maximally inhale and exhale is often a symptom of extrathoracic causes, although patients with severe air trapping associated with BOS and large pleural effusions may have a similar sensation. Also unique to COP is the association with fever, which has been noted in 61% of the cases in a recent report (see subsequent text) [6]. In the setting of normal spirometry and lung volumes, but an abnormal carbon monoxide diffusing capacity (DLCO), other causes of pulmonary symptoms, such as cardiac dysfunction and thromboembolic diseases, should be considered.

Pulmonary Function Testing

Pulmonary function testing plays a major role in assessing changes in lung function and helping to determine which additional test is appropriate. Pulmonary function measurements fall into three main categories: spirometry, lung volumes, and diffusion capacity. Each of these provides unique information which, when combined, provides a comprehensive assessment of lung function.

Spirometry measures the rate of air exhaled by the patient as a function of time, calculated as the rate of volume change over time (liters/second). The forced vital capacity (FVC), the 1 second FEV_1 of the FVC maneuver, and the FEV_1/FVC ratio are the most commonly reported spirometric values. Interpretation of these spirometric results begins by differentiating between an obstructive versus a restrictive physiologic pattern. Although the American Thoracic Society (ATS) defines airflow obstruction as a disproportionate reduction of the FEV_1 to the FVC to below the lower limit of normal, in most pulmonary laboratories, an FEV_1/FVC ratio of ≤ 0.7 is generally accepted as an indicator of the presence of an obstructive spirometric pattern [7]. Once an obstructive pattern is evident, the severity of the obstruction is graded using the FEV_1. If the FEV_1 and the FVC are decreased proportionally, such that the ratio remains in the normal range despite significant reductions of the FEV_1 and FVC, a restrictive physiologic pattern should be suspected and must be confirmed with lung volume measurements (see subsequent text). Another value often assessed is the forced mid-expiratory flow rate (FEF 25%–75%) This measurement represents the average flow rate between 25% and 75% FVC and is intended to reflect the most effort independent portion of the expiratory curve. The terminal peripheral airways are assumed to be the most sensitive to changes in caliber, and are where diseases of chronic airflow obstruction are thought to begin [8, 9]. Although the FEF 25% to 75% is frequently used by clinicians, studies of large cohorts of healthy subjects indicate the FEF 25% to 75% varies widely, such that its sensitivity for detecting disease is very limited [10, 11]. When a significant reduction in airflow is detected, spirometry may be repeated

after inhalation of a short-acting bronchodilator (BD). The ATS defines a significant BD response as an increase in either the FEV_1 or FVC by $\geq 12\%$ and an increase in either the FEV_1 or FVC by ≥ 0.2 L from the pre-BD value [12]. Although a significant BD response may help predict response to therapy for other diseases with airflow obstruction such as asthma, the implications of a significant BD response in a transplantation patient who has developed rapid airflow decline has not been well studied.

There are three main lung volume parameters to consider for most pulmonary function tests (PFTs) [13]. The total amount of gas in the lungs after a full inspiration total lung capacity (TLC), the amount of gas remaining after maximal expiration residual volume (RV), and the amount of gas inhaled from RV to TLC (vital capacity [VC]). Comparable reduction of the FVC and the VC, with a reduction in TLC, confirms the suspicion for a restrictive process suggested by the proportional decrease of the FEV_1 and FVC mentioned in the preceding text. In general, the TLC is reduced when a parenchymal (e.g., fibrosis, COP) or extraparenchymal (e.g., pleural effusion, muscle weakness, sclerodermic changes of the skin) abnormality results in a restrictive pulmonary physiology. Parenchymal disorders typically result in reductions of all the lung volumes. In contrast, a chest wall disorder may reduce the TLC but increase the RV and RV/TLC ratio. In the presence of an obstructive pattern, the RV/TLC ratio may be increased due to air trapping reflected by an increased RV, while maintaining a normal to slightly elevated TLC.

The diffusion capacity, most commonly assessed by the single-breath carbon monoxide method (DLCO) [14], is a measure of the patient's ability to exchange gases at the alveolar capillary interface, reflecting alveolar membrane thickness, hemoglobin level, cardiac output and heterogeneity in the distribution of the diffusion capacity to regional ventilation and perfusion (in patients with pulmonary disease) [15, 16]. Of all of the pulmonary function parameters, DLCO has the most interlaboratory variability. Although an adjustment of the DLCO for hemoglobin is not required, the changes in DLCO, as a function of hemoglobin, are well known [17]. For transplantation patients, whose hemoglobin levels may vary significantly, this correction is particularly important. There are no official recommendations regarding whether the DLCO should be corrected for alveolar volume [18]. However, since it is known that the relationship between a lower alveolar volume and decrease in diffusion capacity is not in a 1:1 proportion [16] current recommendations do not suggest routine corrections of the DLCO for alveolar volume [14].

Chest Imaging

As is important with the clinical assessment, interpretation of chest images should first determine the likelihood of a noninfectious versus infectious etiology for the respiratory symptoms. If there are symptoms suggestive of a sinus infection, this should be confirmed with a sinus computed tomographic (CT) scan. Although a posteroanterior and lateral chest radiograph is generally adequate as an initial assessment, the major non-infectious syndromes related to the transplantation population (e.g., COP and BOS) require CT images for directing additional work-up. At our center, selection of a noncontrasted regular CT versus a high-resolution CT depends upon whether the PFT reveals a restrictive versus obstructive pattern (see subsequent text). However, if the PFT results are not readily available, a high-resolution CT will capture all of the data necessary for differentiating between COP and BOS.

Diagnostic Procedures

The focus of additional diagnostic procedures is also on identifying or ruling out an infectious etiology to the respiratory symptoms. If there are upper respiratory tract symptoms, a sputum specimen and nasopharyngeal aspiration may be adequate for bacterial and viral studies. However, if chest radiographs or CT scans indicate airway or parenchymal abnormalities, a bronchoalveolar lavage via a fiberoptic bronchoscope should be pursued. If the bronchoalveolar lavage is negative but an infectious process remains possible based upon the CT scan abnormalities (e.g., alveolar filling abnormality, nodular changes, diffuse interstitial process), a lung biopsy, preferably obtained via a videoscope (not trasbronchial), should be pursued to confirm a noninfectious process before the initiation of high-dose systemic immunosuppressive therapy.

CRYPTOGENIC ORGANIZING PNEUMONIA

Risk Factors and Epidemiology

Freudenberg et al. from the Fred Hutchinson Cancer Research Center reported on 49 patients with COP after allogeneic transplantation [6]. They reported that both acute and chronic GVHD were significantly more common in patients with histologically confirmed COP than in control subjects. Among subjects with histologic COP, 81% (vs. 56% of controls) developed acute GVHD, which was also more severe than the controls. Patients with COP were more likely to have clinically extensive and progressive chronic GVHD at disease onset and were more likely to have involvement of the gastrointestinal tract and oral mucosa. Other studies have found that patients receiving grafts from unrelated donors have a higher risk of COP when compared to those receiving related grafts [19, 20].

Clinical Manifestation

The clinical manifestations of COP, if there are any, are generally nonspecific and constitutional. According to the Freudenberger study, which represents the largest single collection of transplantation related COP [6], the median day of onset of symptoms was 108 days after transplantation, with a very wide range extending from 5 days to over 4 years after transplantation. The most commonly reported symptoms included fever (61%), dyspnea (45%), nonproductive (43%) and productive (16%) cough. However, 23% were asymptomatic.

Upon physical examination, although 48% of the patients had crackles, 50% did not have any physical examination findings. There was also a strong association between COP and the presence of acute and chronic GVHD. Patients with COP were more likely to have skin involvement with acute GVHD and were more likely to have gut and oral cavity involvement with chronic GVHD.

The predominant pattern found on pulmonary function testing was a restrictive defect. Forty-three percent of the patients with COP had a restrictive pattern. However, 11% had an obstructive pattern and 38% had no abnormalities at all. Three of the patients also had a combined restrictive and obstructive pattern. In our clinical experience, we have also observed this and have pathologic confirmation that both COP and BOS may be present simultaneously. The majority of the patients with COP also had a decrease of the DLCO (64%), which is likely related to the involvement of gas-exchanging units in this syndrome. Although this study did not comment on the prevalence of hypoxia, our clinical experience indicates that significant hypoxia can be present, but this is highly variable, likely due to the duration and severity of the process at presentation. In Table 21.1, we provide a description of the common PFT patterns observed in the setting of COP.

There are three main radiographic patterns associated with COP: multiple or bilateral alveolar airspace opacities, diffuse bilateral infiltrates, and solitary focal infiltrates (Figure 21.1). Unfortunately, all of these patterns may be consistent with an infection. Therefore, it is highly recommended that at minimum, all patients suspected of having COP should receive a bronchoalveolar lavage. However, given that COP is commonly treated with a prolonged course of corticosteroids, it is preferred that all cases of COP are histologically documented, preferably with video-assisted thoracoscopic biopsy.

Diagnostic Criteria

Classic histologic findings of COP include obliteration of terminal bronchioles with fibrotic tissue in the lumen, extending into the alveolar sacs, consistent with organizing pneumonia [21]. Although a histologic diagnosis is always preferred when dealing with a syndrome that requires immunosuppressive therapy, the risks associated with a lung biopsy should always be considered, especially in a patient whose pulmonary function is already compromised. Unfortunately, if a histologic diagnosis is not pursued, there are no current accepted clinical diagnostic criteria for COP. Given the aforementioned discussion, we have developed recommended diagnostic criteria that differentiate between confirmed and probable COP, depending upon whether the diagnosis is supported by pathologic findings (Table 21.2).

Therapy and Outcome

Currently, there are no standard recommendations for the treatment of hematopoietic cell transplantation (HCT)-related COP. However, given the experience with idiopathic COP in

Table 21.1: Typical Pulmonary Function Testing Abnormalities Associated with COP and BOS

Parameter	COP	BOS
FEV_1	↓ or normal	↓ to ↓↓↓, may be reversible with bronchodilators
FVC	↓ or normal	↓ or normal
FEV_1/FVC ratio	normal	↓↓↓
TLC	↓ or normal	Normal
RV	↓ or normal	↑ to ↑↑↑
DLCO	↓ or normal	↓ to ↓↓↓
Overall pattern	Restrictive defect with compromise of alveolar capillary interface	Obstructive defect with air trapping and compromise of alveolar capillary interface

BOS, bronchiolitis obliterans syndrome; COP, cryptogenic organizing pneumonia; DLCO, carbon monoxide method; FEV_1, forced expiratory volume; FVC, forced vital capacity; RV, residual volume; TLC, total lung capacity.

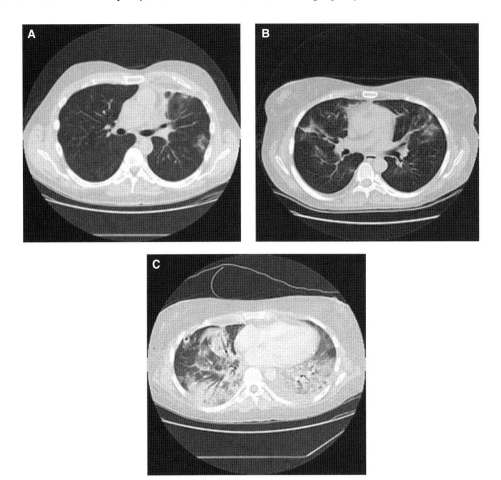

Figure 21.1 Common computed tomographic patterns of cryptogenic organizing pneumonia. A: Focal airspace consolidation with a nodular appearance, B: Multifocal airspace consolidation with a nodular appearance, and C: Bilateral diffuse airspace consolidation.

the nontransplant population, a prolonged course of systemic corticosteroid therapy is commonly used. In the Freudenberg study, 77% of the COP patients received corticosteroids at different doses [6]. Treatment with corticosteroids and corticosteroid dosing strategy did not appear to affect the COP outcome or survival. COP resolved or remained stable in 78%

of cases and progressed in 22% despite corticosteroids with initial doses that ranged from 1 mg/kg/day to 2 g/day. Of these patients with progressive disease, 73% died of respiratory failure secondary to COP. Fifty-five percent survived to 1 year following transplantation with an estimated 5-year survival of 33%. However, in general, it appears that COP and BOS are

Table 21.2: Recommended Clinical Criteria for the Diagnosis of Probable or Definite COP

Probable COP: all of the following must be present
1. Evidence of multiple or bilateral alveolar airspace opacities, diffuse bilateral infiltrates, or solitary focal infiltrates on CT scan
2. No evidence of active infection in the respiratory tract, documented with investigations directed by clinical symptoms, such as radiologic studies (x-rays and/or CT scans) and/or microbiologic cultures (sinus aspiration, upper respiratory tract viral screen, sputum culture, bronchoalveolar lavage, CT guided aspiration, and/or open lung biopsy or video-assisted thoracoscopic biopsy)
3. Complete resolution after treatment with immunosuppressive therapy

Definite COP
- Pathologic changes consistent with COP. Suggest VATS as method of choice for obtaining tissue samples, but transbronchial and CT guided needle biopsies acceptable when adequate tissue specimens are obtained

COP, cryptogenic organizing pneumonia; CT, computerized tomography; VATS, video-assisted thoracic surgery.

not common causes of death in patients undergoing transplantation [22]. There are also some preliminary data on the use of macrolides, particularly azythromycin and erythromycin, suggesting that these drugs improve the pulmonary function on patients with both posttransplant as well as idiopathic COP [23, 24]. However, these reports are anecdotal and further investigation is warranted.

Pulmonary rehabilitation programs may be of value in patients with pulmonary chronic GVHD. If the need for supplemental oxygen is documented (SpO_2 <87% while breathing room air), then the amount of oxygen supplementation should be titrated using a 6-minute walk. Standard 6-minute walk protocols should be conducted according to ATS guidelines [25]. A comprehensive set of recommendations on supportive care for patients with pulmonary involvement by chronic GVHD have been recently published by the National Institutes of Health Consensus Conference on GVHD with the goal of improving the performance of these patients [5].

BRONCHIOLITIS OBLITERANS SYNDROME

Risk Factors and Epidemiology

Depending on the diagnostic criteria employed, the incidence of BOS after transplant varies between studies [4, 26, 27]. Dudek et al. retrospectively analyzed 2,859 patients who received either an autologous or allogeneic hematopoietic cell transplant at the University of Minnesota between 1980 and 1999 [28]. Forty-seven allogeneic transplant patients with a confirmed diagnosis of BOS were identified among 1,789 allogeneic recipients. There were no cases of BOS among the autologous transplant patients. The median time from transplantation to the onset of BOS was 465 days (range, 77–3,212 days). Of 47 BOS patients, 38 were already diagnosed with chronic GVHD before the onset of BOS. The cumulative incidence of BOS among allogeneic transplant patients was 2% at 1 year and 3% at 3 years after transplantation. Among those with chronic GVHD, the incidence of BOS was 6% at 1 year and 7% at 3 years after transplantation. Cox regression analysis identified older donor and recipient age and prior acute GVHD as statistically significant independent predictors of BOS. Type of disease treated with transplantation, type of donor, source of stem cells, and *Cytomegalovirus* (CMV) status

(identified in univariate analysis) were not associated with the development of BOS.

Clinical observation of these patients suggests that severe airflow obstruction observed when BOS develops is preceded by milder airflow obstruction that may be observed earlier on. With this in mind, Chien et al. conducted a 10-year epidemiologic study to determine the prevalence of significant airflow obstruction that may not qualify as BOS at 1 year after transplant and its impact on mortality [29]. This study found that among all patients who receive an allogeneic transplant, 26% developed significant airflow decline, defined as an annualized rate of percent of predicted FEV_1 greater than 5% and an FEV_1/FVC ratio <0.8. Among patients who developed chronic GVHD, 30% had significant airflow decline after transplant. Many risk factors have been found to be associated with an increased risk in developing BOS. These include low immunoglobulin (Ig)G levels, the use of peripheral blood stem cells (that has been linked to the development of GVHD), the use of busulfan or methotrexate during the transplant process, and the intensity of the conditioning employed, pretransplant reduction in FEV_1 and respiratory complications in the first 100 days post transplantation [4, 30–32]. Although some of these associations have not been replicated, the risk factor most consistently found to be associated with an increased risk of developing BOS is the presence of GVHD. In Dudek's study, 81% of all the BOS cases was diagnosed with GVHD before the onset of BOS. In Chien's study, all of the patients who had significant early airflow decline had some form of GVHD at a site other than the lung. However, presence of progressive-onset clinically extensive chronic GVHD conferred only a 1.9-fold increase in risk for significant early airflow decline ($p < 0.001$), suggesting other factors such as genetic predisposition may be important [33]. In the same study, older age at transplant, poor lung function at baseline, and respiratory viral infection within the first 100 days after transplant were also identified as risk factors for early airflow decline. Additional analysis of the early respiratory viral infections revealed that most respiratory viral infections during the first 100 days after HCT results in fixed airflow obstruction at 1 year and lower respiratory tract parainfluenza virus infection was associated with the highest risk for fixed airflow obstruction at 1 year (odds ratio, 17.9 [95% confidence interval, 2.0–160]; $p = 0.01$)[34].

Clinical Manifestation

Early diagnosis of BOS is difficult because most patients remain relatively asymptomatic until the late stages of airflow obstruction (i.e., $FEV_1 < 60\%$) when it is unlikely to be reversible with treatment. The main symptoms of BOS are nonspecific and include dyspnea, dry cough, and wheezing, characteristic of airflow obstruction; however, some patients are asymptomatic for some time [4, 27, 29]. They usually are insidious in nature and rarely (if ever) include fever [4].

Diagnostic Criteria

Histologic samples usually demonstrate bronchiolitis involving the small airways and fibrinous obliteration of the lumen of the respiratory bronchioles, with or without associated interstitial pneumonia, fibrosis, or diffuse alveolar damage; inflammatory cell infiltrates consist of predominantly mononuclear cells in the lumens of the affected bronchioles, and are thought to be more prominent early in the disease process. In the chronic phase, there are variable degrees of intralumenal or peribronchiolar fibrosis, ranging from proliferation of fibroblasts and myofibroblasts to collagen scarring [35]. Although, it is also preferred that BOS is diagnosed based upon histologic confirmation, because the radiographic features of BOS is less consistent with infection (e.g., no airspace or interstitial infiltrates), the risks associated with a lung biopsy are less justified. Therefore, a recent NIH consensus has recommended clinical criteria for diagnosing BOS using PFTs and radiologic testing (Table 21.3) [36]. Unfortunately, if a regular pulmonary function monitoring program is not instituted, most patients will present with a severe obstructive pattern with significant air trapping (Table 21.1). Radiographic assessment of the lungs should include high-resolution CT scans with inspiratory and expiratory images, which are required to visualize the most common radiographic features, which include air trapping, bronchiectasis, and bronchial wall thickening (Figure 21.2) [37]. It should be noted that although the radiographic features of BOS is less likely to be consistent with an infectious etiology, it is recommended that all efforts are made to rule out an infection, including a bronchoalveolar lavage. As discussed previously, presence of a lower respiratory tract viral infection has been associated with a significant increase in risk of subsequent fixed airflow obstruction [29, 34, 38], suggesting that there may be an infectious etiology to this syndrome, and additional immunosuppressive therapy may not be appropriate.

Therapy and Outcome

As in other forms of GVHD, the use of immunosuppression has been advocated for the therapy of patients with BOS. Ratjen et al. reported on the use of high doses of methylprednisolone for the treatment of children with BOS with improvement in oxygen saturations and FEV_1 [39]. Seven out of nine children studied remained stable without lung function deterioration during long-term follow up.

Table 21.3: National Institute of Health Consensus Criteria for Diagnosis of Bronchiolitis Obliterans after Hematopoietic Cell Transplantation

All of the following criteria must be present

1. $FEV_1 \leq 70\%$; FEV_1/FVC ratio ≤ 0.7
2. Presence of active GVHD at least one other site
3. Presence of air trapping on PFTs (residual volume >120% of predicted measured by body plethysmography) **OR**
4. Evidence of air trapping and/or small airway thickening/bronchiectasis on high-resolution chest CT **OR**
5. Pathologic confirmation of constrictive bronchiolitis

FEV_1, forced expiratory volume; FVC, forced vital capacity; GVHD, graft versus host disease; PFT, pulmonary function test.

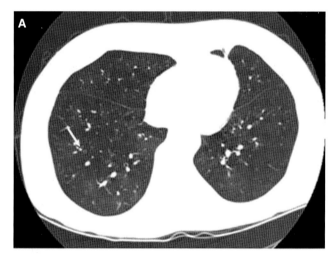
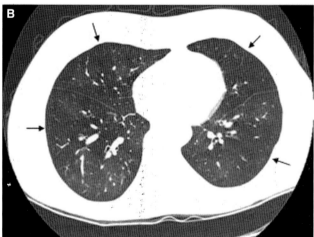

Figure 21.2 Common high-resolution computed tomographic findings of bronchiolitis obliterans organizing pneumonia. A: Inspiratory high-resolution images with bronchial wall thickening (white arrow), which is best visualized in the right lower lobe. B: Expiratory high-resolution images demonstrating patchy lucencies (arrows) indicating air trapping.

In the study by Dudek et al., in 23 of 47 patients, BOS improved after treatment (using antithymocyte globulin [ATG], steroids, cyclosporine, azathioprine, thalidomide); in 8 patients, it remained stable for at least 3 months but later worsened; and in 16 cases, BOS progressively worsened despite treatment [28].

As in COP, it appears that azithromycin may confer a clinical benefit. Khalid et al. reported eight patients with BOS that were given azithromycin 500 mg daily for 3 days, followed by 250 mg three times a week for 12 weeks [40]. Clinically significant improvements were achieved both in FVC and in the FEV_1. However, the data available are very limited in this population. There have also been some reports of lung transplantation for patients with severe end-stage BOS [41, 42]. However, the outcome of these cases have been generally poor and lung transplantation is currently not considered standard practice for treatment of end-stage BOS.

Other treatments have been reported to be beneficial for BOS in uncontrolled studies. Extracorporeal photochemotherapy is a modality that has shown some activity in BOS [43]. Couriel et al. reported on six patients with BOS treated with extracorporeal photochemotherapy, one achieved a complete response with resolution of all the symptoms and normalization of PFTs, and five had partial responses [43]. Fullmer et al. reported a girl treated with tumor necrosis factor-α (TNF-α) blockade with infliximab [44]. Although there have been no major reports, inhaled corticosteroids are now often considered for the treatment of early airflow decline whose severity may not warrant systemic corticosteroid therapy. Symptomatic management with inhaled beta agonists and ipatropium bromide are also suggested given their efficacy in other obstructive airways diseases such as asthma and chronic obstructive pulmonary disease. There have also been some reports of lung transplantation for patients with severe end-stage BOS [41, 42]. However, the outcome of these cases have been generally poor and lung transplantation is currently not considered standard practice for treatment of end-stage BOS. Supportive care for patients with severe BOS should include participation in pulmonary rehabilitation programs and supplemental oxygen when indicated, both of which can significantly improve quality of life. Prophylactic IVIgG does not prevent BOS so its use is not recommended [45].

The outcome of patients with BOS is poor despite the use of steroids, and improvement in pulmonary function is only seen in less than 20% of cases [19, 38, 46]. A rapid decline in FEV_1 is associated with increased mortality, as well as resistance to initial therapy and early onset after transplant [27, 28, 47]. Older patients or those with older donors had responsive disease more frequently [28]. Mortality has been reported to be as high as 100% in patients with BOS, but is not as elevated in all studies [27]. Clark et al. reported a mortality of 65% in patients with chronic GVHD and BOS at 3 years and Dudek et al. reported that only 10% of patients with BOS survived at 5 years [28, 47]. The presence of significant airflow decline at 1 year also has significant clinical implications. Chien et al. found that early airflow decline identified after the first year of transplant independently contributed a 2.3-fold increased risk of mortality

Table 21.4: Evidence-Based Rating System for Ancillary Therapy and Supportive Care Guidelines in Chronic GVHD with pulmonary involvement [5]

Type of Intervention	Rating
Pulmonary function testing	BIIa
Imaging, bronchoscopy and biopsy	BII
Monitoring of oxygen saturation	BIIb
Inhaled corticosteroids and bronchodilators	CIII
Immunosuppression for BOS/COP	BIIa
IVIgG prophylaxis for BOS	EIIa

BOS, bronchiolitis obliterans syndrome; COP, cryptogenic organizing pneumonia; GVHD, graft versus host disease.

following transplant, and the estimated attributable mortality rate associated with this phenotype was 9%, 12%, and 18% at 3-, 5-, and 10-years respectively [29]. Infections and progressive respiratory failure are common causes of death [28] (Table 21.4).

SUMMARY

Pulmonary manifestations of chronic GVHD are underrecognized complications of blood and bone marrow transplantation. Due to its rapidly progressive nature, underrecognized status, and limited therapeutic options, pulmonary GVHD is associated with high morbidity and mortality. Clinical symptoms, imaging studies and pulmonary function testing are very helpful in the diagnosis, but a pathologic diagnosis remains the gold standard, especially given the need for prolonged systemic immunosuppression. It is of paramount importance that patients diagnosed with this complication are enrolled in clinical trials so more can be learned about the treatment of this condition.

REFERENCES

1. Bolaños-Meade J, Hartley E, Jones RJ. Long-term follow-up of allogeneic marrow transplantation for acute myelogenous leukemia after treatment with busulfan and cyclophosphamide. *Biol Blood Marrow Transplant.* 2006;12(3):366–367.
2. Bolaños-Meade J, Ioffe O, Hey JC, Vogelsang GB, Akpek G. Lymphocytic pneumonitis as the manifestation of acute graft-versus-host disease of the lung. *Am J Hematol.* 2005;79(2):132–135.
3. Beschorner WE, Saral R, Hutchins GM, Tutschka PJ, Santos GW. Lymphocytic bronchitis associated with graft-versus-host disease in recipients of bone-marrow transplants. *N Engl J Med.* 1978;299(19):1030–1036.
4. Watkins TR, Chien JW, Crawford SW. Graft versus host-associated pulmonary disease and other idiopathic pulmonary complications after hematopoietic stem cell transplant. *Semin Respir Crit Care Med.* 2005;26(5):482–489.

5. Couriel D, Carpenter PA, Cutler C, et al. Ancillary therapy and supportive care of chronic graft-versus-host disease: national institutes of health consensus development project on criteria for clinical trials in chronic Graft-versus-host disease: V. Ancillary Therapy and Supportive Care Working Group Report. *Biol Blood Marrow Transplant.* 2006;12(4):375–396.

6. Freudenberger TD, Madtes DK, Curtis JR, Cummings P, Storer BE, Hackman RC. Association between acute and chronic graft-versus-host disease and bronchiolitis obliterans organizing pneumonia in recipients of hematopoietic stem cell transplants. *Blood.* 2003;102(10):3822–3828.

7. Lung function testing: selection of reference values and interpretative strategies. American Thoracic Society. *Am Rev Respir Dis.* 1991;144(5):1202–1218.

8. McFadden ER, Jr., Linden DA. A reduction in maximum mid-expiratory flow rate. A spirographic manifestation of small airway disease. *Am J Med.* 1972;52(6):725–737.

9. Cosio M, Ghezzo H, Hogg JC, et al. The relations between structural changes in small airways and pulmonary-function tests. *N Engl J Med.* 1978;298(23):1277–1281.

10. McCarthy DS, Craig DB, Cherniack RM. Intraindividual variability in maximal expiratory flow-volume and closing volume in asymptomatic subjects. *Am Rev Respir Dis.* 1975;112(3):407–411.

11. Cochrane GM, Prieto F, Clark TJ. Intrasubject variability of maximal expiratory flow volume curve. *Thorax.* 1977;32(2):171–176.

12. Miller MR, Hankinson J, Brusasco V, et al. Standardisation of spirometry. *Eur Respir J.* 2005;26(2):319–338.

13. Wanger J, Clausen JL, Coates A, et al. Standardisation of the measurement of lung volumes. *Eur Respir J.* 2005;26(3):511–522.

14. MacIntyre N, Crapo RO, Viegi G, et al. Standardisation of the single-breath determination of carbon monoxide uptake in the lung. *Eur Respir J.* 2005;26(4):720–735.

15. Crapo RO, Forster RE. Carbon monoxide diffusing capacity. *Clin Chest Med.* 1989;10(2):187–198.

16. Yamaguchi K, Mori M, Kawai A, Takasugi T, Oyamada Y, Koda E. Inhomogeneities of ventilation and the diffusing capacity to perfusion in various chronic lung diseases. *Am J Respir Crit Care Med.* 1997;156(1):86–93.

17. Cotes JE, Dabbs JM, Elwood PC, Hall AM, McDonald A, Saunders MJ. Iron-deficiency anaemia: its effect on transfer factor for the lung (diffusion capacity) and ventilation and cardiac frequency during sub-maximal exercise. *Clin Sci.* 1972;42(3):325–335.

18. Pellegrino R, Viegi G, Brusasco V, et al. Interpretative strategies for lung function tests. *Eur Respir J.* 2005;26(5):948–968.

19. Palmas A, Tefferi A, Myers JL, et al. Late-onset noninfectious pulmonary complications after allogeneic bone marrow transplantation. *Br J Haematol.* 1998;100(4):680–687.

20. Patriarca F, Skert C, Sperotto A, et al. Incidence, outcome, and risk factors of late-onset noninfectious pulmonary complications after unrelated donor stem cell transplantation. *Bone Marrow Transplant.* 2004;33(7):751–758.

21. Epler GR. Bronchiolitis obliterans organizing pneumonia. *Semin Respir Infect.* 1995;10(2):65–77.

22. Sharma S, Nadrous HF, Peters SG, et al. Pulmonary complications in adult blood and marrow transplant recipients: autopsy findings. *Chest.* 2005;128(3):1385–1392.

23. Ishii T, Manabe A, Ebihara Y, et al. Improvement in bronchiolitis obliterans organizing pneumonia in a child after allogeneic bone marrow transplantation by a combination of oral prednisolone and low dose erythromycin. *Bone Marrow Transplant.* 2000;26(8):907–910.

24. Stover DE, Mangino D. Macrolides: a treatment alternative for bronchiolitis obliterans organizing pneumonia? *Chest.* 2005;128(5):3611–3617.

25. ATS statement: guidelines for the six-minute walk test. *Am J Respir Crit Care Med.* 2002;166(1):111–117.

26. Yoshihara S, Yanik G, Cooke KR, Mineishi S. Bronchiolitis obliterans syndrome (BOS), bronchiolitis obliterans organizing pneumonia (BOOP), and other late-onset noninfectious pulmonary complications following allogeneic hematopoietic stem cell transplantation. *Biol Blood Marrow Transplant.* 2007;13(7):749–759.

27. Afessa B, Litzow MR, Tefferi A. Bronchiolitis obliterans and other late onset non-infectious pulmonary complications in hematopoietic stem cell transplantation. *Bone Marrow Transplant.* 2001;28(5):425–434.

28. Dudek AZ, Mahaseth H, DeFor TE, Weisdorf DJ. Bronchiolitis obliterans in chronic graft-versus-host disease: analysis of risk factors and treatment outcomes. *Biol Blood Marrow Transplant.* 2003;9(10):657–666.

29. Chien JW, Martin PJ, Gooley TA, et al. Airflow obstruction after myeloablative allogeneic hematopoietic stem cell transplantation. *Amer J Resp Crit Care Med.* 2003;168(2):208–214.

30. Yoshihara S, Tateishi U, Ando T, et al. Lower incidence of Bronchiolitis obliterans in allogeneic hematopoietic stem cell transplantation with reduced-intensity conditioning compared with myeloablative conditioning. *Bone Marrow Transplant.* 2005;35(12):1195–1200.

31. Holland HK, Wingard JR, Beschorner WE, Saral R, Santos GW. Bronchiolitis obliterans in bone marrow transplantation and its relationship to chronic graft-v-host disease and low serum IgG. *Blood.* 1988;72(2):621–627.

32. Santo Tomas LH, Loberiza FR, Jr., Klein JP, et al. Risk factors for bronchiolitis obliterans in allogeneic hematopoietic stem-cell transplantation for leukemia. *Chest.* 2005;128(1):153–161.

33. Chien JW, Zhao LP, Hansen JA, Fan WH, Parimon T, Clark JG. Genetic variation in bactericidal/permeability-increasing protein influences the risk of developing rapid airflow decline after hematopoietic cell transplantation. *Blood.* 2006; 107(5):2200–2207.

34. Erard V, Chien JW, Kim HW, et al. Airflow decline after myeloablative allogeneic hematopoietic cell transplantation: the role of community respiratory viruses. *J Infect Dis.* 2006;193(12):1619–1625.

35. Epler GR, Colby TV. The spectrum of bronchiolitis obliterans. *Chest.* 1983;83(2):161–162.

36. Filipovich AH, Weisdorf D, Pavletic S, et al. National Institutes of Health consensus development project on criteria for clinical trials in chronic graft-versus-host disease: I. Diagnosis and staging working group report. *Biol Blood Marrow Transplant.* 2005;11(12):945–956.

37. Gunn MLD, Godwin JD, Kanne JP, Flowers ME, Chien JW. Correlation of high resolution computed tomography findings and lung function among patients with hematopoietic cell transplantation related airflow obstruction. *J Thoracic Imaging.* 2008;23(4):244–250.

38. Chan CK, Hyland RH, Hutcheon MA, et al. Small-airways disease in recipients of allogeneic bone marrow transplants. An analysis of 11 cases and a review of the literature. *Medicine (Baltimore).* 1987;66(5):327–340.

39. Ratjen F, Rjabko O, Kremens B. High-dose corticosteroid therapy for bronchiolitis obliterans after bone marrow transplantation in children. *Bone Marrow Transplant.* 2005;36(2):135–138.

40. Khalid M, Al SA, Saleemi S, et al. Azithromycin in bronchiolitis obliterans complicating bone marrow transplantation: a preliminary study. *Eur Respir J.* 2005;25(3):490–493.

41. Gascoigne A, Corris P. Lung transplants in patients with prior bone marrow transplants. *Chest.* 1994;105(1):327.

42. Boas SR, Noyes BE, Kurland G, Armitage J, Orenstein D. Pediatric lung transplantation for graft-versus-host disease following bone marrow transplantation. *Chest.* 1994;105(5):1584–1586.

43. Couriel DR, Hosing C, Saliba R, et al. Extracorporeal photochemotherapy for the treatment of steroid-resistant chronic GVHD. *Blood.* 2006;107(8):3074–3080.

44. Fullmer JJ, Fan LL, Dishop MK, Rodgers C, Krance R. Successful treatment of bronchiolitis obliterans in a bone marrow transplant patient with tumor necrosis factor-alpha blockade. *Pediatrics.* 2005;116(3):767–770.

45. Sullivan KM, Storek J, Kopecky KJ, et al. A controlled trial of long-term administration of intravenous immunoglobulin to prevent late infection and chronic graft-vs.-host disease after marrow transplantation: clinical outcome and effect on subsequent immune recovery. *Biol Blood Marrow Transplant.* 1996;2(1):44–53.

46. Crawford SW, Clark JG. Bronchiolitis associated with bone marrow transplantation. *Clin Chest Med.* 1993;14(4):741–749.

47. Clark JG, Crawford SW, Madtes DK, Sullivan KM. Obstructive lung disease after allogeneic marrow transplantation. Clinical presentation and course. *Ann Intern Med.* 1989;111(5):368–376.

22

HEMATOLOGIC COMPLICATIONS OF CHRONIC GRAFT VERSUS HOST DISEASE

Corey Cutler

Chronic graft versus host disease (GVHD) is a frequent, polymorphous complication of stem cell transplantation, with every organ as a possible target of alloimmune attack. The mechanism of reported hematologic chronic GVHD remains a mystery, since the hematopoietic system after transplantation is donor derived, and therefore, any hematologic chronic GVHD must represent aberrant autoimmunity. Alternatively, since immunologic attack against host-derived tumor cells after transplantation is directed against hematopoietically expressed antigenic elements, chronic GVHD may represent an alloimmune effect aberrantly extended to normal elements of the hematopoietic system, perhaps on the basis of newly expressed shared antigenic epitopes. The disordered homeostatic expansion of lymphocytes after transplant-induced lymphopenia or in the context of chronic GVHD may be the cause of such phenomena [1].

The hematologic system is only an infrequent target in chronic GVHD, and, more often than not, cytopenias perceived as manifestations of chronic GVHD have alternate explanations. In this chapter, an approach to the patient with hematologic abnormalities after transplantation is reviewed, as are some of the more commonly seen hematologic manifestations of chronic GVHD.

EVALUATION OF THE PATIENT WITH CYTOPENIAS

There are numerous causes to explain single- or multi-lineage cytopenia seen after transplantation, and many of these causes can overlap temporally with the occurrence of chronic GVHD. Table 22.1 lists the many of the more common causes of cytopenias after transplantation. The most ominous causes of cytopenia after transplantation, usually involving all three blood lines are graft failure and/or rejection, with or without malignant disease relapse. In the absence of a circulating clonal component, only marrow examination is able to diagnose this, although peripheral blood chimerism is an excellent surrogate. A similar clinical scenario can be seen with the marrow aplasia following donor lymphocyte infusions. More

common, however, is an unrecognized toxicity from a drug, and a number of drug classes may be implicated, including prophylactic antibiotics given after transplantation as well as drugs used to prevent or treat chronic GVHD. Infections may suppress hematopoiesis, and there are some viral pathogens that may infect marrow cells directly. Before ascribing cytopenias to chronic GVHD, each of these phenomena must be systematically excluded, either by replacing or stopping potential responsible drugs and ensuring that there is no concomitant infection. In the absence of an obvious cause, marrow evaluation with chimerism analysis is warranted.

COAGULATION SYSTEM ABNORMALITIES: PLATELETS AND CLOTTING FACTORS IN CHRONIC GVHD

Acute bleeding is a significant contributor to the morbidity and mortality of allogeneic stem cell transplantation [2, 3]. In a study of 287 100-day survivors of allogeneic stem cell transplantation, Pihusch et al. demonstrated a 4.2-fold increased risk of any hemorrhagic complication in individuals with chronic GVHD, although the median time to these bleeding events was 33 days from transplantation (Table 22.2). The risk of severe bleeding complications was 10.8-fold higher when compared with patients without chronic GVHD. The majority of these events occurred in organ systems affected by GVHD, and the authors attribute this excess in bleeding to the destruction and fragility of affected tissues and the ensuing hyperperfusion and proliferation of blood vessels in the area [3], although the role of thrombocytopenia cannot be overlooked.

Thrombocytopenia in Chronic GVHD

Thrombocytopenia, defined as a platelet count less than 100,000/μL, is the single most common hematologic abnormality associated with chronic GVHD and has been reported to occur in over 35% of newly diagnosed patients [4]. The mechanism of thrombocytopenia is unknown, although the clinical syndrome of thrombocytopenia is often similar to

Table 22.1: Differential Diagnosis of Cytopenia after Transplantation

Graft/Marrow Related	Immunological	Drugs	Infection
Poor/Partial Engraftment Graft Failure Malignant Relapse	Graft Rejection Post-DLI Persistent Isohemaglutinin* Transfer of Donor Autoimmunity	Antiinfective agents 　Sulfa preparations 　Ganciclovir, Valganciclovir 　Glycopeptides (Vancomycin, Teicoplanin) 　Oxazilidinones (Linezolid) GVHD prevention/therapy 　Mycophenolate mofetil 　Sirolimus 　Chemotherapeutic agents (Pentostatin, 　　Methotrexate) 　Biological therapy (Rituximab, Denileukin 　　Diffitox) Concommitant nontransplant therapeutics Herbal and over-the-counter preparations	Cytomegalovirus Parvovirus B19* Hepatitis B/C Tuberculosis

* Affecting red cell lineage predominantly.
DLI, donor lymphocyte infusion; GVHD, graft versus host disease.

Table 22.2: Coagulation Abnormalities in Chronic GVHD

	After Day 100 Chronic GVHD		Relative Risk
	No n = 114	Yes n = 173	
Any hemostatic event	80 (70.2%)	157 (90.8%)**	4.2 (2.2–8.0)
Bleeding complication	80 (70.2%)	157 (90.8%)**	4.2 (2.2–8.0)
Number (median [range])	1 (0–9)	3 (0–10)**	
Localization			
Skin	39 (34.2%)	80 (46.2%)*	1.7 (1.0–2.7)
Epistaxis	41 (36.0%)	78 (45.1%)	
Mouth	32 (28.1%)	72 (41.6%)*	1.8 (1.1–3.0)
Gastrointestinal	23 (20.2%)	63 (36.4%)*	2.3 (1.3–4.0)
Intracranial	2 (1.8%)	7 (4.0%)	
Urinary bladder	13 (11.4%)	56 (32.4%)**	3.7 (1.9–7.1)
Eye	13 (11.4%)	32 (18.5%)	
Vaginal	6 (5.4%)	8 (4.6%)	
Other	4 (3.5%)	11 (6.4%)	
Severity			
Mild	10 (6.1%)	37 (20.8%)**	4.0 (2.0–8.5)
Severe	1 (0.6%)	11 (6.2%)**	10.8 (1.3–84)
Lethal	1 (0.6%)	4 (2.2%)	
Thrombotic complication			
Catheter thrombosis	–	2 (1.2%)	
Extremity thrombosis-PE	1 (0.9%)	12 (6.9%)*	13.1 (1.7–99)
VOD	1 (0.9%)	–	
MAHA	–	6 (3.5%)	

GVHD, graft versus host disease; MAHA, microangiopathic hemolytic anemia; VOD, veno-occlusive disease.
Adapted from Pihusch R, Salat C, Schmidt E, et al. Hemostatic complications in bone marrow transplantation: a retrospective analysis of 447 patients. *Transplantation.* 2002;74(9):1303–1309.

that of classic idiopathic thrombocytopenic purpura (ITP). In a series of patients with persistent thrombocytopenia and acute or chronic GVHD, platelet-bound autoantibodies were found in five of six affected patients, suggesting a pathophysiology similar to ITP [5]. Since this mechanism certainly does not explain all of the thrombocytopenia noted during chronic GVHD, other pathophysiologic mechanisms have been explored, including the measurement of thrombopoietin (TPO) concentrations in patients with thrombocytopenia and chronic GVHD. Hirayama *et al.* were able to demonstrate in two affected patients that platelet numbers correlated well with TPO concentrations, and that the amount of TPO production in the bone marrow stromal cells decreased throughout the duration of thrombocytopenia [6].

Therapy for ITP occurring in the context of chronic GVHD is very similar to traditional nontransplant ITP, and is responsive to rituximab therapy. Ratanatharathorn *et al.* reported a single case of rituximab-responsive disease [7], while an Italian transplant group has described responses in two of three patients with chronic GVHD associated ITP treated with rituximab [8]. In addition, other traditional therapy for ITP unassociated with transplantation may be effective.

The significance of thrombocytopenia occurring as a manifestation of chronic GVHD has been examined by several groups. In defining a new prognostic scoring system for chronic GVHD, Akpek *et al.* demonstrated a major impact of thrombocytopenia on survival with chronic GVHD, with a hazard ratio between 1.8 and 3.6 for nonrelapse mortality [4]. Other small studies had previously similarly demonstrated that thrombocytopenia was an adverse risk factor for survival with chronic GVHD [9, 10]; however, a more contemporary analysis of several large databases was unable to confirm this fact [11].

Clotting Factors in Chronic GVHD

Evaluation of individual clotting factors during active chronic GVHD has not been performed, although there is evidence that patients with active acute GVHD of the gastrointestinal tract may have depressed levels of Factor XIII, a phenomenon also noted in inflammatory bowel disease [12]. In the study reported by Pihusch *et al.*, no clinically relevant differences in prothrombin time, partial thromboplastin time or serum fibrinogen concentration was noted between chronic GVHD patients with and without bleeding disorders [3].

Factor VIII is a large, complex procoagulant glycoprotein with numerous expressed and unexpressed polymorphisms. It is possible that this protein may act as a minor histocompatibility antigen between disparate donor–recipient pairs, and in fact, the development of an acquired, high Bethesda unit inhibitor to Factor VIII mimicking hemophilia A has been observed in a 50-year-old woman as the sole manifestation of chronic GVHD approximately 13 months after allogeneic transplantation for leukemia (Cutler et al, unpublished observation). This syndrome was responsive to rituximab with corticosteroids and resolved entirely.

Venous Thromboembolism in Chronic GVHD

Venous thrombosis may also be associated with chronic GVHD. In the Pihusch study of hemostatic complications among transplant recipients, the relative risk of an extremity thrombotic event was 13.1 for individuals with chronic GVHD (Table 22.2). In contrast to the excess in bleeding complications, however, these events occurred later after transplantation [3]. A comprehensive investigation of prothrombotic mutations among patients with chronic GVHD did not reveal a relationship between any of the known thrombophilic mutations and thrombotic events among chronic GVHD patients [13]. It has been postulated that the excess of thrombophilia noted among chronic GVHD patients is related to highly thrombogenic microparticles that circulate in chronic GVHD patients [14], or related to endothelial damage from chronic GVHD [3].

RED BLOOD CELL ABNORMALITIES IN CHRONIC GVHD

The red cell system is less frequently involved as a result of chronic GVHD than the platelet system. The two most common pathologic phenomena involving the erythron to have been reported are pure red cell aplasia (PRA) and warm autoimmune hemolytic anemia (AIHA). However, as with any other chronic disease, mild to moderate anemia may occur, and it is likely that chronic GVHD itself may suppress hematopoiesis. Mild to moderate anemia may also be a toxic effect of any number of medications used to treat chronic GVHD or its complications. In addition, complications of transplantation across ABO barriers, graft rejection, malignant relapse, and occult infection must be considered when evaluating anemia in the posttransplant patient (Table 22.1).

Pure red cell aplasia is most commonly associated with persistent isohemaglutinin titres after across ABO-incompatible allogeneic transplantation. Less commonly, it is associated with infection with Parvovirus B19 in the context of prolonged immune suppression. When PRA occurs, a variety of therapeutic maneuvers have been reported to be effective, including the administration of IVIG, plasmapheresis, immunosuppressive medication tapering, and the infusion of donor lymphocytes [15]. When seen as a complication of chronic GVHD, PRA has also been associated with Parvovirus B19 infection where it has been treated successfully with IVIg [16]. Outside of Parvovirus B19 infection, PRA has been treated with some success using rituximab [17, 18].

AIHA, both of the warm and cold variant, may be noted after transplantation in the absence of chronic GVHD, where it may be due to autoantibodies and alloantibodies from red cell transfusion. The incidence may be as high as 3% to 4.4% after transplantation in adult patients [19–21]. In addition, it rarely noted in chronic GVHD [19, 22, 23], where it is often in association with thrombocytopenia (Evans Syndrome) [24, 25]. Therapy for this entity in the presence or absence of chronic GVHD is the same, and consists of corticosteroids, IVIg, rituximab, and other immunomodulatory techniques [26]. Microangiopathic hemolysis may also be associated with chronic GVHD [3], but this may simply be an effect of calcineurin inhibitors used to treat the chronic GVHD.

The role of recombinant erythropoietin therapy has not formally been evaluated in chronic GVHD but may be used in cases of moderate anemia, particularly in cases without an obvious cause and where marrow examination has excluded disease relapse, graft rejection, or infection. This intervention may be particularly useful in patients with renal dysfunction or in spurious cases of low endogenous erythropoietin levels. In addition, folic acid supplementation should be provided.

WHITE BLOOD CELL ABNORMALITIES IN CHRONIC GVHD

The most obvious defect in the leukocyte system during chronic GVHD is the alteration of function in leukocyte subsets, which is associated with an increased incidence of infection when compared with chronic GVHD-free transplant controls. In addition, there are shifts among T-cell subsets, including the regulatory T cells and the subclasses of T helper cells that are associated with the development of chronic GVHD. These lymphocyte cellular subsets, however, are not routinely measured clinically. In addition, there is a failure to reconstitute immunological diversity in the context of chronic GVHD, which is likely more severe than would be expected from immunosuppression alone. Leukopenia has been reported occasionally as a manifestation of chronic GVHD, and there is a reported case of neutropenia coinciding with infection in a patient with chronic GVHD that responded to intravenous gamma globuilin [27]. Infections, immunity, and T-cell function in relation to chronic GVHD are discussed in Chapter 15.

The only major leukocyte subset that is notably altered in the context of chronic GVHD is the eosinophil, which may be increased before clinical signs of chronic GVHD are noted [28–30]. Eosinophil infiltration of affected organs has been reported in chronic GVHD [31, 32] and may be the hallmark of fasciitis after transplantation [33, 34]. In one study, the presence of eosinophils correlated with GVHD severity [35]. The etiology of eosinophilia in chronic GVHD is unclear, although elevated levels of interleukin-5 have been noted in the serum of patients with eosinophilia [36], and within tissue eosinophils at the site of chronic GVHD injury, suggesting an autocrine pathophysiology [35].

The differential diagnosis of eosinophilia in chronic GVHD includes allergy to medications and parasitic infection, and these two etiologies should be excluded before therapy for GVHD on the basis of eosinophilia alone occurs. While tissue eosinophilia in skin biopsy specimens after transplantation is commonly associated with a drug eruption and allergy, this may not always necessarily be the case [37].

CONCLUSIONS

While cytopenias are common after transplantation, the association with chronic GVHD appears limited in the majority of cases, and alternate explanations for the disturbance in hematopoiesis should be sought. However, autoimmune or alloimmune phenomena do occur, and should be treated accordingly, often, with immune suppression. The mechanisms of hematologic chronic GVHD, largely, remains unknown, but may become apparent as the larger story of the pathophysiology of chronic GVHD becomes clearer.

REFERENCES

1. Daikeler T, Tyndall A. Autoimmunity following haematopoietic stem-cell transplantation. *Best Pract Res Clin Haematol.* 2007;20(2):349–360.
2. Nevo S, Swan V, Enger C, et al. Acute bleeding after bone marrow transplantation (BMT)- incidence and effect on survival. A quantitative analysis in 1,402 patients. *Blood.* 1998;91(4):1469–1477.
3. Pihusch R, Salat C, Schmidt E, et al. Hemostatic complications in bone marrow transplantation: a retrospective analysis of 447 patients. *Transplantation.* 2002;74(9):1303–1309.
4. Akpek G, Lee SJ, Flowers ME, S et al. Performance of a new clinical grading system for chronic graft-versus-host disease: a multicenter study. *Blood.* 2003;102(3):802–809.
5. Anasetti C, Rybka W, Sullivan KM, Banaji M, Slichter SJ. Graft-v-host disease is associated with autoimmune-like thrombocytopenia. *Blood.* 1989;73(4):1054–1058.
6. Hirayama Y, Sakamaki S, Tsuji Y, et al. Thrombopoietin concentrations in peripheral blood correlated with platelet numbers in two patients with thrombocytopenia by chronic graft-versus-host disease. *Am J Hematol.* 2003;73(4):285–289.
7. Ratanatharathorn V, Carson E, Reynolds C, et al. Anti-CD20 chimeric monoclonal antibody treatment of refractory immune-mediated thrombocytopenia in a patient with chronic graft-versus-host disease. *Ann Intern Med.* 2000;133(4):275–279.
8. Zaja F, Bacigalupo A, Patriarca F, C et al. Treatment of refractory chronic GVHD with rituximab: a GITMO study. *Bone Marrow Transplant.* 2007;40(3):273–277.
9. Pavletic SZ, Smith LM, Bishop MR, et al. Prognostic factors of chronic graft-versus-host disease after allogeneic blood stem-cell transplantation. *Am J Hematol.* 2005;78(4):265–274.
10. Sullivan KM, Witherspoon RP, Storb R, et al. Prednisone and azathioprine compared with prednisone and placebo for treatment of chronic graft-v-host disease: prognostic influence of prolonged thrombocytopenia after allogeneic marrow transplantation. *Blood.* 1988;72(2):546–554.
11. Lee SJ, Klein JP, Barrett AJ, et al. Severity of chronic graft-versus-host disease: association with treatment-related mortality and relapse. *Blood.* 2002;100(2):406–414.
12. Pihusch R, Salat C, Gohring P, et al. Factor XIII activity levels in patients with allogeneic haematopoietic stem cell transplantation and acute graft-versus-host disease of the gut. *Br J Haematol.* 2002;117(2):469–476.
13. Pihusch M, Lohse P, Reitberger J, et al. Impact of thrombophilic gene mutations and graft-versus-host disease on thromboembolic complications after allogeneic hematopoietic stem-cell transplantation. *Transplantation.* 2004;78(6):911–918.

14. Pihusch R, Wegner H, Salat C, et al. Flow cytometric findings in platelets of patients following allogeneic hematopoietic stem cell transplantation. *Bone Marrow Transplant.* 2002;30(6):381–387.

15. Helbig G, Stella-Holowiecka B, Wojnar J, et al. Pure red-cell aplasia following major and bi-directional ABO-incompatible allogeneic stem-cell transplantation: recovery of donor-derived erythropoiesis after long-term treatment using different therapeutic strategies. *Ann Hematol.* 2007;86(9):677–683.

16. Hsu JW, Czander M, Anders V, Vogelsang G, Brodsky RA. Parvovirus b19-associated pure red cell aplasia in chronic graft-versus-host disease. *Br J Haematol.* 2002;119(1):280–281.

17. Benson DM, Jr., Smith MK, Krugh D, Devine SM. Successful therapy of chronic graft-versus-host disease manifesting as pure red cell aplasia with single-agent rituximab. *Bone Marrow Transplant.* 2007.

18. Zaja F, Bacigalupo A, Patriarca F, et al. Treatment of refractory chronic GVHD with rituximab: a GITMO study. *Bone Marrow Transplant.* 2007;40(3):273–277.

19. Sanz J, Arriaga F, Montesinos P, et al. Autoimmune hemolytic anemia following allogeneic hematopoietic stem cell transplantation in adult patients. *Bone Marrow Transplant.* 2007;39(9): 555–561.

20. Chen FE, Owen I, Savage D, et al. Late onset haemolysis and red cell autoimmunisation after allogeneic bone marrow transplant. *Bone Marrow Transplant.* 1997;19(5):491–495.

21. Drobyski WR, Potluri J, Sauer D, Gottschall JL. Autoimmune hemolytic anemia following T cell-depleted allogeneic bone marrow transplantation. *Bone Marrow Transplant.* 1996;17(6): 1093–1099.

22. Godder K, Pati AR, Abhyankar SH, Lamb LS, Armstrong W, Henslee-Downey PJ. De novo chronic graft-versus-host disease presenting as hemolytic anemia following partially mismatched related donor bone marrow transplant. *Bone Marrow Transplant.* 1997;19(8):813–817.

23. Sevilla J, Gonzalez-Vicent M, Madero L, Diaz MA. Acute autoimmune hemolytic anemia following unrelated cord blood transplantation as an early manifestation of chronic graft-versus-host disease. *Bone Marrow Transplant.* 2001;28(1):89–92.

24. Hartert A, Willenbacher W, Gunzelmann S, et al. Successful treatment of thrombocytopenia and hemolytic anemia with IvIG in a patient with lupus-like syndrome after mismatched related PBSCT. *Bone Marrow Transplant.* 2001;27(3):337–340.

25. Urban C, Benesch M, Sovinz P, Schwinger W, Lackner H. Fatal Evans' syndrome after matched unrelated donor transplantation for hyper-IgM syndrome. *Eur J Haematol.* 2004;72(6):444–447.

26. Raj K, Narayanan S, Augustson B, et al. Rituximab is effective in the management of refractory autoimmune cytopenias occurring after allogeneic stem cell transplantation. *Bone Marrow Transplant.* 2005;35(3):299–301.

27. Khouri IF, Ippoliti C, Gajewski J, Przepiorka D, Champlin RE. Neutropenias following allogeneic bone marrow transplantation: response to therapy with high-dose intravenous immunoglobulin. *Am J Hematol.* 1996;52(4):313–315.

28. Jacobsohn DA, Schechter T, Seshadri R, Thormann K, Duerst R, Kletzel M. Eosinophilia correlates with the presence or development of chronic graft-versus-host disease in children. *Transplantation.* 2004;77(7):1096–1100.

29. Skert C, Patriarca F, Sperotto A, et al. Sclerodermatous chronic graft-versus-host disease after allogeneic hematopoietic stem cell transplantation: incidence, predictors and outcome. *Haematologica.* 2006;91(2):258–261.

30. Kalaycioglu ME, Bolwell BJ. Eosinophilia after allogeneic bone marrow transplantation using the busulfan and cyclophosphamide preparative regimen. *Bone Marrow Transplant.* 1994;14(1):113–115.

31. Daneshpouy M, Facon T, Jouet JP, Janin A. Acute flare-up of conjunctival graft-versus-host disease with eosinophil infiltration in a patient with chronic graft-versus-host disease. *Leuk Lymphoma.* 2002;43(2):445–446.

32. Nonomura A, Kono N, Mizukami Y, Nakanuma Y. Histological changes of the liver in experimental graft-versus-host disease across minor histocompatibility barriers. VIII. Role of eosinophil infiltration. *Liver.* 1996;16(1):42–47.

33. Markusse HM, Dijkmans BA, Fibbe WE. Eosinophilic fasciitis after allogeneic bone marrow transplantation. *J Rheumatol.* 1990;17(5):692–694.

34. Ustun C, Ho G, Jr. Eosinophilic fasciitis after allogeneic stem cell transplantation: a case report and review of the literature. *Leuk Lymphoma.* 2004;45(8):1707–1709.

35. Daneshpouy M, Socie G, Lemann M, Rivet J, Gluckman E, Janin A. Activated eosinophils in upper gastrointestinal tract of patients with graft-versus-host disease. *Blood.* 2002;99(8):3033–3040.

36. Masumoto A, Sasao T, Yoshiba F, et al. [Hypereosinophilia after allogeneic bone marrow transplantation. A possible role of IL-5 overproduction by donor T-cells chronic GVHD]. *Rinsho Ketsueki.* 1997;38(3):234–236.

37. Marra DE, McKee PH, Nghiem P. Tissue eosinophils and the perils of using skin biopsy specimens to distinguish between drug hypersensitivity and cutaneous graft-versus-host disease. *J Am Acad Dermatol.* 2004;51(4):543–546.

23

Neurological Manifestations of Chronic Graft versus Host Disease

Harry Openshaw

INTRODUCTION

Neurological complications from hematopoietic cell transplantation (HCT) often occur from the conditioning regimen (immediate or delayed), from the interval of pancytopenia (infection, bleeding), and from prophylactic drugs for graft versus host disease (GVHD) (particularly calcineurin inhibitors). Less common and more controversial are neurological problems related to chronic graft versus host disease (cGVHD) itself, the topic of this chapter.

With cGVHD defined narrowly as a systemic syndrome mediated by donor T cells, then only polymyositis would qualify as a bone fide neurological manifestation of cGVHD. However, a broader and probably more appropriate perspective would include neurological immune-mediated manifestations that occur in the context of characteristic manifestations of systemic cGVHD or at least in the appropriate time frame of cGVHD. With this broader perspective, myasthenia gravis, possibly immune-mediated polyneuropathies, and a variety of central nervous system (CNS) problems could be considered as instances of "neurological cGVHD."

The obvious difficulty in this interpretation is that cGVHD occurs relatively late in the transplant course (after 3 months) and still later in the course of the hematological malignancy. With multiple intervening therapies and metabolic and infectious complications along the way, it may be problematic to attribute a particular neurological problem directly to cGVHD.

This chapter reviews peripheral nervous system (PNS) manifestations of cGVHD, describes some interesting CNS cases, and proposes criteria that may be appropriate in accepting particular cases as CNS cGVHD. Table 23.1 lists the various entities discussed with estimates of frequency and range of time post-HCT when they most commonly occur. The clinical literature in all these entities is limited almost entirely to individual case reports, only a brief number of which are cited here. Also discussed are other more common and well-accepted, neurological complications that may occur in patients with systemic cGVHD, and need to be considered in the differential diagnosis.

PERIPHERAL NERVOUS SYSTEM MANIFESTATIONS OF cGVHD

Muscle weakness is the common sign in all patients with PNS manifestations of cGVHD. Figure 23.1 shows an approach in differential diagnosis of lower motor neuron weakness using neurophysiological tests [1]. Onset of upper motor neuron weakness (associated with spasticity, increase in deep tendon reflexes, and extensor plantar responses) carries a grave prognosis, usually indicating a brain mass lesion or epidural cord compression. For lower motor neuron weakness, clinical examination usually suffices in localizing the problem to (1) motor nerve roots (segmental weakness and loss of reflexes in a nerve root distribution), (2) peripheral nerves (primarily distal distribution with usually some sensory loss), (3) neuromuscular junction (variable weakness with fatiguability involving eye, bulbar, or proximal muscles), or (4) muscle (proximal distribution). As shown in this figure, neurophysiological tests can also be used for localization depending on whether there is acute denervation (fibrillation potentials or positive sharp waves) on electromyography (EMG), whether there are myopathic or neuropathic motor units on EMG, and whether there are slow nerve conduction velocities (NCVs) (modified from Reference 1). The entities marked by asterisks in the last column of Figure 23.1 will be discussed in this section. In patients with severe neuropathic weakness, nerve conduction tests are particularly important to differentiate demyelinating neuropathies (generally immune mediated) from axonal neuropathies (such as, critical illness polyneuropathy in HCT patients who develop acute respiratory distress syndrome). Weakness in a nerve root distribution suggests a leptomeningeal recurrence or an epidural deposit. Also possible but much less common is segmental zoster motor paresis. Clinical examination of the pattern of weakness in HCT patients with the help of neurophysiological tests allows distinction among weakness of a deconditioned state, myopathic weakness from steroids or cGVHD-associated polymyositis, neuromuscular junction abnormality of myasthenia gravis, and neuropathic weakness of posttransplant demyelinating polyneuropathy.

Table 23.1: Neurological Manifestations of cGVHD

	Incidence of HCT (%)	Onset After HCT	References
Polymyositis	2–3	3–35 mon (median 18 mon)	(2–5)
Myasthenia gravis	0.2	7–60 mon (median 28 mon)	(8–10, 14, 15)
Post-HCT polyneuropathy	≤1	1–16 mon (median 9 mon)	(16, 17, 23–25)
CNS cGVHD	Uncertain	2–31 mon (median 14.5 mon)	(34–36, 41–46, 48)

cGVHD, chronic graft versus host disease; CNS, central nervous system; HCT, hematopoietic cell transplantation; mon, months.

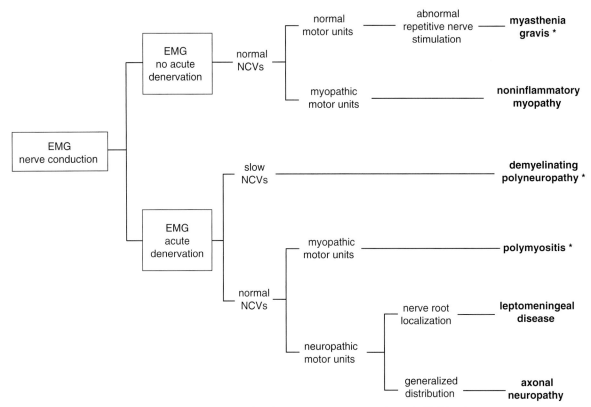

Figure 23.1 Diagnostic approach to lower motor neuron weakness in HCT patients.

Polymyositis

Polymyositis is the most common immunologically mediated neurological complication of transplantation, occurring in 2% to 3% of allogeneic transplants, usually from 1 to 3 years after transplantation [2, 3]. It is a well-recognized part of the syndrome of cGVHD, and rarely it is the sole manifestation of cGVHD [4]. There is at least one report of polymyositis after autologous transplantation, with onset very early in the course (2 months after transplantation) [5]. The proximal muscle weakness from polymyositis may be mild and may go unrecognized for a time (particularly in patients having a slow motor

rehabilitation from the transplant). Rare instances of autoimmune hyperthyroidism during cGVHD may cause proximal weakness that is mistaken for polymyositis [6]. Iatrogenic inflammatory myopathies must also be excluded. For example, a ricin-tagged antibody to CD5 used investigationally for GVHD, has been implicated in cases of myopathy, and cyclosporin-associated rhabdomyolyis has been encountered in transplant patient [7].

The most common diagnostic problem, however, is to exclude steroid myopathy as the cause of proximal muscle weakness. Muscle cramps and tenderness are more characteristic of polymyositis than steroid myopathy, and serum creatine phosphokinase levels generally are normal in steroid myopathy and elevated in polymyositis. In confusing cases, the distinction may depend on muscle biopsy and electromyography (EMG). Polymyositis is confirmed on muscle biopsy by demonstrating necrotic myofibers and mononuclear inflammatory cells (primarily suppressor/cytotoxic T cells) [3]. Also polymyositis and not steroid myopathy characteristically has signs of membrane instability on EMG (positive sharp waves and fibrillation potentials). Muscle weakness in posttransplant polymyositis usually responds to the initiation or dose escalation of prednisone. For patients in whom polymyositis and steroid myopathy may coexist, particular care is needed as the prednisone dose is adjusted.

Myasthenia Gravis

Myasthenia gravis (MG) is an immune-mediated disease of the neuromuscular junction in which autoantibodies to the postsynaptic acetyl choline receptor produce a characteristic pattern of fluctuating weakness involving eye lids, extraocular muscles, and sometimes bulbar and proximal muscles. Post-HCT MG is considered to be set off through the immune dysregulation of cGVHD. However, unlike polymyositis, symptomatic MG tends to be delayed, coming on when immunosuppressant drugs for cGVHD have been tapered or stopped, not at the height of systemic cGVHD [1, 8, 9]. In 15 separate case reports, there is only one patient with onset earlier than 23 months: a 20-year-old man with aplastic anemia who developed MG 7 months after HCT when cyclosporin was stopped [10]. This patient is unique in that there was no other manifestations of cGVHD, antiacetyl choline receptor antibody was negative, and there was prompt complete remission when corticosteroids were started.

Another unusual aspect of post-HCT MG is the marked overrepresentation in patients transplanted for aplastic anemia: 9 of 15 case reports of post-HCT MG are in patients with aplastic anemia. MG also is associated with pure red blood cell dyscrasia in nontransplant patients [11]; and malignant thymomas occur occasionally in both diseases, although thymomas have not been reported in post-HCT MG. Other features of post-HCT MG include relatively young age (median age of 20 in reported cases), overrepresentation of opposite sex donors, and presence of other autoantibodies as well (including antiplatelet antibodies, antinuclear antibody, antimitochondrial antibodies, and antismooth-muscle antibodies). Some patients when assayed retrospectively had antireceptor antibody early in the posttransplant course, well before the first symptoms of MG. Moreover, antireceptor antibody without neurological symptoms has been recognized in hematological malignancies and aplastic anemia [12] and in as many as 40% of transplant patients in the first year [13]; its detection early after HCT does not predict the later development of MG. In autologous transplant patients, antireceptor antibody also occurs but MG has not been reported.

In terms of medical evaluation and management, most patients with post-HCT MG have had a good symptomatic response to anticholinesterase drugs. Low dose or alternate day prednisone can be used and there is some limited experience with mycophenolate mofetil and rituximab [14, 15]. Reported cases have not been sufficiently severe to require plasmapheresis and there has been no experience with thymectomy as treatment of post-HCT MG. Return to higher level of immunosuppressant therapy is generally not recommended.

Posttransplant Peripheral Neuropathy

In contrast to polymyositis and MG, peripheral neuropathy after HCT can occur early in the course, when the patient is medically most vulnerable [16]. Quadriparesis and the need for ventilatory support at this stage may jeopardize the transplant outcome. In a review, 7 of the 12 cases of severe motor neuropathies after HCT had their onset in the first 3 months, usually during the stage of acute GVHD and often following systemic infections [17]. Very early onset neuropathy has rarely occurred with cytarabine conditioning. In a published case, both cerebellar toxicity and demyelinating polyneuropathy began in the first week of transplant, and the polyneuropathy progressed to quadriplegia and the requirement for ventilatory assistance [18]. A few similar nontransplant patients have been reported with severe motor neuropathy attributed to high-dose cytarabine, all having onset of the neuropathy within 2 weeks of the initial dose [19]. More common but clinically delayed and much less severe is the primary sensory axonal neuropathy from etoposide conditioning [20].

There is a known association between inflammatory polyneuropathies and hematological malignancies, particularly Hodgkin's disease [21]. Therefore, transplant centers will occasionally encounter candidates who have prior history or have an active problem with chronic inflammatory demyelinating polyneuropathy (CIDP) . There is a report of two such patients who suffered severe exacerbations of their CIDP leading to quadriplegia and contributing to death after transplant (allogeneic in one patient and autologous in the other) [22]. In both patients, the exacerbation started in the first week of the transplant just after conditioning therapy that included total-body irradiation.

Demyelinating polyneuropathies that occur after the first posttransplant month are presumed to have an immunological mechanism. These patients are quite heterogenous in terms of hematological diagnosis, conditioning therapy, time of neurological onset, and deficit. Although dysesthesias in the feet usually occur first, the fully developed neuropathies are predominately motor and the disability is usually moderate or severe; patients are often not ambulatory and are sometimes quadriplegic, requiring ventilatory support. Only 3 of the 10 allogeneic transplant patients reported with demyelinating polyneuropathy did not have GVHD, including a 28-year-old man who was seen because of a typical course of mild Guillain-Barre syndrome (GBS) 1 year after transplant and who recovered completely without treatment [17]. Two patients had autologous transplantation. In one, signs of autologous GVHD were reported (but no clinical details were given) and in the other patient, it was speculated that an immune-mediated neuropathy may have been the only manifestation of autologous GVHD [17]. In one patient with relapsing polyneuropathy, the clinicians suspected cyclosporin to be responsible because permanent remission occurred only after cyclosporin was stopped [23]. Similarly, there are three liver transplant patients in whom a demyelinating polyneuropathy was attributed to tacrolimus [24]. The presumed mechanism is that partial immunosuppression alters T-cell subsets, increasing the risk for polyneuropathy, analogous to the increased risk of Guillain-Barre syndrome in Hodgkin's disease. In at least two patients, the course of cGVHD and the neuropathy seemed to be parallel, with improvement in neuropathy only after control of the cGVHD. Treatment included adjustment of GVHD immunosuppressant therapy, plasma exchange, and intravenous IgG. Definite steroid responsiveness was noted in some patients.

In an informative case report published in 2007, Suzuki et al. stressed the distinction between the acute, generally monophasic course of GBS and the subacute, progressive course of CIDP [25]. On the basis of the clinical course of 28 published cases, they found that approximately two-thirds of the 19 patients with GBS had onset within the first 3 posttransplant months; whereas, two-thirds of the 9 patients with CIDP had onset after the third month and generally during the course of cGVHD [25]. There is very limited nerve biopsy information on post-HCT polyneuropathy. In two cGVHD patients with late onset polyneuropathy (4–5 years post-HCT), vasculitis was seen in one and decreased myelinated fibers with occasional nerve fasicle T cells in the other patient [26, 27].

Another cause of neuropathy during cGVHD is thalidomide, sometimes used investigationally for treatment or prevention of refractory cGVHD. Onset, usually after at least 2 months of 100 mg/d, is with numbness, burning, and hypesthesia of the feet. Unlike cisplatinum, which affect primarily large diameter fibers, thalidomide involves superficial sensation more than proprioception or vibration. Weakness distally in the feet and depression of the ankle deep tendon reflexes tend to occur late in the course; and on discontinuation, motor signs revert more readily and completely than sensory symptoms. Thalidomide does not cause major motor disability as seen with high-dose cytarabine and immunologically mediated neuropathies. Although clinical characteristics will usually suffice, nerve conduction tests may be helpful in distinguishing thalidomide from milder cases of immunologically mediated neuropathies. In the latter, there is nerve conduction slowing and conduction block, whereas thalidomide neuropathy (an axonal, dying-back neuropathy) is characterized by decreased amplitude, primarily, of sensory nerve action potentials without nerve conduction slowing [28]. Critical illness polyneuropathy occurring in HCT patients in the context of multiorgan failure and prolonged ventilatory assistance also is an axonal neuropathy but with motor nerves primarily involved and usually profound weakness [29]. As shown in Figure 23.1, with axonal neuropathies like critical illness polyneuropathy, nerve conductions are not slowed but there is marked reduction of compound muscle action potential on motor nerve stimulation.

It is uncertain whether scleredermatous cGVHD itself is associated with neuropathy. Indeed, in systemic sclerosis, despite four decades of occasional case reports and small series, controversy remains as to the existence of neuropathy as a real entity, the frequency of neuropathy, and the mechanism (i.e., whether neuropathies are solely compressive from fibrosis of skin and connective tissue or whether there may also be primary involvement of neural sheath). A recent report in 14 unselected systemic sclerosis patients found what many would consider a higher than anticipated frequency of sensory neuropathy, including increase in sensory thresholds by quantitative sensory tests in 57% of patients [30]. Vasculitic neuropathies with mononeuritis multiplex as is seen in polyarteritis nodosa, rheumatoid arthritis, or other rheumatological diseases rarely occur in systemic sclerosis. Rather, the pathology shows reduction of myelinated fibers of all diameters, endoneurial fibrosis, and intimal hyperplasia of epineural vessels without inflammation. Autonomic nervous system symptoms particularly gastric mobility difficulty and signs occur early; but weakness from motor neuropathy is uncommon.

There has not been a similar neuropathy screening study in scleredermatous cGVHD, and one would anticipate that such a study would be difficult to interpret because of high background problem with iatrogenic neuropathy in transplant patients, including prior therapy with vincristine, conditioning with etoposide, use of thalidomide for cGVHD, and the high incidence of prolonged steroid-associated glucose intolerance in patients with cGVHD. However, in analogy to systemic sclerosis, it is likely that there is increased risk of sensory neuropathy, including carpal tunnel syndrome and other entrapment neuropathies in patients with scleredermatous cGVHD.

Central Nervous System cGVHD: A Real Entity?

In long-term HCT survivors, the incidence of MRI white matter abnormalities and abnormalities in neuropsychological tests have been shown to correlate most strongly with cGVHD [31]. This correlation, however, may result from the myriads of associated complications of prolonged immunosuppression and not from a direct CNS effect of cGVHD. The focus of this section is on those rare patients after allogeneic HCT who develop acute or subacute neurological problems that appear to be immune mediated, affecting the brain or spinal cord.

It has been questioned whether CNS cGVHD is a real entity, whether the actual diagnosis of an infectious complication or disease recurrence was missed in these cases. As an example, in 1988 a single case report was published entitled "Graft-versus-host disease in the central nervous system: A real entity?" [32] This paper, still cited in reviews of neurological complications of HCT, gives clinical and autopsy findings in an infant with severe combined immune deficiency (SCID). Almost 10 years after the original case report, the same authors published further immunpathological studies that established the diagnosis of *Epstein Barr virus* (EBV) lymphoproliferative disease in this patient [33].

Kamble et al. in 2007 comment on this particular case, review other cases, and describe two patients of their own in whom a diagnosis of CNS cGVHD seems plausible [34]. Combining other cases from the literature [35, 36], there have been at least 18 reported cases of putative CNS cGVHD between 1990 and 2007. Age range was 9 to 58 (median age 32), there were 10 women and 8 men, and range of time of neurological onset after HCT was 2 to 31 months (median 14.5 months). Hematological diagnoses were non-Hodgkin's lymphomas (NHL) in five, chronic myelocytic leukemia (CML) in five, acute lymphoblastic leukemia (ALL) in four, acute myelocytic leukemia (AML) in three, and aplastic anemia in one. Neurological presentation was most consistent with stroke in seven, encephalopathy in seven (four with seizures as well), myelopathy in two, and progressive motor abnormalities in two. Representative case reports are given in Table 23.2, subdivided under the headings of demyelinative diseases, stroke from vasculitis or angiitis, and immune-mediated encephalitis.

Proposed Diagnostic Criteria to Establish CNS cGVHD as Real Entity

What is helpful in beginning a review of these cases is to establish certain diagnostic criteria which, if met in full, would result in a consensus diagnosis of cGVHD of the CNS. Cases that fall short may still be instances of cGVHD but more open to argument. Table 23.3 proposes six diagnostic criteria, beginning with the requirement of characteristic signs of systemic cGVHD. Although there is precedent for atypical instances of cGVHD to be limited to a single organ (bronchiolitis obliterans, immune thrombocytopenia, and rare patients with polymyositis as the sole manifestation of cGVHD), CNS cGVHD is too controversial, heterogeneous, and rare to accept cases outside the usual time frame or without some typical clinical signs of systemic cGVHD. In analogy with the now outdated Schumacher criteria for the diagnosis of multiple sclerosis, putative cases of cGVHD of the CNS should have abnormal neurological signs on examination, which are localized to white matter of the brain or spinal cord and no other reasonable autoimmune, infectious, or neoplastic explanation for these signs. This requirement would exclude paraneoplastic syndromes that involve specific set of neurons, including cerebellar degeneration associated with lymphomas and the subacute neuronopathy of Hodgkins disease involving spinal cord motor neurons [37, 38]. Brain magnetic resonance imaging (MRI) white matter abnormalities are included in the criteria as well as cerebrospinal fluid abnormality (at least pleocytosis or elevated protein). Figure 23.2 shows various MRI fluid attenuated inversion recovery (FLAIR) sequence brain abnormalities after HCT that may be misinterpreted as immune-mediated CNS disease: posterior leukoencephalopathy from calcineurin inhibitors, methotrexate leukoencephalopathy, and multifocal abnormalities in

EBV encephalitis. Also, the FLAIR or T2 sequence abnormalities in multiple sclerosis and progressive multifocal leukoencephalopathy could be misinterpreted as immune-mediated encephalitis of cGVHD. Neuropathological study of biopsy or post mortem brain would be necessary to show angiitis or perivascular cellular infiltrates. Demonstration of donor T cells, major histocompatibility complex (MHC) class II expression, and activated microglial cells also would provide supporting evidence of an immune-mediated process. Biopsy material may be required to exclude EBV lymphoproliferative disorder, as in the case discussed in the previous paragraph. Finally, clinical response to immunosuppressant therapy is important in establishing the process as immune mediated. Given the lympholytic effect of corticosteroids and the often recognized transient response particularly of CNS lymphomas to corticosteroids, a sustained response in terms of CNS disease activity would be needed to convincingly exclude CNS infection or recurrence of hematological malignancy. Unfortunately, most of the 18 published case reports fall short of meeting these criteria. Only seven had neuropathology from brain biopsy or autopsy, and in some of these seven, clinical details of the patient's neurological presentation or course are scant. Also cerebrospinal fluid polymerase chain reaction (CSF PCR) assays for viral nucleic acid sequences (including PCR for EBV, *Varicella zoster virus* [VZV], *Human herpes virus-6* [HHV-6], JC virus [*John Cunningham* virus]), now considered standard in evaluating HCT patients with unclear neurological problems, were not available or not obtained in many of the older case reports.

cGVHD and CNS Demyelinative Disease

Two patients with recurrent myelopathy have been reported (Patients 1 & 2 in Table 23.2). Both had skin manifestations of cGVHD and one had optic neuritis associated with a myelopathy exacerbations, suggestive of the multiple scleosis variant neuromyelitis optica, but neither of these patients, followed now for over 10 years, have had other demyelinating attacks to suggest remitting and relapsing multiple sclerosis [36]. One patient seen in pre-MRI era had myelograpy; the other patient met five of six criteria in Table 23.3 (no neuropathology).

A recent letter reported immune-mediated optic neuritis in a 34-year-old man after allogeneic HCT for CML, but the onset was early, day 71, before typical onset of cGVHD [39]. There is also a report of optic neuritis with onset 2 months after HCT in a patient with multiple sclerosis who underwent HCT for CML and had full donor chimerism [40].

A more complicated patient with onset of apparent demyelinative disease 13 months after HCT for ALL is shown as Case 3 in Table 23.2. This patient had CSF oligoclonal bands indicative of immunoglobulin formation in the CNS and neurophysiological abnormalities consistent with PNS as well as CNS demyelination [41]. Unfortunately, there was only a partial improvement with immunotherapy and the patient became wheel chair bound. Although there were definite CNS

Table 23.2: Selected Case Reports of Putative CNS cGVHD

Case Report	Age/Sex	Diagnosis	Onset Post-HCT	cGVHD	Clinical Manifestations	CSF Findings	MRI	Neuropathology	Immunotherapy Outcome	Reference
A. Demyelinating disease										
1	38/F	AML	15 mon	Scleredermatous	Myelopathy, exacerbation at 27 mon with optic neuritis	Increase IgG synthesis	None	None	CS, resolved with fixed neurological deficits	Openshaw et al. 1995 [36]
2	40/M	CML	27 mon	Skin	Myelopathy, exacerbations at 28 mon and 40 mon	Pleocytosis	Focal areas of increase signal with enhancement in thoracic cord	None	CS, PE; resolved with no deficit	Openshaw et al. 1995 [36]
3	24/F	T-cell lymphoma	13 mon	Skin and liver	Progressive motor abnormalities	Pleocytosis, oligoclonal bonds	Demyelinative lesions pons, cerebellum, corona radiata	None	CS, PE; partial improvement	Solaro et al. 2001 [41]
B. Angiitis										
4	43/M	CML	19 mon	Skin and liver	Strokes	Elevated protein	Multiple hemorrhages, focal areas increased signal with mild enhancement	Vessel wall and perivascular inflammatory cells, thrombi	CS, CY; remission	Padovan et al. 1999 [33]
5	32/F	AML	28 mon	Skin	Strokes	Normal	Bilateral areas of ischemia	None	CS, CY; initial improvement then massive stroke, herniation	Padovan et al. 1999 [33]
C. Immune-mediated encephalitis										
6	9/F	Aplastic anemia	8 mon	Skin and liver	Seizures, spasticity, reduced sensorium	Not provided	Generalized atrophy	CD3 cell infiltration, panencephalitis	Not provided, persistent severe deficit, death at 20 mon	Iwasaki et al. 1993 [42]
7	44/F	T-cell lymphoma	18 mon	Scleredermatous	Hemiparesis and seizure	Negative	Infiltrative solitary lesion with mild enhancement	Perivascular infiltrate of donor CD3 cells	CS, near-complete resolution of MRI lesion (6 year follow-up)	Kamble et al. 2001 [34]

AML, acute myelogenous leukemia; cGVHD, graft versus host disease; CML, chronic myelogenous leukemia; CNS, central nervous system; CS, corticosteroids; CSF, cerebrospinal fluid; CY, cyclophosphamide; HCT, hematopoietic cell transplantation; Ig, immunoglobulin; mon, months; MRI, magnetic resonance imaging; PE, plasma exchange.

Table 23.3: Criteria for CNS cGVHD

1. Systemic cGVHD
2. Neurological signs of CNS white matter abnormality and no other explanation
3. Corresponding MRI abnormality
4. Abnormal CSF studies
5. Brain biopsy or postmortem examination abnormality
6. Response to immunosuppressive therapy

cGVHD, graft versus host disease; CNS, central nervous system; CSF, cerebrospinal fluid; MRI, magnetic resonance imaging.

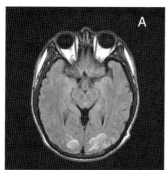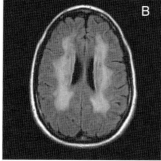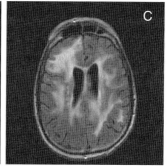

Figure 23.2 Examples of white matter abnormalities in hematopoietic cell transplantation (HCT) patients as visualized on magnetic resonance imaging (MRI) FLAIR (fluid attenuated inversion recovery) sequences. A: Reverible posterior leukoencephalopathy from cyclosporin, B: methotrexate leukoencephalopathy, and C: *Epstein Barr* virus encephalitis.

signs (extensor plantar responses), it is not possible in review of the case to know whether the disability was primarily from the CNS or the PNS. Neither sural nerve or stereotactic brain biopsy was done.

cGVHD and Stroke from Vasculitis or Angiitis

In a mouse model of systemic GVHD to minor H antigens, brain perivascular CD45+ cells were present at day 45 with microglial cells activation and mild changes of angiitis [43]. This experimental model lent support to Padovan's earlier clinical observation of angiitis or suspected angiitis in five patients with cGVHD [35]. Their first patient (shown as Case 4 in Table 23.2) developed right hemiparesis and dysphasia and had hemorrhages and areas of increase signal consistent with multivessel ischemia on brain MRI. Neurological stabilization and improvement occurred with corticosteroids and cyclophosphamide. Typical neuropathological changes of angiitis were still present when the patient died 5 months later from pneumonia. Except for absence of CSF abnormalities, this case report met the criteria set forth in Table 23.3 for CNS cGVHD. Padovan's second patient (Case 5 in Table 23.2) had right hemiparesis and dysphasia, improved with corticosteroids and cyclophosphamide, but then 1 month later suffered a massive infarct in the right anterior circulation with fatal transtentorial herniation. Survival in this patient

was too short to evaluate response to immunotherapy and post mortem brain examination was not done in this case or in the other three patients reported by Padovan et al. There was a single neuropathological case of CNS vasculitis, possibly immune mediated, found in a review of 109 consecutive neuropathological brain examinations from post mortem of HCT patients [44].

In a more recent case report of granulomatous angiitis, brain biopsy documented donor cells in STR (short tandem repeat) analysis of inflamed arteriole walls [45]. The clinical presentation in this patient was more consistent with episodic delirium and progressive cognitive decline, partially corticosteroid-responsive, rather than cerebrovascular disease; and the neurological onset was early for GVHD, 2 months after HCT, although there continued to be neurological worsening 5 months after HCT when the patient had skin cGVHD. Other than two possible exceptions [46, 47], cerebral angiography has not shown typical beading pattern of vasculitis in post-HCT patients suspected of having angiitis, possibly because involvement is primarily in small vessels.

cGVHD and Immune-Mediated Encephalitis

Allogeneic stimulation in a rat model of GVHD leads to MHC I and II expression not only in CNS blood vessels but also in brain parenchyma [48], creating conditions favorable for CNS neuroimmunological process. Case 6 (Table 23.2) summarizes a progressive panencephalitis in a 9-year-old girl with onset 8 months post-HCT for aplastic anemia and pathological findings of widespread brain parenchymal infiltration of CD3 cells at the time of her death 20 months post-HCT. Unfortunately, the case report does not provide information either on CSF tests or on immunotherapy [42]. In contrast, Case 7 in Table 23.2 could best be characterized as a focal left frontoparietal encephalitis with primarily perivascular CD3 and CD4 cells demonstrated on brain biopsy and shown by in situ hybridization to be of donor (male) origin [34]. The patient was a 44-year-old woman with T-cell lymphoma who developed right hemiparesis and seizures 18 months post-HCT. There was improvement following initial methylprednisolone treatment. With persistence of the focal infiltrative MRI lesion 1 year later, a second methylprednisolone course was given; there was then complete resolution of this lesion and no further neurological problem over a 6 year follow-up. CSF studies were normal in this patient, but the other 5 diagnostic criteria outlined in Table 23.3 were met in this case. A thorough evaluation for infection including immunostaining of brain biopsy sections was negative in this patient, and it is difficult to imagine that she had an isolated relapse of CNS T-cell lymphoma post-HCT since only methylprednisolone was given according to the case report. Of the cases reviewed, this patient probably is most convincing as an instance of cGVHD. The second case reported by Kamble et al. died within 6 days of neurological onset (seizures and encephalopathy) and had primarily leptomeningeal and not brain parenchymal lymphocytic infiltration [34].

CONCLUSION

Of the recognized or suspected neurological manifestations of cGVHD, only polymyositis is established as part of cGVHD syndrome, occurring in 2% to 3% of allogeneic HCT and requiring change or adjustment of immunosuppressant therapy. Even more uncommon, MG tends to occur not as part of systemic cGVHD but later when immunosuppressant drugs are tapered or stopped, particularly in patients transplanted for aplastic anemia. Disabling, primarily demyelinating motor neuropathy may occur as often as post-HCT polymyositis; but multiple etiologies are suspected with only about half the patients having onset in the time frame of cGVHD and these patients tending to follow a course of refractory CIDP rather than the usual acute course of GBS. Rare instances of CNS problems occurs post-HCT with characteristics of demyelinating disease, angiitis, or immune-mediated encephalitis that cannot be explained by infection or hematological disease recurrence and by default have been proposed as cases of CNS cGVHD. More experience is needed with these CNS cases before one can be confident that CNS cGVHD is a real entity and before a reasonable estimate of incidence can be made.

REFERENCES

1. Openshaw H, Slatkin NE. Differential diagnosis of neurological complications in bone marrow transplantation, *Neurologist.* 1995;1(4):191–206.
2. Urbano Marquez A, Estruch R, Grau JM, et al. Inflammatory myopathy associated with chronic graft-versus-host disease. *Neurology.* 1986;36(8):1091–1093.
3. Parker P, Chao NJ, Ben Ezra J, et al. Polymyositis as a manifestation of chronic graft-versus-host disease, *Medicine.* 1996; 75:279–85.
4. Pier N, Dubowitz V. Chronic graft versus host disease presenting with polymyositis. *Br Med J (Clin Res Ed).* 1983;286(6383):2024.
5. Schmidley JW, Galloway P. Polymyositis following autologous bone marrow transplantation in Hodgkin's disease, *Neurology.* 1990;40(6):1003–1004.
6. Mulligan SP, Joshua DE, Joasoo A, Kronenberg H. Autoimmune hyperthyroidism associated with chronic graft-versus-host disease, *Transplantation.* 1987;44(3):463–464.
7. Volin L, Jarventie G, Ruutu T. Fatal rhabdomyolysis as a complication of bone marrow transplantation. *Bone Marrow Transplant.* 1990;6(1):59–60.
8. Smith C, Aarlija J, Biberfeld P, et a. Myasthenia gravis after bone marrow transplantation: Evidence of a donor origin. *N Engl J Med.* 1983;309:1565–1568.
9. Bolger GB, Sullivan KM, Spence AM, et al. Myasthenia gravis after allogeneic bone marrow transplantation: relationship to chronic graft-versus-host disease. *Neurology.* 1986;36(8):1087–1091.
10. Baron F, Sadzot B, Wang F, Beguin Y. Myasthenia gravis without chronic GVHD after allogeneic bone marrow transplantation. *Bone Marrow Transplant.* 1998;22(2):197–200.
11. Socinski MA, Ershler WB, Frankel JP, et al. Pure RBC aplasia and myasthenia gravis. Coexistence of two diseases associated with thymoma. *Arch Intern Med.* 1983;143(3):543–546.
12. Lefvert AK, Bjorkholm M. Antibodies against the acetylcholine receptor in hematologic disorders: implications for the development of myasthenia gravis after bone marrow grafting. *N Engl J Med.* 1987;317(3):170.
13. Lefvert AK, Bolme P, Hammarstrom L, et al. Bone Marrow grafting selectively induces the production og acetylcholine receptor antibodies, immunoglobulins bearing related idiotypes, and anti-idiotypes, and anti-idiotypic antibodies. *Ann NY Acad Sci.* 1987;505:825–827.
14. Kotani A, Takahashi A, Koga H, et al. Myasthenia gravis after allogeneic bone marrow transplantation treated with mycophenolate mofetil monitored by peripheral blood OX40 + CD4 + T cells. *Eur J Haematol.* 2002;69(5–6):318–320.
15. Zaja F, Russo D, Fuga G, Perella G, Baccarani M. Rituximab for myasthenia gravis developing after bone marrow transplant. *Neurology.* 2000;55(7):1062–1063.
16. Amato AA, Barohn RJ, Sahenk Z, Tutschka PJ, Mendell Jr. Polyneuropathy complicating bone marrow and solid organ transplantation. *Neurology.* 1993;43(8):1513–1518.
17. Openshaw H. Peripheral neuropathy after bone marrow transplantation. *Biol Blood Marrow Transplant.* 1997;3:202–209.
18. Johnson NT, Crawford SW, Sargur M. Acute acquired demyelinating polyneuropathy with respiratory failure following high-dose systemic cytosine arabinoside and marrow transplantation, *Bone Marrow Transplant.* 1987;2(2):203–207.

19. Openshaw H, Slatkin NE, Stein AS, Hinton DR, Forman SJ. Acute polyneuropathy after high dose cytosine arabinoside in patients with leukemia. *Cancer.* 1996;78(9):1899–1905.

20. Imrie KR, Couture F, Turner CC, Sutcliffe SB, Keating A. Peripheral neuropathy following high-dose etoposide and autologous bone marrow transplantation. *Bone Marrow Transplant.* 1994;13(1):77–79.

21. Lisak RP, Mitchell M, Zweiman B, Orrechio E, Asbury AK. Guillain-Barre syndrome and Hodgkin's disease: three cases with immunological studies. *Ann Neurol.* 1977;1(1):72–78.

22. Openshaw H, Hinton DR, Slatkin NE, Bierman PJ, Hoffman FM, Snyder DS. Exacerbation of inflammatory demyelinating polyneuropathy after bone marrow transplantation, *Bone Marrow Transplant.* 1991;7(5):411–414.

23. Liedtke W, Quabeck K, Beelen DW, Straeten V, Schaefer UW. Recurrent acute inflammatory demyelinating polyradiculitis after allogeneic bone marrow transplantation. *J Neurol Sci.* 1994;125(1):110–111.

24. Wilson JR, Conwit RA, Eidelman BH, Starzl T, Abu-Elmagd K. Sensorimotor neuropathy resembling CIDP in patients receiving FK506. *Muscle Nerve.* 1994;17(5):528–532.

25. Suzuki S, Mori T, Mihara A, et al. Immune-mediated motor polyneuropathy after hematopoietic stem cell transplantation. *Bone Marrow Transplant.* 2007;40(3):289–291.

26. Gabriel CM, Goldman JM, Lucas S, Hughes RA. Vasculitic neuropathy in association with chronic graft-versus-host disease, *J Neurol Sci.* 1999;168(1):68–70.

27. Nagashima T, Sato F, Chuma T, et al. Chronic demyelinating polyneuropathy in graft-versus-host disease following allogeneic bone marrow transplantation. *Neuropathology.* 2002;22(1):1–8.

28. Ochonisky S, Verroust J, Bastuji-Garin S, Gherardi R, Revuz J. Thalidomide neuropathy incidence and clinico-electrophysiologic findings in 42 patients. *Arch Dermatol.* 1994;130(1):66–69.

29. Witt NJ, Zochodne DW, Bolton CF, et al. Peripheral nerve function in sepsis and multiple organ failure. *Chest.* 1991;99(1):176–184.

30. Poncelet AN, Connolly MK. Peripheral neuropathy in scleroderma, *Muscle Nerve.* 2003;28(3):330–335.

31. Booth-Jones M, Jacobsen PB, Ransom S, Soety E. Characteristics and correlates of cognitive functioning following bone marrow transplantation, *Bone Marrow Transplant.* 2005;36(8):695–702.

32. Rouah E, Gruber R, Shearer W, Armstrong D, Hawkins EP. Graft-versus-host disease in the central nervous system. A real entity? *Am J Clin Pathol.* 1988;89(4):543–546.

33. Armstrong D, Hawkins E, Rouah E, Shearer W, Gruber R. Graft-vs-host disease in the central nervous system. *Am J Clin Pathol.* 1997;107(3):379.

34. Kamble RT, Chang CC, Sanchez S, Carrum G. Central nervous system graft-versus-host disease: report of two cases and literature review. *Bone Marrow Transplant.* 2007;39(1):49–52.

35. Padovan CS, Bise K, Hahn J, et al. Angiitis of the central nervous system after allogeneic bone marrow transplantation? Stroke; a *Journal of Cerebral Circulation.* 1999;30(8):1651–1656.

36. Openshaw H, Slatkin NE, Parker PM, Forman SJ. Immune-mediated myelopathy after allogeneic marrow transplantation, *Bone Marrow Transplant.* 1995;15(4):633–636.

37. Bernal F, Shams'ili S, Rojas I, et al. Anti-Tr antibodies as markers of paraneoplastic cerebellar degeneration and Hodgkin's disease, *Neurology.* 2003;60(2):230–234.

38. Schold SC, Cho ES, Somasundaram M, Posner JB. Subacute motor neuronopathy: a remote effect of lymphoma. *Ann Neurol.* 1979;5(3):271–287.

39. Ooi J, Takahashi S, Tajika K, Tojo A, Tani K, Asano S. Immune-mediated optic neuritis after unrelated allogeneic bone marrow transplantation. *Blood.* 1998;91(7):2619.

40. Jeffery ER, Alshami E. Allogenic Bone Marrow Transplantation in Multiple Sclerosis. *Neurology.* 1998;50:A147.

41. Solaro C, Murialdo A, Giunti D, Mancardi G, Uccelli A. Central and peripheral nervous system complications following allogeneic bone marrow transplantation, *Eur J Neurol.* 2001;8(1):77–80.

42. Iwasaki Y, Sako K, Ohara Y, et al. Subacute panencephalitis associated with chronic graft-versus-host disease. *Acta Neuropathol (Berl).* 1993;85(5):566–572.

43. Padovan CS, Gerbitz A, Sostak P, et al. Cerebral involvement in graft-versus-host disease after murine bone marrow transplantation. *Neurology.* 2001;56(8):1106–1108.

44. Mohrmann RL, Mah V, Vinters HV. Neuropathologic findings after bone marrow transplantation: an autopsy study. *Hum Pathol.* 1990;21(6):630–639.

45. Ma M, Barnes G, Pulliam J, Jezek D, Baumann RJ, Berger JR. CNS angiitis in graft vs host disease. *Neurology.* 2002;59(12):1994–1997.

46. Takatsuka H, Okamoto T, Yamada S, et al. New imaging findings in a patient with central nervous system dysfunction after bone marrow transplantation, *Acta Haematol.* 2000;103(4):203–205.

47. Campbell JN, Morris PP. Cerebral vasculitis in graft-versus-host disease: a case report. *AJNR Am J Neuroradiol.* 2005;26(3):654–656.

48. Hickey WF, Kimura H. Graft-vs.-host disease elicits expression of class I and class II histocompatibility antigens and the presence of scattered T lymphocytes in rat central nervous system, *Proc Natl Acad Sci U S A.* 1987;84(7):2082–2086.

24

Rehabilitation Evaluation and Treatment of Patients with Chronic Graft versus Host Disease

Li Li, Leighton Chan, and Lynn H. Gerber

INTRODUCTION TO REHABILITATION AND THE REHABILITATION MODEL

Physical Medicine and Rehabilitation, also known as physiatry, focuses on prevention, diagnosis, and treatment of disabling conditions. Disability is usually the result of a disease process or injury and is associated with a change in life roles or activities. Comprehensive rehabilitation promotes improved functional outcomes and quality of life through the use of physical, occupational, speech, and recreational therapists, psychologists, social workers, vocational counsellors, and specialists in other medical/surgical fields. All members of the rehabilitation team focus on restoring or enhancing functional capacity so that individuals can engage optimally in meaningful and satisfying life activities.

The International Classification of Functioning, Disability and Health (ICF) has become the world standard for identifying the domains that influence health and disability. It provides a conceptual model to view human functioning and disability from the perspective of the body, the individual, and society. Rehabilitation professionals frequently use this in evaluating and developing treatment plans for patients. Its first part classifies functioning and disability and its second part identifies environmental and personal contextual factors. For more specific information, please see www.WHO.org.

Human functioning is the end result of contributors from body structures and their functions, and at the level of the whole person, activities, and participation. Body structures are defined as anatomic parts of the body, such as organs, limbs, and their components; body functions are defined as the physiologic and psychological functions of body systems. An activity is defined as the execution of a task or action by an individual and participation takes the environmental, social, interactive perspective.

Conversely, the concept of disability includes impairments, limitations of activity, and restrictions to participation. Impairments are defined as problems in body structure or function. Activity limitations infer difficulties an individual may have in executing routines and physical activities.

Participation restrictions are used in place of the more negative term, "handicaps."

Contextual factors are grouped into personal factors and environmental factors. Personal factors include the individual's particular attitudes, gender, age, race, vocation, and experience. Environmental factors include the physical, social, and attitudinal environments in which people live and conduct their lives. Disability is not inherent in the individual, but rather it is a product of the interaction of the individual with the environment. It results when mental and physical injury or illness meets an environment that inhibits integration.

This classification system does not provide specific measurements; rather, it provides a conceptual framework about how to approach the evaluation and treatment of individuals with disabilities. It is a method by which to evaluate an individual with life status changes of physical and/or mental function. This chapter approaches the complex problems of chronic graft versus host disease (cGVHD) from this perspective.

Scope of Chapter

Chronic graft versus host disease (cGVHD) may lead to multiple organ system abnormalities, including the skin, musculoskeletal, and pulmonary systems. These abnormalities may be associated with functional sequelae, for example, mobility or self-care problems. In addition, problems related to treatment, such as, steroid myopathy and chemotherapy-related neuropathy can impair function or cause activity limitations.

This chapter discusses the impact of cGVHD and its treatment on an individual's life activities within the context of the ICF. The approach we have used is to examine the specific organ system impairments and relate each to associated functional problems. Finally, we discuss how these conditions may be assessed or treated to maximize an individual's ability to engage in meaningful and satisfying activity. Some of what is presented in this chapter is based on experience the authors obtained at the Clinical Center, National Institutes of Health (NIH). Some of the treatments recommended are, therefore, empirical and have not been tested in clinical trials. Nonetheless, it represents our experience, and the application of well-established principles to this unique population. More planned, prospective, validation, and intervention studies in this field are needed.

Rehabilitation Evaluation

A rehabilitation evaluation should include an evaluation of function. It emphasizes the assessment of the neuromusculoskeletal systems, within the context of function-limiting symptoms such as pain and fatigue. The following standard assessments are typically included in the evaluation: joint range of motion (ROM), muscle strength, muscle tone, sensation and perception, cognition, endurance (stamina), functional activities, and quality of life. Strength is measured on a 0 to 5 scale. Muscle strength of good to normal ($\geq$3/5) is considered necessary for the independent performance of most functional tasks. ROM is a function of joint morphology, capsule and ligament integrity, and muscle/tendon strength. Some limitations in ROM have a more significant impact on function than others. For example, loss of elbow flexion is likely to have a significantly greater impact on function than loss of elbow extension, thereby requiring remediation or adaptive equipment. ROM is measured with a universal goniometer, a device having a pivoting arm attached to a stationary arm divided into 1° intervals. Joints are measured in their planes of movements with the stationary arm parallel to the long axis of the proximal body segment or bony landmark and the moving arm of the goniometer aligned with a bony landmark or parallel to the moving body segment. Factors such as age, sex, physical conditioning, obesity, and genetics can influence ROM. A publication of the American Academy of Orthopedic Surgeons provides normal ROM for the joints of the human body [1].

Functional assessment is a method for measuring a person's abilities and limitations in performing activities of daily life (ADL), leisure and vocational activities, social interactions, and other required behaviors. This can be performed objectively using an observed activity (e.g., measuring how far one can walk in a specified amount of time) or by self-report. It enables accurate diagnosis and quantification of the functional loss, which leads to development of an appropriate and effective rehabilitation program. Some of these measures can be used as treatment outcome measures, as well.

Quality-of-life (QOL) measures are important endpoints in clinical research (Table 24.1). The Bone Marrow Survivor Study (BMT-SS) questionnaire, originally developed for use by the Childhood Cancer Survivor Study, has been modified to address topics specifically related to the hematopoietic cell transplantation (HCT) survivor population and has been validated on a random sample of 100 HCT survivors [2]. It provides self-reported impairments of organ systems, limitations that interfere with daily function and the impact of these impairments and/or functional limitations on daily life either at home, at school, or at work. The Short Form 36 (SF-36) of the Medical Outcomes Version-I also has been used to assess

Table 24.1: Health Status and QOL Measures Frequently Used in Patients with HCT or GVHD

- Karnofsky Scale
- Short Form 36 Health Survey (SF-36)
- Bone Marrow Survivor Study (BMT-SS)
- Functional Assessment of Cancer Therapy-Bone Marrow Transplant Scale (FACT-BMT)
- European Organization of Research and Treatment of Cancer Quality-of-Life Questionnaire (EORTC QOL-C30)

QOL in patients with HCT [3]. The Functional Assessment of Cancer Therapy-Bone Marrow Transplant scale (FACT-BMT), a validated, oncology-specific, QOL instrument has been used in bone marrow transplant (BMT) patients [4]. It has 37 items comprised of four core scales: physical, functional, social, and emotional. It has been reported that the trial of outcome index (TOI) of the FACT-BMT composite of the physical, functional, and transplantation-specific subscales is particularly sensitive to the effects of different medical treatments and sensitive to occurrence to either acute or cGVHD, appearing better able to discriminate between patients who did or did not experience acute or chronic GVHD than SF12 [5]. The European Organization of Research and Treatment of Cancer Quality-of-Life Questionnaire (EORTC QLQ-C30), an internationally validated thirty-item questionnaire, is specifically designed for multidimensional measurement of QOL in cancer patients [6]. It includes five functional scales (physical, role, emotional, cognitive, and social functioning), three symptom scales (fatigue, nausea and vomiting, and pain), six single items (dyspnea, loss of appetite, constipation, diarrhea, sleep disturbance, and financial difficulties), two questions on patient overall QOL and overall physical condition allowing a global QOL score to be obtained. Review of many outcome measures can be obtained from "Measuring health" [7].

REHABILITATION IMPACT OF ORGAN SYSTEM INVOLVEMENT

Frequently Identified Musculoskeletal Problems

The involvement of the musculoskeletal system in cGVHD after allogeneic BMT can be quite extensive and frequently involves the skin, fascia, muscle, tendon, joint capsule, and bone. Musculoskeletal manifestations of cGVHD include joint contractures, fasciitis, polyserositis, arthritis, and polymyositis. Symptoms of myalgia, cramps, weakness, fatigue, balance impairment, and tremor are often reported. The most frequent musculoskeletal abnormalities are soft tissue contractures and limitation in range of motion, fasciitis, steroid-induced myopathy (atrophy), and osteoporosis [8]. Additionally, reduction of glucocorticosteroid dosage might cause polyarthralgia affecting the knees in particular, which often occurs at night, essentially benign and time-limited. Hypomagnesemia, potentiated by cyclosporine, can cause bone pain and hypocalcemia [9].

Arthritis/Arthralgia

In our patient population (NIH cGVHD consultation clinic), approximately 30% of the patients had joint swelling and/or pain. Ankle joints are most frequently involved. Involvement of the wrist joints and all other small joints of the hands are not uncommon. On the basis of our experience, joint symptoms are not usually reported as the most significant disabling condition; they are usually responsive to typical pharmacological treatment.

Fasciitis

Fascia are sheets or bands of fibrous connective tissue that bind or separate soft tissues (organs and muscles) in the body. Fasciitis is an inflammation of this tissue. It is commonly seen in diseases such as ankylosing spondylitis, rheumatoid arthritis, and other inflammatory arthritis. A particular form of fasciitis, eosinophilic fasciitis (EF), also called Shulman's Syndrome [10], is a scleroderma-like process, in which the skin is thickened and edematous, tethered to the subepidermal fascia. It is an uncommon connective tissue process characterized by symmetric inflammatory painful swelling and tightness most frequently involving the medial aspects of the proximal portion of extremities. On biopsy, the fascia is inflamed and there is eosinophilic infiltration of the tissue. Additionally, there is peripheral eosinophilia with elevated erythrocyte sedimentation rate often after an episode of intense physical exertion.

Fasciitis is thought to be due to microtrauma/microlesion, possibly with local ischemia, which develops after intense exertion. This subsequently incites an inflammatory cascade that leads to thickening and fibrosis of the fascia. Cytokines such as transforming growth factor-beta, interleukin (IL)-4, IL-13, and connective tissue growth factor seem to induce an accentuated and persistent fibrogenic response to tissue injury [11].

The first symptom of EF consists of a painful, edematous swelling of the skin, often associated with nonspecific general signs such as arthralgia, fever, pruritus, and weight loss [12]. Meanwhile, a scleroderma-like subcutaneous infiltration or induration, mostly without visible skin changes, develops symmetrically over the distal parts of both arms and legs. Sometimes, orange-peel appearance called *peau d'orange*, erythema, hyperpigmentation, depigmentation, are observed. Extracutaneous involvement may occur within the synovium or tenosynovium. Arthritis, joint contractures, and carpal tunnel syndrome are frequently found and synovitis is not rare [12]. Pain, swelling, and contractures can cause marked functional impairments leading to functional disability. Not all, but many, of these features of EF are shared with the fasciitis of

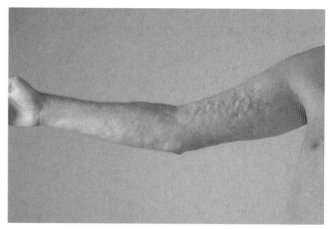

Figure 24.1 cGVHD-associated Fasciitis. See Plate 70 in the color plate section.

cGVHD, and it may be a model for the pathogenesis of the fasciitis commonly seen in cGVHD (Figure 24.1).

It has been reported that fasciitis could be one of the presentations of chronic skin GVHD or the only presentation of cGVHD [13]. Janin et al. reported that 14 patients with cGVHD developed fasciitis in their follow-up course [14]. Half of the patients reported a history of recent strenuous physical activity such as all night dancing, a long bicycle tour, or a football match, and 60% were noted to have peripheral eosinophilia. Partial improvement of cutaneous tightness and contractures and increased mobility were observed in seven patients in response to treatment with corticosteroids. The other patients remained functionally disabled because of skin tightness, severe joint stiffness, loss of muscle mass, contractures, and skin ulceration. Also, six patients had a lymphocytic infiltrate around septal and fascial nerves although none had a documented peripheral neuropathy.

Symptoms of fasciitis are varied and impact on many aspects of one's life. Therefore, a multidisciplinary rehabilitation program might be of benefit to manage fasciitis [15]. While there have been no controlled trials assessing the efficacy of this approach to prevention or treatment of fasciitis in cGVHD, a systematic, comprehensive rehabilitation intervention that addresses prevention, early intervention, and restoration of function may be effective in reducing the disability and symptomatology in cGVHD patients with fasciitis (Table 24.2). We have observed that early intervention for control of edema, strategies for controlling inflammation including pharmacological, such as nonsteroid anti-inflammatory drugs (NSAIDs), and nonpharmacological, to maintain ROM, could be valuable. Thermo-modalities such as continuous ultrasound could be applied, followed by joint mobilization (capsular distraction) techniques, deep friction massage, active range of motion (AROM) exercises, and passive sustained stretching including serial splinting. Patients will benefit from optimal and interdisciplinary pain management, allowing more vigorous therapies to be used. Relaxation and other behavioral pain control techniques are probably useful as well. Individual

Table 24.2: Rehabilitation Program of Fascitis

- Physical therapy
  - Thermo-modalities such as ice, paraffin, or ultrasound to assist in ROM
  - Joint mobilization (capsular distraction) techniques and deep friction massage (in the noninflammatory stage), sustained passive stretching
  - Strengthening exercises (isotonic and isometric)
  - Splint assessment and provision
  - Aquatic therapy
  - Aerobic conditioning
  - Edema management, including wraps, elastic, and inelastic compression garments
- Occupational therapy
  - Activities of daily life (ADL) evaluation and training, adaptive equipment evaluation
  - ROM activities and stretching exercises
  - Fine motor coordination skills
- Others
  - Intraarticular injections of steroids and anesthetic agents
  - Pain management
  - Management of sleep disturbance
  - Psychological therapy
  - Leisure and work-related issues
  - Lifestyle changes to increase activity
  - Vocational counselling

Table 24.3: Nondisease-Specific Risk Factors for Osteoporosis

- Postmenopausal status or estrogen deficiency at an early age
- Elderly age $\geq$65 years
- Low body weight <57.6 kg (especially, low lean mass)
- Tobacco and or excessive alcohol use
- Inadequate dietary vitamin D or calcium intake
- Low physical activity
- History of fracture as an adult
- Family history of osteoporosis
- Drugs: anticonvulsant agents, excess thyroxin, lithium, prolonged unfractionated heparin, methotrexate, and wafarin
- Endocrine disorders: hyperthyroidism, hypogonadism, hyperparathyroidism

Table 24.4: Glucocorticoid-Induced Metabolic Effects Leading to Bone Loss

- Direct effects on bone such as suppression of osteoblast numbers, life span, and function
- Effects of calcium metabolism
- Effects on sex hormones: suppression of adrenal androgen and gonadal hormone release
- Other effects such as decreased muscle mass and strength

psychological therapy to promote healthy adjustment reactions might be needed.

Osteoporosis

Osteoporosis is a disease characterized by low bone mass and deterioration of microarchitecture of bone tissue, which leads to increased bone fragility and fracture risk. Nondisease-specific risk factors for osteoporosis are described in (Table 24.3). Additional factors predisposing to bone loss posttransplant include the high-dose conditioning regimen, cyclosporine and tacrolimus, corticosteroid treatment (Table 24.4), granulocyte colony-stimulating factor, BMT, and GVHD. It has been reported that BMT has adverse effects on bone marrow osteoprogenitors and there may be a direct effect of GVHD on bone cells. Bone marrow function could be impaired by both myeloablative treatment and BMT through the early release of cytokines. The cumulative dose and number of days of glucocorticosteroid therapy and the number of days of cyclosporine A (CsA) or tacrolimus (FK506) therapy have shown significant association with loss of bone marrow density (BMD). Cyclosporine has independent adverse effects that increase bone turnover, and Tacrolimus causes trabecular bone loss in rat. Tacrolimus may cause less bone loss in humans than CsA and also protect the skeleton by reducing glucocorticoid use, however [16, 17].

Osteoporosis occurs in 30%–50% of patients receiving long-term ($\geq$1 year) glucocorticoid therapy. Bone loss is rapid during the first 6 months with glucocorticoid treatment. Trabecular bones including the cortical rim of the vertebral body and proximal femur are more susceptible to deleterious effects of glucocorticoids than the cortical region of long bones. Therefore, the lumbar spine and proximal femur are particularly vulnerable to osteoporosis and related fractures caused by glucocorticoids. Dosages of oral prednisone $\geq$7.5 mg/day produce the most substantial osteoporotic effects, vertebral fracture risk increases to almost threefold and hip fracture risk doubles relative to patients not receiving glucocorticoids [18]. The loss of lean mass in those receiving glucocorticoids may also compound the risk for osteoporosis. The contractile force of muscle, which is necessary for maintaining or increasing bone mineralization, is reduced after muscle atrophy. It has been reported that glucocorticoid-associated adverse effects are not reduced by alternate-day administration [19]; however, local administration (e.g., intraarticular glucocorticoids or intranasal inhaled glucocorticoids) reduces the risk for systemic adverse effects.

Clinical Manifestations of Osteoporosis

The first clinical presentation of osteoporosis will usually be pain or fracture. The most common areas for osteoporotic fractures and pain are the mid-thoracic and upper lumbar spine, hip, and distal forearm. Compression fracture usually results in acute pain, and the spinal deformity caused by vertebral wedging, compression, and secondary ligamentous strain can

Table 24.5: Management of Osteoporosis

- Prevention: modify lifestyle risks for osteoporosis (including smoking, excessive alcohol intake, sedentary behaviors)
- Adequate calcium intake and vitamin D supplementation
- Physical therapy
  - Postural exercises: pelvic tilt and back extension with posture training
  - Range of motion, strengthening program with 1–2 lbs up to 5 lbs as tolerated in each hand, coordination
  - Back extensor strengthening
  - Walking 40 minutes/day as tolerated
  - Aquatic exercises
  - In the presence of clinically significant pain or fracture, strenuous spinal flexion and spinal flexion exercises should be avoided
- Occupational therapy: ADL evaluation and training, home evaluation for adaptation and use of assistive technologies
- Pharmacological intervention

This article was published in *Physical medicine and rehabilitation principles and practice, 3rd edition*, Sinaki M, Chapter 42, pp. 929–949, Copyright Elsevier (2005).

Table 24.6: Guidelines for the Management of Osteoporosis after Organ Transplantation

- Prevention:
  - Baseline dual-energy x-ray absorptiometry (DEXA) scanning, and regular follow-up
  - Rapid resumption of weight-bearing exercises
  - Back extension exercises
  - Calcium 1,000–1,500 mg daily in divided doses and at least 400–800 IU of vitamin D
  - Oral or intravenous bisphosphonates
  - Calcitriol
- Treatment
  Bisphosphonates
  Calcitriol and calcitonin

produce chronic pain due to muscles spasms and abnormalities of motion. Chronic pain can also be due to microfractures that are visible only on bone scanning.

Management of Osteoporosis

Management of osteoporosis requires good nutrition, physical and rehabilitation measures, and pharmacologic interventions (Tables 24.5 and 24.6). All transplant recipients should be considered candidates for early prevention for transplantation osteoporosis. It has been shown that calcitriol can reduce bone loss through suppressing bone resorption indirectly by facilitating intestinal calcium absorption and suppressing parathyroid hormone (PTH) secretion, and second- and third-generation bisphosphonates are very effective in preventing bone loss after transplantation. It was reported that risedrone or intravenous

zoledronate given for 12 months after BMT could prevent spinal and proximal femoral bone loss [20, 21]. In addition, two recent randomized studies demonstrated pamidronate prevented bone loss after BMT [22, 23]. The benefits of pamidronate therapy were restricted to patients receiving an average daily prednisolone dose greater than 10 mg and cyclosporine therapy for more than 5 months within the first 6 months after allogeneic BMT. Most benefits were lost 12 months after stopping pamidronate, however. Although it was reported that 1-year therapy is mandatory following cardiac transplantation, their optimal duration following transplants is unclear, it is undetermined at what level of renal impairment bisphosphonates should be avoided and whether this level is the same for all bisphosphonates. The main short-term side effects associated with nitrogen-containing bisphosphonates are gastrointestinal intolerance with oral administration, flu-like symptoms with intravenous administration [24]. Concerns about a potential for reduced bone quality and strength have been also discussed in the literature [24]. Moreover, there have been reports suggesting an association between bisphosphonate use and an unusual condition called *osteonecrosis of the jaw* (ONJ) in the literature recently. Patients with multiple myeloma and metastatic carcinoma to the skeleton who received intravenous, nitrogen-containing bisphosphates were at greatest risk for osteonecrosis of the jaws [25].

It has been reported that patients with primary osteoporosis who performed back extension exercises had a significantly lower rate of fracture than those who performed spinal flexion exercises or no exercise, and disproportionate weakness in back extensor musculature relative to body weight or flexor strength considerably increases the possibility of compressing vertebrae in the fragile osteoporotic spine [26]. Recognition and improvement of decreased back extensor strength enhance the ability to maintain proper vertical alignment leading to good posture and providing skeletal support. The pain and skeletal deformity associated with vertebral fracture might secondarily reduce muscle strength, which can further exacerbate the postural abnormalities associated with this condition.

Management of Fractures

Spinal compression fractures can be painful and cause functional sequelae. A rehabilitation program might be of benefit to manage the back pain due to vertebral compression fracture (Table 24.7). Vertebroplasty (kyphoplasty) is a new surgical procedure that has been introduced to relieve unremitting pain from vertebral compression fractures. Vertebroplasty involves the injection of acrylic cement into a partially collapsed vertebral body. The treatment of choice for femoral neck fracture and trochanteric hip fracture is surgery [26].

Management of Glucocorticoid-Induced Osteoporosis

The American College of Rheumatology Ad Hoc Committee on glucocorticoid-induced osteoporosis (GIO) for the prevention and treatment of GIO recommended to use a bisphosphonate and, when indicated, hormone replacement therapy in addition to calcium and vitamin D supplementation. Risedronate

Table 24.7: Rehabilitation Management of Back Pain in Patients with Vertebral Fracture

---

Acute pain [26]
- Best rest for 2 days, avoid exercises and spinal strain or minimize spine loading
- Analgesics
- Physical therapy: modalities and stroking massage, isometric muscle contractions of the paraspinal muscles.
- Rigid thoracolumbar orthoses to promote extension of the spine or combination of a kypho-orthosis and lower back support if the rigid orthosis is not tolerable.
- Gait aids if needed
- Adaptive equipment for self-care and ADL

Chronic pain
- Posture training
- Avoid physical activities that exert extreme vertical compression forces on vertebrae
- Back supports
- Physical therapy: modalities, massage, transcutaneous electro-stimulation (TENS), and a therapeutic exercise program
- Biofeedback, relaxation therapy
- Evaluate and treat psychological and social consequences
- Analgesics

This article was published in *Physical medicine and rehabilitation principles and practice, 3rd edition*, Sinaki M, Chapter 42, pp. 929–949, Copyright Elsevier (2005).

and alendronate are the two bisphosphonates recommended for use in GIO in the United States. It has been reported that both alendronate and risedronate are able to reduce vertebral fracture incidence. Risedronate is indicated for the prevention and treatment of GIO in patients treated with 7.5 mg/day of prednisone or equivalent, and alendronate is indicated for GIO in patients who have low BMD receiving ≥7.5 mg/day of prednisone or equivalent.

Avascular Necrosis

Avascular necrosis (AVN) is a prevalent musculoskeletal complication in the cGVHD population [27]. AVN developed in 10% 20% of survivors of allogeneic BMT after a median of 12 months [28, 29]. Enright et al. reported that 10.4% of allo-BMT recipients who received glucocorticoid therapy for GVHD developed avascular bone necrosis at median of 12 months post-BMT [30]. It most frequently involves the femoral head, commonly bilaterally, and the knee. Prolonged post-BMT use of glucocorticoids and CsA for the treatment of GVHD in all BMT recipients is associated with substantial bone loss and a significant albeit small, risk of avascular necrosis of bone. Glucocorticoid treatment of cGVHD is the most important risk factor. It seems to be related to decreased numbers of bone marrow colony forming units-fibroblasts (CFU-f) in vitro,

facilitated by a deficit in bone marrow stromal stem cell regeneration and low osteoblast numbers after stem cell transplantation (SCT). Other risk factors include older age at time of transplantation, total-body irradiation, and an initial diagnosis of aplastic anemia or acute leukemia.

AVN should be suspected when joint pain develops insidiously, especially on weight-bearing. Magnetic resonance imaging is the most sensitive and most specific technique for detecting AVN. When there is evidence of AVN on plain radiology, any chance to prevent joint damage has already been lost.

Treatment for AVN includes protected weight bearing for the lower extremity and use of anti-inflammatory medication. The underlying mechanical factors such as leg length discrepancy should be corrected. In the early stage of the disease, or before any collapse of the femoral head has occurred, surgical core decompression of the femoral head or a vascularized fibular graft inserted into the neck and head of the femur occasionally prevents collapse. Persistent pain, especially nocturnal, along with a significant mechanical disability, will require joint replacement surgery, which carries a good prognosis.

GVHD-Related Neurological Abnormalities

Both central and peripheral nervous systems (CNS and PNS) are at risk for dysfunction following BMT. The etiology of these complications include sequelae of chemotherapy for tumor, impact of immunosuppression and the associated risks for infection and/or tumor recurrence, and inflammatory and GVHD-associated autoimmune processes. The following neurological problems have been reported in patients following BMT: metabolic encephalopathy, CNS infections, stroke, seizure, peripheral neuropathy, and nerve infections with herpes zoster. It has been reported that the most likely causes of CNS dysfunction in patients with GVHD are metabolic encephalopathy and infection [31]. Direct neurological manifestations of cGVHD are uncommon. A few case reports of the CNS involvement by GVHD including transverse myelitis have been published [32, 33].

Regarding the PNS involvement, generalized sensory neuropathy in a patient with cGVHD was first reported in 1990 [34]. A case of a 32-year-old man suffering from cGVHD following an allogeneic BMT developed a demyelinating, motor greater than sensory, polyneuropathy with T lymphocytes being expressed [35]. A case of cGVHD patient presenting with a sensory multiple mononeuropathy considered to be attributed to vasculitis was reported in 1998 [36]. In 1999, Amato et al. reported a generalized polyneuropathy coincident with the occurrence of GVHD in four patients undergoing BMT [37]. In this study, a majority of clinical features of those cases were compatible with chronic inflammatory demyelinating polyneuropathy (CIDP) and met the probable or possible CIDP described by Barohn and Bromberg et al. The pathomechanism of polyneuropathy in GVHD is unknown. It has been speculated that the withdrawal of CsA may trigger an atypical GVHD involving unconventional target organs such as CNS and PNS [38]. The development of polyneuropathy could also be associated with a long-standing disease course in some patients with cGVHD. Vasculitis should be considered as a possible cause of neuropathy or CNS dysfunction in patients with cGVHD.

Symptoms of polyneuropathy include weakness, alterations in sensation or sensory loss, and areflexia/hyporeflexia. The alterations in sensation can lead to wide-based or unsteady gait and ataxia. Polyneuropathy associated impairments can result in activity limitations.

Treatment consists of gait training, possibly with gait aides, balance training, and strengthening exercises. Altered sensation puts the patient at risk for skin breakdown. The patient should avoid use of heat for protracted periods of time onto the affected limbs, and avoid foot trauma. Daily inspection of the affected areas is necessary. Toenails must be cut straight across to prevent ingrown nails. Proper fitting and protective foot wear with appropriate in-shoe orthoses is imperative.

Late Respiratory Complications in Patients with cGVHD

Respiratory complications, the most common life-threatening conditions in cGVHD, occur in 30%–60% of HSCT recipients. Late complications include sinusitis, obliterative bronchiolitis, interstitial pneumonitis, and pulmonary fibrosis. These complications are often associated with dyspnea, wheezing, coughing, air trapping, bronchiectasis, pneumothorax, pneumomediastinum, subcutaneous emphysema, microbial colonization or infection, and obstructive or restrictive changes on pulmonary function tests. Most patients with respiratory complications experience changes in exercise and activity tolerance.

Pulmonary Rehabilitation

Pulmonary abnormalities cause significant functional limitations and reduce the quality of life. Patients may benefit from an educational program aimed at teaching energy conservation (use of adaptive equipment, planning activities to maximize efficiencies, obtaining household and other help), and techniques of breathing (pursed lip and diaphragmatic). An exercise reconditioning program to improve respiratory symptoms, exercise tolerance, will likely increase independent functioning, and sense of well-being, and decrease their depression and anxiety. Depending on the pulmonary function, exercise prescriptions are usually directed toward increasing functional activity rather than aerobic conditioning. The optimal intensity of aerobic exercise for training purposes probably occurs between 57% and 78% of VO2max, which corresponds to 70%–85% heart rate maximum. This is calculated as follows: 220 – age of person in years × % maximum wished to achieve. For example, if a 60-year-old wishes to exercise at 75% of VO2

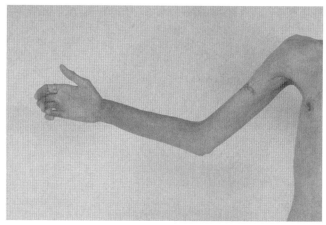

Figure 24.2 cGVHD-associated contractures.
Image reprinted with permission from eMedicine.com, 2008. Available at: http://www.emedicine.com/Med/topic2924.htm. See Plate 71 in the color plate section.

maximum, $(220–60) \times 0.75 = 120$ beats/minute. This level of exercise intensity is usually not tolerated by these patients. It is important to select a program that is well tolerated and the patient experiences as helpful in improving function and valued activities. Patient symptomatology, blood pressure (BP), pulse oximetry, and heart rate during therapy sessions are used to guide the intensity and duration of exercise. Patients, who have adequate pulmonary function for training, should receive aerobic conditioning under supervision and follow a symptom-limited approach. Walking, jogging, and bicycling are the most popular forms of exercises. Possible contraindications to exercise according to the American College of Sports Medicine include unstable angina, resting ST depression >2 mm, uncontrolled dysrhythmias, uncontrolled sinus tachycardia (120 bpm), third-degree A-V block, critical aortic stenosis, uncompensated congestive heart failure, resting systolic blood pressure (SBP) >200 mmHg or diastolic blood pressure (DBP) >110 mmHg, orthostatic BP drop or drop during exercise training of ≥20 mmHg, acute systemic illness or fever, orthopedic problems that prohibit exercise, and uncontrolled diabetes.

FREQUENTLY SEEN SYMPTOMS AND COMPLICATIONS AND THEIR TREATMENTS

Contractures

It has been reported that extensive cGVHD caused contractures in approximately 40% of cases and caused severe disability in a majority of patients (Figure 24.2) [39]. In patients with cGVHD, fibrotic changes of skin and subcutaneous tissue cause loss of skin elasticity, which leads to loss of range of motion/joint contractures, which subsequently results in contractures of deeper soft tissues, including ligaments and joint capsules, tendons, and muscles. Other secondary effects include severe wasting/loss of strength and endurance as well as functional capabilities.

Management

It has been reported that long-term conservative management of joint contractures with physical therapy and orthotics was successful in restoring premorbid functional status in patients with cGVHD-related contractures, but, on the other hand, surgical interventions in the treatment of joint contractures resulting from cGVHD did not appear qualitatively to improve patient's functional status [40]. In fact, all patients treated surgically had a recurrence of contractures within 6 months after the surgical procedure followed by aggressive postoperative management with therapy and orthotics.

The rehabilitation management should be targeted toward prevention and restoration of joint ROM as well as restoration of loss of function. It is important to have stretching and strengthening exercises to prevent loss of strength and ROM from disuse or sclerotic skin changes. Aerobic conditioning is useful in preventing fatigue and restoring cardiopulmonary performance. Therapeutic modalities such as moist heat, paraffin, ultrasound, and techniques to improve or maintain ROM through stretching and splinting could be used, with sclerotic skin changes of cGVHD with or without fascial involvement. Topical treatments, such as heat, emollient lotions, massage, stretching, and application of pressure, can cause the fibrous connective tissue that is forming or has already formed to become thinner, softer, and more elastic [41].

Heat is the most important modality to achieve the goal of increased collagen distensibility. The therapeutic temperature range at which increased collagen extensibility occurs without thermal damage is approximately 40°C to 45.5°C. It can be reached by heating the collagen for approximately 20 minutes, leaving the collagen more distensible for 30 minutes afterward. Paraffin is well tolerated over large surface areas without raising the core temperature and also has the added advantage of not drying the skin. It is easily applied to areas by painting it on the skin with a paintbrush in several layers and covered with transparent wraps and towels to allow it to stay warm long enough to increase collagen extensibility. Ultrasound (US) is the best therapeutic modality for heating deep tissues (>1 cm) and can be used effectively as a prestretching treatment. Precautions and contraindications for its use include the presence of tumor, acute hemorrhage sites, ischemic areas, pacemakers, and infection sites. US is also contraindicated in pregnancy, heart, or brain tissues.

Friction or deep friction massage is perhaps the primary method of preventing or treating adhesion of scar tissue to bone and deeper structures. The purpose of this is to compress and soften fibrotic soft tissue and to reduce adhesions formed between layers, probably allowing loose connective tissue to form where dense connective tissue exists. It is contraindicated when it would cause worsening of a condition, unwanted destruction of tissue, presence of metastatic disease to bone, severe osteoporosis, or spread of the condition such as malignancy, thrombi, atherosclerotic plaques, and infected tissue. Relative contraindications include not fully healed scar tissue, calcified soft tissue, skin grafts, inflamed tissue, atrophic skin, and patients on anticoagulants.

Increased ROM is achieved via the process of stretching most typically. The terms stretching is defined as activity applying a deforming force along the rotational or transitional plane of motion of a joint. It should be applied for at least 15 to 30 seconds and repeated several times in an exercise session, two times per day. The longer the stretch is sustained, the better it is in relieving contracture. The intensity and duration of the stretch are dependent on the patient's tolerance, however. It may be applied through positioning of the patient, with weighted traction, and pulley systems or serial casting. Mechanical passive stretching with equipment or low-intensity external force could be applied over a prolonged period of time (15–30 minutes). When skin is the cause of loss of joint ROM, it is usually necessary to move multiple joints at the same time to achieve effective stretching of the skin. Similarly, when monitoring improvement, it is usually necessary to measure the ROM of ≥ 2 joints at the same time.

Splints may be applied to prevent and restore complications and prevents further contractures.

Fatigue

Fatigue is a multidimensional concept with several modes of expression: physical, cognitive, and emotional, generally thought to involve subjective feeling of tiredness and/or lack of energy and is often associated with inactivity and lack of motivation. Fatigue can be "normal," such as after strenuous activity and relieved by rest. It can be abnormal, in that it is not attributable to any specific cause and not responsive to rest.

Cancer-related fatigue (CRF) is defined as a persistent, subjective sense of tiredness related to cancer or cancer treatment that interferes with usual functioning [42]. It is not caused by specific or strenuous activity, not relieved with rest and is often disturbing. Fatigue symptoms and physical limitations have been found to be prevalent and persistent among cancer patients surviving 3 to 10 years following HSCT. Gielissen et al. reported that 35% of the patients receiving stem cell transplantation experienced severe fatigue [43]. However, the prevalence of fatigue in patients with cGVHD is unclear, although fatigue is a very common symptom experienced by those patients. In our cohort of patients with cGVHD, it is approximately 30%.

Multiple factors contribute to fatigue, including biochemical changes secondary to disease, medical comorbidities, anemia, infection, endocrine disorders, metabolic disorders, nausea/vomiting/nutritional status, pain, deconditioning, inactivity, insomnia or lack of restorative sleep, depression or psychosocial factors, prior cancer treatment, and current medications. Medications that commonly produce fatigue include opioids, benzodiazepines, β-blockers, antiemetics, antihistamines, tricyclic antidepressants, anticonvulsants, thalidomide, α2-adrenergic agonists, and immunosuppressants. Long-term use of corticosteroids can disrupt the sleep–wake cycle, and increase fatigue.

Table 24.8: Interventions for Fatigue

- Correct associated medical causes/contributors (comorbidities and treatments)
- Medications: stimulants such as methylphenidate, antidepressants, cytokine-targeted therapy including nonsteroidal anti-inflammatory agents (NSAIDs)
- Exercise
- Energy conservation
- Psychological/coping

Cytokines such as ILs and interferons are implicated in cancer-related fatigue [44]. Cardiorespiratory and musculoskeletal deconditioning can reduce work capacity; therefore, patients need a higher degree of effort to perform usual activities. The resulting increments in metabolic rate and energy consumption produce tiredness and fatigue. Physical inactivity is known to be associated with an increased risk of obesity and decreased lean body mass, which can be expected to lower the anaerobic threshold in working muscle, produce symptoms of fatigue, diminish physical work capacity, and limit customary physical activities. Physical inactivity or decreased endurance creates a self-perpetuating condition: diminished activity leads to easy fatigability and vice versa [45]. Patients gradually become accustomed to their impaired condition and finally experience it as normal. Furthermore, it was reported that six perpetuating factors of postcancer fatigue appeared to be applicable in SCT cancer survivors as well, including insufficient coping with the experience of cancer, fear of disease recurrence, dysfunctional cognitions concerning fatigue (dysfunctional sense of control in relationship to fatigue complaints), dysregulation of sleep, dysregulation of activity, low social support, and negative social interactions [43]. The patients experiencing severe fatigue had more difficulties in coping with the experience of cancer, more fear of disease recurrence, more dysfunctional cognitions, sleep disturbances, less physical activity, and low social functioning. Prieto et al. reported that depression is the variable most consistently and strongly associated with fatigue, and lower Karnofsky performance status associates with fatigue in hematologic cancer patients receiving SCT [46].

Fatigue reduces the energy, mental capacity, functional status, and psychological resilience, with a profound effect on patients' ability to perform activities of daily living. It results in substantial adverse physical, psychosocial, and economic/occupational consequences, having a major negative effect on the patient's quality of life.

Management

Treatment includes control of specific causes of fatigue, associated symptoms, coping strategies, physical and psychological therapies, using both nonpharmacologic and pharmacologic interventions (Table 24.8). Appropriate treatment of pain, nausea/vomiting, or anemia may be effective in reducing fatigue. Methylphenidate has been used most extensively to treat fatigue in cancer patients. Aerobic conditioning programs have been shown to be effective in reducing symptoms of CRF and other symptoms and maximize functional status. It is important to screen for depression in cancer patients who complain of fatigue. Cognitive behavior therapy (CBT) is a general form of psychotherapy directed at changing condition-related cognitions and behaviors. CBT especially designed for fatigued cancer survivors after conservative treatment can be used in the management of fatigue after SCT [43].

Exercise

While only a few studies have looked at exercise in patients receiving BMT [47], at least 20 studies have been conducted focusing on the effects of exercise on CRF. Exercise has been shown to be the most effective nonpharmacological intervention for CRF [48]. Exercise training at moderate levels was reported to improve adaptive cardiorespiratory responses, increase cardiac output, lower heart rate, decrease fatigue, and improve mood state and sleep quality. Aerobic interval training and low-moderate intensity aerobic exercise programs are best supported by the current available evidence for application to diverse oncology populations. An aerobic training program can break the vicious circle of lack of exercise, impaired performance, and easy fatigability. Aerobic exercise is defined as the rhythmic contraction and relaxation of large muscle groups over a prolonged time. In addition, resistance training exercise either alone or in combination with aerobic exercise could be utilized [49]. Wilson et al. showed that a home-based aerobic exercise program consisting of 20–40 minutes of activity in the target heart rate zone (40%–60% predicted heart rate reserve) delivered in three to five sessions per week for 12 weeks, is an acceptable, safe, and potentially effective intervention for improving physical functioning and fatigue in sedentary HSCT recipients [50]. Dimeo et al. also showed benefit in physical performance and decreases in fatigue in group of early posttransplant patients [47]. Sixteen patients participated in a 6-week program of walking on a treadmill using aerobic interval training pattern, shortly after completing treatment. Interval training was characterized by alternating brief periods of moderate-to high intensity exercise with brief periods of low-intensity exercise. Exercise was withheld only for platelet counts less than 20, 000/mm^3, fever, uncontrolled infection, or multiple complications. No patient in the training group reported significant fatigue or limitations in daily activities due to low physical performance. Moreover, another study demonstrated that a program of bed- or chair-based bicycle ergometer pedaling was found to be safe and effective in reducing fatigue in hospitalized patients undergoing peripheral blood stem cell transplantation (PBSCT), even during hematologic nadir [47].

Edema

Edema is defined as soft tissue swelling due to expansion of the interstitial volume resulting from the imbalance between

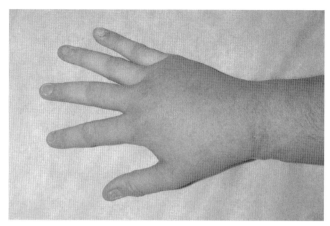

Figure 24.3 cGVHD-associated edema. See Plate 72 in the color plate section.

capillary filtration and lymph drainage, produced by accumulation of fluid in the extra cellular space, filtered plasma proteins, extravascular blood cells, and parenchymal cell products. It can be **localized** or **generalized.**

Causes of generalized edema include congestive cardiac failure, renal failure, hypoalbuminemia, and protein-losing nephropathy. Local edema may result from deep venous thrombosis, cellulitis, interruption or blockage of lymphatic channels, varicose vein, inflammation, and malignancy. Non-pitting edema occurs in certain disorders of the lymphatic system such as lymphedema and patients with hyperthyroidism. In addition, many medications such as vasodilators have been implicated in pedal edema. People undergoing allogeneic stem cell transplantation are at risk for generalized/localized edema if they have one of the risk factors mentioned previously (Figure 24.3). Edema can cause impairments and functional limitations including symptoms of heaviness and dysesthesia, pain, ROM deficits, reduced strength, and difficulty with upper extremity activities.

The goals of management are to (1) prevent its occurrence, if possible, (2) reduce and maintain limb size, (3) alleviate symptoms, (4) educate the patient so that the risk of infection is minimized, and (5) improve overall functional and psychological well-being. Management of edema resulting from any one of these systemic causes includes reversing the underlying disorder if possible, restricting dietary sodium to minimize fluid retention, elevating the lower extremities above the level of the left atrium, using compression garments and diuretic therapy. The selection of diuretic, route of administration, and dosing regimen will vary, on the basis of the underlying disease, its severity, and the urgency of the problem. Angiotensin-receptor blocks and angiotensin-converting enzyme inhibitors seem to be effective in patients with pedal edema.

Localized edema of the upper or lower extremities is best treated early, during the subclinical phase. The patient may not be aware of a volumetric change, during the early phase, hence the health care provider must utilize sensitive measures to detect this and act quickly. The use of water-displacement volumetric measures or electric infrared scanning devices provides early detection methods that can be easily used in the clinic. Once an increase of more than 100 cc of fluid is detected, treatment with compression garments should be provided [51]. It is possible to manage this successfully using a low gradient, off-the-shelf garment. It is more effective to treat lower volumes of fluid (<250 cc) than higher volumes [52].

Recent reports suggest that complex decongestive physiotherapy (CDP), the current international standard of care for lymphedema management, is an effective approach [51, 52]. This technique has two phases [53]. The first phase lasts approximately 4 weeks and aims at reducing the size of the extremity, reversing any distortion in the shape, softening the subcutaneous tissue, and improving the overall health of the skin. This is accomplished via manual lymph drainage (MLD), multilayer compression bandaging, skin and nail care, and exercise. The second phase aims to conserve and optimize the results obtained in phase 1, consisting of compression by a low-stretch elastic stocking or sleeve, skin care, continued exercise, and repeated light massage as needed. MLD is aimed at encouraging the development of collateral drainage routs and increasing the function of the remaining patent routs, to enhance the sequestration and transport of lymphatic fluid. It is a very light superficial massage limited to finger/hand pressures of ideally around 30–45 mm, initially focusing on stimulating lymph flow in the unaffected adjoining quadrants to prepare for the greater volume of fluid to come and moving fluid proximally gradually along the extremity toward an area that has already been "cleared." Relative contraindications to the use of MLD include uncontrolled bacterial infection, acute cellulites, the presence of an inflamed limb because of arterial or venous occlusion, and renal dysfunction.

Compression therapy using compression garments or static, gradient compression devices or short-stretch bandaging increases tissue pressure, improves venous and lymphatic return, facilitates filling of the initial lymph vessels, maintains skin integrity, and protects the limb from potential trauma. Compression also provides counter pressure against the muscle pump and breaks down the protein in the tissue of fibrotic limbs. In phase 1 of CDP, compression bandages should be worn 24 hours/day to prevent reaccumulation of fluid. In general, the highest compression level (approximately 20–60 mmHg) tolerated by the patient is likely to be the most beneficial. Short-stretch bandaging provides a high treating pressure and exerts force when the underlying muscles contract. Static, gradient compression devices could be used for patients who are unable to master appropriate bandaging technique. Medical contraindications for the compression therapy include arterial disease, painful postphlebitic syndrome, and occult visceral neoplasia.

Generally, exercise employing full ROM of the extremity and repetitive activity is encouraged. Resistive training could be beneficial; however, its intensity should produce only to very mild fatigue. *Flexibility activities* can stretch scar and reduce the effect of fibrosis, normalize biomechanics, enhance posture, and facilitate lymph flow. Patients who have specific deficits in stamina or strength are referred for aerobic conditioning, focal strength and endurance training, and ROM activities. Remedial exercises are encouraged because they repeatedly compress the lymph vessels through rhythmic contraction and relaxation of muscles, which trigger smooth muscle contraction within the walls of lymph transport vessels [54]. It should always be performed with some type of external compression on the limb, most commonly garments or bandages. *Aerobic conditioning* stimulates lymph sequestration and transport through a mechanism of elevated sympathetic tone, increasing of the rate of smooth muscle contraction within lymph vessels. External compression must be worn during aerobic activity to optimize those benefits.

Weakness in Patients with cGVHD

Weakness in patients with cGVHD is a common symptom that can result from factors including, but not limited to, immobility or deconditioning, steroid myopathy, polymyositis, and myasthenia gravis. Disuse atrophy occurs in patients who have been immobilized for prolonged periods. Muscle strength decreases at least 1% per day of bed rest or 10%–15% of original strength per week [55]. Reduction in muscle protein synthesis has been considered the main contributor to muscle atrophy. Skeletal muscle protein synthesis is diminished due to both disuse of a given muscle and systemic, insulin-mediated effects causing inhibition of protein synthesis. Immobility can also lead to loss of joint motion/joint contractures, producing a biomechanical disadvantage to muscle performance.

Polymyositis

Polymyositis (PM) occurs in approximately 3% to 8% of patients with established cGVHD [56]. Whether polymyositis is a concurrent finding or a manifestation of cGVHD is controversial. Stevens et al. stated that polymyositis can occur as part of the constellation of manifestations of cGVHD and muscle tissue may be a target for cGVHD in HCT patients [57]. Experimental evidence suggested that allogeneic lymphocytes of particular genetic backgrounds may be engaged in the development of myositis, and an abnormal cellular immune reaction by donor T cells may be causative. Aplastic anemia has been believed to be an important host factor in the development of myositis in patients with cGVHD. It has been noted that pathological findings of polymyositis in cGVHD are similar to those seen in idiopathic polymyositis.

The clinical syndrome of polymyositis associated with GVHD is indistinguishable from that of idiopathic polymyositis. The most common presenting symptoms are moderate to severe proximal muscle weakness and myalgia, with lower extremities more commonly involved. Muscular atrophy and weakness could involve both the distal muscles and the proximal muscles, however [58]. Other signs and symptoms may include

Table 24.9: Diagnostic Criteria for Polymyositis

- Proximal muscle weakness
- Electromyography showing small, short-duration, polyphasic motor unit potentials with spontaneous fibrillations and positive sharp waves
- Muscle biopsy demonstrating endomysial lymphocytic infiltrate surrounding or invading individual nonnecrotic muscle fibers
- Elevated serum muscle enzymes (creatine phosphokinase or CPK, aldolase, transaminases, or lactate dehydrogenase)

* The presence of two criteria is designated "possible PM," three criteria "probable PM" and four criteria "definite PM." [59]

fever, dysphagia, eosinophilia, skin induration over the areas of muscle involvement, and contractures. Majority of the patients do present with elevated creatine phosphokinase (CPK) and aldolase enzymes. The electromyographic features of GVHD-associated polymyositis are identical to idiopathic polymyositis, which include low amplitude, short-duration polyphasic motor unit potentials with early recruitment and spontaneous fibrillation potentials and positive sharp waves (Table 24.9).

There is no established standard therapy for cGVHD-related polymyositis. A combination of steroids and cyclosporine or tacrolimus with subsequent tapering of immunosuppression as tolerated has been widely used. The majority of cases of GVHD-associated polymyositis showed a response to immunosuppressive treatment. The eventual prognosis depends on the activity of cGVHD rather than on the severity of myositis.

Rehabilitation intervention depends on the associated impairments, functional problems, and disabilities present. Rehabilitation goals are to maintain ROM of the joints preventing joint contractures, to increase and regain muscle strength, and to return to functional ADL and mobility and improve quality of life. In general, isometric exercise is appropriate for patients with stable or inactive, mildly or moderately active idiopathic polymyositis. Low-weight concentric isotonic exercise is also appropriated for patients with inactive or mildly active disease following a ROM and isometric program [60].

Myasthenia Gravis

Myasthenia gravis (MG), a neuromuscular disorder, appears to be a rare complication of cGVHD. The specific pathogenesis of GVHD-associated MG remains unclear. However, a long-term elevation of IgM and IgG antiacetylcholine receptor antibodies has been found in patients with cGVHD before the occurrence of clinical manifestations [61]. It has been reported that donor cells may play an important role in the pathogenesis of GVHD-related MG, and differences between the donor and the recipient acetylcholine receptors causing the graft to produce antibodies against recipient receptors may result in myasthenia gravis. Moreover, most cases of MG have been identified in patients following the allogeneic transplantation for aplastic anemia.

Table 24.10: Frequently Affected Organ Systems, Their Associated Impairments and Symptoms, and Rehabilitation Model as It Applies to GVHD

Organ/System	Abnormality/ Impairment	Symptoms	Activity Limitation	Participation Restriction
Musculoskeletal	Scleroderma, fascitis, arthritis, osteoporosis, avascular necrosis, myositis	Loss of range of motion/contracture, weakness, atrophy, pain including arthralgia and myalgia, limb edema, decreased stamina or fatigue	Mobility and self-care problems/decreased ambulation and or decreased self-care	Cannot work or go to school. Impact family
Neurological	Neuropathy, Neuromuscular Junction (NMJ) disorder	Numbness and tingling sensation, weakness, balance problems, neuropathic pain		
Pulmonary	Bronchiolitis Obliterans (BO), Bronchiolitis Obtliterans Organizing Pneumonia (BOOP), interstitial pneumonitis (IP)	Dyspnea, cough		
Metabolic		Fatigue and/or decreased stamina		

The clinical manifestations of GVHD-associated MG do not differ from those seen in classic autoimmune MG. However, common clinical features of all reported cases of MG postallogeineic BMT do include the presence of other manifestations of cGVHD, an association with diminishing immunosuppression, antiacetylcholine receptor antibodies, and the absence of an associated thymoma.

Generally, the onset of GVHD-associated MG is more delayed in most cases, ranging from 26 to 39 months after BMT. Neuromuscular weakness is frequently severe with bulbar weakness and respiratory insufficiency. Elevated acetylcholine receptor antibody levels could be observed and repetitive nerve stimulation may demonstrate a characteristic decremental response.

Standard therapies for idiopathic MG seem to have been effective in the GVHD-associated MG. Responses to edrophonium and oral pyridostigmine as well as to plasma exchange are similar to those in classical autoimmune MG. In contrast to idiopathic MG, the role of thymectomy remains unclear, in the induction of remission and the reduction of need for long-term immunosuppression. The activity of cGVHD determines prognosis of GVHD-associated MG [62].

Steroid Myopathy

Steroid myopathy (SM) is often seen in patients who have taken corticosteroids. It is characterized by type II muscle fiber atrophy, variation in fiber size, and phagocytosis with degeneration and replacement of muscle by fibrous and adipose tissue. The exact incidence is uncertain. The initial clinical symptom is a subtle hip girdle weakness, first noted as difficulty in rising from a squatting position. It is usually associated with normal biochemistry findings. Electromyography may be helpful for differential diagnosis in some patients. Recovery of corticosteroids-induced myopathy can occur with dose reduction. Improvement in strength may occur within 2 or 3 weeks and complete resolution may take from 1 to 4 months up to 1 to 2 years. Steroid-induced weakness can be mediated by ongoing strengthening and endurance exercises. The most realistic goal is preservation of strength and prevention of decline. Low resistance exercises are generally recommended to prevent further muscle breakdown [63]. Special emphasis on strengthening techniques to improve both muscle balance and stabilization of proximal joints should be placed. Strengthening exercise and functional activity can be combined to simulate activities of daily living and ensure optimal carryover.

CONCLUSION/SUMMARY

The following tables were designed to provide the reader with a summary of (1) which organ systems are most likely to be affected by cGVHD, their associated impairments and symptoms (causing functional sequela Table 24.10); (2) which abnormalities are seen in cGVHD, organized using the rehabilitation model to associate the multidimensional aspects of the findings and the rehabilitation interventions frequently used for the abnormalities, symptoms, impairments, functional loss associated with cGVHD (Table 24.11).

Table 24.11: Summary of Rehabilitation for Patients with cGVHD

Problems		Activity	Pharmacological Interventions	Pain Mgmt.	Exercises/Physical Therapy	Occupational Therapy	Surgical Interventions	Psychological Therapy
	Fasciitis		Nonsteroidal anti-inflammatory drugs (NSAIDS)	as needed	Edema management, thermo-modalities, joint mobilization techniques, deep friction message, active ROM exercises, passive sustained stretching including serial splinting, strengthening exercises, endurance training, pool therapy	ADL evaluation and training, adaptive equipment evaluation, fine motor coordination skills		Relaxation, behavioral pain control techniques, psychological therapy
	Osteoporosis	Avoid strenuous spinal flexion and spinal flexion exercises in the presence of fracture	Prevention: Calcium 1,000–1,500 mg daily, calcitriol, second- and third generation biphosphonates Treatment: Bisphosphonates, calcitriol, and calcitonin	in patients with fractures	Postural exercises, ROM and strengthening program, back extensor strengthening, walking or weight-bearing exercises	ADL evaluation and training, assistive device, adaptive equipment	Vertebroplasty and kyphoplasty to relieve unremitting pain from compression fractures	
Musculoskeletal	AVN	Protected weight bearing	NSAIDs as needed	as needed	Correct the underlying mechanical factors such as leg length discrepancy	as needed	core decompression joint replacement	
	Contracture			as needed	Therapeutic modalities, stretching and strengthening exercises, deep friction message, splinting, aerobic conditioning	ADL evaluation and training, adaptive equipment evaluation, splinting	not useful	
	Edema		Reverse the underlying disorder, diuretic therapy	as needed	Elevation of the limb, compression garments, complex decongestive physiotherapy including MLD, flexibility activities, strengthening exercises, aerobic conditioning	ADL evaluation and training, adaptive equipment evaluation		

System	Symptom/Condition	Precautions	Medical management		Physical therapy	Occupational therapy	Other
	Weakness	Isometric exercise/low-weight concentric isotonic excercise/low-resistance excercise	Immunosuppresants/edrophonium and pyridostigmine/discontinuation of the steroid	as needed	Isometric exercise for inactive, mildly or moderately active polymyositis, low-weight concentric isotonic exercise for inactive or mildly active disease; ROM and stretching exercises with strengthening (low resistance)and endurance exercises for steroid myopathy, mobility training	ADL evaluation and training and adaptive equipment evaluation	
Neurological	Polyneuropathy	Avoid use of heat and avoid foot trauma, cut toe nails, proper protective foot wear		Management of pain as needed	Gait training with gait aid as needed, balance training, strengthening exercises	ADL evaluation and training, adaptive equipment evaluation, fine motor coordination skills	
Pulmonary	BO, BOOP, IP				Techniques of breathing (pursed lip and diaphragmatic), aerobic conditioning	Energy conservation	
Metabolic	Fatigue	Energy conservation	Stimulants such as methylphenidate, antidepressants, cytokine-targeted therapy including NSAIDs		Aerobic conditioning	Use of adaptive equipment, planning activities to maximize efficiencies, obtaining assistance	CBT

ADL, activities of daily life; AVN, avascular necrosis; AROM, active range of motion; BO, bronchiolitis obliterans; BOOP, bronchiolitis obliterans organizing pneumonia; CBT, cognitive behavioral therapy; cGVHD, chronic graft versus host disease; IP, interstitial pneumonitis; Mgmt, management.

REFERENCES

1. Greene WB, Heckman, JD. The clinical measurement of joint motion. 1st ed. Copyright © 1994 by the American Academy of Orthopaedic Surgeons.

2. Louie AD, Robison LL, Bogue M, Hyde S, Forman SJ, Bhatia S. Validation of self-reported complications by bone marrow transplantation survivors. *Bone Marrow Transplant.* 2000;25 (11):1191–1196.

3. Syrjala KL, Langer SL, Abrams JR, Storer BE, Martin PJ. Late effects of hematopoietic cell transplantation among 10-year adult survivors compared with case-matched controls. *J Clin Onco.* 2005;23 (27):6596–6606.

4. McQuellon RP, Russell GB, Cella DF, et al. Quality of life measurement in bone marrow transplantation: development of the functional assessment of cancer therapy-bone marrow transplant (FACT-BMT) scale. *Bone Marrow Transplant.* 1997;19(4):357–368.

5. Lee SJ, Kim HT, Ho VT, et al. Quality of life associated with acute and chronic graft-versus-host disease. *Bone Marrow Transplant.* 2006;38 (4):305–310.

6. Aaronson NK, Ahmedzai S, Bergman B, et al. The European organization for research and treatment of cancer QLQ-C30: a quality of life instrument for use in international clinical trials in oncology. *J Natl Cancer Inst.* 1993;85(5):365–376.

7. McDowell I. Measuring Health: a guide to rating scales and questionnaires. 3rd ed. Oxford, England: Oxford University Press, 2006.

8. Couriel D, Carpenter PA, Cutler C, et al. Ancillary therapy and supportive care of chronic graft-versus-host disease: national institutes of healthy consensus development project on criteria for clinical trials in chronic graft-versus-host disease: V. Ancillary Therapy and Supportive Care Working Group Report. *Biol Blood Marrow Transplant.* 2006;12 (4):375–396.

9. Ebeling PR, Thomas DM, Erbas B, Hopper JL, Szer J, Grigg AP. Mechanisms of bone loss following allogeneic and autologous hemopoietic stem cell transplantation. *J Bone Miner Res.* 1999;14 (3):342–350.

10. Shulman LE. Diffuse fasciitis with hypergammaglobulinemia and eosinphilia. A new syndrome? *J Rheumatol.* 1974;1 (Suppl 1):46.

11. Mori Y, Kahari VM, Varga J. Scleroderma-like cutaneous syndromes. *Curr Rheumatol Rep.* 2002;4(2):113–122.

12. Van Den Bergh V, Tricot G, Fonteyn G, Dom R, Bulcke J. Diffuse fasciitis after bone marrow transplantation. *Am J Med.* 1987;83 (1):139–143.

13. Kim KW, Yoon CH, Kay CS, Kim HJ, Lee HE, Park SY. Fasciitis after allogeneic peripheral blood stem cell transplantation in a patient with chronic myelogenous leukemia. *J Clin Rheumato.* 2003;9 (1):33–36.

14. Janin A, Socie G, Devergie A, Aractingi S. Fasciitis in chronic graft-versus-host disease. *Ann Intern Med.* 1994;120:993–998.

15. O'Laughlin TJ, Klima RR, Kenney DE. Rehabilitation of eosinophilic fasciitis. *Am J Phys Med & Rehabil.* 1994;73 (4):286–292.

16. Goffin E, Devogelaer JP, Depresseux G, Squifflet JP, Pirson Y. Osteoporosis after organ transplantation. *Lancet.* 2001;357 (9268):1623.

17. Monegal A, Navasa M, Guañabens N et al. Bone mass and mineral metabolism in liver transplant patients treated with FK506 or cyclosporine A. *Calcif Tissue Int.* 2001;68 (2):83–86

18. Van Staa TP, Leufkens HG, Abenhaim L, Zhang B, Cooper C. Oral corticosteroids and fracture risk: relationship to daily and cumulative doses. *Rheumatology (Oxford)* 2000;39 (12):1383–1389.

19. Rŭegsegger P, Medici TC, Anliker M. Corticosteroid-induced bone loss. A longitudinal study of alternate day therapy in patients with bronchial asthma using quantitative computed tomography. *Eur J Clin Pharmacol.* 1983;25(5):615–620.

20. Tauchmanovà L, Selleri C, Esposito M, et al. Beneficial treatment with risedronate in long-term survivors after allogeneic stem cell transplantation for hematological malignancies. *Osteoporosis Int.* 2003;14 (12):1013–1019.

21. Tauchmanovà L, Ricci P, Serio B, et al. Short-term zoledronic acid treatment increases bone mineral density and marrow clonogenic fibroblast progenitors after allogeneic stem cell transplantation. *J Clin Endocrinol Metab.* 2005;90 (2):627–634.

22. Kananen K, Volin L, Laitinen K, et al. Prevention of bone loss after allogeneic stem cell transplantation by calcium, vitamin D, and sex hormone placement with or without pamidronate. *J Clin Endocrinal Metab.* 2005;90 (7):3877–3885.

23. Grigg AP, Shuttleworth P, Reynolds J, et al.: Pamidronate reduces bone loss after allogeneic stem cell transplantation. *J Clin Endocrinol Metab.* 2006;91 (10):3835–3843.

24. Jeffcoat M, Watts NB. Osteonecrosis of the jaw: balancing the benefits and risks of oral bisphosphonate treatment for osteoporosis. *Gen Dent.* 2008;56 (1):96–102.

25. Woo SB, Hellstein JW, Kalmar JR. Narrative review: bisphosphonates and osteonecrosis of the jaws. *Ann Intern Med.* 2006;144 (10):753–761.

26. Sinaki M. Prevention and treatment of osteoporosis. In: Braddom R, ed. Physical medicine and rehabilitation principles and practice. 3rd ed. W. B. Sauders Company, 2005:929–949.

27. Atkinson K, Cohen M, Biggs J. Avascular necrosis of the femoral head secondary to corticosteroid therapy for graft-versus-host-disease after marrow transplantation: effective therapy with hip arthroplasty. *Bone Marrow Transplant.* 1987;2 (4): 421–426.

28. Tauchmanovà L, De Rosa G, Serio B, Fazioli F, et al. Avascular necrosis in long-term survivors after allogeneic or autologous stem cell transplantation: a single center experience and a review. *Cancer.* 2003;97 (10):2453–2461.

29. Wiesmann A, Pereira P, Böhm P, Faul C, Kanz L, Einsele H. Avascular necrosis of bone following allogeneic stem cell transplantation: MR screening and therapeutic options. *Bone Marrow Transplant.* 1998;22(6):565–569.

30. Enright H, Haake R, Weisdorf D. Avascular necrosis of bone: a common serious complication of allogeneic bone transplantation. *Am J Med.* 1990;89 (6):733–738.

31. Nelson KR, Mcquillen MP. Neurologic complications of graft-versus-host disease. *Neurological Clinics.* 1988;6 (2): 389–403.

32. Richard S, Fruchtman S, Scigliano E, Skerrett D, Najfeld V, Isola L. An immunological syndrome featuring transverse myelitis, Evans syndrome and pulmonary infiltrates after unrelated bone marrow transplant in a patient with severe aplastic anemia. *Bone Marrow Transplant.* 2000;26 (11):1225–1228.

33. Campbell JN Morris PP. Cerebral vasculitis in graft-versus-host disease: a case report. *AJNR Am J Neur Radiol.* 2005;26 9(3):654–656.

34. Greenspan A, Deeg HG, Cottler-Fox M, Sirdofski M, Spitzer TR, Kattah J. Incapacitating peripheral neuropathy as a manifestation of chronic graft versus host disease. *Bone Marrow Transplant.* 1990;5:349–352.

35. Nagashima T, Sato F, Chuma T, Mano Y, et al. Chronic demyelinating polyneuropathy in graft-versus- host disease following allogeneic bone marrow transplantation. *Neuropathology.* 2002;22 (1):1–8.

36. Gabriel CM, Goldman JM, Lucas S, Hughes RA. Vasculitis neuropathy in association with chronic graft versus host disease. *J Neurol Sci.* 1999;168 (1):68–70.

37. Amato AA, Barohn RJ, Sahenk Z, Tutschka PJ, Mendell JR. Polyneuropathy complicating bone marrow and solid organ transplantation. *Neurology.* 1993;43 98):1513–1518.

38. Solaro A, Murialdo A, Giunti D, Mancardi G, Uccelli A. Central and peripheral nervous system complications following allogeneic bone marrow transplantation. *Eur J of Neurol.* 2001;8 (1):77–80.

39. Sullivan KM, Shulman HM, Storb R, et al: Chronic graft-versus-host disease in 52 patients: adverse natural course and successful treatment with combination immunosuppression. *Blood.* 1981;57 (2):267–276.

40. Beredjiklian PK, Drummond DS, Dormans JP, Davidson RS, Brock GT, August C. Orthopaedic manifestations of chronic graft-versus-host disease. *J Pediatr Orthop.* 1998;18 (5):572–575.

41. Currie DM, Ludvigsdottir GK, Diaz CA, Kamani N. Topical treatment of sclerodermoid chronic graft vs host disease. *Am J Phys Med Rehabil.* 2002;81:143–149.

42. Mock V. Cancer related fatigue. In Given CW, Given B, Champion VL, et al. eds. Evidence-based cancer care and prevention: Behavioral interventions. New York: Springer, 2003:242–273.

43. Gielissen MFM, Schattenberg AVM, Verhagen CAHHVM, Rinkes MJ, Bremmers MEJ, Bleijenberg G. Experience of severe fatigue in long-term survivors of stem cell transplantation. *Bone Marrow Transplant.* 2007;39:595–603.

44. Bower JE, Ganz PA, Aziz N, Fahey JL. Fatigue and proinflammatory cytokine activity in breast cancer survivors. *Psychosom Med.* 2002;64(4):604–611.

45. Winningham ML. Strategies for managing cancer-related fatigue syndrome: a rehabilitation approach. *Cancer.* 2001;92 (Suppl 4):988–997.

46. Prieto JM, Jordi B, Atala J, et al. Clinical factors associated with fatigue in haematologic cancer patients receiving stem-cell transplantation. *Eur J of Cancer.* 2006;42 (12):1749–1755.

47. Dimeo FC, Tilmann MHM, Bertz H, Kanz L, Mertelsmann R, Keul J. Aerobic exercise in the rehabilitation of cancer patients after high dose chemotherapy and autologous peripheral stem cell transplantation. *Cancer.* 1997;79:1717–1722.

48. Stricker CT, Drake D, Hoyer KA, Mock V. Evidence-based practice for fatigue management in adults with cancer: exercise as an intervention. *Oncol Nurs Forum.* 2004;31(5):963–974.

49. Coleman EA, Coon S, Hall-Barrow J, Richards K, Gaylor D, Stewart B. Feasibility of exercise during treatment for multiple myeloma. *Cancer Nurs.* 2003;26(5):410–419.

50. Wilson RW, Jacobsen PB, Fields KK. Pilot study of a home-based aerobic exercise program for sedentary cancer survivors treated with hematopoietic stem cell transplantation. *Bone Marrow Transplant.* 2005;35:721–727.

51. Gergich NLS, Pfalzer LA, McGarvey C, et al. Pre-operative assessment enables early diagnosis and successful treatment of lymphedema. *Cancer.* 2008 in press.

52. Ramos SM, O'Donnell LS, Kinght G. Edema volume, not timing, is the key to success in lymphedema treatment. *AM. J. Surg.* 1999;178 (4):311–315.

53. Gary DE. Lymphedema diagnosis and management. *J Am Acad Nurse Pract.* 2007;19 (2):72–78.

54. Cheville AL, McGarvey CL, Petrek JA, Russo SA, Taylor ME, Thiadens RJ. Lymphedema management. *Seminars in Radiation Oncology.* 2003;13:290–301.

55. Germain P, Guell A, Marini JF. Muscle strength during bed rest with and without muscle exercise as a countermeasure. *Eur J Appl Physiol.* 1995;71:342–348.

56. Parker P, Chao NJ, Ben-Ezra J, et al. Polymyositis as a manifestation of chronic graft-versus-host disease. *Medicine.* 1996 Sep;75 (5):279–285.

57. Stevens AM, Sullivan KM, Nelson JL. Polymyositis as a manifestation of chronic graft-versus-host disease. *Rheumatology (Oxford)* 2003;42 (1):34–39.

58. Takahashi K, Kashihara K, Shinagawa K, Yoshino T, Abe K, Harada M. Myositis as a manifestation of chronic graft-versus-host disease. *Intern Med.* 2000;39 (6):482–485.

59. Bohan A, Peter JB. Polymyositis and dermatomyositis. *N Eng L Med.* 1975;292 (8):403–407.

60. Shepard RJ, Shek PN. Autoimmune disorders, physical activity and training with particular reference to rheumatoid arthritis. *Exerc Immunol Rev.* 1997;3:53–67.

61. Smith CI, Aarli JA, Biberfeld P, et al. Myasthenia gravis after bone-marrow transplantation. Evidence for a donor origin. *N Engl J Med.* 1983;309 (25):1565–1568.

62. Tse S, Sunders EF, Silverman E, Vajsar J, Becker L, Meaney B. Myasthenia gravis and polymyositis as manifestations of chronic graft-versus-host-disease. *Bone Marrow Transplant.* 1999;23 (4):397–399.

63. Grant J, Young MA, Pidcock FS, Christensen JR. Physical medicine and rehabilitation management of chronic graft versus host disease. Rehabilitation Oncology. 1997;15 (3): 13–15.

25

INFECTIONS

Juan Gea-Banacloche and Michael Boeckh

Infection is a common complication of chronic graft versus host disease (cGVHD), and it contributes significantly to the mortality of this condition. As an example, in a prospective cohort study of 159 patients with cGVHD from the University of Minnesota, 42 of the 67 deaths were attributed to infection [1]. Studies from other institutions provide similar data. Accordingly, most authorities emphasize the need for appropriate infection prophylaxis and management [2, 3]. The Guidelines for Supportive Care in cGVHD provide specific recommendations for prophylaxis, and emphasize the lack of direct evidence to support many of them [4]. This chapter will present a review of the infectious syndromes commonly found in cGVHD and will offer recommendations regarding prevention of the different pathogens.

GENERAL CONCEPTS ABOUT INFECTION IN CGVHD

Infection was identified as an important problem in cGVHD since the original descriptions of the disease [5–9]. Six patients described by Graze and Gale in 1979 experienced six episodes of bacteremia/septicemia, six pneumonias (three viral, two bacterial, one *Aspergillus*), four episodes of zoster and a variety of other infections [6]. Shulman et al., in their description of the "cGVHD syndrome" in 20 patients out of the 227 transplanted at the Fred Hutchinson Cancer Research Center (FHCRC) between 1969 and 1976 reported seven deaths caused by infection [8]. Early on, these investigators had identified cGVHD as the main risk factor for non-*Varicella zoster* virus (VZV) infection late after transplantation [5]. The increased risk of infection and infection-related death in patients with cGVHD has been confirmed in subsequent studies [1, 10].

Several factors seem to contribute to the high infectious risk:

1. Immune dysregulation
2. Delayed immune reconstitution
3. Functional hyposplenism
4. Treatment of GVHD (corticosteroids and other immunosuppressive agents)

The importance of each one of these factors in individual patients is difficult to assess. Studies of immune function have identified a variety of problems, with abnormalities involving, among others, decreased thymic function [11], restricted T-cell repertoire [12], decreased CD4 T-cell number [13], decreased regulatory T cells [14], decreased B cells [15], or increased immature B cells [16]. Decreased splenic size and functional hyposplenism are well documented [17–19] (Figure 25.1) and may contribute significantly to the increased risk in bacterial infections. Delayed immune reconstitution may be compounded by the type of transplant. For example, the Unrelated Donor Marrow Transplantation Trial documented higher frequency of infections in cGVHD patients who had received T-cell depleted transplants [10]. However, within the same type of transplant procedure, the presence of cGVHD results in delayed immune reconstitution [20–22]. Of the variety of immunosuppressive treatments used in cGVHD, systemic corticosteroids have been identified as the most important risk factor for infection in recent series [23], but this could be a reflection of the severity of the disease and the fact that steroid use is easier to quantify than other factors.

Bacterial infections are most common, followed by viral and fungal infections in most series [5, 6, 10, 13, 23–32]. Overall, the risk of infection decreases steadily after the first 6 months. In a prospective cohort of 149 patients with cGVHD enrolled between 1987 and 1993 and followed-up for a median of 8.4 years, researches at the University of Minnesota reported an incidence density of infection of 7 of 1,000 patient-days at 6 months, 2.4 of 1,000 patient-days at 1 year and 0.3 of 1,000 patient-days at 2 years [1]. Parallel decreases were observed in bacterial, fungal, and viral infections. Individual factors (e.g., intensive immunosuppressive treatment of a flare of GVHD) may alter the infectious risk in a particular patient, but in general infections become less and less frequent over time.

SYNDROMIC APPROACH TO THE PATIENT WITH cGVHD

When examining a patient with cGVHD, one of the most important tasks of the clinician is to make an accurate assessment of

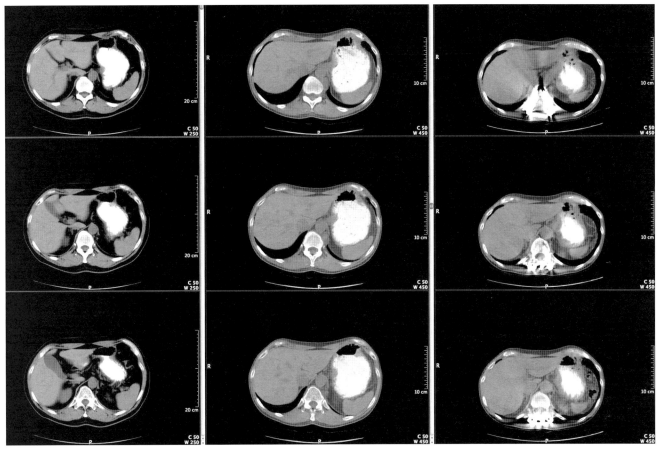

Figure 25.1 Decreasing splenic size in the course of chronic extensive GVHD. A 45-year-old man with multiple myeloma underwent allogeneic transplant in 2001. He did not develop cGVHD until 2003, following a DLI after recurrence of his disease. The series shows decreasing splenic size over the 2 years of his cGVHD. From left to right, the columns show abdominal CTs from December 2001, March 2003 and May of 2005. He did not suffer significant infectious complications, but his blood smear showed signs of hyposplenism.

the risk of infection. The global statistics mentioned in the preceding text have limited applicability in the individual case. The range of cGVHD is broad, from patients with limited disease receiving topical treatment with oral corticosteroids and artificial tears to patients with uncontrolled chronic extensive disease on high-dose corticosteroids, a calcineurin inhibitor, and one or more experimental agents like fludarabine, pentostatin, or rituximab, often with a history of past or currently active opportunistic infections. These two hypothetical individuals present different diagnostic and therapeutic challenges. This section will present a summary of the diagnostic and (when appropriate) empirical therapeutic approach to different clinical syndromes.

General Approach to the Patient with cGVHD and Fever of Acute Onset

Fever in cGVHD is almost always caused by infection, although some less common possible etiologies should be kept in mind: drug fever, relapse of the malignancy, *Epstein–Barr virus* (EBV)-related immunoproliferative disease, and some of the pulmonary noninfectious complications of allogeneic hematopoietic cell transplantation (HCT). Adrenal insufficiency may be particularly easy to miss in patients with cGVHD, and it occasionally presents with full-blown adrenal crisis with fever and refractory hypotension in response to a minor stress or a viral infection. Conversely cGVHD *per se* is an unlikely cause of fever, and infection should remain the working hypothesis.

Bacterial infections are the most common, particularly pneumonia and bacteremia/sepsis, as well as the more rapidly lethal [23, 30, 31], so empirical administration of antibacterial agents should be considered early. As in other immunocompromised patients, multiple infections may be present at the same time or follow each other. The immunosuppressive agents used to treat c GVHD may mask the signs of infection and make control of the pathogen difficult.

A detailed history should include current medication use (emphasis on immunosuppressive agents and antiinfective prophylactic agents), as well as previous infections and drug toxicities. A thorough physical examination should pay special attention to skin, mouth, lungs, and catheter exit site if one is present. Blood cultures should always be drawn. Other cultures (sputum, urine, stool) should be obtained as indicated by history and physical. Tests to rule out *Cytomegalovirus* (CMV) reactivation should be ordered if the patient is at high risk. This is sometimes overlooked when the transplant took

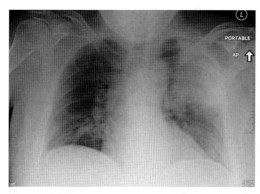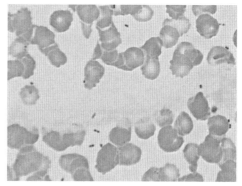

Figure 25.2 Pneumococcal pneumonia and overwhelming sepsis in cGVHD. A 59-year-old man with chronic GVHD presented with a history of 36 hours of shortness of breath and fever. On admission he was on florid septic shock. The chest radiograph showed left upper lobe pneumonia (A). His peripheral blood smear showed intracellular and extracellular diplococci. (B: Giemsa stain). The blood cultures grew *Streptococcus pneumoniae*, partially susceptible to penicillin. The patient suffered cardiorespiratory arrest and resuscitation was ineffective.

The patient had received a reduced-intensity matched-sibling allo-HCT for CLL 5 years earlier, and was in complete remission. He had suffered chronic extensive GVHD involving skin, eyes, mouth, and liver, but at the time of the event he was not on any systemic immunosuppressive therapy. He had received the pneumococcal vaccine (23-valent). He had been on penicillin VK, but more than a year had passed since the last time he had refilled his prescription. See Plate 73 in the color plate section.

place several months earlier and weekly monitoring has been discontinued. Imaging should include at a minimum a chest x-ray, as pneumonia is particularly common. Noninfectious pulmonary complications of HCT are often in the differential diagnosis, and computerized tomography (CT) is often a more useful diagnostic modality for these [33].

The antimicrobial prophylaxis needs to be assessed, because the presence or absence of specific agents modifies the risk of particular infections and hence may determine the management. If there are no localizing signs or symptoms, given that these patients often have functional hyposplenism and are at risk for overwhelming infection with *Streptococcus pneumoniae* [34]. *Hemophilus influenzae, Neisseria* sp. [35], and other encapsulated pathogens, antibiotics active against these organisms are commonly initiated (Figure 25.2). Bacteremia is related to a central venous catheter only half the time [23, 27], which means a high degree of suspicion should be maintained even in the absence of a catheter. Decreased splenic function was demonstrated in most patients with chronic extensive GVHD [19], but milder defects have been identified in patients with less severe forms of the disease [17], and spleen size as determined by ultrasound is decreased even in patients with limited cGVHD [36]. From the practical standpoint, the safer approach is to consider any patient with cGVHD and an acute febrile illness possibly hyposplenic. Besides *Streptococcus, Neisseria,* and *Hemophilus,* other bacteria occasionally mentioned as potential pathogens in patients with asplenia include Group B *Streptococcus, Staphylococcus aureus, Klebsiella,* and *Capnocytophaga canimorsus* [37].

Not related to hyposplenism, but rather to a defect in T-cell immunity, *Listeria monocytogenes* is another bacterial infection

that may present as primary septicemia without focal signs or symptoms, and its frequency seems to be increased after HCT, particularly in the presence of lymphopenia [38].

Regarding empirical antibacterial therapy, considering the range of bacterial pathogens, ceftriaxone or a fluoroquinolone with activity against *S. pneumoniae* may be chosen, depending on the local patterns of pneumococcal resistance and current antibacterial prophylaxis used by the patient.

Although the acute onset of fever suggests bacterial infection, respiratory viruses after HCT may also present similarly, but most patients have respiratory symptoms [39]. It should be emphasized, however, that many respiratory viral infections in HCT recipients are accompanied by significant copathogens, including *Aspergillus* [40]. In our experience, finding a respiratory virus does not always end the infectious diseases work-up.

In the case of subacute processes, the likelihood of bacteremia is lower and a diagnosis should be established before initiating empirical treatment. The variety of infectious and noninfectious complications that may present with fever is so broad that no universal safe and effective empirical antimicrobial regimen can be recommended.

Respiratory Infections in cGVHD

The respiratory tract is the most common site of severe infection in cGVHD in most series [23, 26, 31]. Of the 44 infectious late deaths in 668 patients at Karolinska University Hospital, 30 (68%) were pneumonias [30]. In their study of late pneumonia in a cohort of 1,359 patients transplanted at the FHCRC between January 1992 and January 1997, investigators reported a cumulative incidence of pneumonia of 34%–39% at 4 years in recipients of allogeneic transplants (the higher number in unrelated or mismatched recipients, as opposed to human leukocyte antigen [HLA]-matched related) [41]. The cumulative incidence of cGVHD among the patients with pneumonia was 67%, and indeed cGVHD was an independent risk factor for pneumonia in the multivariate analysis, together with age and donor type [41].

Chronic GVHD patients with respiratory symptoms and radiographic findings may be suffering from pneumonia caused by bacterial, viral, and fungal pathogens (including *Pneumocystis*, now classified as a non-mould fungus), but noninfectious entities should be considered. Some of these "late non-infectious pulmonary complications" of allo-HCT, seem to be associated with cGVHD and may be temporarily related to donor lymphocyte infusions (DLIs). The list includes diffuse alveolar hemorrhage (uncommon late complication, it is more common early after HCT), chronic organizing pneumonia (also known as bronchiolitis obliterans organizing pneumonia or BOOP), bronchiolitis obliterans syndrome (also known as obliterative bronchiolitis) and idiopathic pneumonia syndrome (also typically seen earlier after HCT) [42–45]. Besides these classic late-onset pulmonary complications one must consider drug toxicity, caused by imatinib [46], dasatinib [47], or sirolimus (a cause of several pulmonary syndromes [48]).

Diagnostic Work-Up

An assessment of the likely pathogens is based on prior history, current immunosuppressive and prophylactic therapies and radiographic findings (e.g., focal vs. disseminated process). Given the potential for bacterial pneumonia and overwhelming pneumococcal sepsis, empirical broad-spectrum antibiotics should be started early, but an etiologic diagnosis should be aggressively pursued. In selected cases (e.g., patients who are clinically stable with limited cGVHD, no active immunosuppression and focal findings in the chest radiograph) a slightly modified version of the standard management algorithm of community-acquired pneumonia may be applied [49]. For these patients a chest radiograph, blood cultures, and sputum Gram stain and culture will be obtained and empirical treatment against *S. pneumoniae* and other agents of community-acquired pneumonia initiated with a "respiratory" fluoroquinolone (moxifloxacin, gemifloxacin, or levofloxacin) or a beta-lactam plus a macrolide. In patients receiving systemic immunosuppression, a broader regimen may be chosen to ensure coverage of pathogens like methicillin-resistant *Staphylococcus aureus* (MRSA) or *Pseudomonas*, and further diagnostic procedures are appropriate. Frequently, a CT will be obtained (to better define the anatomy of distribution of the disease process) and bronchoscopy with bronchoalveolar lavage (BAL) will be indicated from the outset [50]. The general concept is that the more immunocompromised the patient is, the more critical the determination of the true pathogen or pathogens is, and hence the more aggressive the evaluation should be. The presence of more than one pathogen is common.

Laboratory Tests: Bronchoalveolar Lavage, Blood, and Urine

The infectious disease workup from the BAL fluid should include the necessary stains, cultures and molecular testing to rule out conventional and opportunistic respiratory pathogens. The following list is an example: Gram stain and respiratory culture, fungal stain and culture, modified acid-fast bacilli (AFB) stain (for *Nocardia*) and *Nocardia* culture, AFB stain and culture, stains for *Pneumocystis*, viral culture or polymerase chain reaction (PCR) for respiratory virus, CMV rapid culture and herpes virus cultures. Part of the BAL should be submitted for cytopathologic studies to look for viral cytopathic effect and perform silver stain and other special stains for microorganisms. New microbiological techniques in the analysis of bronchoalveolar lavage, including PCR for *Legionella*, *Pneumocystis* as well as determination of aspergillus galactomannan antigen [51–53] offer considerable promise to minimize the need for more invasive procedures in the future. Their value is not universal, however. Many molecular techniques are "home-brew" assays that have not been generally validated. There are preliminary indications that, besides galactomannan antigen for *Aspergillus*, *Pneumocystis* or *Aspergillus* or panfungal PCR may be of value, whereas, CMV PCR in the BAL fluid is often misleading or useless [54] (Figure 25.3).

Some blood and urine tests may occasionally be useful for the diagnosis of pneumonia. The urine should be sent for determination of *S. pneumoniae* and *Legionella pneumophila* antigens [49]. Histoplasma antigen may be found in the urine in disseminated histoplasmosis, but this infection seems to be uncommon after HCT [55]. Determination in serum of the fungal antigens galactomannan (polysaccharide antigen of *Aspergillus* released during infection and detectable in serum by enzyme-liked immunoassay) and beta-D-glucan (a polysaccharide component of the fungal cell wall of several fungi, including *Candida*, *Aspergillus*, and *Pneumocystis*) may be used to try to rule out invasive aspergillosis (see subsequent text). PCR in the blood for *Adenovirus* may be suggestive of disseminated adenovirus disease in the right setting (e.g., severe GVHD, lymphopenia, intense immunosuppression), as blood PCR for VZV may be helpful in cases of VZV without cutaneous lesions. A rising level of EBV in the blood as determined by PCR is suggestive of posttransplant lymphoproliferative disease. Of note, for several of these tests (galactomannan and beta-D-glucan antigens and EBV and adenovirus PCR) utility is greatly improved when they are obtained serially over time, and one single isolated result obtained to evaluate a new pulmonary process may be misleading. In select cases mycobacterial and fungal blood cultures may be appropriate.

The BAL is the accepted diagnostic modality for pneumonia in immunocompromised patients. The routine need for transbronchial biopsy is controversial, as it adds considerable morbidity and questionable infectious disease yield [56]. In cases of diffuse parenchymal processes undiagnosed by other means, a transbronchial biopsy may be helpful. Nodular infiltrates are better diagnosed by fine-needle biopsy [57], but the invasive diagnostic test of choice may vary depending on the

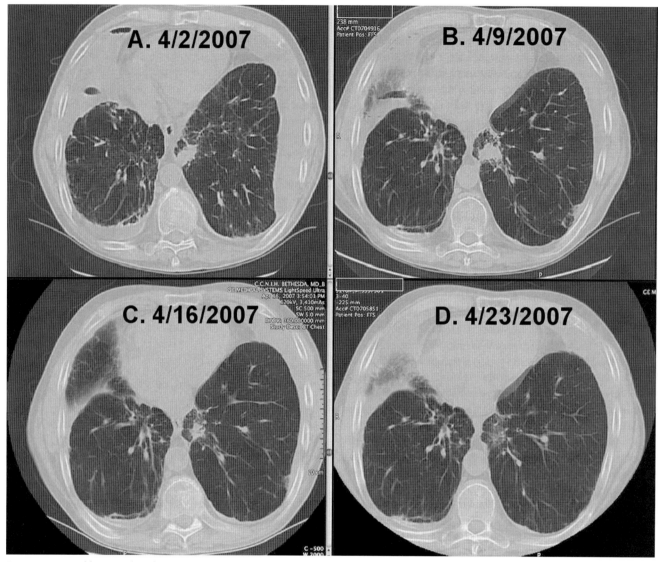

Figure 25.3 Possible PCP Identified by PCR. A 52-year-old man, s/p nonmyeloablative allo-HCT for CML in July 2000 had chronic extensive GVHD (mouth, eyes, skin, and liver) for several years. Since his transplant he has been admitted at least once a year with respiratory infection (influenza in 2002, RSV in 2003, *Moraxella* in 2004, *Streptococcus pneumoniae* (resistant to penicillin) in 2005, *Staphylococcus aureus* in 2006, *Hemophilus influenzae* pneumonia in 2007). After his last pneumonia, a new nodule was found on the follow-up CT (A). He has severe COPD on treatment with fluticasone and salmeterol inhalers and cGVHD on treatment with prednisone 60 mg PO every other day and hydroxychloroquine 200 mg PO every other day. His prophylactic antimicrobials included itraconazole 200 mg PO twice daily (recent levels in the therapeutic range), dapsone 100 mg PO daily and valacyclovir 500 mg PO daily. At the time of the first image, he was still on oral levofloxacin 500 mg PO daily for his recent bacterial infection. The location of the nodule and his underlying pulmonary disease made his doctors choose a BAL as initial diagnostic procedure. All the studies were negative except for a positive PCR for *Pneumocystis*. The patient had been stated empirically on posaconazole after the bronchoscopy, but when the PCR results were known a repeat CT was obtained and atovaquone added. After the introduction of atovaquone, the nodule started improving and posaconazole was discontinued. Atovaquone was maintained for 3 weeks and itraconazole reintroduced. The nodule resolved completely.

facilities available and the overall risk for the patient (location of the lesion, thrombocytopenia, coagulation abnormalities). A surgical biopsy (i.e., VATS), despite its considerable morbidity, may be the diagnostic test of choice in an immunocompromised patient with worsening pulmonary infiltrates despite broad-spectrum empirical antimicrobial therapy and negative BAL work-up. Some series have failed to show significant changes in therapy or improved outcome with biopsy, whereas, others report significant treatment changes in up to two-thirds of patients. From our standpoint, in patients with cGVHD surgical lung biopsy may be invaluable to identify some of the noninfectious late pulmonary complications [44].

BACTERIAL PNEUMONIA

S. pneumoniae is the most commonly isolated bacterial pathogen in pneumonia in cGVHD, but many others have been reported, including *Klebsiella pneumoniae, S. aureus,* and *Haemophilus influenzae* [23, 30, 31, 41, 58]. Lobar infiltrates, patchy consolidation, and even interstitial patterns may be seen with bacterial pneumonia. As is often the case in community-acquired pneumonia, a significant fraction of the episodes respond to antibiotics but no pathogen is identified. *Pseudomonas* and MRSA are not known to be more frequent in cGVHD than in other patients with close contact with a health-care setting with community-acquired pneumonia [23, 30, 41, 58].

Nocardia infections are not common after HCT, but they tend to occur late and in patients with active cGVHD [59, 60]. The patients are often on pneumocystis pneumonia (PCP) prophylaxis other than trimethoprim/sulfamethoxazole (TMP/SMX), which has made some investigators suggest that TMP/SMX prophylaxis may be effective to prevent Nocardia [60]; this hypothesis is not substantiated by other studies [59]. The presentation is usually subacute with fever and pulmonary infiltrates that may be nodular and cavitate, suggesting mould infection. Blood cultures are positive only infrequently, but dissemination is common, particularly to the CNS [61, 62]. BAL and fine-needle aspirate are effective diagnostic modalities; when *Nocardia* is suspected, a modified-acid-fast stain is recommended. The results of cytopathology may allow earlier diagnosis, as *Nocardia* tends to grow slowly. Special stains for microorganisms (GMS and Fite) should be requested. The nomenclature of the genus *Nocardia* has been revised [63], and many older articles may be misleading regarding the species causing disease. Currently the most helpful classification separates the different species in "antibiotic groups," which results in the clinician finding out the predictable susceptibilities of the pathogen that has been isolated. There are no comparative trials to guide therapy. Most experience is with TMP/SMX, but ceftriaxone, imipenem and meropenem, minocycline, and moxifloxacin have also been used. Amikacin may be added in severe cases. Linezolid is effective [64], but long-term administration may result in unacceptable toxicity, and the treatment of nocardiosis usually requires 6 months to 1 year.

TUBERCULOSIS (TB) AND NONTUBERCULOUS MYCOBACTERIA

TB is relatively infrequent after allo-HCT, although its incidence is higher than in the general population [65]. It is a late infection after HCT. Corticosteroid use, total body irradiation and cGVHD have been identified as risk factors [66], but only half the patients are reported to have cGVHD when they are diagnosed with TB [67–69]. Most series emphasize the diagnostic difficulties, with a delay between symptoms and diagnosis of 30 to 45 days. The presentation is usually with fever and cough. Constitutional syndrome, dyspnea and hypoxemia are found in less than one-third of patients. Nonspecific interstitial infiltrates are more common than cavitary lesions, and normal chest radiographs are well documented [68, 69]. The tuberculin skin is characteristically negative during cGVHD [70]. Bronchoscopy with BAL is the preferred diagnostic modality, but biopsies may be necessary as the sensitivity of the AFB smear from a BAL in proven tuberculosis has sometimes been as low as 40% [71].

Nontuberculous mycobacteria are occasionally isolated from the sputum or the BAL of patients with cGVHD [68], often in patients with abnormal lung parenchyma secondary to radiation, chemotherapy, chronic organizing pneumonia, and obliterative bronchiolitis. The interpretation of these isolates is not always straightforward, even in immunocompromised patients, and careful consideration must be given to the species isolated, the radiographic appearance and the pulmonary function tests. The American Thoracic Society published guidelines in 2007 that address in detail many of the difficulties of the diagnosis and make recommendations for treatment on the basis of the species and severity of the disease [72].

VIRAL PNEUMONIA

CMV

Cytomegalovirus (CMV) used to be the most common viral cause of late pneumonia after HCT [26, 30, 41, 73]. The decreasing presence of CMV pneumonia in recent studies [23, 31] is likely related to the use of preemptive therapy. General risk factors for late CMV disease include early CMV antigenemia, lymphopenia, absolute CD4 count lower than 50, corticosteroid use, GVHD [74], as well as the type of transplant (more common in unrelated, cord, haploidentical, or T-cell-depleted transplants). Most cases of late CMV pneumonia occur in patients who have received T–cell-depleted grafts, have chronic extensive GVHD requiring intense immunosuppression, or both [75]. Interestingly, in the largest reported series of late CMV pneumonitis more than half the patients had significant copathogens identified [75]. The isolation of CMV in the BAL fluid may represent asymptomatic shedding, and deciding that it is causing disease may be a challenge when other pathogen is detected (Figure 25.4). The recommended treatment of CMV pneumonia is with ganciclovir 5 mg/kg IV q 12 hours for 2 to 3 weeks, often followed by another 2 weeks of maintenance therapy, with intravenous immunoglobulin (IVIG) or CMV-specific immunoglobulin (CMV-Ig) during the first 2 to 3 weeks [76]. The addition of IVIG or CMV-Ig to ganciclovir is based on early nonrandomized studies that showed much higher efficacy of the combination compared with historical controls, although more recent studies have suggested that current outcomes are not influenced by IVIG [77].

RESPIRATORY VIRUSES

Community respiratory viruses (*Influenza, Parainfluenza, Respiratory syncytial* virus (RSV), *Adenovirus, Picornavirus, Metapneumovirus,* and others) are common infections after HCT [78]. Early after transplant, progression from upper respiratory infection to pneumonia and respiratory failure seems to be related to neutropenia, lymphopenia and, at least for parainfluenza 3, the use of corticosteroids [40]. Late infections do not progress to pneumonia so readily, but may have significant long-term effects on respiratory function [79]. The interaction of respiratory virus infections and late airflow obstruction may be bidirectional since preexisting airflow obstruction may be a risk for progression to lower respiratory tract disease late after

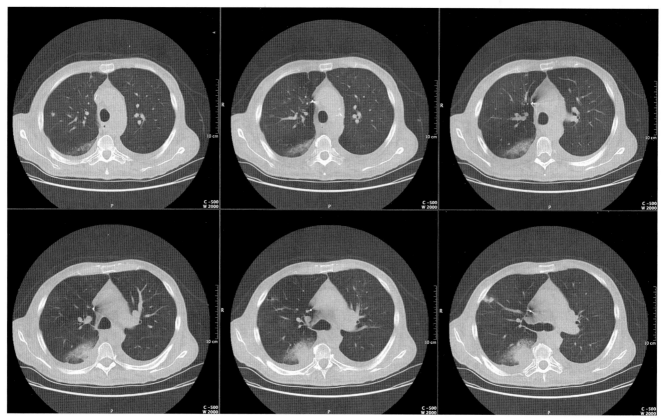

Figure 25.4 CMV isolated from the BAL without causing disease. A 67-year-old man s/p allo-HCT for primary cutaneous large cell T-cell lymphoma came for his 9-month follow-up. He had chronic extensive GVHD and was on prednisone 40 mg PO daily and cyclosporine A. He was found to be febrile and hypoxemic during a routine follow-up visit. The chest CT is shown. A bronchoalveolar lavage was performed, and *Nocardia farcinica*, *Legionella pneumophila* serogroup 3 and *Stenotrophomonas maltophilia* grew in culture. CMV was also isolated by rapid culture from the BAL. However, the CMV PCR in blood was low positive (at the limit of detection of the assay, less than 250 genome equivalents per mL of blood) and the CT findings were considered inconsistent with CMV pneumonia. Antibacterial treatment was initiated, with improvement and, eventually, complete resolution. A repeat CMV PCR the following week was negative.

HCT. Late RSV pneumonia seems to be uncommon, but the reported cases suggest cGVHD as a potential risk factor. [80] Early intervention with inhaled ribavirin during RSV upper respiratory infection may result in less pneumonia, although the evidence is inconclusive [81]. The patient's individual risk factors for progression to pneumonia should be considered before recommending inhaled ribavirin for every cGVHD patient with RSV (Figure 25.5). Influenza has sometimes been reported as an early infection [82], whereas, other study documented cGVHD in 11 of 19 patients who developed the infection after day 100 [83]. The early use of neuraminidase inhibitors seems to result in good outcomes [83, 84].

FUNGAL DISEASE

Fungal pneumonia, particularly due to *Aspergillus*, accounts for a sizable fraction of late infections after HCT. In most cases it is related to active immunosuppression for the treatment of cGVHD, particularly corticosteroids [85]. Comprehensive guidelines for the management of aspergillosis are regularly published by the Infectious Disease Society of America [86]. When invasive fungal infection (IFI) is suspected (e.g., in patients receiving corticosteroids), a chest CT is the preferred radiologic modality [86]. Nodules >1 cm and halo sign seem to be preferentially associated with IFIs [87, 88]. However, most cases of late invasive aspergillosis show nonspecific broncho-pneumonia-like infiltrates [89]). The diagnosis of IFI remains challenging, as the yield of the BAL seldom exceeds 40% with standard detection methods (and is probably less in cases of mucormycosis [90]). Galactomannan determination in the BAL may improve the diagnostic yield. The reported sensitivity for invasive aspergillosis of galactomannan antigen in the BAL is in the 60% range [51], although a study in neutropenic patients suggested 100% sensitivity and specificity [91].

In contrast to the determinations in the BAL fluid, galactomannan and beta-D-glucan determinations in the serum have been validated as monitoring tools during the time at risk for infection, particularly during neutropenia [92, 93], rather than as ad hoc tests that may rule in or rule out the diagnosis during an individual episode. In a retrospective study at the University of Minnesota, Foy et al. found a sensitivity of 0.50 and a specificity of 0.94 [94]. Marr et al. described increased sensitivity by decreasing the cutoff value of the test [95]; however, this and the previous study address mainly neutropenic or early transplant patients.

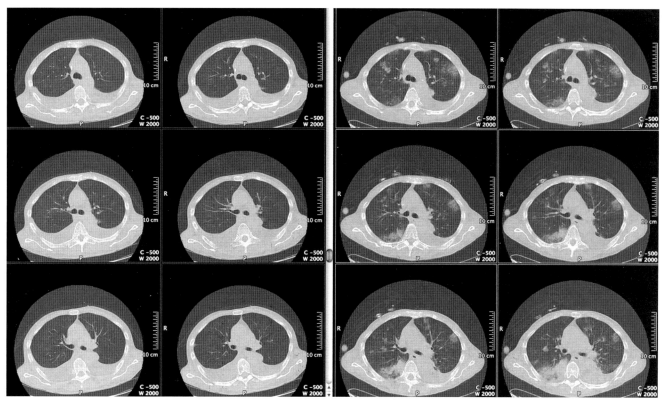

Figure 25.5 Multiple pathogens in refractory cGVHD. A 55-year-old man was admitted with chronic extensive GVHD refractory to corticosteroids 1 year after matched-sibling HCT. Before initiating intensive immunosuppression with infliximab and daclizumab, a BAL was obtained after the CT form March 11 A: His only respiratory complaint was chronic cough, persistent after an episode of RSV a few months prior. The BAL showed moderate neutrophils and many gram-negative bacilli, and had heavy growth of *Stenotrophomonas maltophilia*. The fungal stain showed few branching septate hyphae, and grew moderate *Aspergillus fumigatus*. The viral culture grew RSV. The cytologic examination showed ciliocytophthoria and rare septate hyphae. The PCR for *Pneumocystis* was positive. Preemptive treatment with TMP/SMX, levofloxacin, caspofungin and voriconazole was initiated. After starting infliximab and daclizumab, however, he developed progressive shortness of breath and worsening pulmonary infiltrates B: The addition of inhaled ribavirin coincided with acute pulmonary decompensation and fatal respiratory failure. The autopsy showed no evidence of invasive aspergillosis or *Pneumocystis*, but multifocal areas of diffuse alveolar damage with hemorrhage and exudates.
RSV, *Respiratory syncitial* virus; TMP/SMX, trimethoprim/sulfomethoxazole.

At the present time the serum galactomannan and beta-D-glucan tests have unknown value in the diagnosis of a patient with cGVHD and possible pneumonia. Regardless of what the true sensitivity and specificity of these tests turns out to be, non-aspergillus mould infections may still be present when the results are negative. Given the limitations of each agent in the current antifungal armamentarium, a typical pressing question is if the probable IFI is aspergillosis and requires treatment with voriconazole [96] (alone or combined with an echinocandin [97]) or if it is mucormycosis and requires a lipid formulation of amphotericin B. The best empirical strategy to solve this dilemma is not known. Posssible options include early biopsy, empirical treatment with voriconazole (given the relative rarity of mucormycosis), or empirical treatment with a combination of amphotericin and an echinocandin. The best approach may vary depending on the local diagnostic capabilities and prevalence of mucormycosis. Even if empirical management is a reasonable option in stable patients, we think biopsy should be considered early, particularly when risk factors for non-aspergillus mould infection are present (the most important of which seems to be the use of voriconazole [98]). The prognosis of invasive aspergillosis after HCT has improved over the past decade, but late onset and high-dose corticosteroids (=2 mg/kg/d of prednisone equivalent) remain significant risk factors for death [99].

Other pulmanory mould infections present similarly to invasive aspergillosis during cGVHD (for reviews, see Varkey and Perfect [100] and Walsh et al [101]). Basic principles of management include (1) decrease the immunosuppression (particularly the corticosteroids), (2) identify the organism, (3) consider surgery for nondisseminated disease, (4) check for drug interactions [102], (5) administer the drug of choice to achieve optimal therapeutic levels as soon as possible (posaconazole does not reach therapeutic levels for several days [103]), (6) in case of unexpected worsening, consider obtaining drug levels, which are quite variable in the case of voriconazole, particularly when administered orally long term [104, 105].

PNEUMOCYSTIS JIROVECI

Most cases of *Pneumocystis jiroveci* (PCP) after HCT are late pneumonias associated with discontinuation of prophylaxis or suboptimal prophylaxis (i.e., prophylaxis other than TMP/SMX); chronic extensive GVHD is present in the majority of cases [106–109]. Seven of thirteen patients described by De Castro et al. had cGVHD, six of them were on steroids but one was receiving only cyclosporine. All had discontinued prophylaxis, mainly because of concern with hematologic toxicity. All the patients had CD4 lymphopenia (<200 /μL or <10% of lymphocytes) [107]. In the series reported by Souza and Torres, breakthroughs happened on low-dose dapsone (50 mg bid three times per week) [108] or pentamidine (inhaled or IV) [109]. The clinical presentation seems to be relatively typical, with fever, hypoxemia, and interstitial infiltrates, but the very frequent presence of coinfections (often CMV and aspergillosis) may result in atypical radiographic patterns, including nodules and pleural effusions [109] (Figure 25.3). The relatively uncommon granulomatous form of the disease has been reported after HCT [110]. In this form, the characteristic presentation is single or multiple nodules without hypoxemia and with normal LDH. The treatment of choice for PCP is TMP/SMX (15–20 mg/kg based on the trimethoprim dose), even for the rare patient who develops disease as a breakthrough of TMP/SMX prophylaxis. Intravenous pentamidine, 4 mg/kg/d, is the second choice for severe disease. The guidelines for treating PCP in AIDS recommend all patients with an arterial $pO_2 < 70$ mmHg receive concomitant corticosteroids (prednisone 40 mg by mouth twice a day for days 1–5, 40 mg daily for days 6–10, and 20 mg daily for days 11–21) [111]. For mild to moderate disease, other treatment options that can be considered include atovaquone suspension (750 mg PO bid with food); dapsone (50 mg PO twice daily or 100 mg PO once a day); dapsone and trimethoprin (dapsone 100 mg PO daily and TMP 15 mg/kg/d PO in three divided doses) or primaquine and clindamycin (primaquine 15–30 mg base PO daily and clindamycin 600–900 mg/6–8 hours IV or 300–450 mg/6–8 hours PO). None of these treatments have been systematically analyzed in HCT recipients.

SINUSITIS

Sinusitis may be particularly common in cGVHD [112, 113]. It is bacterial more often than fungal. but microbiological studies should be performed, as the clinical presentation may be similar. CT of the sinuses and ENT consultation should be obtained. Fiberoptic examination allows obtaining samples and biopsy of suspicious arcas. In cases of bacterial sinusitis the pathogens isolated are often gram-negative bacilli (including *Pseudomonas*) and *S. aureus*, although frequently the cultures are negative [114]. Isolation of moulds in culture is not sufficient to establish the diagnosis of invasive fungal sinusits; a biopsy should be obtained for this purpose. Most reported cases of invasive fungal sinusitis late after HCT had severe cGVHD and were receiving immunosuppression, particularly corticosteroids. Of note, some patients have developed fungal sinusitis with relatively uncommon moulds such

as *Exserohilum* or *Scedosporium* (instead of aspergillosis or mucormycosis) that later may go on to cause disseminated disease and death [115, 116]. Invasive fungal sinusitis in severely immunocompromised patients should be considered medical-surgical emergencies. The combination of extensive debridement, discontinuation or decrease of the immunosuppression and antifungal agents is necessary for a successful outcome.

An association between the presence of chronic sinusitis and the development of airway obstruction has been postulated [117], so an aggressive management with antibiotics and ENT consultation is often advocated, although there is no study formally evaluating this approach

Skin and Soft Tissue Infections

The major infection involving the skin in patients with cGVHD is shingles. Reactivation of VZV with clinical disease happens in approximately 30% of HCT recipients within the first year [118, 119]. The diagnosis should be entertained in any case of vesicular rash, and in any maculopapular rash with a radicular distribution. It is important to consider VZV also in the differential diagnosis of abdominal pain, facial palsy and a variety of pain syndromes. Cutaneous disease is easy to diagnose by obtaining a scraping of the base of a vesicle and performing a direct fluorescence assay (DFA). When herpes sine herpete is suspected in an immunocompromised patient, the diagnosis may be established by VZV PCR in the peripheral blood [120, 121]. It is worth noting that *Herpes simplex virus* (HSV) lesions may be clinically indistinguishable from VZV; the etiology should be determined by DFA, culture (for HSV) or molecular methods. Treatment of VZV disease should include the early institution of antiviral therapy (valacyclovir, acyclovir, or famciclovir) and the appropriate management of bacterial superinfection if present. The association of VZV with Group A Streptococcus infection, including the development of necrotizing fasciitis is well documented in children and has also been documented in immunocompromised patients, and a high index of suspicion is appropriate. Regarding the choice of antiviral agent, disseminated VZV is best treated with acyclovir IV 10 to 15 mg/kg every 8 hours. Nonimmunocompromised patients with localized shingles may be treated with oral valacyclovir of famciclovir. Patients with cGVHD may be closer to one or the other end of this clinical spectrum depending on the severity of their disease and degree of immunosuppression, but we tend to err on the side of the more conservative approach with IV acyclovir, at least initially.

Bacterial infections of the skin would be expected in patients with cGVHD and scleroderma-like skin involvement or those with cutaneous ulcers. The original descriptions of cGVHD did report a significant number of skin infections ("boils" and paronychia) [5, 24], but this category is often not mentioned in more recent series. We have seen a variety of skin infections, most commonly secondary to their GVHD of the skin creating an appropriate portal of entry for potential pathogens from the skin flora (typically erysipelas or impetigo caused by *S. aureus* or *Streptococcus pyogenes*) (Figure 25.6),

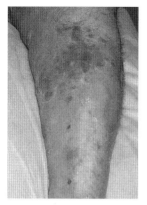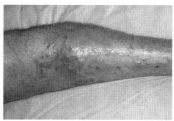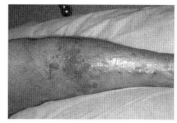

Figure 25.6 Secodarily infected skin ulcers in a patient with chronic extensive GVHD. See Plate 74 in the color plate section.

but occasionally related to bacteremia with subsequent seeding of the skin.

Skin lesions may represent the portal of entry of infection and also be the first manifestation of systemic infections. Fungal, mycobacterial, and nocardia infections may present a so-called sporotrichoid distribution consisting of subcutaneous nodules following a lymphangitic spread from a portal of entry. Disseminated bacterial infections may present with erythematous macules or papules that become necrotic in ecthyma gangrenosum (classically associated with *Pseudomonas aeruginosa*, but described also with *Aeromonas*, other gram-negative bacilli, *S. aureus*, and several moulds [122]). Such lesions should be biopsied. Disseminated candidiasis occasionally presents with nontender, nonblanching erythematous macules, papules, or nodules. These lesions are nonspecific and may be similar to a drug rash. In general, a low threshold for obtaining a skin biopsy should be maintained in immunocompromised patients.

Gastrointestinal Infections in cGVHD

There is limited information available regarding the incidence and epidemiology of infectious diarrhea late after HCT and during cGVHD in particular. The differential diagnosis includes GVHD of the bowel, pancreatic insufficiency [123], drug toxicity (particularly mycophenilate mofetil [MMF]), and infectious causes. Infections may be bacterial (*Clostridium difficile, Salmonella, Shigella, Campylobacter, Vibrio, Aeromonas*), viral (CMV, adenovirus, VZV, rotavirus, norovirus, astrovirus) or parasitic (*Giardia, Cryptosporidium*).

CMV gastrointestinal (GI) disease is the most important GI infection during cGVHD. Its incidence varies significantly depending on the kind of transplant and the preventive strategy in place. In a prospective study of 42 GI complications in 273 allogeneic transplants, (equally divided sibling and matched-unrelated donor), none of the 15 GI complications that happened after day 100 was caused by CMV [124]. In another report, CMV colitis or enteritis was documented in only 1 of 145 patients with cGVHD following HLA-matched related or unrelated HCT [23] and in 2 of 196 survivors of HLA-matched related transplant [31]. In a different kind of study, however, van

Burik and her colleagues documented 46 cases of CMV enteritis over 10 years of transplants at the University of Minnesota, 20 of which happened in patients with cGVHD [125].

The diagnosis of CMV GI disease requires endoscopy and biopsies, which should be processed both for rapid viral culture and histopathology with CMV-specific immunostains, because the combination of both techniques is more sensitive than either alone [125]. Regarding treatment, most published experience is with ganciclovir 5 mg/kg IV q12h for several weeks (the optimal duration is uncertain) but foscarnet 90 mg/kg IV q 12h is assumed to be equivalent. There are no data supporting the use of IVIG for the treatment of CMV GI disease.

Central Nervous System Infections in cGVHD

Central nervous system (CNS) infections are not common in cGVHD. Bacterial meningitis is the most commonly reported CNS infection in these patients [23, 24, 30, 31]. *S. pneumoniae* is the most common single bacterial etiology, occasionally resistant to penicillin [126]. *Herpes simplex* and VZV encephalitis, as well as CNS disease due to aspergillus and toxoplasma have been described. Given the defective T-cell immunity associated with cGVHD and its treatment *Listeria* should be expected, but it is reportedly uncommon [127].

In a patient with cGVHD presenting with signs or symptoms of CNS infection, empirical treatment for bacteria including penicillin-resistant *S. pneumoniae* and *L monocytogenes* should be started without delay (i.e., ceftriaxone 2 g q12h IV, ampicillin 4 g q 4h IV and vancomycin 1 g q 12h IV). The management of presumed CNS infection involves imaging and obtaining cerebrospinal fluid (CSF). MRI is a much better diagnostic modality than CT for infectious etiologies. Meningeal enhancement, characteristic of bacterial meningitis, mass lesions or abscesses (*Aspergillus* or other moulds, toxoplasmosis, *Nocardia*, other bacteria), nonenhancing white matter lesions (progressive multifocal leukoencephalopathy [PML]) and abnormalities characteristic of viral encephalitis may be seen (Figure 25.7). Meningeal involvement by the primary malignancy as well as mass lesion suggestive of CNS lymphoma may be identified. The CSF should be sent for bacterial,

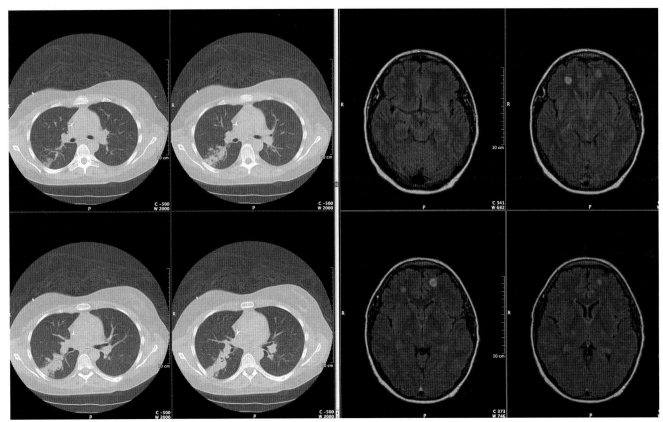

Figure 25.7 Late aspergillosis, disseminated to the CNS. A 32-year-old woman underwent nonmyeloablative T-cell-depleted transplant form a matched sibling in December of 2001. The immediate posttransplant period was uneventful. She developed acutely de novo cGVHD involving her skin and gut in May 2002, and was started on methylprednisolone 2 mg/kg/d. After 2 weeks of treatment she markedly improved on prednisone 60 mg/d when she developed fever and chest pain. The chest CT showed an infiltrate and the BAL grew *Aspergillus fumigatus*. An MRI was obtained for screening, although she had no neurological signs or symptoms, and showed one round lesion on each frontal lobe. The lung infiltrate and the brain lesions resolved on voriconazole and caspofungin.

fungal, and mycobacterial culture as well as for PCR for viruses including HSV, VZV, CMV, EBV, and JC virus, depending on the prophylactic antivirals the patient is receiving at the time of presentation. For patients at risk (known positive toxoplasma serology) toxoplasma PCR should be sent. The pathogenic potential of *Human Herpes virus-6* (HHV-6) late after transplant remains to be defined, although early after HCT it has been associated with a syndrome of amnesia and seizures (posttransplant acute limbic encephalitis [PALE]) [128] as well as possibly other CNS signs and symptoms [129].

RECOMMENDED INFECTION PROPHYLAXIS IN CGVHD

Immunizations

Immunizations should be a routine part of every HCT program. Recommendations regarding immunizations have been made by the CDC/ASBMT and the Infectious Diseases Working Party of the EBMT [130, 131]. Table 25.1 is a summary adapted from the current recommendations (Table 25.1 and Table 25.2).

Response to immunizations is impaired during cGVHD, even in the absence of immunosuppressive treatments, although this impairment varies for different vaccines. The response to inactivated polio vaccine does not seem to be affected by the presence of cGHVD [132]. Response to the polysaccharide pneumococcal vaccine is particularly poor [133]. The implication is that patients may not be adequately protected, and complementary measures have to be instituted. For instance, a patient may not develop a protective immune response to the influenza vaccine, but vaccination of his immediate family combined with a low threshold for initiating prophylactic or empirical treatment with oseltamivir during influenza outbreaks may result in very effective protection [83, 134].

Prevention of Bacterial Infections

Intravenous Immunoglobulin

There is no evidence that universal administration of IVIG is beneficial for allo-HCT recipients [135]. However, some experts recommend its use in patients who remain hypogammaglobulinemic (IgG <400 mg/dL) following transplant and who have repeated or severe infections [4]. Some patients with

Table 25.1: Suggested Recommendations for Immunizations in HCT Recipients (for information see [131, 130]

	6 months	12 months	14–18 months	24 months
Bacterial				
DTaP[1]		✓	✓	✓
Pneumococcal conjugate[2]	✓	✓	✓	✓
Hemophilus influenzae type b conjugate		✓	✓	✓
Meningococcal[3]		✓		
Viral				
Influenza[4]	✓			
Polio (inactivated)		✓	✓	✓
Hepatitis B	✓	✓	✓	
MMR[5]				✓
Hepatitis A[6]		✓	✓	
Varicella[7]				✓

[1] DTaP: Diphtheria and Tetanus Toxoids and Acellular Pertussis vaccine, Absorbed. Acellular pertussis vaccine is preferable, but the whole-cell pertussis vaccine should be used if it is the only pertussis vaccine available.

[2] The 7-valent pneumococcal conjugate vaccine is preferable; the polysaccharide vaccine can be given subsequently as a fourth dose to broaden the immune response.

[3] Follow recommendations for general population in each country.

[4] Lifelong, seasonal, starting before HSCT and resuming after 4 to 6 months.

[5] Measles, mumps, and rubella vaccine, live or attenuated; only given if the patient is immunocompetent at 24 months, that is, NOT on immune suppression and no GVHD for 6 months. Two doses are favored in the first 2 years posttransplant and in individuals who have never received an MMR vaccine. For persons <18 years of age, two doses are favored.

[6] Follow recommendations for general population in each country; Ig should be administered to hepatitis A-susceptible HSCT recipients who anticipate hepatitis A exposure (e.g., during travel to endemic areas) and for postexposure prophylaxis.

[7] There is limited data regarding safety and efficacy. It should only be given to seronegative patients. Given only if patients are immunocompetent at 24 months, that is, not on immune suppression and no GVHD for 6 months; If patients were vaccinated, revaccinate; If patients were never vaccinated with positive serology, do not vaccinate; If patients were never vaccinated with negative serology, vaccinate; Pediatric patients ages 12 months to12 years receive a single dose; persons aged ≥ 13 years should receive two doses, 4 to 8 weeks apart.

cGVHD would fulfill these criteria. This recommendation would be an extrapolation of the favorable effect of replacement immunoglobulin administered in other hypoglobulinemic states, including Bruton's agammaglobulinemia, common variable immunodeficiency, chronic lymphocytic leukemia (CLL) and multiple myeloma. The use of IVIG has not been adequately studied in cGVHD, however.

Prophylactic Antibiotics

Given that bacterial infections are the most common during cGVHD, prophylactic antibiotics are often recommended. Evidence supporting the efficacy of some of these practices is limited, and frequently derives from retrospective case series or clinical trials performed in other diseases or patient populations. Additionally, compliance is a significant issue in a chronic disease that is frequently characterized by polypharmacy and mood disorders including anxiety and depression. A prescription for penicillin should not be a substitute for advising patients to be seen promptly by a physician when they develop a febrile illness.

The more widespread recommendation is Penicillin VK (250–500 mg PO twice daily) aiming to prevent *S. pneumoniae* invasive disease. The incidence of invasive pneumococcal disease was found to be much higher in patients with cGVHD (18.85/1,000 transplants) than in patients without it (8.25/1,000) in a survey by the Infectious Diseases Working Party of the European Bone Marrow Transplantation [136]. One-third of the cases of *S. pneumoniae* infection in HCT recipients reported by investigators from the M.D. Anderson Cancer Center had cGVHD [137]. Most series of infections in cGVHD have significant numbers of pneumococcal bacteremia, pneumonia, and meningitis [23, 24, 30, 31]. The high risk of pneumococcal disease has been attributed to functional hyposplenism, impaired immunoglobulin production, decrease production of antipneumococcal antibodies and decreased opsonization. The evidence supporting the use of penicillin derives from its successful use to prevent pneumococcal disease in children with sickle cell disease [138] and from retrospective case series in which fatal outcome of invasive pneumococcal disease after transplant is associated with lack of prophylaxis. Kulkarni et al. reported 31 cases of invasive pneumococcal disease after allo-HCT, with all seven deaths taking place in patients who had not been taking prophylaxis [34]. This study did not provide incidence data on patients receiving and not receiving prophylaxis, and consequently cannot address the question of the effectiveness of the intervention. The aforementioned EBMT Survey documented that only 4 of 44 cases of invasive pneumococcal disease had received penicillin prophylaxis before the episode, and emphasized the issue of compliance [136]. A possible argument against penicillin prophylaxis (besides lack of compliance) is the increasing prevalence of penicillin-resistant strains of *S. pneumoniae* [126]. However, no study so far demonstrates that resistance is a problem in the HCT setting. The decreasing susceptibility of *S. pneumoniae*, the limited antibacterial spectrum of penicillin VK and the frequency of non-pneumococcal bacterial infection in cGVHD beg the question if a different antibiotic should be chosen. Regardless, penicillin VK 250 to 500 mg PO bid seems relatively inexpensive and safe, and is widely recommended.

For penicillin-allergic patients the options include azithromycin 250 mg PO daily or TMP/SMX 1 SS tablet PO bid, which has the advantage of providing *Pneumocystis* prophylaxis. The resistance of *S. pneumoniae* to either of azithromycin and TMP/SMX agents remains around 30% in the United States (vs. 12%

Table 25.2: Suggested Infectious Disease Prophylaxes for Patients with Chronic GVHD

Kind of Pathogen/ Disease	First Choice	Alternative	Duration	Comment
Bacterial	Penicillin VK 500 mg PO bid	Trimethoprim/sulfamethoxazole 80/400 mg (1 SS tablet) PO bid Azithromycin 250 mg PO bid	Indefinite	Efficacy of prophylaxis unproven. Prompt management of fever important
Fungal	Posaconazole 200 mg PO tid[1]	Voriconazole 200 mg PO bid Fluconazole 400 mg PO daily	As long as the patient is on more than 0.8 mg/kg qod of prednisone equivalent	Fluconazole has no activity against moulds, which are the main concern during cGVHD receiving corticosteroids
PCP	Trimethoprim-sulfamethoxazole (TMP/SMX), 1 double-strength tablet PO daily or 1 single-strength tablet PO daily or 1 double-strength tablet PO 3 times/week	Dapsone, 50 mg by mouth 2 times/day or 100 mg by mouth daily or pentamidine, 300 mg every 3–4 weeks by Respirgard II™ nebulizer	Six months after the patient has discontinued active immunosuppression	Consider desensitization to TMP/SMX
HSV and VZV	Acyclovir 800 mg PO bid OR valacyclovir 500 mg PO bid		Safe and effective for at least 1 year. Continue for at least 6 moths after stopping immunosuppression	VZV reactivation happens predictably in 30% of patients after stopping prophylaxis
CMV	Preemptive management with ganciclovir, valganciclovir or foscarnet. Induction doses: ganciclovir 5 mg/kg IV q12h; valganciclovir 900 mg PO bid; foscarnet 60 mg/kg IV q12h; Maintenance dose: ganciclovir 5 mg/kg IV daily 5–6 days/week or foscarnet 60 mg/kg daily	Universal prophylaxis with valganciclovir 900 po daily (adjusted to renal function)	Until CMV PCR has been negative × 3 AND the patient is receiving no more immunosuppression than prednisone 0.5 mg/kg	Preemptive therapy is initiated with CMV >1,000 copies/mL

[1] The role of antifungal prophylaxis during chronic graft versus host disease (cGVHD) is unclear. Posaconazole may be recommended based on a single randomized trial that included many patients with cGVHD, but its use did not result in improved outcome nor did it show a statistically significant reduction in IFIs in the subgroup of patients with cGVHD

to 20% resistance to penicillin) [139]. Both azithromycin and TMP/SMX have been shown to be effective to prevent severe bacterial infections in other immunocompromised patient populations, namely HIV-infected children [140] and children with chronic granulomatous disease [141]. Some investigators report using levofloxacin 500 mg PO daily, but there are insufficient data regarding efficacy, safety, and tolerability of long-term use (probably years) of a broad-spectrum fluoroquinolone in this setting.

The duration of prophylaxis is unclear. Published guidelines suggest continuing prophylaxis for as long as treatment for cGVHD is given; other investigators suggest life-long prophylaxis [134]. It is worth considering that many of the immune defects that make patients susceptible to bacterial infections (and particularly to *S. pneumoniae*) do not necessarily disappear upon cessation of active administration of

immunosuppressive drugs; thus prophylaxis should be continued for at least 6 additional months

Antifungal Prophylaxis

There is insufficient evidence to decide which patients with cGVHD should receive antifungal prophylaxis and for how long. The frequency of reported IFIs in prospective series of patients cGVHD is relatively low and seems associated mainly with the use of corticosteroids [1, 23, 24, 26]. However, in the largest studies of risk factors for IFI after transplant, chronic extensive GVHD remains an independent risk factor in multivariate analysis [85, 142, 143]. Smaller studies tend to find corticosteroid use (variably described as ≥1 mg/kg/d of prednisone equivalent for more than 3 weeks) is the independent risk factor [144]. Late after transplant aspergillosis seems to be more frequent than candidiasis [23, 85, 142]. Consequently, the goal of antifungal prophylaxis during cGVHD should be to prevent mould infections. Some experts recommend antifungals only for patients with chronic extensive GVHD who are receiving active immunosuppression, mainly corticosteroids. The specifics regarding how much corticosteroids and for how long vary considerably. There are three systemic antifungal classes of agents currently available: polyenes (amphotericin B deoxycholate and lipid formulations of amphotericin B), echinocandins (caspofungin, micafungin, and anidulafungin) and azoles (fluconazole, itraconazole, voriconazole, and posaconazole). The randomized controlled trial of antifungal prophylaxis that included most patients with cGVHD receiving corticosteroids (patients with cGVHD were eligible if they were receiving corticosteroids at ≥0.8 mg/kg of prednisone equivalent every other day) showed that posaconazole was superior to fluconazole to prevent invasive aspergillosis [145]. There was less aspergillosis in the posaconazole group (5.3% in the posaconazole group vs. 9% in the patients who received fluconazole), but the study did not show a survival advantage, and most cases of aspergillosis were diagnosed by galactomannan antigenemia. With these results it is possible to argue that a strategy of fluconazole prophylaxis and frequent galactomannan antigenemia testing could be a valid alternative. However, if one prefers to rely on the antifungal agent, posaconazole should be preferred to fluconazole when the patient is considered at risk. It is conceivable that other antifungals with activity against moulds (itraconazole and voriconazole, or any of the echinocandins) could we substituted. In fact, there are data suggesting voriconazole is effective to prevent invasive aspergillosis after transplant [146], and is better tolerated than itraconazole, which also is effective [147, 148], We have successfully used voriconazole prophylaxis in patients with cGVHD who were receiving corticosteroids (prednisone equivalent ≥1 mg/kg/d), but some of the patients have experienced severe phototoxicity that has complicated the management of their skin cGVHD. This is a well-described complication of long-term voriconazole treatment [149], which may be of particular importance in patients with severe skin cGVHD.

A possible alternative to universal antifungal prophylaxis being proposed by some experts is monitoring by using serological markers, namely galactomannan antigen or beta-D-glucan. These tests have been used successfully in "proof of principle" studies during neutropenia [92, 93]. In these studies, serial monitoring of the fungal antigens in the serum resulted in early detection of many cases of IFI as well as the appropriate withholding of empirical antifungal therapy. Although these strategies remain promising, their role (if any) during cGVHD remains to be determined.

Pneumocystis jiroveci *prophylaxis*

Pneumocystis jiroveci (PCP) is a significant concern in patients with cGVHD, typically associated with early discontinuation of prophylaxis or prophylaxis other than TMP/SMX [106–109]. This infection is easy to prevent by using TMP/SMX; several doses seem to provide protection and have not been compared in HCT recipients: 1 double-strength (800 mg/160 mg) tablet by mouth daily or 1 single-strength tablet by mouth daily or 1 double-strength tablet by mouth three times/week. The alternatives include dapsone, 50 mg by mouth two times/day or 100 mg by mouth daily or pentamidine, 300 mg every 3 to 4 weeks by Respirgard II™ nebulizer [130]. Atovaqone 1,500 mg PO daily has been used successfully in HIV-infected patients [150], but breakthrough cases in HCT have been reported. TMP/SMX is clearly the most effective agent and an attempt should be made to continue it rather than to change. In case of allergy, desensitization may be attempted. As an alternative, dapsone 100 mg daily can be substituted [151]. Lower doses are associated with high failure rates [108]. Inhaled pentamidine has the advantage of eliminating compliance issues, but has been associated with high failure rates and risk of other infections [152].

Antiviral Prophylaxis

CMV PROPHYLAXIS

Late CMV disease presents most commonly as pneumonia or gastrointestinal disease [74]. These two manifestations do not differ significantly from their presentation before day +100. An uncommon manifestation, apparently associated with cGVHD, is retinitis, which was diagnosed in nine allo-HCT recipients over 14 years at the FHCRC [153]. Eight of the nine patients had chronic extensive GVHD. Retinitis occurred between day 106 and 356 posttransplant, and presented with decreased or blurred vision or floaters, most commonly unilateral. Except for one patient who developed retinitis as a manifestation of primary CMV infection (he and his donor were CMV-negative), all had had CMV reactivation or disease before.

Risk factors for late CMV disease include early CMV antigenemia, lymphopenia, absolute CD4 count lower than 50 and GVHD [74]. CMV-specific immunodeficiency seems to be the underlying problem. Monitoring and management of late CMV infection present special challenges. The patients may not be in close proximity to the transplant center, and it is unclear for which patients monitoring should be continued and for how long. Continuation of weekly CMV antigenemia or PCR surveillance is advocated in patients with cGVHD who are CMV seropositive or have a seropositive donor and had CMV infection or disease before day 100. The level of CMV reactivation that should trigger intervention is poorly defined. If plasma PCR is used, the authors recommend a level of greater than 1,000 copies per mL [154]. When surveillance can be discontinued has not been formally studied. The authors stop surveillance when the steroid dose is less than 0.5 mg/kg prednisone per day and at least three negative tests have been documented. If the level of immunosuppression increases, surveillance should be resumed.

The recommended doses of antivirals for preemptive management are as follows: ganciclovir: 5 mg/kg q 12h for 1 week (induction) followed by 5 mg/kg daily 5 days/week for 2 weeks. Valganciclovir may be an alternative, based on the results of a randomized comparison of universal valganciclovir administration (900 mg PO daily) with preemptive treatment initiated for CMV DNA >1,000 copies/mL in patients at risk which showed both strategies to be similar regarding a composite endpoint CMV disease, bacterial or fungal infection or death [154]. Foscarnet (60 mg/kg q 12h for 1 week followed by 60 mg/kg/daily) seems to be as effective, with a different toxicity profile.

Prophylaxis of Varicella zoster virus and Herpes simplex virus

Varicella zoster virus (VZV) and Herpes simplex virus reactivation may be prevented by continuing acyclovir prophylaxis for at least 1 year, as demonstrated in a randomized controlled trial [119]. A retrospective analysis of different strategies of acyclovir administration after transplant suggests that prevention of VZV reactivation is associated with decreased mortality of all causes [155]. No "rebound" VZV was seen after discontinuation of acyclovir. The continued use of acyclovir 800 mg PO bid or valacyclovir 500 mg PO bid in patients requiring immunosuppression resulted in continued low rates of VZV reactivation, although compliance seemed to become an issue and occasional breakthroughs were seen during the second year [155]. Given that acyclovir and valcyclovir are known to be safe at these dosages, we think it is reasonable to continue them, at least as long as cGVHD patients remain on immunosuppression. Lower acyclovir dose regimens (e.g., 400 mg BID) have also been reported to effectively prevent VZV in uncontrolled trials [156] but whether these doses prevent HSV reactivation disease as well has not been studied.

Prophylaxis of Community-Acquired Respiratory Viruses with Antiviral Agents

Influenza may be prevented during outbreaks by the administration of neuraminidase inhibitors (oseltamivir 75 mg PO daily or zanamavir). These drugs have shown to be safe and effective in immunocompetent hosts, but the experience on immunocompromised patients (much less in patients with cGVHD) is limited, although favorable so far [134]. RSV is a common cause of severe upper respiratory tract infection in adults, and may progress to pneumonia particularly during the peri-engraftment period or in the presence of profound lymphopenia. Inhaled ribavirin has been used in allo-HCT recipients with RSV-associated upper respiratory infection to prevent the development of pneumonia [81].

INFECTIONS RELATED TO SPECIFIC IMMUNOSUPPRESSIVE TREATMENTS

As mentioned earlier, the initial series of patients with cGVHD reported mainly bacterial infections and VZV. A significant part of the risk associated with opportunistic infections seems related to immunosuppressive treatment of the disease. Of the many agents used, corticosteroids are probably the principal infectious risk factor. Increase in bacterial infections is well documented with corticosteroids at a dose of 20 mg of prednisone daily for more than a few weeks; the risk of aspergillosis

seems to increase significantly as soon as 2 weeks of 1 mg/kg of prednisone equivalent is administered, and viral infections are also known to be more common and or more severe in the presence of corticosteroids [157].

Calcineurin inhibitors are seldom given as the only immunosuppressive agents in any setting, and consequently the risk of infection they bring about is less well defined. They clearly increase the risk of PCP in the animal model of Pneumocystis, and experience for the solid organ transplant literature suggest they increase the risk of BK virus reactivation [158].

For chronic extensive GVHD refractory to corticosteroids and calcineurin inhibitors, a variety of approaches are used [159, 160], typically in combination, which complicates the attribution of risks. The associations that follow should be taken as a guide of what has been reported rather than as a "cause and effect" relationship [161].

Mycophenolate mofetil (MMF) is frequently added to the combination prednisone-calcineurin inhibitor [162]. There is some evidence from the solid organ transplant literature suggesting MMF-containing regimens result in more infections (particularly CMV reactivation or disease) than alternative regimens, including progressive multifocal leukoencephalopathy [163].

Rituximab, a monoclonal antibody against CD20 that targets all cells of the B lineage except plasma cells is increasingly used in cGVHD [164–166]. The well-established infectious complication associated with rituximab is hepatitis B reactivation. Multiple other associations including PCP and progressive multifocal leukoencephalopathy have been reported, but their significance is uncertain. It seems likely that the highest risk is for patients already severely immunocompromised [167]. A small fraction of patients who receive rituximab for the treatment of lymphoma develop late neutropenia, an even smaller percentage develop long-lasting hypogammaglobulinemia. In the largest experience of rituximab use in cGVHD reported to date, 4 of 38 patients experienced severe infections and three of them died [165]. Other published series do not show an unexpectedly high rate of infections.

Alemtuzumab, a humanized monoclonal antibody directed against CD52, results in prolonged, profound lymphocytopenia, and it also targets monocytes and NK cells. There are few reports of its use in refractory cGVHD [168]. Alemtuzumab has been associated with a variety of opportunistic and nonopportunistic severe infections, particularly when used in the treatment of malignancy [169]. In particular, CMV reactivation after alemtuzumab treatment seems to be extremely common in any setting [170, 171], and alemtuzumab use has been identified as a risk factor for late CMV reactivation after HCT [172]. In 15 patients with refractory acute GVHD, 11 experienced CMV reactivation after being treated with alemtuzumab [173].

Infliximab, an anti-tumor necrosis factor (TNF) monoclonal antibody, has been used, alone or in combination with daclizumab (a humanized monoclonal against the IL-2 receptor), mainly for acute steroid-refractory GVHD, but also in cases of cGVHD [174]. Fungal infections have clearly been a problem in some studies of anti-TNF agents for acute GVHD [175,

176], and prophylaxis against mould has been recommended by groups using this approach successfully [177]. Daclizumab alone has also been associated with unacceptably high number of infections when used in acute GVHD [178].

Pentostatin (2'-deoxycoformycin), a potent inhibitor of adenosine deaminase, is being actively evaluated for steroid-refractory cGVHD [179, 180]. Pentostatin is known to result in very prolonged CD4 lymphocytopenia (2–4 years when used in hairy cell leukemia) [181], and it has been associated to opportunistic infections like cryptococcosis, PCP, and listeriosis [182]. The experience in cGVHD has suggested that bacterial and fungal infections are also increased [183].

In summary, patients with steroid-refractory chronic GVHD who receive second-line agents are at even greater risk of infection. There may be true differences in the kind of infections (e.g., anti-TNF agents seem to predispose to IFIs whereas alemtuzumab seems to increase the risk of CMV) but not enough to recommend distinct prophylactic strategies. In general, a high degree of vigilance (including renewed CMV monitoring) should be established, and antifungal prophylaxis active against moulds should be considered, even if its benefit has not been convincingly demonstrated. Finally, as the duration of action of some monoclonal agents and pentostatin is quite long, it is reasonable to extend the duration of prophylaxis for several months, even if no active immunosuppression is continued. The use of CD4$^+$ T-cell count as a surrogate global measure of immune function has been advocated, but there is no evidence supporting any specific CD4 number or percentage to discontinue antiinfective prophylaxis in cGVHD.

SUMMARY

Chronic GVHD is a prime example of a disease characterized by a long, debilitating course intercalated with life-threatening emergencies, many of them infections. A multitude of risk factors combine to make these individuals extremely susceptible to infection. The use of immunizations of the patients and their surroundings as well as the judicious use of antiinfective prophylaxis may contribute to decrease the incidence of infections and increase their quality of life. However, not all episodes of infection are preventable. Prompt use of antimicrobial agents, guided by the ever increasing number of diagnostic procedures available will undoubtedly result in steady improvement in the outcome of established infections.

REFERENCES

1. Arora M, Burns LJ, Davies SM, et al. Chronic graft-versus-host disease: a prospective cohort study. Biol Blood Marrow Transplant. 2003;9:38–45.
2. Fraser CJ, Baker KS. The management and outcome of chronic graft-versus-host disease. British Journal of Haematology. 2007;138:131–145.
3. Vogelsang GB. How I treat chronic graft-versus-host disease. Blood. 2001;97:1196–1201.
4. Couriel D, Carpenter PA, Cutler C, et al. Ancillary therapy and supportive care of chronic graft-versus-host disease: national institutes of health consensus development project on criteria for clinical trials in chronic Graft-versus-host disease: V. Ancillary Therapy and Supportive Care Working Group Report. Biol Blood Marrow Transplant. 2006;12:375–396.
5. Atkinson K, Storb R, Prentice RL, et al. Analysis of late infections in 89 long-term survivors of bone marrow transplantation. Blood. 1979;53:720–731.
6. Graze PR, Gale RP. Chronic graft versus host disease: a syndrome of disordered immunity. Am J Med. 1979;66:611–620.
7. Shulman HM, Sale GE, Lerner KG, et al. Chronic cutaneous graft-versus-host disease in man. Am J Pathol. 1978;91:545–570.
8. Shulman HM, Sullivan KM, Weiden PL, et al. Chronic graft-versus-host syndrome in man. A long-term clinicopathologic study of 20 Seattle patients. Am J Med. 1980;69:204–217.
9. Sullivan KM, Shulman HM, Storb R, et al. Chronic graft-versus-host disease in 52 patients: adverse natural course and successful treatment with combination immunosuppression. Blood. 1981;57:267–276.
10. Pavletic SZ, Carter SL, Kernan NA, et al. Influence of T-cell depletion on chronic graft-versus-host disease: results of a multicenter randomized trial in unrelated marrow donor transplantation. Blood. 2005;106:3308–3313.
11. Atkinson K, Incefy GS, Storb R, et al. Low serum thymic hormone levels in patients with chronic graft-versus-host disease. Blood. 1982;59:1073–1077.
12. Matsutani T, Yoshioka T, Tsuruta Y, et al. Restricted usage of T-cell receptor alpha-chain variable region (TCRAV) and T-cell receptor beta-chain variable region (TCRBV) repertoires after human allogeneic haematopoietic transplantation. Br J Haematol. 2000;109:759–769.
13. Storek J, Gooley T, Witherspoon RP, Sullivan KM, Storb R. Infectious morbidity in long-term survivors of allogeneic marrow transplantation is associated with low CD4 T cell counts. Am J Hematol. 1997;54:131–138.
14. Zorn E, Kim HT, Lee SJ, et al. Reduced frequency of FOXP3+ CD4+CD25+ regulatory T cells in patients with chronic graft-versus-host disease. Blood. 2005;106:2903–2911.
15. Storek J, Witherspoon RP, Webb D, Storb R. Lack of B cells precursors in marrow transplant recipients with chronic graft-versus-host disease. Am J Hematol. 1996;52:82–89.
16. Greinix HT, Pohlreich D, Kouba M, et al. Elevated numbers of immature/transitional CD21- B lymphocytes and deficiency of memory CD27+ B cells identify patients with active chronic graft-versus-host disease. Biol Blood Marrow Transplant. 2008;14:208–219.
17. Cuthbert RJ, Iqbal A, Gates A, Toghill PJ, Russell NH. Functional hyposplenism following allogeneic bone marrow transplantation. J Clin Pathol. 1995;48:257–259.
18. Dahut W, Georgiadis M. Pneumococcal arthritis and functional asplenia after allogeneic bone marrow transplantation. Bone Marrow Transplant. 1995;15:161.
19. Kalhs P, Panzer S, Kletter K, et al. Functional asplenia after bone marrow transplantation. A late complication related to extensive chronic graft-versus-host disease. Ann Intern Med. 1988;109:461–464.
20. Abrahamsen IW, Somme S, Heldal D, Egeland T, Kvale D, Tjonnfjord GE. Immune reconstitution after allogeneic stem cell

transplantation: the impact of stem cell source and graft-versus-host disease. Haematologica. 2005;90:86–93.

21. Hazenberg MD, Otto SA, de Pauw ES, et al. T-cell receptor excision circle and T-cell dynamics after allogeneic stem cell transplantation are related to clinical events. Blood. 2002;99:3449–3453.

22. Poulin JF, Sylvestre M, Champagne P, et al. Evidence for adequate thymic function but impaired naive T-cell survival following allogeneic hematopoietic stem cell transplantation in the absence of chronic graft-versus-host disease. Blood. 2003;102:4600–4607.

23. Yamasaki S, Heike Y, Mori S, et al. Infectious complications in chronic graft-versus-host disease: a retrospective study of 145 recipients of allogeneic hematopoietic stem cell transplantation with reduced- and conventional-intensity conditioning regimens. *Transpl Infect Dis*. 2008;10:252–259.

24. Atkinson K, Farewell V, Storb R, et al. Analysis of late infections after human bone marrow transplantation: role of genotypic nonidentity between marrow donor and recipient and of non-specific suppressor cells in patients with chronic graft-versus-host disease. Blood. 1982;60:714–720.

25. Sullivan KM, Mori M, Sanders J, et al. Late complications of allogeneic and autologous marrow transplantation. Bone Marrow Transplant. 1992;10 (Suppl 1):127–134.

26. Ochs L, Shu XO, Miller J, et al. Late infections after allogeneic bone marrow transplantations: comparison of incidence in related and unrelated donor transplant recipients. Blood. 1995;86:3979–3986.

27. Romano V, Castagnola E, Dallorso S, et al. Bloodstream infections can develop late (after day 100) and/or in the absence of neutropenia in children receiving allogeneic bone marrow transplantation. Bone Marrow Transplant. 1999;23:271–275.

28. Socie G, Stone JV, Wingard JR, et al. Long-term survival and late deaths after allogeneic bone marrow transplantation. Late Effects Working Committee of the International Bone Marrow Transplant Registry. N Engl J Med. 1999;341:14–21.

29. Weinthal JA, Goldman SC, Rosenfeld CS, Hooker M, Henderson D, Lenarsky C. Early and late infectious complications following unrelated cord blood transplantation (UCBT). Blood. 2001;98:362B-363B.

30. Bjorklund A, Aschan J, Labopin M, et al. Risk factors for fatal infectious complications developing late after allogeneic stem cell transplantation. Bone Marrow Transplant. 2007;40:1055–1062.

31. Robin M, Porcher R, De Castro Araujo R, et al. Risk factors for late infections after allogeneic hematopoietic stem cell transplantation from a matched related donor. Biol Blood Marrow Transplant. 2007;13:1304–1312.

32. Safdar A, Rodriguez GH, De Lima MJ, et al. Infections in 100 cord blood transplantations – Spectrum of early and late post-transplant infections in adult and pediatric patients 1996–2005. Medicine. 2007;86:324–333.

33. Worthy SA, Flint JD, Muller NL. Pulmonary complications after bone marrow transplantation: high-resolution CT and pathologic findings. Radiographics. 1997;17:1359–1371.

34. Kulkarni S, Powles R, Treleaven J, et al. Chronic graft versus host disease is associated with long-term risk for pneumococcal infections in recipients of bone marrow transplants. Blood. 2000;95:3683–3686.

35. Elias M, Bisharat N, Goldstein LH, Raz R, Saliba W. Pneumococcal sepsis due to functional hyposplenism in a bone marrow transplant patient. Eur J Clin Microbiol Infect Dis. 2004;23:212–214.

36. Picardi M, Selleri C, Rotoli B. Spleen sizing by ultrasound scan and risk of pneumococcal infection in patients with chronic GVHD: preliminary observations. Bone Marrow Transplant. 1999;24:173–177.

37. Cunha BA. Infections in nonleukopenic compromised hosts (diabetes mellitus, SLE, steroids, and asplenia) in critical care. Crit Care Clin. 1998;14:263–282.

38. Rivero GA, Torres HA, Rolston KV, Kontoyiannis DP. Listeria monocytogenes infection in patients with cancer. Diagn Microbiol Infect Dis. 2003;47:393–398.

39. Bowden RA. Respiratory virus infections after marrow transplant: the Fred Hutchinson Cancer Research Center experience. Am J Med. 1997;102:27–30; discussion 42–3

40. Nichols WG, Corey L, Gooley T, Davis C, Boeckh M. Parainfluenza virus infections after hematopoietic stem cell transplantation: risk factors, response to antiviral therapy, and effect on transplant outcome. Blood. 2001;98:573–578.

41. Chen CS, Boeckh M, Seidel K, et al. Incidence, risk factors, and mortality from pneumonia developing late after hematopoietic stem cell transplantation. Bone Marrow Transplant. 2003;32:515–522.

42. Duncker C, Dohr D, Harsdorf S, et al. Non-infectious lung complications are closely associated with chronic graft-versus-host disease: a single center study of incidence, risk factors and outcome. Bone Marrow Transplant. 2000;25:1263–1268.

43. Sakaida E, Nakaseko C, Harima A, et al. Late-onset noninfectious pulmonary complications after allogeneic stem cell transplantation are significantly associated with chronic graft-versus-host disease and with the graft-versus-leukemia effect. Blood. 2003;102:4236–4242.

44. Palmas A, Tefferi A, Myers JL, et al. Late-onset noninfectious pulmonary complications after allogeneic bone marrow transplantation. Br J Haematol. 1998;100:680–687.

45. Patriarca F, Skert C, Sperotto A, et al. Incidence, outcome, and risk factors of late-onset noninfectious pulmonary complications after unrelated donor stem cell transplantation. Bone Marrow Transplant. 2004;33:751–758.

46. Ohnishi K, Sakai F, Kudoh S, Ohno R. Twenty-seven cases of drug-induced interstitial lung disease associated with imatinib mesylate. Leukemia. 2006;20:1162–1164.

47. Radaelli F, Bramanti S, Fantini NN, Fabio G, Greco I, Lambertenghi-Deliliers G. Dasatinib-related alveolar pneumonia responsive to corticosteroids. Leuk Lymphoma. 2006;47: 1180–1181.

48. Pham PT, Pham PC, Danovitch GM, et al. Sirolimus-associated pulmonary toxicity. Transplantation. 2004;77:1215–1220.

49. Mandell LA, Wunderink RG, Anzueto A, et al. Infectious Diseases Society of America/American Thoracic Society consensus guidelines on the management of community-acquired pneumonia in adults. Clin Infect Dis. 2007;44 (Suppl 2):S27-S72.

50. Jain P, Sandur S, Meli Y, Arroliga AC, Stoller JK, Mehta AC. Role of flexible bronchoscopy in immunocompromised patients with lung infiltrates. Chest. 2004;125:712–722.

51. Musher B, Fredricks D, Leisenring W, Balajee SA, Smith C, Marr KA. Aspergillus galactomannan enzyme immunoassay and quantitative PCR for diagnosis of invasive aspergillosis with bronchoalveolar lavage fluid. J Clin Microbiol. 2004;42:5517–5522.

52. Meersseman W, Lagrou K, Maertens J, et al. Galactomannan in bronchoalveolar lavage fluid: a tool for diagnosing aspergillosis in intensive care unit patients. Am J Respir Crit Care Med. 2008;177:27–34.

53. Nguyen MH, Jaber R, Leather HL, et al. Use of bronchoalveolar lavage to detect galactomannan for diagnosis of pulmonary aspergillosis among nonimmunocompromised hosts. J Clin Microbiol. 2007;45:2787–2792.

54. Hohenthal U, Itala M, Salonen J, et al. Bronchoalveolar lavage in immunocompromised patients with haematological malignancy–value of new microbiological methods. Eur J Haematol. 2005;74:203–211.

55. Vail GM, Young RS, Wheat LJ, Filo RS, Cornetta K, Goldman M. Incidence of histoplasmosis following allogeneic bone marrow transplant or solid organ transplant in a hyperendemic area. Transpl Infect Dis. 2002;4:148–151.

56. Hofmeister CC, Czerlanis C, Forsythe S, Stiff PJ. Retrospective utility of bronchoscopy after hematopoietic stem cell transplant. Bone Marrow Transplant. 2006;38:693–698.

57. Clark BD, Vezza PR, Copeland C, Wilder AM, Abati A. Diagnostic sensitivity of bronchoalveolar lavage versus lung fine needle aspirate. Mod Pathol. 2002;15:1259–1265.

58. Lossos IS, Breuer R, Or R, et al. Bacterial pneumonia in recipients of bone marrow transplantation. A five-year prospective study. Transplantation. 1995;60:672–678.

59. van Burik JA, Hackman RC, Nadeem SQ, et al. Nocardiosis after bone marrow transplantation: a retrospective study. Clin Infect Dis. 1997;24:1154–1160.

60. Daly AS, McGeer A, Lipton JH. Systemic nocardiosis following allogeneic bone marrow transplantation. Transpl Infect Dis. 2003;5:16–20.

61. Bhave AA, Thirunavukkarasu K, Gottlieb DJ, Bradstock K. Disseminated nocardiosis in a bone marrow transplant recipient with chronic GVHD. Bone Marrow Transplant. 1999;23:519–521.

62. Machado CM, Macedo MC, Castelli JB, et al. Clinical features and successful recovery from disseminated nocardiosis after BMT. Bone Marrow Transplant. 1997;19:81–82.

63. Brown-Elliott BA, Brown JM, Conville PS, Wallace RJ, Jr. Clinical and laboratory features of the Nocardia spp. based on current molecular taxonomy. Clin Microbiol Rev. 2006;19:259–282.

64. Moylett EH, Pacheco SE, Brown-Elliott BA, et al. Clinical experience with linezolid for the treatment of nocardia infection. Clin Infect Dis. 2003;36:313–318.

65. Yuen KY, Woo PC. Tuberculosis in blood and marrow transplant recipients. Hematol Oncol. 2002;20:51–62.

66. Ip MS, Yuen KY, Woo PC, et al. Risk factors for pulmonary tuberculosis in bone marrow transplant recipients. Am J Respir Crit Care Med. 1998;158:1173–1177.

67. Martino R, Martinez C, Brunet S, Sureda A, Lopez R, Domingo-Albos A. Tuberculosis in bone marrow transplant recipients: report of two cases and review of the literature. Bone Marrow Transplant. 1996;18:809–812.

68. Cordonnier C, Martino R, Trabasso P, et al. Mycobacterial infection: a difficult and late diagnosis in stem cell transplant recipients. Clin Infect Dis. 2004;38:1229–1236.

69. de la Camara R, Martino R, Granados E, et al. Tuberculosis after hematopoietic stem cell transplantation: incidence, clinical characteristics and outcome. Spanish Group on Infectious Complications in Hematopoietic Transplantation. Bone Marrow Transplant. 2000;26:291–298.

70. Rouleau M, Senik A, Leroy E, Vernant JP. Long-term persistence of transferred PPD-reactive T cells after allogeneic bone marrow transplantation. Transplantation. 1993;55:72–76.

71. Conde MB, Soares SL, Mello FC, et al. Comparison of sputum induction with fiberoptic bronchoscopy in the diagnosis of tuberculosis: experience at an acquired immune deficiency syndrome reference center in Rio de Janeiro, Brazil. Am J Respir Crit Care Med. 2000;162:2238–2240.

72. Griffith DE, Aksamit T, Brown-Elliott BA, et al. An official ATS/IDSA statement: diagnosis, treatment, and prevention of nontuberculous mycobacterial diseases. Am J Respir Crit Care Med. 2007;175:367–416.

73. Meyers JD, Flournoy N, Thomas ED. Nonbacterial pneumonia after allogeneic marrow transplantation: a review of ten years' experience. Rev Infect Dis. 1982;4:1119–1132.

74. Boeckh M, Leisenring W, Riddell SR, et al. Late cytomegalovirus disease and mortality in recipients of allogeneic hematopoietic stem cell transplants: importance of viral load and T-cell immunity. Blood. 2003;101:407–414.

75. Nguyen Q, Champlin R, Giralt S, et al. Late cytomegalovirus pneumonia in adult allogeneic blood and marrow transplant recipients. Clin Infect Dis. 1999;28:618–623.

76. Boeckh M, Nichols WG, Papanicolaou G, Rubin R, Wingard JR, Zaia J. Cytomegalovirus in hematopoietic stem cell transplant recipients: Current status, known challenges, and future strategies. Biol Blood Marrow Transplant. 2003;9:543–558.

77. Machado CM, Dulley FL, Boas LS, et al. CMV pneumonia in allogeneic BMT recipients undergoing early treatment of pre-emptive ganciclovir therapy. Bone Marrow Transplant. 2000;26:413–417.

78. Kim YJ, Boeckh M, Englund JA. Community respiratory virus infections in immunocompromised patients: hematopoietic stem cell and solid organ transplant recipients, and individuals with human immunodeficiency virus infection. Semin Respir Crit Care Med. 2007;28:222–242.

79. Erard V, Chien JW, Kim HW, et al. Airflow decline after myeloablative allogeneic hematopoietic cell transplantation: the role of community respiratory viruses. J Infect Dis. 2006;193:1619–1625.

80. Khushalani NI, Bakri FG, Wentling D, et al. Respiratory syncytial virus infection in the late bone marrow transplant period: report of three cases and review. Bone Marrow Transplant. 2001;27:1071–1073.

81. Boeckh M, Englund J, Li Y, et al. Randomized controlled multicenter trial of aerosolized ribavirin for respiratory syncytial virus upper respiratory tract infection in hematopoietic cell transplant recipients. Clin Infect Dis. 2007;44:245–249.

82. Nichols WG, Gooley T, Boeckh M. Community-acquired respiratory syncytial virus and parainfluenza virus infections after hematopoietic stem cell transplantation: the Fred Hutchinson Cancer Research Center experience. Biol Blood Marrow Transplant. 2001;7 Suppl 1:11S–15S.

83. Machado CM. Influenza infections after hematopoietic stem cell transplantation. Clin Infect Dis. 2005;41:273–274.

84. Nichols WG, Guthrie KA, Corey L, Boeckh M. Influenza infections after hematopoietic stem cell transplantation: risk factors, mortality, and the effect of antiviral therapy. Clin Infect Dis. 2004;39:1300–1306.

85. Fukuda T, Boeckh M, Carter RA, et al. Risks and outcomes of invasive fungal infections in recipients of allogeneic hematopoietic stem cell transplants after nonmyeloablative conditioning. Blood. 2003;102:827–833.

86. Walsh TJ, Anaissie EJ, Denning DW, et al. Treatment of aspergillosis: clinical practice guidelines of the Infectious Diseases Society of America. Clin Infect Dis. 2008;46:327–360.

87. Escuissato DL, Gasparetto EL, Marchiori E, et al. Pulmonary infections after bone marrow transplantation: high-resolution

CT findings in 111 patients. AJR Am J Roentgenol. 2005; 185:608–615.

88. Gasparetto TD, Escuissato DL, Marchiori E. Pulmonary infections following bone marrow transplantation: High-resolution CT findings in 35 paediatric patients. Eur J Radiol. 2008;66:117–121.

89. Kojima R, Tateishi U, Kami M, et al. Chest computed tomography of late invasive aspergillosis after allogeneic hematopoietic stem cell transplantation. Biol Blood Marrow Transplant. 2005;11:506–511.

90. Kontoyiannis DP, Wessel VC, Bodey GP, Rolston KV. Zygomycosis in the 1990s in a tertiary-care cancer center. Clin Infect Dis. 2000;30:851–856.

91. Becker MJ, Lugtenburg EJ, Cornelissen JJ, Van Der Schee C, Hoogsteden HC, De Marie S. Galactomannan detection in computerized tomography-based broncho-alveolar lavage fluid and serum in haematological patients at risk for invasive pulmonary aspergillosis. Br J Haematol. 2003;121:448–457.

92. Maertens J, Theunissen K, Verhoef G, et al. Galactomannan and computed tomography-based preemptive antifungal therapy in neutropenic patients at high risk for invasive fungal infection: a prospective feasibility study. Clin Infect Dis. 2005;41:1242–1250.

93. Senn L, Robinson JO, Schmidt S, et al. 1,3-Beta-D-glucan antigenemia for early diagnosis of invasive fungal infections in neutropenic patients with acute leukemia. Clin Infect Dis. 2008;46:878–885.

94. Foy PC, van Burik JA, Weisdorf DJ. Galactomannan antigen enzyme-linked immunosorbent assay for diagnosis of invasive aspergillosis after hematopoietic stem cell transplantation. Biol Blood Marrow Transplant. 2007;13:440–443.

95. Marr KA, Balajee SA, McLaughlin L, Tabouret M, Bentsen C, Walsh TJ. Detection of galactomannan antigenemia by enzyme immunoassay for the diagnosis of invasive aspergillosis: variables that affect performance. J Infect Dis. 2004;190:641–649.

96. Herbrecht R, Denning DW, Patterson TF, et al. Voriconazole versus amphotericin B for primary therapy of invasive aspergillosis. N Engl J Med. 2002;347:408–415.

97. Marr KA, Boeckh M, Carter RA, Kim HW, Corey L. Combination antifungal therapy for invasive aspergillosis. Clin Infect Dis. 2004;39:797–802. Epub 2004 Aug 27.

98. Trifilio SM, Bennett CL, Yarnold PR, et al. Breakthrough zygomycosis after voriconazole administration among patients with hematologic malignancies who receive hematopoietic stem-cell transplants or intensive chemotherapy. Bone Marrow Transplant. 2007;39:425–429.

99. Upton A, Kirby KA, Carpenter P, Boeckh M, Marr KA. Invasive aspergillosis following hematopoietic cell transplantation: outcomes and prognostic factors associated with mortality. Clin Infect Dis. 2007;44:531–540.

100. Varkey JB, Perfect JR. Rare and emerging fungal pulmonary infections. Semin Respir Crit Care Med. 2008;29:121–131.

101. Walsh TJ, Groll A, Hiemenz J, Fleming R, Roilides E, Anaissie E. Infections due to emerging and uncommon medically important fungal pathogens. Clin Microbiol Infect. 2004;10 (Suppl 1):48–66.

102. Marty FM, Lowry CM, Cutler CS, et al. Voriconazole and sirolimus coadministration after allogeneic hematopoietic stem cell transplantation. Biol Blood Marrow Transplant. 2006;12:552–559.

103. Zonios DI, Bennett JE. Update on azole antifungals. Semin Respir Crit Care Med. 2008;29:198–210.

104. Trifilio S, Pennick G, Pi J, et al. Monitoring plasma voriconazole levels may be necessary to avoid subtherapeutic levels in hematopoietic stem cell transplant recipients. Cancer. 2007;109:1532–1535.

105. Mulanovich V, Lewis RE, Raad, II, Kontoyiannis DP. Random plasma concentrations of voriconazole decline over time. J Infect. 2007;55:e129-e130.

106. Lyytikainen O, Ruutu T, Volin L, et al. Late onset Pneumocystis carinii pneumonia following allogeneic bone marrow transplantation. Bone Marrow Transplant. 1996;17:1057–1059.

107. De Castro N, Neuville S, Sarfati C, et al. Occurrence of Pneumocystis jiroveci pneumonia after allogeneic stem cell transplantation: a 6-year retrospective study. Bone Marrow Transplant. 2005;36:879–883.

108. Souza JP, Boeckh M, Gooley TA, Flowers ME, Crawford SW. High rates of Pneumocystis carinii pneumonia in allogeneic blood and marrow transplant recipients receiving dapsone prophylaxis. Clin Infect Dis. 1999;29:1467–1471.

109. Torres HA, Chemaly RF, Storey R, et al. Influence of type of cancer and hematopoietic stem cell transplantation on clinical presentation of Pneumocystis jiroveci pneumonia in cancer patients. Eur J Clin Microbiol Infect Dis. Jun 2006;25(6):382–388.

110. Gal AA, Plummer AL, Langston AA, Mansour KA. Granulomatous Pneumocystis carinii pneumonia complicating hematopoietic cell transplantation. Pathol Res Pract. 2002;198:553–558; discussion 559–61

111. Benson CA, Kaplan JE, Masur H, Pau A, Holmes KK. Treating opportunistic infections among HIV-infected adults and adolescents: recommendations from CDC, the National Institutes of Health, and the HIV Medicine Association/ Infectious Diseases Society of America. MMWR Recomm Rep. 2004;53:1–112.

112. Ortiz E, Sakano E, De Souza CA, Vigorito A, Eid KA. Chronic GVHD: predictive factor for rhinosinusitis in bone marrow transplantation. Rev Bras Otorrinolaringol (Engl Ed). 2006;72:328–332.

113. Savage DG, Taylor P, Blackwell J, et al. Paranasal sinusitis following allogeneic bone marrow transplant. Bone Marrow Transplant. 1997;19:55–59.

114. Imamura R, Voegels R, Sperandio F, et al. Microbiology of sinusitis in patients undergoing bone marrow transplantation. Otolaryngol Head Neck Surg. 1999;120:279–282.

115. Machado CM, Martins MA, Heins-Vaccari EM, et al. Scedosporium apiospermum sinusitis after bone marrow transplantation: report of a case. Rev Inst Med Trop Sao Paulo. 1998;40:321–323.

116. Togitani K, Kobayashi M, Sakai M, et al. Ethmoidal sinusitis caused by Exserohilum rostratum in a patient with malignant lymphoma after non-myeloablative allogeneic peripheral blood stem cell transplantation. Transpl Infect Dis. 2007;9:137–141.

117. Ralph DD, Springmeyer SC, Sullivan KM, Hackman RC, Storb R, Thomas ED. Rapidly progressive air-flow obstruction in marrow transplant recipients. Possible association between obliterative bronchiolitis and chronic graft-versus-host disease. Am Rev Respir Dis. 1984;129:641–644.

118. Locksley RM, Flournoy N, Sullivan KM, Meyers JD. Infection with varicella-zoster virus after marrow transplantation. J Infect Dis. 1985;152:1172–1181.

119. Boeckh M, Kim HW, Flowers ME, Meyers JD, Bowden RA. Long-term acyclovir for prevention of varicella zoster virus disease after allogeneic hematopoietic cell transplantation–a

randomized double-blind placebo-controlled study. Blood. 2006;107:1800–1805.

120. Rogers SY, Irving W, Harris A, Russell NH. Visceral varicella zoster infection after bone marrow transplantation without skin involvement and the use of PCR for diagnosis. Bone Marrow Transplant. 1995;15:805–7

121. de Jong MD, Weel JF, van Oers MH, Boom R, Wertheim-van Dillen PM. Molecular diagnosis of visceral herpes zoster. Lancet. 2001;357:2101–2102.

122. Wolf JE, Liu HH, Rabinowitz LG. Ecthyma gangrenosum in the absence of Pseudomonas bacteremia in a bone marrow transplant recipient. Am J Med. 1989;87:595–597.

123. Radu B, Allez M, Gornet JM, et al. Chronic diarrhoea after allogenic bone marrow transplantation. Gut. 2005;54:161, 174.

124. Schulenburg A, Turetschek K, Wrba F, et al. Early and late gastrointestinal complications after myeloablative and nonmyeloablative allogeneic stem cell transplantation. Ann Hematol. 2004;83:101–106.

125. van Burik JA, Lawatsch EJ, DeFor TE, Weisdorf DJ. Cytomegalovirus enteritis among hematopoietic stem cell transplant recipients. Biol Blood Marrow Transplant. 2001;7: 674–679.

126. Haddad PA, Repka TL, Weisdorf DJ. Penicillin-resistant Streptococcus pneumoniae septic shock and meningitis complicating chronic graft versus host disease: a case report and review of the literature. Am J Med. 2002;113:152–155.

127. Safdar A, Papadopoulous EB, Armstrong D. Listeriosis in recipients of allogeneic blood and marrow transplantation: thirteen year review of disease characteristics, treatment outcomes and a new association with human cytomegalovirus infection. Bone Marrow Transplant. 2002;29:913–916.

128. Seeley WW, Marty FM, Holmes TM, et al. Post-transplant acute limbic encephalitis: clinical features and relationship to HHV6. Neurology. 2007;69:156–165.

129. Zerr DM, Corey L, Kim HW, Huang ML, Nguy L, Boeckh M. Clinical outcomes of human herpesvirus 6 reactivation after hematopoietic stem cell transplantation. Clin Infect Dis. 2005;40:932–940.

130. Guidelines for preventing opportunistic infections among hematopoietic stem cell transplant recipients. MMWR Recomm Rep. 2000;49:1–125, CE1–7.

131. Ljungman P, Engelhard D, de la Camara R, et al. Vaccination of stem cell transplant recipients: recommendations of the Infectious Diseases Working Party of the EBMT. Bone Marrow Transplant. 2005;35:737–746.

132. Ljungman P, Duraj V, Magnius L. Response to immunization against polio after allogeneic marrow transplantation. Bone Marrow Transplant. 1991;7:89–93.

133. Hammarstrom V, Pauksen K, Azinge J, Oberg G, Ljungman P. Pneumococcal immunity and response to immunization with pneumococcal vaccine in bone marrow transplant patients: the influence of graft versus host reaction. Support Care Cancer. 1993;1:195–199.

134. Machado CM, Boas LS, Mendes AV, et al. Use of Oseltamivir to control influenza complications after bone marrow transplantation. Bone Marrow Transplant. 2004;34:111–114.

135. Cordonnier C, Chevret S, Legrand M, et al. Should immunoglobulin therapy be used in allogeneic stem-cell transplantation? A randomized, double-blind, dose effect, placebo-controlled, multicenter trial. Ann Intern Med. 2003; 139:8–18.

136. Engelhard D, Cordonnier C, Shaw PJ, et al. Early and late invasive pneumococcal infection following stem cell transplantation: a European Bone Marrow Transplantation survey. Br J Haematol. 2002;117:444–450.

137. Youssef S, Rodriguez G, Rolston KV, Champlin RE, Raad, II, Safdar A. Streptococcus pneumoniae infections in 47 hematopoietic stem cell transplantation recipients: clinical characteristics of infections and vaccine-breakthrough infections, 1989–2005. Medicine (Baltimore). 2007;86:69–77.

138. Gaston MH, Verter JI, Woods G, et al. Prophylaxis with oral penicillin in children with sickle cell anemia. A randomized trial. N Engl J Med. 1986;314:1593–1599.

139. Jenkins SG, Brown SD, Farrell DJ. Trends in antibacterial resistance among Streptococcus pneumoniae isolated in the USA: update from PROTEKT US Years 1–4. Ann Clin Microbiol Antimicrob. 2008;7:1.

140. Hughes WT, Dankner WM, Yogev R, et al. Comparison of atovaquone and azithromycin with trimethoprim-sulfamethoxazole for the prevention of serious bacterial infections in children with HIV infection. Clin Infect Dis. 2005;40:136–145.

141. Seger RA. Modern management of chronic granulomatous disease. Br J Haematol. 2008;140:255–266.

142. Jantunen E, Ruutu P, Niskanen L, et al. Incidence and risk factors for invasive fungal infections in allogeneic BMT recipients. Bone Marrow Transplant. 1997;19:801–808.

143. Marr KA, Carter RA, Boeckh M, Martin P, Corey L. Invasive aspergillosis in allogeneic stem cell transplant recipients: changes in epidemiology and risk factors. Blood. 2002;100: 4358–4366.

144. Grow WB, Moreb JS, Roque D, et al. Late onset of invasive aspergillus infection in bone marrow transplant patients at a university hospital. Bone Marrow Transplant. 2002;29:15–19.

145. Ullmann AJ, Lipton JH, Vesole DH, et al. Posaconazole or fluconazole for prophylaxis in severe graft-versus-host disease. N Engl J Med. 2007;356:335–347.

146. Wingard JR, Carter SL, Walsh TJ, et al. Results of a Randomized, Double-Blind Trial of Fluconazole (FLU) vs. Voriconazole (VORI) for the Prevention of Invasive Fungal Infections (IFI) in 600 Allogeneic Blood and Marrow Transplant (BMT) Patients. ASH Annual Meeting Abstracts. 2007;110:163

147. Winston DJ, Maziarz RT, Chandrasekar PH, et al. Intravenous and oral itraconazole versus intravenous and oral fluconazole for long-term antifungal prophylaxis in allogeneic hematopoietic stem-cell transplant recipients. A multicenter, randomized trial. Ann Intern Med. 2003;138:705–713.

148. Marr KA, Crippa F, Leisenring W, et al. Itraconazole versus fluconazole for prevention of fungal infections in patients receiving allogeneic stem cell transplants. Blood. 2004;103:1527–1533.

149. Vandecasteele SJ, Van Wijngaerden E, Peetermans WE. Two cases of severe phototoxic reactions related to long-term outpatient treatment with voriconazole. Eur J Clin Microbiol Infect Dis. 2004;23:656–657.

150. Kaplan JE, Masur H, Holmes KK. Guidelines for preventing opportunistic infections among HIV-infected persons–2002. Recommendations of the U.S. Public Health Service and the Infectious Diseases Society of America. MMWR Recomm Rep. 2002;51:1–52.

151. Sangiolo D, Storer B, Nash R, et al. Toxicity and efficacy of daily dapsone as Pneumocystis jiroveci prophylaxis after hematopoietic stem cell transplantation: a case-control study. Biol Blood Marrow Transplant. 2005;11:521–529.

152. Vasconcelles MJ, Bernardo MV, King C, Weller EA, Antin JH. Aerosolized pentamidine as pneumocystis prophylaxis after bone marrow transplantation is inferior to other regimens and is associated with decreased survival and an increased risk of other infections. Biol Blood Marrow Transplant. 2000;6:35–43.

153. Crippa F, Corey L, Chuang EL, Sale G, Boeckh M. Virological, clinical, and ophthalmologic features of cytomegalovirus retinitis after hematopoietic stem cell transplantation. Clin Infect Dis. 2001;32:214–219.

154. Boeckh M, Nichols G, Chemaly R, et al. Prevention of Late CMV Disease after HCT: A Randomized Double-Blind Multicenter Trial of Valganciclovir (VGCV) Prophylaxis Versus PCR-Guided GCV/VGCV Preemptive Therapy. BMT Tandem Meetings. San Diego: ASBMT, CIBMTR, 2008.

155. Erard V, Guthrie KA, Varley C, et al. One-year acyclovir prophylaxis for preventing varicella-zoster virus disease after hematopoietic cell transplantation: no evidence of rebound varicella-zoster virus disease after drug discontinuation. Blood. 2007;110:3071–3077.

156. Thomson KJ, Hart DP, Banerjee L, Ward KN, Peggs KS, Mackinnon S. The effect of low-dose aciclovir on reactivation of varicella zoster virus after allogeneic haemopoietic stem cell transplantation. Bone Marrow Transplant. 2005;35:1065–1069.

157. Klein NC, Go CH, Cunha BA. Infections associated with steroid use. Infect Dis Clin North Am 2001;15:423–432, viii.

158. Singh N. Infectious complications in organ transplant recipients with the use of calcineurin-inhibitor agent-based immunosuppressive regimens. Curr Opin Infect Dis. 2005;18:342–345.

159. Jacobsohn DA. Emerging therapies for graft-versus-host disease. Expert Opin Emerg Drugs. 2003;8:323–338.

160. Lee SJ, Vogelsang G, Flowers ME. Chronic graft-versus-host disease. Biol Blood Marrow Transplant. 2003;9:215–233.

161. Koo S, Baden LR. Infectious complications associated with immunomodulating monoclonal antibodies used in the treatment of hematologic malignancy. J Natl Compr Canc Netw. 2008;6:202–213.

162. Mookerjee B, Altomonte V, Vogelsang G. Salvage therapy for refractory chronic graft-versus-host disease with mycophenolate mofetil and tacrolimus. Bone Marrow Transplant. 1999;24:517–520.

163. Bernabeu-Wittel M, Naranjo M, Cisneros JM, et al. Infections in renal transplant recipients receiving mycophenolate versus azathioprine-based immunosuppression. Eur J Clin Microbiol Infect Dis. 2002;21:173–180.

164. Cutler C, Miklos D, Kim HT, et al. Rituximab for steroid-refractory chronic graft-versus-host disease. Blood. 2006;108:756–762.

165. Zaja F, Bacigalupo A, Patriarca F, et al. Treatment of refractory chronic GVHD with rituximab: a GITMO study. Bone Marrow Transplant. 2007;40:273–277.

166. Mohty M, Marchetti N, El-Cheikh J, Faucher C, Furst S, Blaise D. Rituximab as salvage therapy for refractory chronic GVHD. Bone Marrow Transplant. 2008;41:909–911.

167. Venhuizen AC, Hustinx WN, van Houte AJ, Veth G, van der Griend R. Three cases of Pneumocystis jirovecii pneumonia (PCP) during first-line treatment with rituximab in combination with CHOP-14 for aggressive B-cell non-Hodgkin's lymphoma. Eur J Haematol. 2008;80:275–276.

168. Ruiz-Arguelles GJ, Gil-Beristain J, Magana M, Ruiz-Delgado GJ. Alemtuzumab-induced resolution of refractory cutaneous chronic graft-versus-host disease. Biol Blood Marrow Transplant. 2008;14:7–9.

169. Martin SI, Marty FM, Fiumara K, Treon SP, Gribben JG, Baden LR. Infectious complications associated with alemtuzumab use for lymphoproliferative disorders. Clin Infect Dis. 2006;43:16–24.

170. Scheinberg P, Fischer SH, Li L, et al. Distinct EBV and CMV reactivation patterns following antibody-based immunosuppressive regimens in patients with severe aplastic anemia. Blood. 2007;109:3219–3224.

171. Peleg AY, Husain S, Kwak EJ, et al. Opportunistic infections in 547 organ transplant recipients receiving alemtuzumab, a humanized monoclonal CD-52 antibody. Clin Infect Dis. 2007;44:204–212.

172. Asano-Mori Y, Kanda Y, Oshima K, et al. Clinical features of late cytomegalovirus infection after hematopoietic stem cell transplantation. Int J Hematol. 2008;87:310–318.

173. Gomez-Almaguer D, Ruiz-Arguelles GJ, del Carmen Tarin-Arzaga L, et al. Alemtuzumab for the treatment of steroid-refractory acute graft-versus-host disease. Biol Blood Marrow Transplant. 2008;14:10–15.

174. Rodriguez V, Anderson PM, Trotz BA, Arndt CA, Allen JA, Khan SP. Use of infliximab-daclizumab combination for the treatment of acute and chronic graft-versus-host disease of the liver and gut. Pediatr Blood Cancer. 2007;49:212–215.

175. Marty FM, Lee SJ, Fahey MM, et al. Infliximab use in patients with severe graft-versus-host disease and other emerging risk factors of non-Candida invasive fungal infections in allogeneic hematopoietic stem cell transplant recipients: a cohort study. Blood. 2003;102:2768–2776.

176. Couriel D, Saliba R, Hicks K, et al. Tumor necrosis factor-alpha blockade for the treatment of acute GVHD. Blood. 2004;104:649–654.

177. Srinivasan R, Chakrabarti S, Walsh T, et al. Improved survival in steroid-refractory acute graft versus host disease after non-myeloablative allogeneic transplantation using a daclizumab-based strategy with comprehensive infection prophylaxis. Br J Haematol. 2004;124:777–786.

178. Perales MA, Ishill N, Lomazow WA, et al. Long-term follow-up of patients treated with daclizumab for steroid-refractory acute graft-vs-host disease. Bone Marrow Transplant. 2007;40:481–486.

179. Goldberg JD, Jacobsohn DA, Margolis J, et al. Pentostatin for the treatment of chronic graft-versus-host disease in children. J Pediatr Hematol Oncol. 2003;25:584–588.

180. Jacobsohn DA, Chen AR, Zahurak M, et al. Phase II study of pentostatin in patients with corticosteroid-refractory chronic graft-versus-host disease. J Clin Oncol. 2007;25:4255–4261.

181. Cheson BD. Infectious and immunosuppressive complications of purine analog therapy. J Clin Oncol. 1995;13:2431–2448.

182. Samonis G, Kontoyiannis DP. Infectious complications of purine analog therapy. Curr Opin Infect Dis. 2001;14:409–413.

183. Jacobsohn DA, Montross S, Anders V, Vogelsang GB. Clinical importance of confirming or excluding the diagnosis of chronic graft-versus-host disease. Bone Marrow Transplantation. 2001;28:1047–1051.

26

ENDOCRINE AND METABOLIC EFFECTS OF CHRONIC GRAFT VERSUS HOST DISEASE

Paul A. Carpenter and Jean E. Sanders

All recipients of hematopoietic cell transplantation (HCT) are at risk for late endocrine and metabolic dysfunction as a complication of the chemoradiotherapy given before HCT. However, these disturbances are often multifactorial. This chapter will focus on the endocrine and metabolic problems that arise predominantly as a result of chronic graft versus host disease (cGVHD) or therapies used to treat cGVHD (Table 26.1).

BONE METABOLISM

The two major iatrogenic complications of cGVHD that involve the skeleton are reduced bone mineral density and avascular bone necrosis (AVN).

Osteopenia and Osteoporosis

Definitions and Incidence

Dual energy x-ray absorptiometry (DEXA) is now the most common method for measuring bone mineral density (BMD). In adults, osteopenia is present when BMD in g/cm^2 equates to a T-score of –1.0 to –2.4 standard deviations (SD) below mean BMD values for healthy young adults. Osteoporosis is present when the T-score is less than or equal to –2.5. In children, T-scores are not used because the DEXA scan will detect area-related increases in BMD associated with increased bone volume during normal growth and development leading to over diagnosis of osteoporosis. Instead, SD scores for children must be normalized according to age-related mean BMD values, giving rise to z-scores.

One prospective study found that 46% of adults had osteopenia or osteoporosis at 12 months after HCT [1]. Other studies have shown that half of children have reduced BMD after HCT [2]. Loss of BMD is particularly concerning in children, since the attainment of peak bone mass during adolescence and early adulthood is an important determinant of long-term bone health that corresponds with the risk for involutional fractures. To detect and treat loss of BMD, a reasonable standard practice is to evaluate BMD at 3 months after allogeneic HCT with an initial follow-up DEXA scan at 1 year [3]. If BMD at 1 year is within the normal range and the patient is not receiving steroids, the monitoring schedule may revert to general population recommendations. However, if BMD is low or decreasing or prolonged steroid use is anticipated, then annual follow-ups are recommended.

Pathophysiology and Risk Factors

Bone loss may result from impaired bone mineralization through disturbances of calcium and vitamin D homeostasis, imbalanced osteoblast and osteoclast function, and deficiencies in growth or gonadal hormone secretion. Factors responsible for these disturbances include glucocorticoid therapy, cranial or total body irradiation (TBI), and other cytotoxic agents given before HCT. The leading cause of reduced BMD after HCT is prolonged glucocorticoid therapy for GVHD. Bone loss is most rapid during the initial 6 months of glucocorticoid therapy and may occur with daily prednisone doses as low as 5 mg.

Treatment

The National Institutes of Health (NIH) Consensus recommendations for management of bone loss in adults with cGVHD are based on evidence derived from large studies of patients, although not transplant survivors (Level Ib) [4, 5]. Supplemental calcium is generally prescribed for patient's receiving glucocorticoid therapy whenever daily calcium losses are increased, or when elemental calcium intake is less than the recommended daily intake of 800 mg, 1,200 mg, or 1,500 mg, respectively, for ages 1 to 5 years, 6 to 8 years, or greater than 9 years [6]. Oral vitamin D supplements are indicated whenever dietary vitamin D intake is less than 400 international units (IU) per day for ages 1 to 8 years or 400 to 800 IU per day for age greater than 9 years. It is reasonable to check the serum calcium, magnesium, and 1,25-hydroxyvitamin D level in patients who have osteoporosis. Because supplementation with calcium, vitamin D, and weight-bearing exercise has not by itself prevented osteopenia, osteoporosis, or fractures, additional therapy is necessary to prevent or reverse steroid-induced bone loss [6, 7].

Table 26.1: Endocrine and Metabolic Complications of cGVHD or its Therapy

Complication

Bone metabolism
  Osteopenia and osteoporosis
  Avascular necrosis
Iatrogenic Cushing's syndrome and adrenal insufficiency
Metabolic syndrome components
  Hyperlipidemia
  Hypertension
  Hyperglycemia
  Obesity
Pancreatic insufficiency*
Abnormal thyroid function
Disturbed growth and development

* Pancreatic insufficiency discussed in Chapter 20.

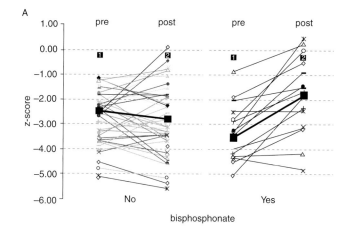

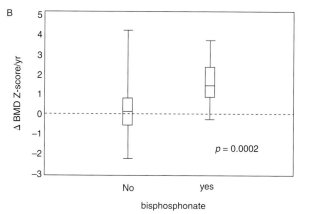

Figure 26.1 Annualized bone mineral density at baseline and after follow-up. Shown for the patients treated without (*n* = 48) and with (*n* = 18) bisphosphonate are as follows: A: the BMD *z*-scores for each patient, together with the median *z*-score (■), at baseline (pre) and at follow-up (post), and B: the median, 25th and 75th percentiles (box), and range of the rates of change of *z*-scores (whiskers). Reproduced with permission from Elsevier (2007) Carpenter et al. *Biology of Blood and Marrow Transplantation*, 13:683–690. See Plate 75 in the color plate section.

Gonadal failure may predate or exacerbate steroid-induced osteoporosis. Hormone replacement therapy can increase BMD in both women and men [8]. However, women beyond age 50 years should consult with a gynecologist first due to potential adverse risks associated with hormone replacement [8, 9]. In children, growth hormone [10–12] and/or estrogen or testosterone replacement therapy can improve BMD but coordination of these therapies is best managed by a pediatric endocrinologist.

Pharmacotherapy with bisphosphonates is necessary when hormone replacement therapy is inappropriate due to patient age, otherwise contraindicated, or does not ameliorate reduced BMD. They act primarily through effects on enzymatic pathways in osteoclasts to inhibit bone resorption but may also stimulate osteoblasts to promote bone formation [13]. The oral forms, alendronate and risedronate, and intravenous formulations, pamidronate and zoledronic acid, have been used widely for this purpose. They have also been administered after HCT for prevention of bone metastases in myeloma, and more recently for prevention and treatment of osteoporosis. One retrospective analysis compared baseline and follow-up DEXA scans of 48 children (controls) who received calcium and vitamin D to 18 children who also received bisphosphonate therapy [3]. Bisphosphonate therapy led to an annualized median change in BMD *z*-score per year of +1.43 (−0.29 to +3.72) whereas, the change in *z*-score for controls was only +0.12 (−2.28 to +4.24, *p* = .0002, Figure 26.1). This degree of improvement allowed one-third of the children to shift from the categories of osteoporosis or osteopenia to normal BMD, and more than half of the remaining children improved from osteoporosis to osteopenia or less severe osteoporosis.

Assumptions about the efficacy of bisphosphonate therapy in HCT recipients to reduce fracture rates are based on extrapolations from other populations [13–19]. A controlled study to show a reduction in fracture rate from a baseline cumulative incidence of 8% at 5 years is probably not feasible in the HCT population. However, it is reasonable to assume that gains in BMD z-scores of more than 1 standard deviation are clinically relevant. Bisphosphonate therapy is given until normal BMD is achieved and glucocorticoid therapy is discontinued. Bisphosphonates are generally well tolerated although oral formulations need to be taken with water, while sitting or standing, and in a fasting state to prevent esophagitis. This may pose practical limitations for small children. The compliance with a weekly or monthly dose regimen may limit the efficacy of oral formulations relative to less frequently administered IV formulations. Osteonecrosis of the jaw is a well recognized and potentially serious but rare complication of amino bisphosphonate therapy in adults (reviewed in Reference 20), mostly occurring when bisphosphonates are administered intravenously and monthly to adults for the management of bone malignancy, and in the setting of recent dentoalveolar

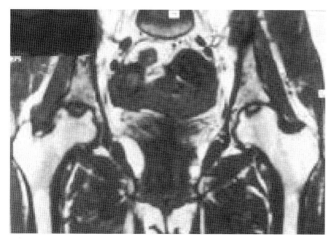

Figure 26.2 T1-weighted image showing decreased signal intensity in both femoral heads. Consistent with avascular necrosis. Image reprinted with permission from eMedicine.com, 2008. Available at: www.emedicine.com/Med/topic2924.htm.

trauma [20, 21]. There have been no reports of ONJ in children who received pamidronate for osteogenesis imperfecta [22]. Physicians need to be aware that characteristic transverse bands of osteosclerosis appear on plain film radiographs during bisphosphonate therapy have no clinical consequence and disappear over time [23].

Avascular Necrosis

Definition and Incidence

Avascular necrosis develops in 4% to 10% of allogeneic HCT survivors at a median of 12 months (range 2 to 132 months) after transplantation. The hip is most frequently affected although multiple joints may be involved [24]. AVN should be suspected if there is persistent or progressive pain in a typically affected joint in a patient who is at risk. Joint involvement is often bilateral and more severe in glucocorticoid-associated AVN compared to idiopathic AVN. Magnetic resonance imaging (MRI) imaging offers high sensitivity and specificity for detecting the earliest lesions of AVN (Figure 26.2) and forms the basis of radiological staging used for prognosis. Early, and often, asymptomatic Stage I lesions (abnormal MRI or bone scan, normal radiograph or computerised tomography [CT] scan) and symptomatic Stage II (diagnostic MRI abnormalities and abnormal radiographs) are potentially reversible and more treatable stages of hip AVN. More advanced lesions show progression to subchondral (Stage III) or more extensive collapse of the femoral head and even secondary osteoarthritis (Stage IV to VI) [25].

Pathophysiology and Risk Factors

The exact pathogenesis of AVN is poorly understood but the final common pathway is bone ischemia due to any combination of factors that include obliterative arteritis, thrombophilia, hyperlipidemia and fat embolism, repeated microfractures of weight-bearing bone, and increased intramedullary pressure

that is possibly secondary to increased intramedullary fat (reviewed in Reference 26). In animal studies glucocorticoid therapy increases intramedullary fat content and, when combined with an immunological insult, caused AVN in experimental animals.

Risk factors include age older than 16 years, an initial diagnosis of aplastic anemia or acute leukemia, and cGVHD [24]. Glucocorticoid therapy has been the factor most associated with increased risk for developing AVN among adult long-term survivors of HCT at Fred Hutchinson Cancer Research Center but increased duration of steroid use does not provide additional risk [27]. Alternate-day prednisone therapy combined with cyclosporine for cGVHD was less likely to result in AVN than alternate-day prednisone alone (13% vs. 22%, $p = .04$) suggesting that steroid-sparing approaches may be helpful [28].

Treatment

Treatment of AVN includes a variety of interventions that are based on the severity of symptoms, radiological staging, and a provisional level of evidence rating that follows the NIH consensus criteria. Pain relief is essential and sometimes difficult to achieve; often prompting referral to experts in pain management. Unfortunately, at least 50% of patients require surgical treatment within 3 years of diagnosis [24, 26] and this has prompted some interest in the use of bisphosphonates and statins for the prevention and treatment of early AVN [29–34]. Early referral to an orthopedic surgeon with experience in treating patients who have AVN as a complication of allograft procedures is recommended so that the timing and outcome of the various surgical procedures can be optimized (Table 26.2).

In children and young adults it is preferable to avoid early replacement with artificial joints that have a finite life span. In an attempt to avoid or delay joint replacement, a core decompression procedure has been used to promote revascularization of the femoral head based upon the hypothesis that AVN results from bone ischemia secondary to an intramedullary compartment syndrome. The procedure decompresses the medullary space by opening the area of the dead bone from the outside thereby restoring blood circulation to the necrotic bone and relieving pain. Variations include removal of dead bone and replacement with autologous fresh bone chips that provide bone morphogenic protein hormones. Uncontrolled studies show that core decompression is a well-tolerated, short-stay procedure that provides excellent and immediate pain relief in 50% to 80% with Stage I and 20% to 35% with Stage II AVN [35, 36]. Two small randomized studies confirmed that core decompression was better than nonoperative therapy for providing prompt pain relief in symptomatic early stage AVN [37, 38]. However, core decompression does not alter the progression of AVN in Stage II hips and is not appropriate for advanced stage AVN.

An advancement of the hip core decompression procedure involves filling the decompressed medullary space with a viable strut of autologous fibula. The blood supply is connected to vessels in the hip area to allow ongoing nourishment to newly placed bone chips. In expert hands the success rate approaches 80% in selected patients. However, the long procedure requires

Table 26.2: Management of Avascular Necrosis in Patients with cGVHD

Intervention	Indication/Comments	Rating*
Pain medication	Any symptoms	AIII
Prednisone reduction	Any stage	BIII
Statins	Prevention or early stage	CIIa
Bisphosphonates	Early stage (precollapse)	CIa/IIa
	Goal is to prevent progression of AVN. The potential for benefit in advanced stage AVN is even less clear	
Limited weight-bearing with crutches	Mild symptoms/early stage AVN	BIII
	Useful if involved segment is <15% and far from weight-bearing region	
Immobilization (brace)	Moderate to severe symptoms/intermediate state AVN	BIII
	Helpful for distal femur or tibia	
Core decompression	Early stage (precollapse)/symptomatic Late stage	CIa-IIa/DIIa
Osteochondral allograft	Advanced stage/symptomatic	CIII
Nonvascularized	Useful for AVN of distal femur	DIII
	Not generally useful for hip AVN	
Vascularized	Generally considered too morbid for patients with cGVHD	EIII
Resurfacing	Intermediate stage (early collapse)/symptomatic	
Partial (hemi)/total†	Helpful in younger patients	BIII
Total joint arthroplasty	Advanced stage/symptomatic	AIa

* Provisional rating based on National Institute of Health (NIH) consensus guidelines (for definitions see Chapter 15).
† 5-year pain relief rates are 80% to 90% for hip hemi-resurfacing but this drops to 60% to 70% at 10 years as the originally intact acetabular cartilage is worn out by contact with the metallic femoral cap which necessitates conversion to total hip arthoplasty. Approximately 90% of patients are satisfied at 10 years after revised total hip replacements.
AVN, avascular bone necrosis; cGVHD, chronic graft versus host disease.

both orthopedic and vascular microsurgeons, is technically demanding and is generally considered too morbid for a patient with cGVHD. Recovery takes months, and pain and weakness associated with removal of the fibula graft can occur.

Most patients with advanced AVN eventually require total joint replacement (arthroplasty), which provides excellent pain relief for many years, although most young patients require repeat surgery. Total hip arthroplasty involves amputation of the whole femoral head, insertion of a metal stem inside the marrow cavity of the femur and resurfacing the hip socket with a metal-on-metal cup. A less invasive but efficacious procedure for patients with more superficial damage of joint surfaces is partial or total hip resurfacing, which caps the head of the femur with a metal shell and lines the acetabulum socket, if necessary (total resurfacing), with a congruent metal cup. Hip resurfacing preserves the femoral head and neck, which is especially attractive for young, active patients who are likely to require more than one total joint arthroplasty during their lifetime. Selected knee joints are also amenable to the resurfacing approach.

IATROGENIC CUSHING'S SYNDROME AND ADRENAL INSUFFICIENCY

Cushingoid appearance may result from prolonged prednisone therapy to treat cGVHD. The cosmetic changes are troubling for patients, and especially for teenagers who are often already dealing with major changes of body image. Cushing's syndrome is generally more manageable once alternate-day steroid dosing can be achieved. It is important to counsel patients that Cushing's syndrome is reversible, especially in younger patients, given enough time off steroids.

Definition and Incidence

Abrupt withdrawal of steroids may provoke symptoms of secondary adrenal insufficiency, which should be anticipated in any patient treated for more than 3 weeks with daily glucocorticoid doses exceeding 7.5 mg of prednisone or equivalent. Chronic suppression of the hypothalamic-pituitary-adrenal (HPA) axis causes adrenocortical atrophy and inability to generate sufficient cortisol. This blunted cortisol response may be life threatening when stress responses are needed. Because when mineralocorticoid deficiency is not present hyperkalemia does not usually occur but hyponatremia may occur due to compensatory vasopressin secretion. Symptoms of adrenal insufficiency may be difficult to distinguish from a flare of GVHD or steroid withdrawal syndrome (Table 26.3).

A diagnosis of adrenal insufficiency may be confirmed by showing that the serum cortisol at 0700 to 0900 hours is <3.6 mcg/dL or the serum cortisol at 30 or 60 minutes does not increase above 19 mcg/dL in response to a standard cosyntropin test (250 mcg IV) [39–41]. Using this definition, approximately half of the patients tested at FHCRC for suspected adrenal insufficiency after allogeneic HCT had a positive test; 30% with

Table 26.3: Differential Diagnosis of Secondary Adrenal Insufficiency in Patients with cGVHD

Symptom or Sign	Secondary Adrenal Insufficiency	Steroid Withdrawal Syndrome	GVHD Flare
Weakness, tiredness, fatigue	++/+++	+	+
Anorexia	+++	+	++/+++
Nausea, vomiting	++/+++	+	++/+++
Constipation/abdominal pain	+/++	±	±
Diarrhea	+	±	++/+++
Weight loss, failure to thrive	+++	++	++/+++
Arthralgias, myalgias	+	++/+++	+
Dizziness	+	–	±
Adrenal crisis risk	+++	–	–
Hyponatremia	+	–	+
Hyperkalemia	–	–	–
Fever	+	+	+
Hypoglycemia	+	–	–
Low AM cortisol or abnormal Cortrosyn test	+++	–	–

low baseline cortisol and another 20% who failed the stimulation test (PC unpublished observations). If one also considers patients who were not tested, the estimated incidence of adrenal insufficiency in the total population is approximately 5%. The median time to diagnosis of adrenal insufficiency is 3 months after HCT and the range extends out to 13 months. Outside of this time frame, symptomatic adrenal insufficiency is uncommon at our center when steroids are tapered cautiously, and when preemptive adrenal axis testing is done as prednisone doses approach 0 mg on alternate-day dose regimens, or less than or equal to 5 mg of prednisone given daily.

Treatment

Hydrocortisone 5 mg/m² to 10 mg/m² per day is the preferred therapy to replace the deficient production of adrenal cortisol. The total dose is usually divided into two to three daily doses, with half to two-thirds of the daily dose administered in the morning to mimic the physiological cortisol secretion pattern. An adult might receive 10 mg upon waking and 5 mg at 1700 to 1800 hours. The exact dose regimen is adjusted according to symptoms and signs suggestive of over or under-replacement. Although prednisone is recommended for the treatment of primary adrenal insufficiency, the longer biological half-life of prednisone compared to hydrocortisone makes it more likely to suppress the HPA axis. Therefore, hydrocortisone is preferable for replacement therapy in secondary adrenal insufficiency. Stress dose steroids should be considered for illnesses that include fever, vomiting, diarrhea, major surgery, or trauma. Recovery of the HPA axis varies from days to several months which must be considered when a taper of replacement therapy is attempted.

METABOLIC SYNDROME AND ITS INDIVIDUAL COMPONENTS

Definition and Incidence

Metabolic syndrome (MS) is defined by the constellation of abdominal obesity, dyslipidemia, hypertension, insulin resistance, and prothrombotic or inflammatory states. In the general population, metabolic syndrome [42, 43] is associated with an increased risk of cardiovascular disease and Type II diabetes [44]. Transplant survivors appear to have an increased frequency of diabetes, hypertension, and dyslipidemia [45–48], which is of particular concern given the possible combined effects of MS and cardiotoxic or endothelial damage caused by prior cancer therapy and conditioning [49, 50]. The largest follow-up study to date does not appear to confirm the predicted increase in arterial disease, myocardial infarction or stroke events. However, serious cardiovascular events may be underestimated by the relatively short follow-up and young age of the study population [48]. Several case reports have documented premature and fatal coronary artery disease (CAD) in HCT recipients [51–55]. At Fred Hutchinsons Cancer Research Center (FHCRC), at least 30 patients who underwent HCT between 1973 and 1998 at a median age of 35 years (range 3.7 to 52 years), died at a median of 7.5 years after transplant due to CAD or heart failure of unspecified etiology (P. Carpenter, unpublished). Hyperlipidemia was present in the majority of these patients who had serum lipid levels documented beyond 90 days after HCT. Because the earliest successful HCTs were performed in younger patients just over 30 years ago, it is possible that the prevalence of premature CAD (<age 55 years) might start to increase as these earlier transplant survivors mature.

Table 26.4 Assessment and Management of Metabolic Syndrome (MS) Components after HCT

MS Component	Assessment	Intervention/Comments	Rating*
Central obesity	Waist circumference Body mass index	Therapeutic lifestyle modifications (ATP III/NCEP) Diet and exercise	AIa
Hyperlipidemia	Fasting LDL, HDL and triglycerides	Therapeutic lifestyle modifications (ATP III/NCEP) NCEP Step 1 diet and exercise	AIa
		Statins (atovastatin, simvastatin, pravastatin) Treatment of choice for lowering LDL (also raise HDL) First line for mixed hyperlipidemias Caution with high dose when on calcineurin inhibitors	BIII
		Fibrates (gemfibrozil/fenofibrate) Well established for isolated hypertriglyceridemia Caution when combined with statins	CIII
		Fish oil supplements Alternative first line for isolated hypertriglyceridemia Currently one FDA approved product (Omacor) Prefer USP-verified over-the-counter supplements	CIII
Hypertension	Blood pressure	Antihypertensive medication	AIII
		Angiotensin-converting enzyme (ACE) inhibitors and Angiotensin-receptor blockers (ARBs) are preferred.	CIII
Diabetes mellitus and Insulin resistance	Fasting glucose	Insulin therapy First line therapy for patients with preprandial glucose >130 mg/dL or posprandial glucose >180 mg/dL	AIII
		Sliding scale insulin is generally inappropriate	EIII
		Scheduled basal intermediate or long-acting	BIII
		Prandial short or rapid acting bolus before meals	AIII
		Noninsulin therapies Meglitinides, incretin mimetics and dipeptidyl peptidase IV inhibitors need further study	DIII
Inflammatory states	C-reactive protein	Needs further study	-

* Provisional rating based on National Institute of Health (NIH) consensus guidelines (for definitions see Chapter 15).
ATP, adult treatment panel; FDA, Food and Drug association; HDL, high density lipoproteins; LDL, low density lipoproteins; NCEP, National Cholesterol Education Program.

Risk Factors

The systemic immunosuppressive therapy (IST) used to treat cGVHD may promote the development of hyperlipidemia, hypertension, and hyperglycemia, or aggravate preexisting risk factors for premature cardiovascular disease. It remains unclear to what extent the usual three or more years of IST contributes to late morbidity or mortality by promoting components of the MS. One study has found that allogeneic HCT, but not cGVHD per se, was associated with the development of diabetes and hypertension but hyperlipidemia was not assessed [48]. It is appropriate to consider each component of the MS when developing a comprehensive management plan for all patients with cGVHD (Table 26.4).

Hyperlipidemia

The incidence of hyperlipidemia as a late effect after HCT in children has been reported as 28% to 39% [45, 47]. By 75 to 100 days after HCT more than half of all patients appear to develop hypercholesterolemia and 4.8% of adults and 8.1% of

children developed elevation of serum triglycerides >750 mg.dL (Table 26.5).

National (NCEP ATP III) guidelines for prevention of cardiovascular disease target lower serum LDL-C levels and higher HDL-C levels. HMG-CoA reductase inhibitors (statins) effectively reduce serum total cholesterol, protect against premature cardiovascular disease, and improve survival in adults with a wide range of cholesterol levels whether they have a history of CAD or not [56–59]. Statins also can also be used safely and effectively to lower serum lipid levels in adults and children and, in several larger studies, improve survival in solid organ transplant recipients [60–71]. By extrapolation, it is reasonable to use statins to target lower LDL-C in HCT recipients when therapeutic lifestyle modifications are ineffective or not feasible. In general the lowest dose possible is used to minimize the potential for adverse drug interactions between statins and other medications. Finally, the pleiotropic effects of statins may extend to improvement in renal function, hypertension, bone mineral density, reduced incidence of avascular necrosis, and even improved control of GVHD [29, 30, 72–78].

Table 26.5: Hyperlipidemia in Recipients of Allogeneic HCT at FHCRC between 2002 and 2003.

	Hypercholesterolemia			Hypertriglyceridemia		
	Before HCT	Day 75–100	%Δ	Before HCT	Day 75–100	%Δ
Adults (n = 293)						
Median	167	225	+34	160	264	+65
Range	54–283	69–463		30–730	54–4211	
Children (n = 62)						
Median	140	204	+45	106	239	+125
Range	68–322	109–597		54–2196	54–2196	

Retrospective analysis (unpublished data).
FHCRC, Fred Hutchinsons Cancer Research Center; HCT, hematopoietic cell transplantation.

Insulin Resistance and Diabetes Mellitus

Two large studies suggest that the prevalence of Type II diabetes after HCT is 6% to 8%, which is higher than in the general population [46, 48]. Reported risk factors include a diagnosis of leukemia, non-Hispanic white ethnicity, family history of diabetes and asparaginase toxicity [46]. In one study, the risk factors of allogeneic HCT and total-body irradiation were somewhat interrelated [48]. Patients at risk should be educated and monitored accordingly.

Hypertension

The incidence of idiopathic chronic kidney disease (ICKD) after HCT varies from 17.5% after myeloablative conditioning to 66% after nonmyeloablative conditioning [79]. The role of hypertension in the development of ICKD after HCT is unclear. Nonetheless it is important to control blood pressure in patients with cGVHD on prednisone and a calcineurin inhibitor. The major risk factors for ICKD are acute and cGVHD, acute renal failure, and after nonmyeloablative regimens, additional risk factors include long-term use of calcineurin inhibitors and previous autologous HCT. Although hypertension after HCT has most commonly been treated with a long-acting calcium channel blocker, blockade of the renin-angiotensin axis using angiotensin-converting enzyme inhibitors (ACEI) alone or in combination with angiotension II receptor blockers (ARB) may be a better choice for treatment of hypertension in patients with ICKD. This concept is based upon studies using ACEI and ARBs in animal models of radiation-induced injury, and upon recent clinical experience [79, 80]. In addition to controlling blood pressure, it may be that ACEI and ARB exert additional positive affects by reducing inflammation and inflammatory markers [79, 80]. There is evidence in patients with diabetes and albuminuria that treatment with an ACEI or an ARB slows the progression of chronic kidney disease (CKD) [81, 82]. Extrapolating from studies in the diabetic population in conjunction with the observation that albuminuria is frequent after HCT [83] raises the possibility that these agents might be beneficial in patients with albuminuria after HCT. Controlled trials using ACEI or ARB after HCT are needed [79, 80].

Obesity

Obesity as an isolated component of MS is itself becoming increasingly prevalent in the general population [84–86]. Prolonged and sometimes recurrent courses of glucocorticoid therapy coupled with lower activity levels as a result of physical or other limitations associated with cGVHD often exacerbate this more general lifestyle problem. A MS of obesity combined with hyperinsulinemia, low HDL cholesterol levels, and reduced spontaneous growth hormone secretion was shown to be significantly increased in 8 of 50 childhood cancer survivors compared to none of the 50 age- and sex-matched controls [86].

ABNORMAL THYROID FUCTION

Abnormal thyroid function after HCT is most often a late effect associated with conditioning regimens that include irradiation which results in compensated or overt hypothyroidism. Transient sick euthyroid syndrome (SES) is a well-recognized, possibly adaptive response to severe systemic nonthyroidal illness and after HCT is more common in adults compared to children. SES is characterized by reduced free T3 or T4, reduced-total thyroxine and a normal thyroid stimulating hormone (TSH). Compared to patients with a normal thyroid function panel patients with SES were receiving higher glucocorticoid doses when thyroid function was tested but it is unclear to what extent high-dose glucocorticoid therapy and acute GVHD were interdependent [87]. Thyroid hormone-replacement is not indicated for SES. Isolated case reports and small case series have documented "auto"-immune hyperthyroidism and hypothyroidism after allogeneic HCT and in many of these cases adoptive transfer of abnormal donor lymphocyte clones has been suggested as a possible mechanism but immune dysregulation associated with concomitant cGVHD might be a contributing factor [88, 89]. Treatment of overt hypothyroidism or hyperthyroidism in these cases is identical to nontransplant situations. Although the clinical significance of antithyroid microsomal antibodies is unclear it is of interest that these have been detected in 5% to 40% of patients with cGVHD [90, 91].

DISTURBED GROWTH AND DEVELOPMENT

Growth in children and the attainment of normal adult height is a complex process that requires an appropriate balance of nutritional, genetic, endocrine, and other physical and psychosocial factors. During infancy, growth is highly dependent on nutrition and thyroid hormone. During childhood, growth hormone (GH) predominates, and in puberty the synergistic interplay of GH and sex steroids are critical for attainment of final adult height [92]. During all stages, any prolonged disturbance of physical or psychosocial well-being may adversely impact growth and development [92–95]. For the child with cGVHD such disturbances may include the delayed hormonal and direct skeletal effects of pretransplant total-body and/or cranial irradiation, chronic glucocorticoid therapy and periods of time when GVHD activity is inadequately controlled. It is important to realize that daily prednisone doses exceeding 5 mg/m^2 for prolonged periods will inhibit growth by several complex mechanisms which may include impaired secretion of GH [96, 97]. Excessive doses of glucocorticoids may cause pubertal delay via inhibition of gonadotropin release or direct inhibition of sex steroid secretion from the gonads in normal persons, but this effect is difficult if not impossible to determine in a population where more than 50% will have primary gonadal failure secondary to the preparative regimen. Close consultation with a pediatric endocrinologist is advised to optimize these critical aspects of care in children with cGVHD who have delayed growth and development. There is no threshold dose of glucorticoids above which the growth response to GH clearly and predictably declines [96]. However, the best growth responses to GH therapy appear to occur when prednisone is given as a single dose of ≤0.5 mg/kg given on alternate-days [98, 99]. A reasonable approach is to wait until prednisone therapy is at every other day dosing or at least below a daily dose of 5 mg/m^2 before GH testing and/or replacement therapy are undertaken. Testosterone or estrogen therapy for pubertal delay must be coordinated with GH therapy so that premature closure of epiphyses is avoided. Interestingly, seven obese prepubertal boys who received 6 months of GH therapy, without additional dietary or exercise modifications, experienced a 5% increase in lean body mass which lends support to the hypothesis that GH may provide other benefits in addition to promoting height growth [100]. Whether GH therapy might reverse aspects of the MS remains to be studied.

CASE PRESENTATION

The following four cases illustrate how endocrine and metabolic complications may be diagnosed and managed in patients with cGVHD.

CASE 1

A 18-year-old young woman is seen in clinic 14 months after a matched related donor PBSC transplant from her HLA-identical sister for chronic myeloid leukemia (CML). cGVHD involving the skin and gastrointestinal tract is currently quiescent on prednisone which has tapered recently from 1 mg/kg every other day, cyclosporine and mycophenolate mofetil. For the past 2 months she has received monthly infusions of pamidronate for osteopenia. Over the past 2 weeks she has developed new and severe pain in multiple joints and has been taking oxycodone every 4 hours. MRI scans show AVN at both distal femoral epiphyses and distal tibial diaphyses. Orthopedics recommend a core decompression procedure of the right knee if she discontinues prednisone. In the interim she is provided with a brace and crutches. The Pain Service prescribes and monitors methadone therapy, which provides good pain relief. One month later her pain occurs only with weight-bearing and she uses a wheelchair if she has to take more than a few steps. Over the next 3 months her methadone requirements gradually increase and she requires a cocktail of medications to relieve constipation. Psychiatry is consulted regarding her progressive depression and insomnia and follow-up continues with the Pain Service every 2 weeks by phone. Prednisone was discontinued 2 months later. Over the course of the next 4 years she undergoes multiple orthopedic procedures for the following developments. Initially she has serial core decompressions on the right and left distal femurs and left proximal femur. Each core decompression provided significant pain relief and improved her mobility. However, she later developed left hip pain and recurrent right knee pain at age 20 years which was treated successfully with a fresh allograft to replace the right knee lateral condyle at age 22 years. The left femoral head collapsed approximately 1 year after the core decompression and was resurfaced, 3 years later this was converted to a left femoral hemiarthroplasty after she developed persistent pain in the groin.

Discussion: This case illustrates the potential complexity and extent of morbidity in a patient who develops multifocal AVN as a consequence of glucocorticoid therapy. Although there is little evidence that accelerated discontinuation of prednisone has any bearing on the natural history of AVN; the general principle is to taper steroids wherever possible but not at the expense of loss of control of GVHD. Consultation with Orthopedic surgeons who have particular expertise in treating AVN in these patients is necessary. Interventions that buy time are often necessary as in this case, to defer definitive total joint arthroplasty until these are age appropriate for the patient given the finite lifespan of artificial joints. Consultation with experts in pain management and other services (Psychiatry, Occupational and Physical therapy) may be helpful in alleviating symptoms and improving functionality.

CASE 2

A 44-year-old man received a marrow transplant 84 days ago from an unrelated donor for severe aplastic anemia. He developed hyperacute GVHD on day 10 and subsequently was successfully treated for steroid-refractory grade III acute GVHD of the skin and intestine. Screening evaluations for cGVHD recently confirmed mild involvement of the mouth at a time when his prednisone dose exceeded 0.5 mg/kg/day. He now continues cyclosporine, topical beclomethasone and budesonide, a prednisone taper, and his extracorporeal photopheresis therapy has just been reduced to a monthly regimen. Over the past 21 days the prednisone dose has been tapered from 60 mg daily down to 60 mg alternating with 0 mg, with a goal to maintain this dose for 2 to 3 months. During the past 11 days he has intermittently verbalized that his "bones hurt" and during the last 3 days since ondansetron was discontinued he has vomited up to twice daily. Appetite is satisfactory. Stools are firm. No fevers. The *review of systems* is otherwise unremarkable but he did comment that he is not quite himself. On *physical examination* he appeared Cushingoid with generalized hirsuitism but otherwise well. Vital signs were satisfactory. Weight 60 kg. No rash or skin erythema. Anicteric sclera and noninjected conjunctivae. Chapped lower lips. Oropharynx notable for mild buccal hyperkeratotic changes and prominent linea albae. Abdomen soft and protuberant, nontender with normoactive bowel tones. Remainder of examination was normal.

Relevant Investigations

Complete blood count:	WBC 6.1, ANC 4.0, Hematocrit 38%, platelets **95,000**
Liver function tests:	Bilirubin 0.5 mg/dL, AST 24 IU, ALT 19 IU, alkaline phosphatase 97 IU,
Creatinine/electrolytes:	0.9 mg/dL, magnesium 2.2 mg/dL.
Cyclosporine level:	285 ng/mL
Cortisol (serum):	Baseline 0800 h 60 minutes after Cortrosyn **0.4** mcg/dL (4.5–23) **2.6** mcg/dL

Discussion The patient has mild cGVHD in the context of severe steroid-refractory acute GVHD that resulted in almost 10 weeks of daily steroid therapy. While recurrent GVHD could account for the vomiting and general malaise, these same symptoms could equally be anticipated with secondary adrenal insufficiency. Pain in the extremities could also be part of this latter symptom constellation or otherwise might simply represent a rebound effect, which is the body's exaggerated response to rapid removal of prednisone, or so-called steroid withdrawal syndrome.

Supportive Care

He began therapy on the days that he does not take prednisone with 15 mg of hydrocortisone in the morning and 5 mg at approximately 5 to 6 PM to attempt to facilitate recovery of the adrenal axis over time. Adults generally require a total dose of 20 mg per day to approximate physiological cortisol replacement of 5 to 10 mg/m² per day, recognizing that the total daily dose may need to be increased by up to 10-fold and divided every 8 hours during times of stress.

CASE 3

A 12-year-old girl is seen in clinic 3 years after myeloablative conditioning and peripheral blood transplant for ALL. She has completed a total of 35 months of multimodality therapy for sclerodermatous cGVHD, which has almost completely resolved. Extracorporeal photopheresis was discontinued 3 months ago and sirolimus was discontinued 1 month ago. She continues tacrolimus and tapering doses of prednisone; currently at 6 mg every other day. She is doing well and has no complaints. Apart from infrequent mild oral sensitivities the *review of systems* is unremarkable. On *physical examination* she was appearing well with normal vital signs. Height 134.8 cm (<5th percentile), Weight 35.1 kg (85th percentile). Tanner stage I. There is minimal

residual fixed flexion deformity at the elbows, wrists and 3rd to 5th digits of the hands but she is now able to play the violin. Remainder of the examination was essentially normal.

Relevant Investigations

Complete blood count:	WBC 7.1, ANC 5.0, Hematocrit 39%, platelets 390,000
Liver function tests:	Bilirubin 0.3 mg/dL, ALT 20 IU, alkaline phosphatase 67 IU,
Creatinine/electrolytes:	0.8 mg/dL, magnesium 2.0 mg/dL.
DEXA scan Z-scores:	Now 1 year ago, 2 years ago
(Lumbar spine)	**−1.1** −0.6 **−1.9**
Height velocity:	**1.8** cm/year (<3rd percentile)
Overnight GH monitoring:	7 peaks (1 at 6.6 ng/mL and 6 at <4 ng/mL), **subnormal**
Clonidine GH stimulation:	**subnormal**
Bone age:	**9.5** years (chronological age 12.0)
IGF-1	245 ng/mL (163–771).
Follicle stimulating hormone:	**63** miU/mL (normal <15)
Luteinizing Hormone:	20 miU/mL
Estradiol:	<20 pg/mL
Free thyroxine:	0.8 (0.8–1.8)
Thyroid stimulating hormone:	1.21 (0.4–5.0)

Discussion: The patient has a history of severe cGVHD that responded to chronic IST which continues to be tapered. As a consequence of a prior cranial irradiation and TBI, she has delayed linear growth. GH testing indicates GH deficiency and it is important to note that testing was deferred until her prednisone dose was below 0.5 mg/kg every other day to allow for reliable results. The delayed bone age, pubertal staging, and mild elevation of serum FSH suggest hypogonadism. Her moderately severe osteopenia had previously responded to monthly infusions of pamidronate but the change to an every-other-month schedule last year has been associated with the redevelopment of osteopenia. At this visit she was advised to continue tacrolimus and to continue to taper prednisone. Supportive care recommendations most pertinent to this chapter include the following:

Supportive Care

1. Resume monthly pamidronate (1 mg/kg) therapy until the BMD is normal or at least until prednisone is discontinued if GH and/or estrogen therapy are begun in the next several months [3].
2. Dietary intake of calcium and vitamin D was reviewed and deemed sufficient.
3. Because her prednisone dose is now < 0.5 mg/kg every other day follow-up is scheduled with a pediatric endocrinologist to discuss GH therapy to address her delayed linear growth and potential estrogen replacement therapy to promote puberty.

Monitoring

1. Repeat DEXA scan in 12 months to determine progress.

2. Maintain close follow-up with pediatric endocrinologist regarding potential growth and hormone therapies.

Key Points

▪ Osteopenia or osteoporosis develops in approximately 50% of patients after HCT and is primarily the result of prolonged glucocorticoid therapy and may occur with daily prednisone doses as low as 5 mg.

▪ Prevention or treatment of reduced BMD in patients with cGVHD involves the provision of adequate calcium and vitamin D intake and individualized therapy with hormone-replacement and/or bisphosphonates as appropriate.

▪ Avascular bone necrosis develops in 4% to 10% of the survivors of allogeneic HCT at a median of 12 months after transplantation.

▪ The therapy of moderate to severe AVN for younger patients involves narcotic analgesia followed by a variety of temporizing surgical interventions but total joint replacement is most often the treatment of choice for older patients.

▪ Secondary adrenal insufficiency should always be considered during the taper of glucocorticoid therapy because the symptoms and signs may be misinterpreted as a flare of cGVHD.

▪ Hypertension should be controlled in patients with cGVHD particularly because there is a high incidence of idiopathic chronic kidney disease and ACE inhibitors might provide protection against chronic kidney disease.

▪ Hyperlipidemia is common in patients receiving chronic systemic immunosuppressive therapy after HCT and generally warrants pharmacotherapy in addition to lifestyle modification.

▪ Abnormal thyroid function is considered to be a late effect of conditioning but in isolated cases it can be shown to be an autoimmune manifestation of cGVHD.

▪ Prednisone therapy may contribute to the blunting of growth and development in childhood that is an expected complication of preparative regimens that contain high-dose total-body irradiation or high-dose busulfan.

▪ GH therapy for children with cGVHD should be delayed until prednisone doses are below 0.5 mg/kg every other day.

REFERENCES

1. Stern JM, Sullivan KM, Ott SM, et al. Bone density loss after allogeneic hematopoietic stem cell transplantation: a prospective study. *Biol Blood Marrow Transplant.* 2001;7:257–264.

2. Kaste SC, Shidler TJ, Tong X, et al. Bone mineral density and osteonecrosis in survivors of childhood allogeneic bone marrow transplantation. *Bone Marrow Transplant.* 2004; 33:435–441.

3. Carpenter PA, Hoffmeister P, Chesnut CH, III, et al. Bisphosphonate therapy for reduced bone mineral density in children with chronic graft-versus-host disease. *Biol Blood Marrow Transplant.* 2007;13:683–690.

4. Schimmer AD, Minden MD, Keating A. Osteoporosis after blood and marrow transplantation: clinical aspects (Review). *Biol Blood Marrow Transplant.* 2000;6:175–181.

5. Couriel D, Carpenter PA, Cutler C, et al. Ancillary therapy and supportive care of chronic graft-versus-host disease: National Institutes of Health consensus development project on criteria for clinical trials in chronic graft-versus-host disease: V. Ancillary Therapy and Supportive Care Working Group report. *Biol Blood Marrow Transplant.* 2006;12:375–396.

6. Anonymous. Recommendations for the prevention and treatment of glucocorticoid-induced osteoporosis. American College of Rheumatology Task Force on Osteoporosis Guidelines. *Arthritis Rheum.* 1996;39:1791–1801.

7. Stallings VA. Calcium and bone health in children: a review (Review). *Am J Ther.* 1997;4:259–273.

8. Rossouw JE, Anderson GL, Prentice RL, et al. Risks and benefits of estrogen plus progestin in healthy postmenopausal women: principal results from the Women's Health Initiative randomized controlled trial. *JAMA.* 2002;288:321–333.

9. Beral V, Million Women SC. Breast cancer and hormone-replacement therapy in the Million Women Study [erratum appears in Lancet. 2003 Oct 4;362(9390):1160]. *Lancet.* 2003;362:419–427.

10. Ohlsson C, Bengtsson BA, Isaksson OG, Andreassen TT, Slootweg MC. Growth hormone and bone (Review). *Endocr Rev.* 1998;19:55–79.

11. Wüster C, Abs R, Bengtsson B-A, et al. The influence of growth hormone deficiency, growth hormone replacement therapy, and other aspects of hypopituitarism on fracture rate and bone mineral density. *J Bone Miner Res.* 2001;16:398–405.

12. Mauseth RS, Kelly BE, Sanders JE. Bone mineral density (BMD) in pediatric marrow transplant patients. *Pediatr Res.* 49 (part 2) [6], 82A, #P1–488. 2001. (Abstract)

13. Lindsay R. Modeling the benefits of pamidronate in children with osteogenesis imperfecta. *J Clin Invest.* 2002;110:1239–1241.

14. Glorieux FH, Bishop NJ, Plotkin H, Chabot G, Lanoue G, Travers R. Cyclic administration of pamidronate in children with severe osteogenesis imperfecta. *N Engl J Med.* 1998;339:947–952.

15. Gatti D, Antoniazzi F, Prizzi R, et al. Intravenous neridronate in children with osteogenesis imperfecta: a randomized controlled study. *J Bone Miner Res.* 2005;20:758–763.

16. Thornton J, Ashcroft DM, Mughal MZ, Elliott RA, O'Neill TW, Symmons D. Systematic review of effectiveness of bisphosphonates in treatment of low bone mineral density and fragility fractures in juvenile idiopathic arthritis (Review). *Arch Dis Child.* 2006;91:753–761.

17. Delmas PD. Treatment of postmenopausal osteoporosis (Review). *Lancet.* 2002;359:2018–2026.

18. Kananen K, Volin L, Laitinen K, Alfthan H, Ruutu T, Valimaki MJ. Prevention of bone loss after allogeneic stem cell transplantation by calcium, vitamin D, and sex hormone replacement with or without pamidronate. *J Clin Endocrinol Metab.* 2005;90:3877–3885.

19. Adachi JD, Bensen WG, Brown J, et al. Intermittent etidronate therapy to prevent corticosteroid-induced osteoporosis. *N Engl J Med.* 1997;337:382–387.

20. Sambrook P, Olver I, Goss A. Bisphosphonates and osteonecrosis of the jaw (Review). *Aust Fam Physician.* 2006;35:801–803.

21. Woo SB, Hellstein JW, Kalmar Jr. Narrative review: bisphosphonates and osteonecrosis of the jaws (Review) [erratum appears

in *Ann Intern Med.* 2006 Aug 1;145(3):235]. *Ann Intern Med.* 2006;144:753–761.

22. Biophosphonates and the risk of osteonecrosis of the jaw (ONJ) in osteogenesis imperfecta. http://www oif org/site/PageServer?pagename=BisphosphonatesArticle 2006.

23. Land C, Rauch F, Glorieux FH. Cyclical intravenous pamidronate treatment affects metaphyseal modeling in growing patients with osteogenesis imperfecta. *J Bone Miner Res.* 2006;21:374–379.

24. Socié G, Cahn JY, Carmelo J, et al. Avascular necrosis of bone after allogeneic bone marrow transplantation: analysis of risk factors for 4388 patients by the Societe Francaise de Greffe de Moelle (SFGM). *Br J Haematol.* 1997;97:865–870.

25. Tofferi JK, Gilliland W. Avascular necrosis. WebMD 2006;http://www.emedicine.com/med/topic2924.htm.

26. Arlet J. Nontraumatic avascular necrosis of the femoral head. Past, present, and future (Review). *Clin Orthopaed Related Res.* 1992;277(4):12–21.

27. Fink JC, Leisenring WM, Sullivan KM, Sherrard DJ, Weiss NS. Avascular necrosis following bone marrow transplantation: a case-control study. *Bone.* 1998;22:67–71.

28. Koc S, Leisenring W, Flowers MED, et al. Therapy for chronic graft-versus-host disease: a randomized trial comparing cyclosporine plus prednisone versus prednisone alone. *Blood.* 2002;100:48–51.

29. Pritchett JW. Statin therapy decreases the risk of osteonecrosis in patients receiving steroids. *Clin Orthop Relat Res.* 2001;173–178.

30. Pritchett JW. Statins and dietary fish oils improve lipid composition in bone marrow and joints. *Clin Orthop Relat Res.* 2007;456:233–237.

31. Nishii T, Sugano N, Miki H, Hashimoto J, Yoshikawa H. Does alendronate prevent collapse in osteonecrosis of the femoral head? *Clinical Orthopaedics & Related Research.* 2006;443:273–279.

32. Lai KA, Shen WJ, Yang CY, Shao CJ, Hsu JT, Lin RM. The use of alendronate to prevent early collapse of the femoral head in patients with nontraumatic osteonecrosis. A randomized clinical study. *J Bone Joint Surg Am.* 2005;87:2155–2159.

33. Ramachandran M, Ward K, Brown RR, Munns CF, Cowell CT, Little DG. Intravenous bisphosphonate therapy for traumatic osteonecrosis of the femoral head in adolescents. *J Bone Joint Surg Am.* 2007;89:1727–1734.

34. Agarwala S, Jain D, Joshi VR, Sule A. Efficacy of alendronate, a bisphosphonate, in the treatment of AVN of the hip. A prospective open-label study [erratum appears in *Rheumatology.* (Oxford). 2005 Apr;44(4):569]. *Rheumatology.* 2005;44:352–359.

35. Castro FPJ, Barrack RL. Core decompression and conservative treatment for avascular necrosis of the femoral head: a meta-analysis. *Am J Orthop.* (Chatham, Nj) 2000;29:187–194.

36. Mont MA, Carbone JJ, Fairbank AC. Core decompression versus nonoperative management for osteonecrosis of the hip (Review). *Clin Orthop Relat Res.* 1996;324(3):169–178.

37. Stulberg BN, Davis AW, Bauer TW, Levine M, Easley K. Osteonecrosis of the femoral head. A prospective randomized treatment protocol. *Clin Orthop Relat Res.* 1991;268(7):140–151.

38. Koo KH, Kim R, Ko GH, Song HR, Jeong ST, Cho SH. Preventing collapse in early osteonecrosis of the femoral head. A randomised clinical trial of core decompression. *J Bone Joint Surg Br.* 1995;77:870–874.

39. Arlt W, Allolio B. Adrenal insufficiency. *Lancet.* 2003;361:1881–1893.

40. Krasner AS. Glucocorticoid-induced adrenal insufficiency. *JAMA.* 1999;282:671–676.

41. Oelkers W. Adrenal insufficiency (Review). *N Engl J Med.* 1996;335:1206–1212.

42. Ford ES, Giles WH, Mokdad AH. Increasing prevalence of the metabolic syndrome among U.S. adults. *Diabetes Care.* 2004;27:2444–2449.

43. Weiss R, Dziura J, Burgert TS, et al. Obesity and the metabolic syndrome in children and adolescents. *N Engl J Med.* 2004;350:2362–2374.

44. Ford ES, Giles WH, Dietz WH. Prevalence of the metabolic syndrome among US adults: findings from the third National Health and Nutrition Examination Survey. *JAMA.* 2002;287:356–359.

45. Taskinen M, Saarinen-Pihkala UM, Hovi L, Lipsanen-Nyman M. Impaired glucose tolerance and dyslipidaemia as late effects after bone-marrow transplantation in childhood. *Lancet.* 2000;356:993–997.

46. Hoffmeister PA, Storer BE, Sanders JE. Diabetes mellitus in long-term survivors of pediatric hematopoietic cell transplantation. *J Pediatr Hematol Oncol.* 2004;26:81–90.

47. Shalitin S, Phillip M, Stein J, Goshen Y, Carmi D, Yaniv I. Endocrine dysfunction and parameters of the metabolic syndrome after bone marrow transplantation during childhood and adolescence. *Bone Marrow Transplant.* 2006;37:1109–1117.

48. Baker KS, Ness KK, Steinberger J, et al. Diabetes, hypertension, and cardiovascular events in survivors of hematopoietic cell transplantation: a report from the bone marrow transplantation survivor study. *Blood.* 2007;109:1765–1772.

49. Nuver J, Smit AJ, Postma A, Sleijfer DT, Gietema JA. The metabolic syndrome in long-term cancer survivors, an important target for secondary preventive measures (Review). *Cancer Treat Rev.* 2002;28:195–214.

50. Mertens AC, Yasui Y, Neglia JP, et al. Late mortality experience in five-year survivors of childhood and adolescent cancer: the Childhood Cancer Survivor Study. *J Clin Oncol.* 2001;19:3163–3172.

51. Chan KW, Taylor GP, Shepherd JD, Shepherd WE. Coronary artery disease following bone marrow transplantation. *Bone Marrow Transplant.* 1989;4:327–330.

52. Gatt ME, Liebster D, Leibowitz D, Matzner Y. Acute myocardial infarction after bone marrow transplantation: an unsuspected late complication. *Ann Hematol.* 2003;82:136–138.

53. Ghobrial IM, Bunch TJ, Caplice NM, Edwards WD, Miller DV, Litzow MR. Fatal coronary artery disease after unrelated donor bone marrow transplantation. *Mayo Clin Proc.* 2004;79:403–406.

54. Kupari M, Volin L, Suokas A, Timonen T, Hekali P, Ruutu T. Cardiac involvement in bone marrow transplantation: electrocardiographic changes, arrhythmias, heart failure and autopsy findings. *Bone Marrow Transplant.* 1990;5:91–98.

55. Wang B, Cao LX, Liu HL, Jiang M, Hu LD. Myocardial infarction following allogeneic bone marrow transplantation. *Bone Marrow Transplant.* 1996;18:479–480.

56. Prevention of cardiovascular events and death with pravastatin in patients with coronary heart disease and a broad range of initial cholesterol levels. The Long-Term Intervention with Pravastatin in Ischaemic Disease (LIPID) Study Group. *N Engl J Med.* 1998;339:1349–1357.

57. Shepherd J, Blauw GJ, Murphy MB, et al. Pravastatin in elderly individuals at risk of vascular disease (PROSPER): a randomised controlled trial. *Lancet.* 2002;360:1623–1630.

58. Shepherd J, Cobbe SM, Ford I, et al. Prevention of coronary heart disease with pravastatin in men with hypercholesterolemia. West of Scotland Coronary Prevention Study Group. *N Engl J Med.* 1995;333:1301–1307.

59. Strandberg TE, Pyorala K, Cook TJ, et al. Mortality and incidence of cancer during 10-year follow-up of the Scandinavian Simvastatin Survival Study (4S). *Lancet.* 2004;364:771–777.

60. Ong CS, Pollock CA, Caterson RJ, Mahony JF, Waugh DA, Ibels LS. Hyperlipidemia in renal transplant recipients: natural history and response to treatment. *Medicine.* 1994;73:215–223.

61. Keogh A, Simons L, Spratt P, et al. Hyperlipidemia after heart transplantation. *J Heart Transplant.* 1988;7:171–175.

62. Seipelt IM, Crawford SE, Rodgers S, et al. Hypercholesterolemia is common after pediatric heart transplantation: initial experience with pravastatin. *J Heart Lung Transplant.* 2004;23:317–322.

63. O'Rourke B, Barbir M, Mitchell AG, Yacoub MH, Banner NR. Efficacy and safety of fluvastatin therapy for hypercholesterolemia after heart transplantation: results of a randomised double blind placebo controlled study. *Int J Cardiol.* 2004;94:235–240.

64. Kobashigawa JA, Katznelson S, Laks H, et al. Effect of pravastatin on outcomes after cardiac transplantation. *N Engl J Med.* 1995;333:621–627.

65. Wenke K, Meiser B, Thiery J, et al. Simvastatin initiated early after heart transplantation: 8-year prospective experience. *Circulation.* 2003;107:93–97.

66. Holdaas H, Fellstrom B, Jardine AG, et al. Effect of fluvastatin on cardiac outcomes in renal transplant recipients: a multicentre, randomised, placebo-controlled trial. *Lancet.* 2003;361:2024–2031.

67. Cosio FG, Pesavento TE, Pelletier RP, et al. Patient survival after renal transplantation III: the effects of statins. *Am J Kidney Dis.* 2002;40:638–643.

68. Del Castillo D, Cruzado JM, Manel DJ, et al. The effects of hyperlipidaemia on graft and patient outcome in renal transplantation. *Nephrol Dial Transplant.* 2004;19 (Suppl 3):iii67–iii71.

69. Chin C, Gamberg P, Miller J, Luikart H, Bernstein D. Efficacy and safety of atorvastatin after pediatric heart transplantation. *J Heart Lung Transplant.* 2002;21:1213–1217.

70. Mahle WT, Vincent RN, Berg AM, Kanter KR. Pravastatin therapy is associated with reduction in coronary allograft vasculopathy in pediatric heart transplantation. *J Heart Lung Transplant.* 2005;24:63–66.

71. Argent E, Kainer G, Aitken M, Rosenberg AR, Mackie FE. Atorvastatin treatment for hyperlipidemia in pediatric renal transplant recipients. *Pediatr Transplant.* 2003;7:38–42.

72. Prasad GV, Ahmed A, Nash MM, Zaltzman JS. Blood pressure reduction with HMG-CoA reductase inhibitors in renal transplant recipients. *Kidney Int.* 2003;63:360–364.

73. Borghi C, Dormi A, Veronesi M, Sangiorgi Z, Gaddi A, Brisighella Heart Study Working Party. Association between different lipid-lowering treatment strategies and blood pressure control in the Brisighella Heart Study. *Am Heart J.* 2004;148:285–292.

74. Tsiara S, Elisaf M, Mikhailidis DP. Early vascular benefits of statin therapy (Review). *Curr Med Res Opin.* 2003;19:540–556.

75. Mach F. Statins as immunomodulatory agents. *Circulation.* 2004;109:II15-II17.

76. Fehr T, Kahlert C, Fierz W, et al. Statin-induced immunomodulatory effects on human T cells in vivo. *Atherosclerosis.* 2004;175:83–90.

77. Prasad GV, Chiu R, Nash MM, Zaltzman JS. Statin use and bone mineral density in renal transplant recipients. *Am J Transplant.* 2003;3:1320–1321.

78. Wang GJ, Cui Q, Balian G. The Nicolas Andry award. The pathogenesis and prevention of steroid-induced osteonecrosis. *Clin Orthop Relat Res.* 2000;295–310.

79. Hingorani S. Chronic kidney disease in long-term survivors of hematopoietic cell transplant: epidemiology, pathogenesis and treatment. *J Am Soc Nephrol.* 2006;17:1995–2005.

80. Vincent F, Costa MA, Rondeau E. Chronic renal failure: a non-malignant late effect of allogeneic stem cell transplantation (Letter to the Editor). *Blood.* 2003;102:2695–2696.

81. Barnett AH, Bain SC, Bouter P, et al. Angiotensin-receptor blockade versus converting-enzyme inhibition in type 2 diabetes and nephropathy [erratum appears in *N Engl J Med.* 2005 Apr 21;352(16)1731]. *N Engl J Med.* 2004;351:1952–1961.

82. Strippoli GF, Craig M, Deeks JJ, Schena FP, Craig JC. Effects of angiotensin converting enzyme inhibitors and angiotensin II receptor antagonists on mortality and renal outcomes in diabetic nephropathy: systematic review (Review). *BMJ.* 2004;329:828.

83. Hingorani SR, Aneja T, Seidel K, Lindner A, McDonald G. Albuminuria in hematopoietic cell transplant (HCT) patients: prevalence and risk factors. *J Am Soc Nephrol.* 17, 218a, #TH-PO818. 2006. (Abstract)

84. Rocchini AP. Childhood obesity and a diabetes epidemic. *N Engl J Med.* 2002;346:854–855.

85. Silink M. Childhood diabetes: a global perspective. *Horm Res.* 2002;57 (Suppl 1):1–5.

86. Strauss R. Perspectives on childhood obesity. *Curr Gastroenterol Rep.* 2002;4:244–250.

87. Vexiau P, Perez-Castiglioni P, Socié G, et al. The 'euthyroid sick syndrome': incidence, risk factors and prognostic value soon after allogeneic bone marrow transplantation. *Br J Haematol.* 1993;85:778–782.

88. Karthaus M, Gabrysiak T, Brabant G, et al. Immune thyroiditis after transplantation of allogeneic CD34+ selected peripheral blood cells. *Bone Marrow Transplant.* 1997;20:697–699.

89. Lee V, Cheng PS, Chik KW, Wong GW, Shing MM, Li CK. Autoimmune hypothyroidism after unrelated haematopoietic stem cell transplantation in children. *J Pediatr Hematol Oncol.* 2006;28:293–295.

90. Patriarca F, Skert C, Sperotto A, et al. The development of autoantibodies after allogeneic stem cell transplantation is related with chronic graft-vs-host disease and immune recovery. *Exp Hematol.* 2006;34:389–396.

91. Lortan JE, Rochfort NC, el Tumi M, Vellodi A. Autoantibodies after bone marrow transplantation in children with genetic disorders: relation to chronic graft-versus-host disease. *Bone Marrow Transplant.* 1992;9:325–330.

92. *Textbook of Pediatrics.* 15th ed. Philadelphia: W.B. Saunders Company, 1996.

93. Powell GF, Brasel JA, Blizzard RM. Emotional deprivation and growth retardation simulating idiopathic hypopituitarism. I. Clinical evaluation of the syndrome. *N Engl J Med.* 1967;276:1271–1278.

94. Powell GF, Brasel JA, Raiti S, Blizzard RM. Emotional deprivation and growth retardation simulating idiopathic hypopituitarism. II. Endocrinologic evaluation of the syndrome. *N Engl J Med.* 1967;276:1279–1283.

95. Albanese A, Hamill G, Jones J, Skuse D, Matthews DR, Stanhope R. Reversibility of physiological growth hormone secretion

in children with psychosocial dwarfism. *Clin Endocrinol.* 1994;40:687–692.

96. Allen DB, Julius JR, Breen TJ, Attie KM. Treatment of glucocorticoid-induced growth suppression with growth hormone. National Cooperative Growth Study. *J Clin Endocrinol Metab.* 1998;83:2824–2829.

97. Tejani A, Butt KM, Rajpoot D, et al. Strategies for optimizing growth in children with kidney transplants. *Transplantation.* 1989;47:229–233.

98. Broyer M, Guest G, Gagnadoux MF. Growth rate in children receiving alternate-day corticosteroid treatment after kidney transplantation. *J Pediatr.* 1992;120:721–725.

99. Reimer LG, Morris HG, Ellis EF. Growth of asthmatic children during treatment with alternate-day steriods. *J Allergy Clin Immunol.* 1975;55:224–231.

100. Kamel A, Norgren S, Elimam A, Danielsson P, Marcus C. Effects of growth hormone treatment in obese prepubertal boys. *J Clin Endocrinol Metab.* 2000;85:1412–1419.

27

OTHER MANIFESTATIONS OF CHRONIC GRAFT VERSUS HOST DISEASE

Kristin Baird and Andrew L. Gilman

INTRODUCTION

Chronic graft versus host disease (cGVHD) is a multisystem alloimmune and autoimmune disorder characterized by immune dysregulation, immunodeficiency, impaired organ function, and decreased survival. cGVHD is characterized by the development of features reminiscent of various autoimmune or immunologic disorders, such as scleroderma, Sjogren's syndrome, chronic immunodeficiency, and bronchiolitis obliterans. cGVHD typically involves the skin and dermal appendages, mouth, eyes, genitalia, gastrointestinal tract, liver, lungs, musculoskeletal system, and hematopoietic system. More rarely, cGVHD can involve the heart or kidneys, or manifest as vasculitis, serositis, or myasthenia gravis (MG). These unusual manifestations are rare and other causes such as drug toxicity and postirradiation effects should be considered.

MYASTHENIA GRAVIS

Incidence

Myasthenia gravis is an autoimmune disease resulting from the production of autoantibodies that bind to the acetylcholine receptor (anti-AchR Ab) of the neuromuscular endplate. This binding causes impaired transmission at the neuromuscular junction, leading to skeletal muscle weakness and fatigue. Despite the fact that approximately 20% of patients with cGVHD show anti-AchR Ab [1, 2], the frequency of clinically apparent MG after hematopoietic stem cell transplantation (HSCT) is relatively low. There are only a few case reports describing MG following HSCT in the literature [3–17]. MG has been reported as far out as 9 years following HSCT [17] and only one patient has developed MG without evidence of cGVHD [11]. MG has been reported in children [8, 13] as well as adults and there appears to be no gender predilection [17]. Currently there are no markers that indicate which patients are at most risk of developing MG, although the development of MG may be associated with patients transplanted for aplastic anemia [18], patients that express human leukocyte antigen (HLA) Cw1,

Cw7, and DR2 antigens [17], and increased peripheral blood OX40 + CD4+ T-cell concentration [16].

Clinical Course

In 1997 Mackey et al. reported the case of a 23-year-old female who developed MG 100 months post allo-HSCT after discontinuation of immunosuppression for cGVHD. Originally, the patient's cGVHD involved the skin, gastrointestinal tract, and lacrimal glands. Eleven months after discontinuing immunosuppression, the patient developed severe, progressive dysphagia initially attributed to esophageal candidiasis. The patient went on to develop muscle weakness, ptosis, and dysphonia. The diagnosis of MG was confirmed by elevated anti-AchR Ab's and a positive edrophonium challenge. The patient was initially treated with prednisone and pyridostigmine to which she responded. A thymectomy was performed and did not reveal evidence of thymoma. The patient required maintenance immunosuppression with prednisone to control symptoms. This case exemplifies the typical features of MG post allo-HSCT. The onset of clinical symptoms usually develops after decreasing or discontinuing immunosuppression. Other typical features include the presence of cGVHD, positive anti-AchR Ab's, and the absence of an associated thymoma. They also identified that HLA Cw1, Cw7, and DR2 were found at increased frequencies above that expected from HLA-antigen prevalence studies, and may be markers for increased risk of developing MG. Interestingly, these are not the HLA antigens associated with idiopathic MG. Reinstitution of immunosuppression and standard therapies for MG were effective in this case, as occurs in the majority of these patients [17].

CASE VIGNETTE 1

A 14-year-old female with aplastic anemia had an HLA identical matched sibling marrow transplant from her sister. GVHD prophylaxis included cyclosporine and methotrexate. She tolerated the transplant well with no significant peri-transplant complications other than grade II skin aGVHD, which responded well to a short course of steroids. Five months following transplant, approximately 6 weeks following discontinuation of all immunosuppression, the patient developed erythematous skin changes, lichenoid oral mucosal changes, and dry eyes. She was reinitiated on steroid therapy and cyclosporine. Symptoms were well controlled; however, the patient's symptoms flared with each attempt to wean steroids. The patient continued steroid therapy for an additional 12 months, when they were eventually successfully weaned off. The patient developed increasing fatigue and muscle weakness during the steroid wean, which was thought to be secondary to a steroid-induced myopathy and the pace of her wean was heightened. Approximately 2 weeks after her steroids were discontinued the patient presented to the emergency room in respiratory distress. The patient's mother noted that the patient had increasing weakness, clumsiness, and "sleepy eyes" over the past couple of weeks. The diagnosis of myasthenia was suspected and confirmed by elevated anti-AchR Ab's and a positive edrophonium challenge. The patient was treated with prednisone and pyridostigmine to which she responded well.

Diagnosis

The diagnosis of MG is based on clinical suspicion and evaluation of a patient with progressive symptoms of muscle weakness and relies on the presence of elevated anti-AchR Ab's and a positive edrophonium challenge. Diagnosis is further supported by electrodiagnostic testing.

Site-Specific Therapy

Standard treatments for idiopathic MG (i.e., prednisone, pyridostigmine, cyclosporine, azathioprine, and plasmapheresis) appear to work in the allo-HSCT setting as well. There is also one case report of a patient with refractory MG who achieved complete regression of neurological symptoms and disappearance of the anti-AchR Ab's after treatment with Rituximab [19] and one patient successfully treated with mycophenolate mofetil (MMF) [16]. Although there is a strong link between idiopathic MG and thymoma, with approximately 15% of MG patients having thymoma, this association has not been reported post-HSCT. Therefore thymectomy, which is used as treatment for idiopathic MG is not generally recommended in this situation [17, 20].

Prevention

No measures have been reported to prevent the development of MG in association with cGVHD.

Future Directions

Although a rare manifestation, clinical suspicion for MG in the posttransplant setting must remain high, as this can be a serious and fatal complication. More studies are needed to help delineate the risk factors and pathophysiology associated

with the development of MG. Investigators encountering these patients should be vigilant in investigating and reporting these patients. Though not yet investigated in relation to cGVHD, murine models mimicking idiopathic MG exist and may provide a platform on which to model this very unusual complication of cGVHD.

Text Box 27.1 Myasthenia Gravis

Signs and symptoms of myasthenia gravis
- Fatigue
- Muscle weakness
- Dysphagia
- Ptosis
- Diplopia

Recommended myasthenia gravis evaluations
- Serum evaluation for antiacetylcholine receptor antibody
- Edrophonium chloride challenge
- Electromyogram
- Pulmonary functions tests (nondiagnostic)

Treatment for myasthenia gravis (rating)
- Prednisone (BIII)
- Pyridostigmine (AIII)
- Cyclosporine (BIII)
- Azathioprine (BIII)
- Plasmapheresis (BIII)

VASCULITIS

Incidence

The incidence of vasculitis as a manifestation of cGVHD is unknown, but this is a relatively rare entity and has been reported as several case reports and small case series [21–26]. Systemic vasculitis, an inflammatory necrotizing disease that targets the blood vessel walls, can either be idiopathic or more commonly, seen secondary to autoimmune and connective tissue diseases. Vasculitis is also frequently seen as a manifestation of graft rejection in the allograft transplant setting. Several autoimmune diseases which cGVHD mimics, such as systemic Lupus and Sjogren's syndrome, have associated vasculitides. Cell-mediated inflammation, immune complex-mediated inflammation, and autoantibody-mediated inflammation all have been implicated in the initiation of systemic vasculitis [27]. The cause of cGVHD-associated vasculitis is unclear, although arterial changes similar to those found in allograft vasculopathy have been demonstrated in patients with cGVHD [28].

Clinical Course

There does not appear to be uniformity in the development or clinical course of vascular involvement of GVHD. There are only limited reports of systemic vasculitis, which may be due to underreporting of this condition. More commonly, reports of vascular involvement of cGVHD are organ specific, in particular there have been several reports of cerebral vasculitis

[21, 22, 26]. Cerebral vasculitis can be a potentially treatable cause of progressive neurologic decline after HSCT. Padovan et al. described the clinical and diagnostic features of five HSCT patients with cGVHD and suspected cerebral angiitis. Patients presented with focal neurological signs and neuropsychological abnormalities including confusion, aphasia, hemiparesis, seizures, vertigo, and hemianopsia [26]. In most patients, these symptoms occurred approximately 2 years after HSCT [21, 26].

In 2002, Ysebaert et al. reported a case of polyarteritis in an 18-year-old female 2 years following allo-HSCT. The clinical manifestations were similar to those of polyarteritis nodosa (PAN) with several organs involved including life-threatening cardiac and mesenteric problems. The patient had initially developed stage 3 cutaneous acute GVHD (aGVHD), which was successfully treated with steroids. The patient subsequently developed chronic skin and liver GVHD. Over a period of time, the patient developed visual impairment due to central retinal vein occlusion, followed months later by a worsening ischemic syndrome associated with abdominal pain, diarrhea, and weight loss related to thrombosis of the inferior mesenteric artery. Concomitantly, myocardial infarction was documented on coronary arteriography and scintigraphy after ST segment elevation had been noted. The patient also had a painful soft tissue swelling of the left shoulder. Muscle biopsy revealed severe myogenic pathology, with a lymphohistiocytic infiltrate, plasma cell, and eosinophilia associated with angiitis. The patient showed no evidence of immune dysfunction, thrombotic microangiopathy, or a prothrombotic condition. Circulating immune complexes were detected. Of note, there was no evidence of renal or lung impairment. She was treated with intravascular immunoglobulin (IVIG), pulses of methylprednisolone, and azathioprine to which she responded well. The patient was weaned to a maintenance schedule, however, exacerbations in the abdominal angina continued to occur over a 1½ year time period, but responded to short pulse steroid therapy [24].

Diagnosis

Campbell et al. found angiographic changes in one patient with cerebral vasculitis; however, the diagnosis is usually made on clinical presentation and magnetic resonance imaging (MRI) findings. MRI can show periventricular white matter lesions, lacunar or territorial infarctions, leukoencephalopathy, and hemorrhages [21]. A case presented by Ma et al. showed only nonspecific findings on MRI and required histologic confirmation of central nervous system (CNS) granulomatous angiitis in a child [22]. The diagnosis of non-CNS vasculitis is dependent on histopathology.

Site-Specific Therapy

In the Padovan series, three patients received cyclophosphamide and steroids (two improved, one died), one patient improved after steroids alone, and one patient without immunosuppressive

therapy deteriorated further [26]. The patient described by Campbell et al. responded to tacrolimus, which was chosen specifically for greater CNS penetration [21].

Prevention

No measures have been reported to prevent vascular involvement of cGVHD.

Future Directions

In 2002, Biedermann et al. postulated that the development of tissue fibrosis in the setting of cGVHD may be a result of endothelial vascular damage. They hypothesized that cytotoxic T-cell mediated vascular injury leads to progressive loss of microvessels causing tissue ischemia and ultimately tissue fibrosis. They assessed skin biopsy samples for the extent of vascular injury by counting microvessels and for evidence of ongoing immune-mediated vascular injury in patients with acute (n = 9) and chronic (n = 10) GVHD. von Willebrand factor (vWF) was measured in plasma as a possible marker of vascular endothelial cell damage, as vWF is released from endothelial cells when injured. The authors found extensive loss of microvessels in affected target tissues and high concentrations of circulating vWF in patients with both acute and chronic GVHD, when compared to controls status post allo-HSCT without GVHD. They further observed that perivascular CD8 T-cell infiltrates in skin correlated with vWF plasma concentrations in patients with GVHD ($p = 0.01$). Activated cytotoxic T lymphocytes and endothelial injury were also present in the skin biopsy samples. They concluded that vWF is released from vascular endothelial cells injured by cytotoxic T lymphocytes and could serve as an early maker for patients as risk of developing cGVHD [23].

Sostak et al. utilized a murine bone marrow transplantation (BMT) model to investigate the pathophysiology of CNS complications following allo-HSCT. Because of the role of cellular adhesion molecules (CAMs) in the recruitment of leukocytes into the CNS, they evaluated the expression of intercellular adhesion molecule-1 (ICAM-1) and vascular cell adhesion molecule-1 (VCAM-1) on cerebral endothelium following allo-HSCT. They compared this expression to that seen after syngeneic transplantation in both wild-type and ICAM-1-knockout mice. As an indicator of enhanced apoptotic cell death, they examined the cerebral expression of Fas antigen, the occurrence of the poly-ADP (adenosine phosphate) ribose polymerase p85 fragment, and the distribution of TUNEL positive-stained cells. When comparing allogeneic recipients to syngeneic animals without GVHD and unmanipulated controls, the authors found cerebral endothelial upregulation of ICAM-1 and in particular of VCAM-1. Immunohistologic staining showed diffuse brain parenchymal infiltration in the allogeneic recipients, but not in the syngeneic recipients, ICAM-1 – knockout mice or the unmanipulated controls. The parenchymal cellular infiltration consisted primarily of lymphocytes (41%), activated microglial cells (44%), and monocytes (7%). In the allogeneic animals, perivascular infiltration was detectable in 27% of arterioles and in 9% of capillaries, whereas, in controls and syngeneic animals only 2% of vessels were infiltrated. The authors therefore concluded that CAMs, VCAM-1 in particular, may promote leukocyte recruitment into the CNS of animals with cGVHD and may help define the mechanism through which CNS vasculitis occurs [29].

Text Box 27.2 Vasculitis

Signs and symptoms of vasculitis
- ▪ Highly variable and specific to involved organ(s)
  - Cerebral vasculitis: confusion, aphasia, seizures, hemiparesis, vertigo
  - Mesenteric: abdominal pain, weight loss, diarrhea
  - Ocular: impaired vision
  - Renal: hypoproteinemia, hematuria, proteinuria, glomerulonephritis, edema
  - General: muscle and joint pain, rash, fever, fatigue, weakness, headache

Recommended vasculitis evaluations
- ▪ Highly variable and specific to involved organ(s)
  - Biopsy (skin, kidney)
  - MRI
  - CT scan
  - Angiogram
  - Ophthalmologic evaluation
  - Urinalysis

Treatment for vasculitis (rating)
- ▪ Prednisone (BIII)
- ▪ Other immunosuppressants, e.g., tacrolimus, cyclophosphamide (BIII)

SEROSITIS

Incidence

In 1980, Shulman et al. reported the outcomes of a long-term clinicopathologic study of 20 Seattle transplant recipients with cGVHD. On autopsy sections of 4 of 18 patients, they found generalized lymphoplasmacytic serositis and fibrosis in the fibroareolar tissue of the breast, epicardium, aorta, adrenal glands, thyroid capsule, and mesentery. Although they found histopathologic evidence of serosal involvement, the occurrence of clinically evident effusions were not reported [28]. In 1988, the Seattle group further reported the outcomes of a comparison study of prednisone and placebo versus prednisone and azathioprine as early treatment of extensive cGVHD. In this study that evaluated 164 patients, 2% were reported to have serosal involvement [30]. Despite the significant numbers of patients with serosal involvement in this report on patients with cGVHD, the incidence in larger populations of unselected BMT patients was unknown. In 1996, Seber et al. published a large retrospective review of the Minnesota BMT Database over a 20-year period. The authors found only seven of 1905 (0.4%) patients with "unexplained" effusions. They identified those patients with effusions involving two or more of the pleural, pericardial, or peritoneal cavities. Patients with

potential confounding causes of serositis (veno-occlusive disease, infections, cardiac insufficiency, tumor relapse, and GM-CSF toxicity) were excluded. All had the onset of symptoms following engraftment and almost all occurred before day 100. These unexplained multiple effusions were observed in recipients of allogeneic transplants but were not seen with autologous transplants and were found only in patients with acute and/or chronic GVHD. They also noted a strong association with *Cytomegalovirus* (CMV) infection, with five of the seven patients having documented CMV disease (pneumonitis and retinitis). The authors concluded that multiple effusions appear to be part of the presentation of severe acute or chronic GVHD [31]. The majority of cases in the literature are isolated case reports and small case series 32–38. Several studies have identified serositis (with or without) vascular leak syndrome as the sole manifestation of cGVHD [33, 37].

To assess the incidence of pericardial effusion and subsequent cardiac tamponade among pediatric HSCT recipients, Rhodes et al. retrospectively examined cardiac effusions occurring over an 11-year period in their institution. Clinically significant pericardial effusions were identified in 9 of 205 patients (4.4%), two patients (1%) had received autologous transplants, five patients (2.4%) had aGVHD and two patients (1%) had extensive cGVHD at the time of the pericardial effusion [36]. Of note, pericardial effusions are associated with the development of organ rejection in the cardiac transplant setting. Though common in many patients following cardiac transplantation, pericardial effusion is twice as likely in those patients with acute rejection [39].

Clinical Course

In 1997, Toren and Nagler reported an 11-year-old boy 20 months post BMT with extensive cGVHD involving the skin, liver, eyes, and mouth who developed a pericardial effusion in association with severe polyserositis including pleural effusion, ascites, and polyarthritis. The child's course started with a several kilogram weight gain and dyspnea. On examination, the patient had abdominal distension and tenderness, tachypnea, tachycardia, distant heart sounds with a pulsus paradoxus, bilateral dullness on percussion, and decreased air entry on both sides. The patient also developed acute arthritis of the major joints. Electrocardiogram (ECG) showed low QRS complexes with flattened T waves. Echocardiogram demonstrated a massive pericardial effusion. Chest x-rays revealed bilateral pleural effusions. Abdominal computerised tomography (CT) scan revealed a moderate amount of ascites. Fluid was subsequently drained from the pericardium, pleural space, and joints. The pericardial fluid had exudative characteristics with fluid/serum dehydrogenase (LDH) ratio of 0.64 and fluid/serum albumin levels of 0.68. Glucose level was 6 mmol/l, protein 4 g/dL, WBC 350 cells/mm³ with no malignant cells. Cultures for bacteria, fungi, tuberculosis, and viruses were all negative. The pleural and synovial fluids had similar characteristics. He was treated with corticosteroids and partially responded with a decrease in fluid content in all involved sites [32].

Following this previous report several additional case reports have followed. In 2000, Ueda et al. presented the case of a 10-year-old girl presenting with massive pericardial/pleural effusion with anasarca 216 days after HSCT as the sole manifestation of cGVHD. The patient had elevated antinucleolar antibody in the blood and the pleural fluid. Additionally, the lymphocytes in the effusions were mostly CD8+/HLA-DR+, and a majority of CD8+ cells in the blood expressed CD57. These data supported that the patient was manifesting cGVHD despite lacking classical diagnostic findings of cGVHD. In this patient, immunosuppressive therapy including prednisolone, cyclosporine A, high-dose methylprednisolone, tacrolimus, and methotrexate had no effect, and the patient subsequently died of infectious complications. Although it had not been previously described, the authors concluded that isolated serositis with edema should be recognized as a clinical feature of cGVHD [33].

Diagnosis

When clinically suspected, effusions can be confirmed by several imaging modalities including ultrasound, echocardiogram, chest x-ray (pleural effusions), and CT scanning. Other causes of serositis must be excluded and can include infection, malignant effusion, veno-occlusive disease, hepatic/portal thromboembolism, and cardiac insufficiency.

Site-Specific Therapy

Mechanical removal of the fluid, when clinically indicated, through pericardiocentesis, pleuracentesis, and paracentesis. Of the nine patients reported in the Rhodes pediatric series, seven patients (78%) required pericardiocentesis or surgical creation of a pericardial window. No patient died as a complication of the effusion or the therapeutic procedures [36]. Immunosuppression using prednisone alone or with other agents (tacrolimus) has been shown to result in partial or complete resolution of pericardial effusions [32, 36–38] but not in all cases [33, 35]. One patient treated with methylprednisolone and tacrolimus had rapid response of skin GVHD and resolution of the pericardial effusion. In addition, the investigators found reductions in cytokine levels [38].

Prevention

No measures have been reported to prevent the development of serositis in patients with cGVHD.

Future Directions

The true incidence and clinical impact of serositis in the cGVHD setting is unknown. Clinically significant pericardial effusions appear to be more common than previously reported in pediatric HSCT recipients, although they are more frequently seen in the setting of aGVHD [36]. In 2005, Saito et al. reported that the pericardial fluid of their patient contained numerous

CD8+/HLA-DR+ lymphocytes. Tumor necrosis factor-α (TNF-α) and sFas were also significantly elevated in the patient's serum and pericardial fluid, while interferon-γ (IFN-γ), interleukin (IL)-2, IL-4, and IL-10 were undetectable. This cytokine profile differs from that seen in infectious pericarditis, where levels of IFN-γ, IL-2, IL-10, and TNF-α are typically high. Their review of several published case reports and their own case revealed that patients with pericardial cGVHD uniformly show high antinuclear antibody (ANA) titers. They note that Ueda et al. also reported lymphocytes found in the pericardial fluid from their patient were predominantly CD8+/HLA-DR+ [33]. Pericardial cGVHD is a rare but potentially fatal complication and can be difficult to distinguish from infection. The authors concluded that cytotoxic T cells play a role in inducing pericarditis in cGVHD and that evaluation of pericardial fluid, especially lymphocyt and cytokine profiles, may provide useful information in diagnosing and monitoring disease activity [38].

Text Box 27.3 Serositis

Signs and symptoms of serositis
- Dyspnea
- Tachypnea
- Tachycardia
- Chest pain
- Weight gain
- Abdominal pain or distension
- Edema

Recommended serositis evaluations
- Chest x-ray
- Echocardiogram
- ECG
- CT scan
- Ultrasound
- Laboratory evaluation of effusion for cytology and culture to rule out recurrent malignancy or infection, when indicated

Treatment for serositis (rating)
- Pericardiocentisis, pleuracentesis, or paracentesis when clinically indicated
- Creation of a pericardial window when clinically indicated
- Prednisone (BIII)
- Other immunosuppressants (tacrolimus) (BIII)

CARDIAC INVOLVEMENT

Incidence

Cardiac involvement associated with cGVHD has been reported in single patient case reports and one case series [40–45]. Cardiac involvement is likely rare, but there is no prospective data collection currently available to provide a determination of the incidence. Of note, almost all cases reported to date are in children. It is unclear if children are more at risk for this complication, or if cardiac involvement has been more readily recognized in children because they are much less likely to have cardiac disease due to other causes than adults.

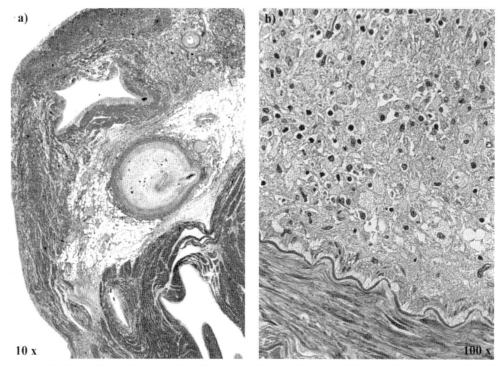

Figure 27.1 Figure shows atherosis with a fibrous cap of connective tissue. Masson trichrome stain of A: left coronary artery showing significant concentric luminal narrowing due to intimal proliferation of foamy macrophages (atherosis cells); B: higher magnification showing inflammatory cells and mesenchymal cells. Reprinted by permission from Macmillan Publishers Ltd: Bone Marrow Transplantation, 2004 [44].

Presentation

Cardiac involvement that has been reported with cGVHD has included arrhythmias [40, 41], myocarditis [42, 43], and coronary artery disease [44, 45]. Although these manifestations are rare and there is skepticism as to whether these manifestations are related to GVHD, there are two facts that strongly support such a link. First, the manifestations and histological findings described with cGVHD are very similar to those reported with graft rejection after cardiac transplantation. In particular, chronic cardiac allograft rejection has been associated with bradyarrhythmias and coronary artery disease [46, 47]. Second, most cases of arrhythmias associated with cGVHD resolved with steroid therapy, and several recurred following weaning of immunosuppression and improved again after increasing immunosuppression. Pericardial effusion is a well-described manifestation of polyserositis associated with cGVHD [31] and is discussed previously.

Ten patients have been reported with bradyarrhythmias that occurred with aGVHD (aGVHD) or with acute flares of cGVHD [41, 42]. Eight of the ten had bradycardia and cGVHD. Bradyarrhythmias occurred from 1 week to 17 months (median 3 months) after transplant. Three patients had asymptomatic mild bradycardia. Three patients had moderate bradycardia, which was asymptomatic in one, associated with worsening hypoxia in one, and associated with intermittent

lightheadedness in one. Two patients had complete heart block and one had sinus node failure. The patients with complete heart block presented with rapid progression of bradycardia. The patient with sinus node failure had significant but asymptomatic bradycardia for days prior to onset, and sinus node failure was precipitated by induction of anesthesia for surgery.

Coronary artery disease has been reported in two patients [44, 45]. Both had sudden death. The only prior suggestion of a cardiac problem was persistent tachycardia in one patient. Histological findings included marked concentric luminal narrowing due to intimal proliferation of foamy macrophages and new connective tissue and slight perivascular cellular infiltrates (Figure 27.1). These findings are similar to those reported in graft rejection after cardiac transplantation [47].

Three patients with lymphocytic infiltrates of the myocardium (myocarditis) in association with cGVHD have been reported. One patient had lymphohistiocytic infiltrates of the atrial and ventricular myocardium associated with myocardial necrosis and scarring [42]. This patient also had complete heart block (discussed in the preceding text) associated with lymphohistiocytic infiltrates of the atrioventricular node, bundle of His, and right and left bundle branches. One patient had myocardiolysis and sudden death. Histology showed mild lymphocytic infiltration and recent microthrombi in cardiac capillaries. Lymphocytic infiltrates with endothelial damage and thrombi are also seen in graft rejection after cardiac transplantation [48]. A third patient presented with dyspnea and had a left ventricular restrictive filling pattern associated with left ventricular wall thickening and focal hypodense areas by MRI. The hypodense areas were felt to represent lymphocytic infiltrates and resolved with an increase in steroid dose [43]. Of note, there are two reports of massive lymphocytic infiltration and myocardial cell necrosis with aGVHD, one manifested by low cardiac output syndrome and both associated with ventricular fibrillation and sudden death [49, 50]. One of the patients had lymphocytic infiltration of the atrioventricular node as well. Interestingly, in cardiac transplantation, acute graft rejection is associated with tachyarrhythmias and chronic graft rejection is associated with bradyarrhythmias [46]. This may parallel the manifestations described in patients with GVHD.

Significance for Prognosis and Clinical Course

Patients that presented with bradyarrhythmias had variable courses, ranging from persistent asymptomatic bradycardia to complete heart block and sinus node failure resulting in cardiac arrest. All patients with bradyarrhythmias were treated with steroids or increased immunosuppression for other manifestations of GVHD, and most had resolution of bradycardia, occurring within 2 to 16 days. The patient with sinus node failure and one patient with complete heart block had complete recovery following intensification of immunosuppression. The former required treatment with beta agonists temporarily, and the latter had a temporary pacemaker until recovery. The other patient with complete heart block had a permanent pacemaker placed, so recovery could not be assessed. The occurrence of bradycardia did not appear to impact the course of GVHD except for the more severely affected patients. However, the presence of bradycardia correlated with GVHD activity and appeared to serve as an easily assessed manifestation for the evaluation of disease response and exacerbation.

Two patients with myocarditis died from this complication, one with sudden death. The other patient had complete resolution with an increase in steroid dose. Both patients with coronary artery disease had sudden death.

CASE VIGNETTE 2

A 4-month-old boy with severe combined immunodeficiency had a T cell-depleted BMT from his haplo-identical father. He had hyperacute GVHD of the skin and GI tract that was associated with fever, respiratory failure, and low output cardiac failure. All of this resolved with immunosuppression. Two months after transplant, he had rapid tapering of his immunosuppression, followed by rash, emesis, diarrhea, hypoxia, and fever. He had progression of GVHD despite an increase in his steroid dose. On day +72 after BMT, he developed intermittent second degree heart block that rapidly progressed to complete atrioventricular block. He had several episodes of asystole, and he required beta agonists to maintain an adequate ventricular heart rate. His methylprednisolone dose was increased to 6 mg kg/day. He had a temporary pacemaker placed on day +74. He had a normal sinus rhythm intermittently on day +78, and his rhythm became normal on day +79. His GVHD resolved. His pacemaker was removed. He never had recurrence of arrhythmias and has done well since.

Diagnosis

Patients with bradyarrhythmias should be evaluated for other causes of arrhythmias including electrolyte abnormalities, drug toxicity, viral infections, and fungal infections involving the coronary arteries [41]. The presence of a viral infection doesn't exclude the presence of concurrent GVHD involvement, as viral infections are known to be associated with GVHD [51, 52]. An association of viral infections (adenovirus, CMV, and enterovirus) with graft rejection and coronary artery disease has also been reported after cardiac transplantation [53]. In rare cases of patients with bradycardia without other manifestations of cGVHD, electrophysiological testing, and endomyocardial biopsy to look for lymphocytic infiltrates could be considered. Another possible approach would be a therapeutic trial of steroid therapy to see if the bradycardia resolves. The use of this approach depends on the likelihood of another cause in a given patient.

Standard cardiac evaluation of patients with cardiac symptoms is prudent in patients after stem cell transplantation, even those without obvious risk factors, because coronary artery disease and myocarditis has been associated with cGVHD.

Site-Specific Therapy

No site-specific therapy has been reported.

Prevention

No measures have been reported to prevent cardiac involvement by cGVHD.

Future

An interesting report of a murine GVHD model demonstrated that the programmed death-1(PD-1)/PD-1 ligand pathway is involved in suppressing alloreactivity of heart infiltrating T cells [54]. There was a significantly increased expression of PD-1 ligand in the heart compared to the ileum. PD-1 ligand expression on lymphoid cells, endothelial cells, and dendritic cells in the heart was upregulated during GVHD. This could explain why cardiac involvement with GVHD is so uncommon.

Also, TNF has been suggested to play a role in cardiac manifestations associated with cGVHD [41]. A patient has been reported whose bradycardia responded to infliximab (Remicade, Centocor, Malvern, PA, USA) [41].

Text Box 27.4 Cardiac cGVHD

Signs and symptoms of cardiac cGVHD
- Fatigue
- Edema
- Dyspnea
- Tachypnea
- Tachycardia
- Arrythmias (sinus bradycardia, sinus node failure, atrio-ventricular block)
- ECG changes associated with coronary artery disease (occlusion)
- Myocarditis (+/− thrombi in myocardial capillaries)

Recommended cardiac evaluations
- Chest x-ray
- Echocardiogram
- ECG
- Consider endomyocardial biopsy

Treatment for cardiac cGVHD (rating)
- Prednisone (BIII)
- Other immunosuppressants (infliximab) (BIII)
- Supportive care (i.e., antihypertensives, afterload reducers, antiarrhythmics)

RENAL INVOLVEMENT

Incidence

Renal impairment has been found in 41% of HSCT patients at 1 year, in 31% at 3 years and in 11% 7 years after HSCT. This impairment is seen in autologous and allogeneic transplant recipients and in some reports is highly associated with total-body irradiation (TBI) exposure [55]. The Seattle group recently published a large cohort study identifying risk factors associated with chronic kidney disease among long-term survivors of HSCT. They reviewed 1,635 patients who survived minimally to day +131 post transplant. Chronic kidney disease was defined as a glomerular filtration rate <60 mL/min/m² on two occasions separated by at least 30 days between days 100 and 540 post transplant. They found that 376 patients (23%) developed chronic kidney disease at a median of 191 days post transplant. They found increased risk of chronic kidney disease with acute renal failure, aGVHD and cGVHD. This group, however, did not find TBI to be associated with chronic kidney disease [56].

Despite the high rates of renal dysfunction post HSCT, renal involvement of cGVHD was thought to be quite rare and has not been widely recognized. Until recently, there had been only several small sporadic case series of renal involvement in cGVHD, with a reported incidence of GVHD-induced nephrotic syndrome (NS) occurring in less than 1% of transplant patients [57]. Recently, however, two larger retrospective studies have reported much higher cumulative incidences of GVHD-induced NS of 6.1% [58] and 8% [59], suggesting this manifestation may be more frequently encountered than previously thought. The first of these studies found that all patients who developed NS had received nonmyeloablative conditioning, whereas, patients receiving myeloablative transplants at

the same institute during the same period had no reported NS. These patients suffered significant morbidity including thromboembolic complications and progressive renal failure and were unlikely to respond to immunosuppression [58]. The second study found no differences between conditioning regimens, but rather saw an association with stem cell source with an increased probability of NS in patients receiving with peripheral blood stem cells (PBSCs) versus bone marrow (BM). All patients in this study responded to immunosuppressive therapy [59].

Clinical Course

Renal GVHD clinically manifests as glomerular lesions with NS. This type of renal disease is a distinct entity from the nephropathy that develops as a result of renal injury that commonly occurs with HSCT or from cumulative toxic insult. In 2006, Brukamp et al. described four cases of renal involvement of cGVHD from their institution and performed an extensive review of the literature. They evaluated 42 cases in the literature that linked allogeneic HSCT and glomerular kidney disease. What they observed was a close temporal association between the development of NS to the cessation of immunosuppression and to the diagnosis of cGVHD. The reviewed cases described several glomerular histologies and included membranous glomerulonephritis (MGN) in approximately two-thirds of patients and minimal change disease (MCD) in nearly one quarter of patients. Glomerular disease was associated with GVHD in nearly half of patients overall and NS followed the diagnosis of GVHD within 5 months in 60% of cases. A decrease in immunosuppressive medication was linked to NS occurrence within 9 months in 63% of patients. Of the two histologies, MCD occurred earlier after HSCT, was diagnosed sooner after weaning of immunosuppression, and exhibited a better prognosis in comparison with MGN [60]. Colombo et al. described six patients who developed NS following HSCT, with a median time to onset of 23 months. The most commonly reported symptoms were fatigue and lower extremity edema. Patient evaluations revealed hypoalbuminemia with creatinine within the normal range. This time of onset was within the range reported throughout the literature, which ranges from 4 to 34 months [59].

The largest case series from Reddy et al. reported the development of NS in 9 patients of 896 HSCT recipients (1% overall incidence, 1.8% incidence in those patients with cGVHD). The development of the NS symptoms (progressive edema and nephrotic range proteinuria) was a late-occurring event with a median onset of approximately 24 months post HSCT. The amount of proteinuria in 24-hour urine collections ranged from 3.6 to 27 grams. Seven of the nine patients also had evidence of hypercholesterolemia at the time NS was diagnosed. A detailed analysis of the coagulation factors was performed in two patients and both were negative at the time of diagnosis and no thrombotic complications were reported in this study. Serum albumin levels ranged from 1.1 to 2.4g/dL. Seven patients had previously been diagnosed and treated for symptomatic cGVHD before the development of NS. However, two patients developed NS without clinical evidence of cGVHD. Of the seven patients who had a history of cGVHD, all had either completed or were in the process of tapering immunosuppression at the onset of NS. Eight of the patients had hypertension requiring therapeutic intervention at the time of onset of NS or upon the initiation of corticosteroids. All patients responded to therapy (rituximab in two patients, corticosteroids +/− additional immunosuppression in the remainder). Two patients died from infectious complications [61].

Diagnosis

Because of the high incidence of multifactorial renal dysfunction in HSCT patients, it is important to delineate the effects of cGVHD on the kidney. The diagnosis of cGVHD in the kidney is based on clinical findings of peripheral edema, laboratory evidence of proteinuria and hypoalbuminemia, and biopsy-proven, histological confirmation whenever possible.

Site-Specific Therapy

In the majority of reported cases in the literature, NS is typically responsive to therapy with most patients showing complete responses. The backbone of the treatment regime consists of corticosteroids with or without other immunosuppressant therapy (cyclosporine, MMF, rituximab, and chlorambucil) [59, 61–63].

The case series published in 2005 by Srinivasan et al. is the one study that showed poor response to immunosuppression. This group of patients, overall, had a high incidence of NS (6.1%) with a median onset of 318 days post HSCT. These patients all received a nonmyeloablative conditioning regimen. Of the four patients biopsied, all had histologies of membranous nephropathy with immune complex deposition along the glomerular basement membrane. Only two of seven patients with NS had complete responses to immunosuppression and three patients developed progressive renal failure [58].

Prevention

No measures have been reported to prevent renal involvement by cGVHD.

Future Directions

The specific pathophysiology of this manifestation of cGVHD is unclear thus far and warrants further investigation. Renal involvement in cGVHD is more commonly seen in murine allograft models than in humans. However, the pathologic findings in both humans and mice are similar. There is evidence of immune complex deposition comparable to renal manifestations of autoimmune diseases such as systemic lupus [64]. Humoral immunity and B-cell dysregulation are thought to be an important component in the development of NS, but whether this is primarily an antibody mediated phenomenon,

or whether this is a consequence of allo-reactive T cells is unknown. T-cell infiltration [65] and high levels of INF-γ and TNF-α have been associated with the development of NS [66].

Text Box 27.5 Renal cGVHD

Signs and symptoms of renal cGVHD
- Fatigue
- Edema
- Hypoproteinemia/hypoalbumenia
- Glomerulonephritis, hematuria, proteinuria

Recommended renal evaluations
- Serum creatinine
- Urinalysis
- Serum proteins
- Consider renal biopsy

Treatment for renal cGVHD (rating)
- Prednisone (BIII)
- Other immunosuppressants, e.g., tacrolimus, cyclosporine, mycophenylate mofetil, rituximab (BIIIa,b)

RETROPERITONEAL FIBROSIS

Incidence

There has been only a single case report of retroperitoneal fibrosis reported in the literature occurring in 36-year-old female patient following HSCT [67].

Clinical Course

In nontransplanted patients, retroperitoneal fibrosis is a rare disorder characterized by an excess of fibrous tissue, which typically surrounds the abdominal aorta and the iliac arteries, and extends into the retroperitoneum enveloping neighboring structures such as the ureters. Retroperitoneal fibrosis is generally idiopathic, but can also be secondary to the use of certain drugs, malignant diseases, infections, and surgery. Idiopathic disease is thought to be a manifestation of a systemic autoimmune or inflammatory disease. Steroids are normally used to treat idiopathic retroperitoneal fibrosis, although, other immunosuppressants are available [68]. The disorder may cause chronic unilateral or bilateral obstructive uropathy, which occurs when the fibrous mass blocks the ureters, and may ultimately lead to end-stage renal failure. Symptoms include dull pain in the abdomen that may increase with time, lower extremity edema, decreased lower extremity circulation leading to pain and discoloration, and possibly severe abdominal pain with hemorrhage due to ischemic bowel. Symptoms that can occur later as the condition progresses includes decreased urine output, anuria, with subsequent nausea, vomiting, and mental status changes associated with renal failure.

The patient reported by Nanda et al. presented after conditioning with TBI, cyclophosphamide, and Ara-C. Her initial posttransplant course was complicated by acute low grade skin GVHD and hemorrhagic cystitis, which required nephrostomy tubes and ureteral stents. Subsequently, the patient developed persistent nausea and vomiting, multiple urinary tract infections, and renal insufficiency. A CT scan revealed ureteral compression secondary to retroperitoneal fibrosis. The patient was eventually successfully treated with coticosteroids [67].

Diagnosis

The diagnosis of retroperitoneal fibrosis is made by a combination of evaluations. Patients will present with elevated serum BUN and creatinine. The diagnosis is confirmed by radiographic imaging. Hydronephrosis and a mass can be visualized by renal ultrasound. However, an abdominal CT scan or MRI is most likely to confirm the diagnosis.

Site-Specific Therapy

In the case where corticosteroid treatment is ineffective, a biopsy should be done to confirm the diagnosis. If confirmed, other immunosuppressants, such as azathioprine, cyclophosphamide, mycophenolate mofetil, methotrexate, and cyclosporine can be utilized. Although the mechanism of action is unclear, tamoxifen, the nonsteroidal antiestrogen, has been successfully used [69, 70]. When immunosuppression is unsuccessful, surgery, and stents may be needed.

Prevention

No measures have been reported that prevent the development of retroperitoneal fibrosis in patients with cGVHD.

Text Box 27.6 Retroperitoneal Fibrosis

Signs and symptoms of retroperitoneal fibrosis
- Pain
- Weight loss
- Fever
- Nausea and vomiting, anorexia, constipation
- Polyuria/polydipsia
- Oliguria, hematuria
- Hypertension
- Lower extremity edema, thrombophlebitis

Recommended retroperitoneal fibrosis evaluations
- Serum BUN and creatinine
- Renal ultrasound
- Excretory urography
- Biopsy
- Abdominal MRI
- Abdominal CT scan
- Urinalysis

Treatment for retroperitoneal fibrosis (rating)
- Prednisone (BIII)
- Other immunosuppressants (BIII)
- Surgery, ureteral stent placement when clinically indicated- BUN, blood urea nitrogen

CONCLUSIONS

Because of the extreme rarity of these unusual complications, investigators should be vigilant in exploring and reporting these manifestations. Regular monitoring of patients after transplantation must include close follow-up of renal and cardiac function and prompt evaluation should be given to any symptoms of organ dysfunction. In addition, a low threshold of suspicion for cGVHD-associated complications should be employed for these patients whether they manifest other symptoms of cGVHD. In particular, complications that may have other potential causes, such as cardiac manifestations in the older patient or renal insufficiency in a patient on chronic immunosuppression, warrant investigation of cGVHD as a possible causative or contributing factor. In cases where infectious etiologies are reasonably excluded and biopsy may not be possible, a therapeutic trial of steroids would be considered. As is the case in the more commonly encountered cGVHD symptoms, most reported cases of these unusual disease manifestations will be responsive to steroids as well.

REFERENCES

1. Smith CI, Hammarstrom L, Lefvert AK. Bone-marrow grafting induces acetylcholine receptor antibody formation. *Lancet.* 1985;1(8435):978.
2. Smith CI, Norberg R, Moller G, Lonnqvist B, Hammarstrom L. Autoantibody formation after bone marrow transplantation. Comparison between acetylcholine receptor antibodies and other autoantibodies and analysis of HLA and Gm markers. *Eur Neurol.* 1989;29(3):128–134.
3. Smith CI, Aarli JA, Biberfeld P, et al. Myasthenia gravis after bone-marrow transplantation. Evidence for a donor origin. *N Engl J Med.* 1983;309(25):1565–1568.
4. Bolger GB, Sullivan KM, Spence AM, et al. Myasthenia gravis after allogeneic bone marrow transplantation: relationship to chronic graft-versus-host disease. *Neurology.* 1986;36(8):1087–1091.
5. Atkinson K, Bryant D, Delprado W, Biggs J. Widespread pulmonary fibrosis as a major clinical manifestation of chronic graft-versus-host disease. *Bone Marrow Transplant.* 1989;4(1):129–132.
6. Grau JM, Casademont J, Monforte R, et al. Myasthenia gravis after allogeneic bone marrow transplantation: report of a new case and pathogenetic considerations. *Bone Marrow Transplant.* 1990;5(6):435–437.
7. Shimoda K, Gondo H, Harada M, et al. Myasthenia gravis after allogeneic bone marrow transplantation. *Bone Marrow Transplant.* 1994;14(1):155–156.
8. Adams C, August CS, Maguire H, Sladky JT. Neuromuscular complications of bone marrow transplantation. *Pediatr Neurol.* 1995;12(1):58–61.
9. Hayashi M, Matsuda O, Ishida Y, Kida K. Change of immunological parameters in the clinical course of a myasthenia gravis patient with chronic graft-versus-host disease. *Acta Paediatr Jpn.* 1996;38(2):151–155.
10. Zaja F, Barillari G, Russo D, et al. Myasthenia gravis after allogeneic bone marrow transplantation. A case report and a review of the literature. *Acta Neurol Scand.* 1997;96(4):256–259.

11. Baron F, Sadzot B, Wang F, Beguin Y. Myasthenia gravis without chronic GVHD after allogeneic bone marrow transplantation. *Bone Marrow Transplant.* 1998;22(2):197–200.

12. Koski SL, Mackey JR, Mackey DS. Myasthenia gravis post allogeneic bone marrow transplantation revisited. *Bone Marrow Transplant.* 1998;22(4):403–404.

13. Tse S, Saunders EF, Silverman E, et al. Myasthenia gravis and polymyositis as manifestations of chronic graft-versus-host-disease. *Bone Marrow Transplant.* 1999;23(4):397–399.

14. Dowell JE, Moots PL, Stein RS. Myasthenia gravis after allogeneic bone marrow transplantation for lymphoblastic lymphoma. *Bone Marrow Transplant.* 1999;24(12):1359–1361.

15. Yanagihara C, Nakaji K, Tanaka Y, Yabe H, Nishimura Y. A patient of chronic graft-versus-host disease presenting simultaneously with polymyositis and myasthenia gravis. *Rinsho Shinkeigaku.* 2001;41(8):503–506.

16. Kotani A, Takahashi A, Koga H, et al. Myasthenia gravis after allogeneic bone marrow transplantation treated with mycophenolate mofetil monitored by peripheral blood OX40+ CD4+ T cells. *Eur J Haematol.* 2002;69(5–6):318–320.

17. Mackey JR, Desai S, Larratt L, Cwik V, Nabholtz JM. Myasthenia gravis in association with allogeneic bone marrow transplantation: clinical observations, therapeutic implications and review of literature. *Bone Marrow Transplant.* 1997;19(9):939–942.

18. Horowitz MM, Rowlings PA. An update from the International Bone Marrow Transplant Registry and the Autologous Blood and Marrow Transplant Registry on current activity in hematopoietic stem cell transplantation. *Curr Opin Hematol.* 1997;4(6):395–400.

19. Zaja F, Bacigalupo A, Patriarca F, et al. Treatment of refractory chronic GVHD with rituximab: a GITMO study. *Bone Marrow Transplant.* 2007;40(3):273–277.

20. Sherer Y, Shoenfeld Y. Autoimmune diseases and autoimmunity post-bone marrow transplantation. *Bone Marrow Transplant.* 1998;22(9):873–881.

21. Campbell JN, Morris PP. Cerebral vasculitis in graft-versus-host disease: a case report. *AJNR Am J Neuroradiol.* 2005;26(3):654–656.

22. Ma M, Barnes G, Pulliam J, et al. CNS angiitis in graft vs host disease. *Neurology.* 2002;59(12):1994–1997.

23. Biedermann BC, Sahner S, Gregor M, et al. Endothelial injury mediated by cytotoxic T lymphocytes and loss of microvessels in chronic graft versus host disease. *Lancet.* 2002;359(9323):2078–2083.

24. Ysebaert L, Deconinck E, Larosa F, et al. Polyvisceral arteritis in chronic graft-versus-host disease: antiphospholipid-negative thrombotic syndrome mimicking polyarteritis nodosa. *Bone Marrow Transplant.* 2002;29(10):873–874.

25. Selby DM, Rudzki JR, Bayever ES, Chandra RS. Vasculopathy of small muscular arteries in pediatric patients after bone marrow transplantation. *Hum Pathol.* 1999;30(7):734–740.

26. Padovan CS, Bise K, Hahn J, et al. Angiitis of the central nervous system after allogeneic bone marrow transplantation? *Stroke.* 1999;30(8):1651–1656.

27. Guillevin L, Dorner T. Vasculitis: mechanisms involved and clinical manifestations. *Arthritis Res Ther.* 2007;9 (Suppl 2):S9.

28. Shulman HM, Sullivan KM, Weiden PL, et al. Chronic graft-versus-host syndrome in man. A long-term clinicopathologic study of 20 Seattle patients. *Am J Med.* 1980;69(2):204–217.

29. Sostak P, Reich P, Padovan CS, et al. Cerebral endothelial expression of adhesion molecules in mice with chronic graft-versus-host disease. *Stroke.* 2004;35(5):1158–1163.

30. Sullivan KM, Witherspoon RP, Storb R, et al. Prednisone and azathioprine compared with prednisone and placebo for treatment of chronic graft-v-host disease: prognostic influence of prolonged thrombocytopenia after allogeneic marrow transplantation. *Blood.* 1988;72(2):546–554.

31. Seber A, Khan SP, Kersey JH. Unexplained effusions: association with allogeneic bone marrow transplantation and acute or chronic graft-versus-host disease. *Bone Marrow Transplant.* 1996;17(2):207–211.

32. Toren A, Nagler A. Massive pericardial effusion complicating the course of chronic graft-versus-host disease (cGVHD) in a child with acute lymphoblastic leukemia following allogeneic bone marrow transplantation. *Bone Marrow Transplant.* 1997;20(9):805–807.

33. Ueda T, Manabe A, Kikuchi A, et al. Massive pericardial and pleural effusion with anasarca following allogeneic bone marrow transplantation. *Int J Hematol.* 2000;71(4):394–397.

34. Silberstein L, Davies A, Kelsey S, et al. Myositis, polyserositis with a large pericardial effusion and constrictive pericarditis as manifestations of chronic graft-versus-host disease after nonmyeloablative peripheral stem cell transplantation and subsequent donor lymphocyte infusion. *Bone Marrow Transplant.* 2001;27(2):231–233.

35. Ivanov V, Faucher C, Bilger K, et al. Massive ascites of donor T-cell origin in a patient with acute GVHD after a reduced-intensity allograft for CLL. *Bone Marrow Transplant.* 2003;32(9):961–963.

36. Rhodes M, Lautz T, Kavanaugh-Mchugh A, et al. Pericardial effusion and cardiac tamponade in pediatric stem cell transplant recipients. *Bone Marrow Transplant.* 2005;36(2):139–144.

37. Gyger M, Rosenberg A, Shamy A, et al. Vascular leak syndrome and serositis as an unusual manifestation of chronic graft-versus-host disease in nonmyeloablative transplants. *Bone Marrow Transplant.* 2005;35(2):201–203.

38. Saito Y, Matsushima T, Doki N, et al. Pericardial graft vs. host disease in a patient with myelodysplastic syndrome following peripheral blood stem cell transplantation. *Eur J Haematol.* 2005;75(1):65–67.

39. Sun JP, Abdalla IA, Asher CR, et al. Non-invasive evaluation of orthotopic heart transplant rejection by echocardiography. *J Heart Lung Transplant.* 2005;24(2):160–165.

40. Gilman AL, Kooy NW, Atkins DL, et al. Complete heart block in association with graft-versus-host disease. *Bone Marrow Transplant.* 1998;21(1):85–88.

41. Rackley C, Schultz KR, Goldman FD, et al. Cardiac manifestations of graft-versus-host disease. *Biol Blood Marrow Transplant.* 2005;11(10):773–780.

42. Rouah E, Gruber R, Shearer W, Armstrong D, Hawkins EP. Graft-versus-host disease in the central nervous system. A real entity? *Am J Clin Pathol.* 1988;89(4):543–546.

43. Cereda M, Trocino G, Pogliani EM, Schiavina R. A case of cardiac localization of graft-versus-host disease after allogenic bone marrow transplantation. *Ital Heart J.* 2003;4(1):60–63.

44. Prevost D, Taylor G, Sanatani S, Schultz KR. Coronary vessel involvement by chronic graft-versus-host disease presenting as sudden cardiac death. *Bone Marrow Transplant.* 2004;34(7):655–656.

45. Chan KW, Taylor GP, Shepherd JD, Shepherd WE. Coronary artery disease following bone marrow transplantation. *Bone Marrow Transplant.* 1989;4(3):327–330.

46. Park JK, Hsu DT, Hordof AJ, Addonizio LJ. Arrhythmias in pediatric heart transplant recipients: prevalence and association

with death, coronary artery disease, and rejection. *J Heart Lung Transplant*. 1993;12(6 Pt 1):956–964.

47. Addonizio LJ, Hsu DT, Smith CR, Gersony WM, Rose EA. Late complications in pediatric cardiac transplant recipients. *Circulation*. 1990;82(Suppl 5):IV295-IV301.

48. Lower RR, Kosek JC, Kemp VE, et al. Rejection of the cardiac transplant. *Am J Cardiol*. 1969;24(4):492–499.

49. Platzbecker U, Klingel K, Thiede C, et al. Acute heart failure after allogeneic blood stem cell transplantation due to massive myocardial infiltration by cytotoxic T cells of donor origin. *Bone Marrow Transplant*. 2001;27(1):107–109.

50. Roberts SS, Leeborg N, Loriaux M, et al. Acute graft-versus-host disease of the heart. *Pediatr Blood Cancer*. 2006;47(5):624–628.

51. Lonnqvist B, Ringden O, Wahren B, Gahrton G, Lundgren G. Cytomegalovirus infection associated with and preceding chronic graft-versus-host disease. *Transplantation*. 1984;38(5):465–468.

52. Soderberg C, Larsson S, Rozell BL, et al. Cytomegalovirus-induced CD13-specific autoimmunity – a possible cause of chronic graft-vs-host disease. *Transplantation*. 1996;61(4):600–609.

53. Shirali GS, Ni J, Chinnock RE, et al. Association of viral genome with graft loss in children after cardiac transplantation. *N Engl J Med*. 2001;344(20):1498–503.

54. Schilbach K, Schick J, Wehrmann M, et al. PD-1-PD-L1 pathway is involved in suppressing alloreactivity of heart infiltrating t cells during murine GVHD across minor histocompatibility antigen barriers. *Transplantation*. 2007;84(2):214–222.

55. Gronroos MH, Bolme P, Winiarski J, Berg UB. Long-term renal function following bone marrow transplantation. *Bone Marrow Transplant*. 2007;39(11):717–723.

56. Hingorani S, Guthrie KA, Schoch G, Weiss NS, McDonald GB. Chronic kidney disease in long-term survivors of hematopoietic cell transplant. *Bone Marrow Transplant*. 2007;39(4):223–229.

57. Imai H, Oyama Y, Miura AB, Endoh M, Sakai H. Hematopoietic cell transplantation-related nephropathy in Japan. *Am J Kidney Dis*. 2000;36(3):474–480.

58. Srinivasan R, Balow JE, Sabnis S, et al. Nephrotic syndrome: an under-recognised immune-mediated complication of non-myeloablative allogeneic haematopoietic cell transplantation. *Br J Haematol*. 2005;131(1):74–79.

59. Colombo AA, Rusconi C, Esposito C, et al. Nephrotic syndrome after allogeneic hematopoietic stem cell transplantation as a late complication of chronic graft-versus-host disease. *Transplantation*. 2006;81(8):1087–1092.

60. Brukamp K, Doyle AM, Bloom RD, et al. Nephrotic syndrome after hematopoietic cell transplantation: do glomerular lesions represent renal graft-versus-host disease? *Clin J Am Soc Nephrol*. 2006;1(4):685–694.

61. Reddy P, Johnson K, Uberti JP, et al. Nephrotic syndrome associated with chronic graft-versus-host disease after allogeneic hematopoietic stem cell transplantation. *Bone Marrow Transplant*. 2006;38(5):351–357.

62. Oliveira JS, Bahia D, Franco M, et al. Nephrotic syndrome as a clinical manifestation of graft-versus-host disease (GVHD) in a marrow transplant recipient after cyclosporine withdrawal. *Bone Marrow Transplant*. 1999;23(1):99–101.

63. Terrier B, Delmas Y, Hummel A, et al. Post-allogeneic haematopoietic stem cell transplantation membranous nephropathy: clinical presentation, outcome and pathogenic aspects. *Nephrol Dial Transplant*. 2007;22(5):1369–1376.

64. Bruijn JA, van Elven EH, Hogendoorn PC, et al. Murine chronic graft-versus-host disease as a model for lupus nephritis. *Am J Pathol*. 1988;130(3):639–641.

65. Romagnani P, Lazzeri E, Mazzinghi B, et al. Nephrotic syndrome and renal failure after allogeneic stem cell transplantation: novel molecular diagnostic tools for a challenging differential diagnosis. *Am J Kidney Dis*. 2005;46(3):550–556.

66. Seconi J, Watt V, Ritchie DS. Nephrotic syndrome following allogeneic stem cell transplantation associated with increased production of TNF-alpha and interferon-gamma by donor T cells. *Bone Marrow Transplant*. 2003;32(4):447–450.

67. Nanda A, Rizzo JD, Vogelsang GB. A case of retroperitoneal fibrosis in a patient following HSCT. *Bone Marrow Transplant*. 2005;35(11):1125–1126.

68. Vaglio A, Salvarani C, Buzio C. Retroperitoneal fibrosis. *Lancet*. 2006;367(9506):241–251.

69. Clark CP, Vanderpool D, Preskitt JT. The response of retroperitoneal fibrosis to tamoxifen. *Surgery*. 1991;109(4):502–506.

70. Vaglio A, Greco P, Buzio C. Tamoxifen therapy for retroperitoneal fibrosis. *Ann Intern Med*. 2006;144(8):619; author reply 619–620.

28

Psychosocial Issues in Chronic Graft versus Host Disease

Loretta A. Williams and Karen L. Syrjala

OVERVIEW: PSYCHOSOCIAL ISSUES IN CHRONIC GRAFT VERSUS HOST DISEASE

Chronic graft versus host disease (cGVHD) is a serious late complication of allogeneic (allo-) hematopoietic stem cell transplantation (HSCT) and the leading cause of nonrelapse deaths more than 2 years after allo-HSCT. Patients who develop cGVHD have an increased risk of death from complications of cGVHD and its treatment and have an impaired quality of life [1, 2]. cGVHD increases the risk of serious medical conditions such as hypothyroidism, osteoporosis, cardiopulmonary problems, and neurological deficits [2].

HSCT is one of the most stressful treatments in modern cancer care. Changes in life, the impact of long-lasting treatment, and side effects are the greatest sources of stress [3]. Onset of cGVHD further lengthens the treatment window for patients following HSCT [4]. Patients' and caregivers' lives remain disrupted, recovery is delayed, and physical and psychological side effects increase. cGVHD has an unpredictable course with waxing and waning symptoms, unpredictable organ involvement and treatment response, and side effects that may become permanent.

Treatments for cGVHD, such as long-term administration of corticosteroids, photopheresis, calcineurin inhibitors, and other immunosuppressants, can have variable efficacies that contribute to the uncertainty of the disease course [5]. These treatments are associated with physical and psychological side effects that can be more devastating than cGVHD itself.

A number of descriptive studies have reported the long-term consequences and effects of allo-HSCT on quality of life, but few studies have tested interventions to treat negative psychosocial sequelae. Likewise, few studies have focused specifically on psychosocial aspects of cGVHD. Some of the studies of allo-HSCT report the number of patients with cGVHD, but few report the specific psychosocial consequences of cGVHD.

The purpose of this chapter is to report what is currently known about the psychosocial aspects of cGVHD, including effects on a patient's mood, cognitive abilities, and social skills. Patients with cGVHD need help in management of psychological and social issues that they face. Clinicians must understand the psychosocial needs of the patient. In this chapter, interventions that may be useful in treating negative psychosocial consequences of cGVHD will be graded according to the level of evidence supporting their effectiveness.

DEMANDS OF MANAGING CONTINUING TREATMENT AND ITS SIDE EFFECTS

Patients with cGVHD often require ongoing therapy, which may necessitate frequent clinic visits for monitoring or administration, besides increasing the financial burden of HSCT. In addition, cGVHD and side effects from its treatment can further interfere with return to normal activities for patients and their families [6]. Patients may also be reluctant to resume normal activities or plan for the future for fear of their cGVHD worsening unexpectedly or their underlying malignancy returning [7].

Activity Limitations and Work Change

cGVHD is the most significant factor for activity limitations following allo-HSCT [8]. Patients' activities are limited by the need to avoid physical encounters that may activate or worsen cGVHD or increase toxicities associated with the treatment of cGVHD [6]. Outdoor elements, such as sun and wind, can activate or worsen cGVHD of the skin or eyes. Certain medications also increase patient sun-sensitivity. In addition, patients may have dietary restrictions if cGVHD is present in the gastrointestinal (GI) tract or liver, or if patients are receiving certain medications such as monoamine oxidase inhibitors (MAOIs) [5]. In addition, patients may have to forgo activities in which they would normally participate in order to keep physician and treatment appointments [9].

The main killer of patients with cGVHD is bacterial infection [10]. Activity and social restrictions can not only prevent exposure to bacteria but also create distressing feelings of isolation. For many patients, the need to limit attendance at church services and religious functions is especially devastating, because spirituality is often an important source of support for patients [11, 12].

cGVHD and its treatment also limit physical activity by effects on the musculoskeletal system. Prolonged immunosuppressive therapy for cGVHD significantly increases a patient's risk for bone loss and osteoporosis [13]. cGVHD can also decrease range of motion, which further limits activity [5]. Activity limitations impact usual functions including work, social interactions, recreational pursuits, and, when severe, even self-care activities. Loss of the ability to engage in normal activities can cause depression, decreased self-image, loss of self-esteem, and feelings of helplessness and worthlessness [8].

Patients may have difficulty returning to their previous jobs or full-time employment because of physical limitations or cognitive dysfunction from cGVHD and its treatment [9, 14–16]. In addition, the need to be absent from work frequently for physician and clinic appointments can cause problems in the work place for patients [9]. Many patients or caregivers are dependent on continued employment to provide health insurance to meet the expenses of continued treatment as well as income to pay expenses not covered by health insurance. Patients often face employment discrimination because they are not able to function as they previously did [9, 16], because of frequent absences from work, or because of their altered physical appearance. Employment difficulties and uncertainties create stress for patients and their families.

Family Burden

Management of continued therapy for cGVHD and its side effects also places burdens on the patient's family. Family members may miss work because they must care for the patient or accompany the patient to clinic visits. Worry and uncertainty about the effectiveness of therapy, worsening of cGVHD, or disease recurrence are additional stresses for family members as well as patients. Family caregivers report yearning for return to a normal life, which continued therapy and its side effects prevents [17, 18].

Setbacks in Recovery and Sustained Uncertainty about Transplant Outcomes

A hallmark of cGVHD is its variable onset, unpredictable episodes of waxing and waning, and often inconsistent response to therapies. Uncertainty about disease, treatment, and outcomes has been found to be a major predictor of stress for patients [19, 20]. Uncertainty challenges a patient's sense of mastery, confidence, and personal control of a situation leading to emotional distress [21, 22].

REACTIVE EMOTIONS IN RESPONSE TO cGVHD

Pain, isolation, and activity restrictions following HSCT can lead to generalized anxiety [2, 19, 23], mild depression [2, 19], sleep problems [19], and feelings of helplessness, withdrawal, anger, and hostility [2]. The development of cGVHD extends the time that patients are susceptible to these reactions. HSCT recipients have a higher level of mood disturbances when compared to groups of solid tumor cancer patients [24]. In a longitudinal study of transplant survivors, 15% to 25% patients suffered from psychological distress [25]. However, the level of psychological distress is negatively correlated with severity of cGVHD, possibly because patients who have significant physical problems are less aware of feelings and emotions [26].

Patients with cGVHD are at risk for numerous reactive emotional responses depending on personality, situational, disease, and treatment factors. These responses are related and often overlap or take place concurrently. However, research shows that there are differences between them [27], which may have implications for effectively intervening to control these reactions now or in the future. These reactive emotions produce negative moods and psychological distress if not adequately managed [28].

Anxiety

Anxiety is a feeling of fear, dread, or apprehension associated with the expectation of a diffuse and certain danger [29]. Almost 50% of patients report elevated levels of anxiety during the first year post-HSCT [26]. The unpredictability of HSCT is the primary factor in the development of anxiety [19]. Various studies have found that anxiety begins to diminish somewhere between 3 months [14] and 12 months [6] following HSCT, possibly as patients return home and begin to resume normal activities. However, some patients are still reporting increased levels of anxiety up to 10 years post-HSCT [6]. Patients with cGVHD were not found to be at increased risk of experiencing anxiety when compared to patients who never had cGVHD or who had resolved cGVHD [6].

Worry

Worry has been reported as the most prevalent and distressing symptom experienced by patients prior to HSCT [30]. Worry declines in severity following transplant, but patients continue to worry about transplant outcomes such as disease recurrence [31]. Recent research has shown that patients with cancer worry about the future, physical problems and symptoms, and interpersonal problems. Cancer-related worry is distinct from anxiety and depression [27]. Patients with cGVHD face considerable uncertainty about the future, experience numerous physical problems and symptoms, and are at risk for interpersonal problems. Further research is needed to delineate the relationship of cGVHD to worry.

Helplessness

The loss of mastery and sense of control due to an inability to affect disease and treatment outcomes can lead to feelings of helplessness in patients following HSCT. Patients' self-concepts may alter as disease and treatment demands cause lifestyle disruptions. Patients begin to view themselves as ineffective and to feel helpless because of their inability to resume normal activities. cGVHD is correlated with the development of a negative self-concept following HSCT, increasing the chances that patients with cGVHD may experience helpless [32]. Patients who display personality characteristics of self-blame, viewing negative situations as unremitting, and globally attributing negative outcomes to all aspects of life are also more likely to experience helplessness that develops into depression [33].

Uncertainty

Uncertainty is the inability to accurately predict illness outcomes based on a person's subjective interpretation of illness-related events. Situations, such as cGVHD, that are ambiguous, complex, unpredictable, and where information is unavailable or inconsistent frequently lead to uncertainty [28].

Chronic illness places a patient in a situation of unremitting uncertainty [28]. The unpredictability of the HSCT course is a major psychological stressor [19]. All patients post-HSCT face the uncertainty that the graft may fail or that their original disease may recur. Patients without cGVHD do not know if cGVHD may develop. Feelings of uncertainty may decrease with time because the longer the time from HSCT, the less likely these events are to occur.

Patients with cGVHD experience the additional uncertainties of when cGVHD may improve or worsen, what organs might be involved, the extent and permanence of the involvement, what therapy may be needed, and how the disease will respond to treatment. Because cGVHD causes increased functional impairments and activity limitations [5], patients also face the uncertainty about when they may be able to resume normal activities or if they will be able to continue normal activities.

COGNITIVE EFFECTS OF TREATMENT

In general, cancer treatment has negative effects on executive function, verbal memory [34], visual memory, and information-processing speed [35]. Physical problems such as renal failure, liver failure, sedation from analgesics, drug interactions, sepsis, hypoxia, and cerebrovascular problems can produce cognitive impairment [36]. Cognitive impairments that appear after HSCT include learning difficulties, problems with school or work performance, impairment in concentration and memory [2, 37], slowed reaction time, clumsiness, reduced attention, and difficulties in reasoning and problem solving [38]. Changes in brain morphology, such as cortical atrophy and ventricular enlargement, which occur in some patients after HSCT conditioning chemotherapy or total body irradiation, are associated with memory, attention, and information-processing deficits [39]. In addition, mycophenolate mofetil and the calcineurin inhibitors, cyclosporine and tacrolimus, can cause leukoencephalopathy and a variety of neurological symptoms in patients following allo-HSCT [40].

Patients' cognitive functioning is less than normal at baseline [39, 41], most likely due to disease and treatment factors prior to HSCT. Cognitive changes that occur after HSCT are usually temporary [39]. Most patients return to pre-HSCT baseline levels of processing speed, learning, visual-motor ability, verbal fluency, and verbal memory by 1-year following HSCT [15, 39]. More than a third of patients still experience significant decreases in sustained attention and verbal memory when compared to norms more than a year after HSCT [41]. Lower educational levels and underemployment or unemployment are correlated with cognitive deficits more than a year post-HSCT [41]. Most patients are able to return to work within 2 years post-HSCT [26]. There is a critical period, approximately 1 to 2 years post-HSCT, in which most cognitive improvements are made. Success during this time period is a predictor of future cognitive recovery.

Statistically significant impairment in motor dexterity and grip strength is still present 1 year post-HSCT. Receiving immunosuppressive therapy with mycophenolate mofetil, cyclosporine, or tacrolimus for the treatment of cGVHD increases the chance that a patient will have manual dexterity deficits at a year post-HSCT [39]. The use of glucocorticoids for immunosuppression avoids this impairment in manual dexterity.

Memory

Prior to HSCT, between 20% and 40% of patients are found to have significant memory deficits when compared to standard norms [39, 42, 43]. Patients who have not received previous chemotherapy (except hydroxyurea) are less likely to display impaired cognition [39]. Difficulties with memory may impair patients' self-care abilities, such as the ability to self-administer a complex schedule of medication, and threaten patient safety [42]. Most studies have found that memory function returned to baseline within 12 months of HSCT [39, 44]. However, one study found that 20% of patients who had normal memory function at baseline had memory deficits 8 months after HSCT [45]. These deficits were not related to inattention, emotional distress, psychoactive drug administration, or psychiatric disturbances. Two to seven years following HSCT, almost 28% of patients reported moderate to severe memory problems that interfered with daily activities. These patients scored significantly lower on tests of visual and long-term verbal memory than norms. There was a significant positive correlation between impaired memory and unemployment, but there was no correlation between cGVHD and impaired memory [37]. Additional research is needed to confirm the influence of cGVHD and its treatments on memory.

Concentration

Prior to HSCT, 4% to 25% of patients have measurable impairment in attention and executive functioning when compared to expected norms [42, 44], while approximately 20% of patients report subjective mild to moderate problems concentrating [44]. While attention and executive function may decline in the first several months following HSCT [39], they return to baseline levels or higher by 1 year post-HSCT [39, 44, 45]. By 2 to 7 years post-HSCT, attention and executive function are two of the cognitive functions that are most impaired when compared to normal levels with over 15% of patients having moderate impairments that interfere with daily activities. A gradual, time-dependent decline in attention occurs over the years following HSCT [37]. Lower levels of education [42], older age [46], and impairment in attention prior to HSCT [41] have been found to be related to impairments in attention and executive function following HSCT.

It has been suggested that the occurrence of acute or chronic GVHD or the use of medications to treat GVHD may cause impairments in attention and executive function [37, 39, 43]; however, this has not been found to be the case [37, 39]. Further research is needed to confirm these findings.

Mood

Cognitive dysfunction occurs primarily because of changes in subcortical white matter, which produce deficits that can include mood changes [47]. White matter changes detected 1 year after HSCT may be related to cGVHD or immunosuppression [48]. Long-term survivors of HSCT have a higher level of mood disturbances when compared to historical samples of cancer patients [49]. In another longitudinal study of survivors of HSCT, 15% to 25% patients suffered from psychological distress [25]. Several studies have found relationships between mood and cognitive function in patients undergoing HSCT. Cognitive function at baseline is negatively correlated with anxiety and depression 8 months after HSCT, and pretransplant anxiety is associated with poorer cognitive outcomes after HSCT [45]. In addition, positive mood was associated with better cognitive outcomes [37]. No research has addressed the influence of cGVHD on the relationship between mood and cognitive functioning in survivors of HSCT.

PSYCHIATRIC EFFECTS OF TREATMENT

During HSCT, between 37% and 53% of patients experience mental disorders that meet the diagnostic criteria for psychiatric illness [50, 51]. The most common diagnosis is mixed anxiety and depressive reaction [51].

There is little literature about psychiatric illnesses during cGVHD. Pharmacological therapies for cGVHD, such as corticosteroids and tacrolimus, are known to cause mood disturbances and psychiatric illnesses. In addition, treatment for cGVHD is often stressful because the effectiveness of the therapy may be uncertain, the cost may present a financial burden, and treatment demands may disrupt personal and family schedules. Mood disturbances occur more frequently in patients receiving HSCT than in other types of cancer patients [49]. In a longevity study of transplant survivors, 15% to 25% patients suffered from psychological distress [25].

Mania

Most reports of mania following HSCT are single case reports describing patients with a psychiatric history prior to HSCT

or steroid-induced mania. Standard treatment for cGVHD includes systemic corticosteroids [52], and mania or other severe mood disturbances can occur during the first days to weeks of corticosteroid therapy. Steroid-induced mania is dose dependent and reversible when the dose is decreased or the drug discontinued [53]. Psychiatric illness is rare (1.3%) when the dose is less than 40 mg/day of prednisone, but the incidence increases remarkably (18.4%) when the dose is more than 80 mg/day of prednisone [54]. Approximately, 25% of patients without previous psychiatric illnesses have been found to develop mania when started on a short-course of high-dose steroids [55]. Depression is a much less common side effect of corticosteroid therapy, occurring in about 10% of patients, and possibly related to other factors in addition to corticosteroid therapy [55, 56].

Depression

Depression is a common psychiatric sequela of HSCT and the associated stresses of frequent outpatient visits, prophylactic medication for GVHD and infections, repeated blood tests and bone marrow biopsies, fatigue, and decreased stamina. Concerns about relapse, integration of home responsibilities, disability, return to work, and transition from a day-to-day to long-term survival mindset can cause depression [19].

Following HSCT, patients may experience clinical depression. This depression can be long lasting [9]. Previously diagnosed depression can also increase following transplantation [2, 57]. However, within 1 year post-HSCT, depression levels decline and stabilize at baseline levels. Five years after transplant, there is no statistically significant difference in depression between HSCT survivors and the general population [58].

Agitation

Tacrolimus is a standard treatment for cGVHD [52]. Agitation, along with other neuropsychiatric symptoms of anxiety, restlessness, fidgetiness, and tremors, is reported by patients receiving tacrolimus. The agitation occurring with tacrolimus has been investigated in a group of liver transplant recipients and was found to be related more to anxiety than akathisia. Severity of agitation and other neuropsychiatric symptoms was dose dependent. Patients with mean tacrolimus trough levels of 0.56 ng/mL had significantly lower severity scores for a number of neuropsychiatric symptoms than a group of patients with mean tacrolimus trough levels of 1.5 ng/mL [59]. More severe neuropsychiatric symptoms of cognitive impairment and delirium can occur when tacrolimus levels are >3.0 ng/mL [60, 61]. Patients with a history of central nervous system damage are at greater risk of experiencing agitation and other neuropsychiatric symptoms from tacrolimus than are patients with no such history. Agitation resolves when peak tacrolimus trough levels decline. Beta blockers and benzodiazepines do not seem to have an effect on tacrolimus-induced agitation [59].

SOCIAL ASPECTS

Some of the most common problems reported by long-term survivors of HSCT are vocational and social adjustment [62]. HSCT survivors report community reintegration problems, such as changes in roles, loss of job, resuming social relationships, and stigmatization [9]. Social relationships with the opposite sex may be abandoned or avoided due to the psychosexual problems that can accompany cGVHD [19, 62, 63]. Separation from social network due to cGVHD may make reintegration even more difficult [62].

Extended Caregiver Demands

Caregiving demands adjustments in the caregiver's time management, social life, and lifestyle [64]. Research in caregivers of persons with chronic illnesses has produced mixed results about the effect of the length of caregiving on the caregiver. Some caregivers, primarily adult daughters caring for parents and mothers caring for children, have negative health effects due to stress [65] and disruption of social contacts the longer the caregiving persists [66]. Other caregivers, primarily spouses, have been found to develop positive adaptational responses with extended caregiving [66, 67].

There is no research on caregivers of patients with cGVHD, except as a subset of caregivers of patients undergoing HSCT. Beginning 6 months following HSCT, family caregivers report becoming physically and mentally exhausted because of the continued care needs of the patient [68]. Most caregivers report that they had expected the patient to have resumed normal activities and roles by this time [17, 68]. These unmet expectations may be a factor in the caregivers' emotional distress. Caregiving responsibilities also create additional stress for caregivers who have resumed work and possibly childcare responsibilities. Social readjustment is the number one priority reported by caregivers 1 to 6 years following HSCT [17]. The development of cGVHD may extend the time that the patient will require care and increase any negative effects that caregiving is having for the caregiver.

Disruption of Social Networks

Patients undergoing HSCT have often been sick for many months or years prior to the HSCT. They may have had to leave their communities to receive treatment or may have had to limit social contacts because of risk of infection. They may have had to quit work or alter work schedules significantly. The HSCT itself is a lengthy process that may require further time away from home or work and limited social contacts to minimize infectious exposures. All of these factors can cause significant disruption of patients' social networks.

Social support has been found to be critical for the wellbeing of persons with cancer [62, 69, 70], but the exact mechanism by which it exerts this effect has not been defined. It is possible that social support directly improves health or that it affects stress appraisal to decrease the negative effects of

stress on health [71–73]. In women with breast cancer receiving therapy, social support has been found to decrease mood disturbance both directly and through its effect on stress perception [74]. Social support both before and during HSCT is associated with less distress and better cognitive functioning in the first year following HSCT [45, 75].

In the years following HSCT, persons who had received an HSCT had poorer social functioning than persons who had not received an HSCT [76–78]. Physical and emotional limitations were responsible for continued disruption of social, work, and family roles [78]. The effect of HSCT on marital relationships is less clear, with some studies finding no effect [78], and other studies finding a negative effect on dyadic adjustment [76]. While cGVHD is a risk factor for poorer outcomes following HSCT [78], the one study that looked at the effect of cGVHD on social and role function did not find a difference between patients with and without cGVHD [77]. Further research is needed to determine how cGVHD might affect social functioning.

Altered Physical Appearance

Skin and connective tissue changes that resemble systemic autoimmune diseases, such as scleroderma and systemic lupus erythematosus, occur frequently with cGVHD [79]. In addition, cGVHD may cause a wasting syndrome, and long-term glucocorticoid therapy can cause Cushingnoid changes and muscle wasting [7]. Treatment with calcineurin inhibitors can produce tremors [60]. All of these complications of cGVHD and its treatment can drastically alter a patient's physical appearance and body image. Changes in body image can cause significant distress and interfere with patient's social reintegration and sexual functioning [19, 63].

Disfiguring changes in physical appearance and body image have been identified as one of the six universal problems encountered by adults undergoing HSCT [9, 19]. More than a year following HSCT, patients remain dissatisfied with their bodily appearance and physical strength [80], and patients with a poorer body image report more feelings of distress [19]. In a group of long-term male survivors of HSCT, 20.7% reported that their body image was altered since the HSCT [63]. Patients with cGVHD are more dissatisfied with their appearance than patients without cGVHD [62, 80].

SEXUALITY

Sexual dysfunction is a common and enduring problem following HSCT [78]. Sexual dysfunction and dissatisfaction are reported by up to 3/4 of patients following HSCT [63, 76, 78, 81]. Women report more problems than men, and women's problems are more likely to increase over time while men's problems tend to resolve [78]. Depression pre-HSCT and lack of discussion of sexual problems with health care providers increase the risk of sexual dysfunction for patients [81]. Sexual dysfunction that occurs after HSCT includes infertility, decreased sexual interest, inability to achieve an erection, inability to ejaculate, difficulty with arousal, decreased frequency, and decreased satisfaction. cGVHD is associated with more sexual dysfunction in females than in males [7].

Body Image

Both men and women are concerned about physical appearance and attractiveness following HSCT [82]. Worry about appearance continues to increase for sexually active men up to 3 years post-HSCT, while worry over appearance is less concerning for women at 3 years post-HSCT [81]. Married survivors of HSCT are more concerned about changes in body image than unmarried survivors [19]. The changes in physical appearance specific to cGVHD contribute to this concern about body image and appearance. Loss of a positive body image can lead to a decreased libido and sexual dysfunction [7].

Genital and Gonadal Effects

Patients may experience permanent ovarian insufficiency or spermatogenesis damage from high doses of chemotherapy drugs or total body irradiation. The majority of patients undergoing HSCT will become infertile [83]. Infertility often creates feelings of embarrassment and distress and may further interfere with sexual performance.

cGVHD that affects the skin can cause open sores on the genitals, making sex uncomfortable, if not impossible. In addition to vaginal dryness, an effect of infertility, vaginal strictures from cGVHD can make intercourse painful or impossible for women [7, 23].

Lack of Libido

Lack of libido is a common cause of sexual dysfunction following HSCT, reported to occur in approximately 40% of long-term survivors [63]. Loss of sexual desire may be related to decreased hormone levels from gonadal damage, change in body image, or fear of disease recurrence [7]. The effect of glucocorticoids on endocrine function in the treatment of cGVHD can decrease libido [84].

PEDIATRIC ISSUES

While offering hope for a cure, allogeneic HSCT is a high-risk procedure and an extremely stressful experience for children with life-threatening illnesses and their families. Because of growth and development issues that are superimposed on HSCT therapy, children and families can experience some unique psychosocial issues. Because the number of pediatric HSCTs performed each year is small and children are at decreased risk for the development of cGVHD, much less is known about the psychosocial effects of cGVHD in pediatric HSCT.

Dependency and Overprotection

Parents may experience varying levels of anxiety and depression related to fear and uncertainty about outcomes of the child's disease and HSCT [85]. While reactions may vary, some parents will experience distress that persists for a prolonged period after the HSCT [86]. Unremitting fear and uncertainty can eventually lead to feelings of guilt as parents may find themselves wishing for a resolution to the child's illness, even if that resolution is death [87].

The concepts of parental overprotection and perceived child vulnerability have been linked, but research has shown that they are not identical or completely correlated [88]. Parents may perceive children as vulnerable if the parents have ever been told by a health care provider that the child may die soon or if the parents perceive that is what will happen [89]. This view of the child as likely to die soon persists even after the immediate health crisis has passed [89]. Viewing the child as chronically vulnerable to death causes parents to experience prolonged anxiety and grief that may eventually turn to guilt and finally anger [89]. During HSCT, cGVHD by itself was not found to be a risk factor for parental distress. However, transfer to an intensive care unit or multiple hospitalizations, either of which can be triggered by cGVHD, are risk factors for parental distress [85]. When children are perceived as vulnerable, parents may become overprotective.

While the desire to protect a child from harm is a normal parental reaction, overprotection becomes extreme [89]. Parents of younger children who have lower educational level and who were overprotected as children themselves are more likely to be overprotective [88, 90]. Overprotection is characterized by highly vigilant, controlling behavior in a parent, who excessively supervises a child and discourages age-appropriate independence [91]. There is often extreme physical or social contact between the parent and child, prolonging of infantile behaviors, and either extreme strictness or complete lack of parental control. Lack of parental control is most likely to occur if parents view children as vulnerable [87].

Children who are overprotected because they are viewed as vulnerable by their parents often become overly dependent, irritable, argumentative, and uncooperative. They may exhibit behaviors that are inappropriate and embarrassing to their parents, but the parents lack control of the children [87]. These children may have low self-esteem, decreased social competence, low school achievement, chronic mild depression, anxiety disorders, and inability to form close interpersonal relationships as adults [89, 90, 92].

Cognitive Development

Theoretical concerns have been raised that total body irradiation (TBI) or immunosuppressive drugs used to prevent and treat GVHD may cause damage to developing neural tissues and permanent cognitive declines in children receiving HSCT [93, 94]. Initial small studies showed mixed results about the effect of HSCT on cognitive development in children. Some

Table 28.1: Recommendations for Managing Demands of Continuing cGVHD Treatment and Treatment Side Effects

Type of Intervention	Rating
Activity Limitations	
Assess patient preferences and ability to keep clinic and treatment appointments based on fatigue level, employment, and transportation and caregiver resources; schedule appointments to match patient preferences and abilities if at all possible	CIII
Select treatments that minimize need for clinic appointments	CIII
Teach patients or family caregivers to administer medications and other treatments at home or utilize home nursing services	CIII
Refer to occupational therapy to advise patient on alternatives to outdoor activities	CIII
Teach patient effective methods of protecting skin from sun and wind when outdoors	AIII
Refer to nutritionist to advise patient on managing dietary restrictions	BIII
Refer to physical therapy for range of motion exercises	AIII
Calcium and vitamin D replacement in patients with, or at, high risk for deficiencies and postmenopausal women	AIb
Antiresorptive therapy for patients on corticosteroid therapy for >3 months	AIIb
Suggest methods to stay in contact with coworkers, family, and friends that do not involve face-to-face contact, such as telephone, e-mail, computer video conferencing, and so on	CIII
Refer to religious advisor or chaplain; suggest other methods of observing/participating in religious services, such as radio, television, computer video conferencing, and so on	CIII
Cognitive behavioral therapy, counseling, psychotherapy, behavioral therapy, and social support for depression	AIb
Antidepressant medications	AIb
Relaxation therapy for depression	BIIb
Work Change	
Refer to social work and patient advocacy organizations to assist patient with identifying financial resources	CIII
Refer to program or organization that assists patients with maintaining a positive appearance	CIII
Cognitive behavioral therapy, counseling, psychotherapy, behavioral therapy, and/or social support to improve self-image and self-esteem	CIIb
Neuropsychological assessment of cognitive function	BIII
Evaluation for correctable causes of cognitive dysfunction such as endocrine or metabolic disorders	AIII
Stimulant therapy, such as methylphenidate or monafidil, for patients diagnosed with attention difficulties, processing-speed deficits, and fatigue	BIb
Refer to neuropsychologist for cognitive rehabilitation	CIII
Refer to occupational therapy to advise patient on workplace accommodations, alternative occupations, and opportunities for rehabilitation/retraining	CIII
Family Burden	
Psychoeducational group programs provide information, identify resources, and promote problem-solving and coping skills	BIIb
Psychotherapy for caregiver distress	BIIb
Individual teaching of problem-solving and coping skills	BIIb
Combination programs including education, support, psychotherapy, and respite care	BIIb
Setbacks in Recovery and Sustained Uncertainty about Transplant Outcomes	
Individual or group psychoeducational counseling to manage uncertainty and improve problem solving	AIb
Cognitive behavioral therapy, counseling, psychotherapy, behavioral therapy, and social support for stress	AIb
Relaxation therapy for stress	BIIb

* The full instruction about this rating is included in Table 28.9.

studies showed that children who had received HSCT had decreased cognitive skills [95] and poorer academic performance [96] than children who had not received HSCT. Younger age at time of HSCT and TBI as part of the conditioning regimen were identified as risk factors for cognitive deficits [95]. Other studies showed that children who had received HSCT preformed as well or better cognitively or academically than children who had not received HSCT [97, 98].

More recent, larger studies that have compared pre- to post-HSCT intelligence quotient (IQ) scores have shown that HSCT carries minimal risk for cognitive impairment [94, 99].

Analysis at 3 years post-HSCT found that children <6 years of age at the time of HSCT, especially if they were <3 years old or had received TBI, had some cognitive decline [100]. However, by 5 years post-HSCT, there were no significant differences from pre-HSCT IQ scores in any age group of children who had undergone HSCT [94]. Children who had received TBI or who had acute GVHD still did show small cognitive declines. The effect of cGVHD could not be determined because the number of children with cGVHD was too small to reach any conclusions [94]. Although some children post-HSCT do have identifiable learning disabilities, they seem able to adapt and

Table 28.2: Recommendations for Managing Reactive Emotions from cGVHD and Its Treatment

Type of Intervention	Rating
Psychoeducational interventions providing information about disease, treatment, symptom management, and self-care strategies such as exercise and relaxation to manage anxiety	AIb
Cognitive behavioral therapy to teach distraction techniques, thought monitoring, cognitive restructuring, coping, or mental imagery exercises	AIb
Individual or group psychotherapy to manage anxiety	AIb
Support-group meetings that teach anxiety management techniques and coping skills	AIb
Antianxiety medications	BIIb
Massage therapy to relieve anxiety	BIIb
Individual or group psychoeducational counseling to manage uncertainty and improve problem solving	AIb

Table 28.3: Recommendations for Managing Cognitive Effects of cGVHD and Its Treatment

Type of Intervention	Rating
Neuropsychological assessment of cognitive function	BIII
Evaluation for correctable causes of cognitive dysfunction such as endocrine or metabolic disorders	AIII
Stimulant therapy, such as methylphenidate or monafidil, for patients diagnosed with attention difficulties, processing-speed deficits, and fatigue	BIb
Refer to neuropsychologist for cognitive rehabilitation	CIII
Cognitive behavioral therapy, counseling, psychotherapy, behavioral therapy, and/or social support for mood disturbance	AIb
Antidepressant medications	AIb
Relaxation therapy or meditation for mood disturbance	BIIb
Minimize dose of systemic corticosteroids, calcineurin inhibitors, and mycophenolate mofetil	BIII

Table 28.4: Recommendations for Managing Psychiatric Effects of cGVHD and Its Treatment

Type of Intervention	Rating
Mania	
Decrease dose of systemic corticosteroids to prednisone <40 mg/ day if possible	BIII
Antimanic, antipsychotic, or anticonvulsant agents such as lithium, olanzapine, quetiapine, haloperidol, or carbamazepine	BIIa
Depression	
Cognitive behavioral therapy, counseling, psychotherapy, behavioral therapy, and social support for depression	AIb
Antidepressant medications	AIb
Relaxation therapy for depression	BIIb
Agitation	
Decrease dose or discontinue tacrolimus	BIII
Benzodiazepines or beta blockers to decrease agitation	DIII

Table 28.5: Recommendations for Managing Social Aspects of cGVHD and Its Treatment

Type of Intervention	Rating
Extended Caregiver Demands	
Psychoeducational group programs to provide information, identify resources, and promote problem-solving and coping skills	BIIb
Psychotherapy for caregiver distress	BIIb
Individual teaching of problem-solving and coping skills	BIIb
Combination programs including education, support, psychotherapy, and respite care	BIIb
Disruption of Social Networks	
Suggest alternate methods to stay in contact with family and friends, such as telephone, e-mail, computer video conferencing, and so on	CIII
Refer to social work to assist patient with identifying social resources	CIII
Psychoeducational group programs for spouses or other family caregivers to provide information, identify resources, and promote problem-solving and coping skills	BIIb
Altered Physical Appearance	
Refer to program or organization that assists patients with maintaining a positive appearance	CIII
Supportive and cognitive behavioral interventions to cope with body image changes	BIII

Table 28.6: Recommendations for Managing Psychosocial Issues of Sexuality in Patients with cGVHD

Type of Intervention	Rating
Body Image	
Refer to program or organization that assists patients with maintaining a positive appearance	CIII
Cognitive behavioral interventions to cope with body image changes	BIII
Genital and Gonadal Effects	
Supportive and cognitive behavioral interventions for distress related to infertility	BIII
Use water-based lubricants to avoid discomfort during intercourse	BIII
Topical estrogen with/without dilator for vaginal symptoms	BIII
Topical therapy, such as corticosteroids or calineurin inhibitors, for genital cGVHD	BIIb
Lack of Libido	
Evaluate for hormonal insufficiencies	CIII
Hormonal replacement	CIII
Supportive and cognitive behavioral interventions for distress that may be interfering with libido	CIII
Decrease dose of systemic corticosteroids if possible	CIII

function academically at or above expected levels [92]. The two most significant factors that predict cognitive functioning post-HSCT appear to be pre-HSCT cognitive functioning and socioeconomic status [94, 101].

Table 28.7: Recommendations for Managing Psychosocial Issues of Pediatric Patients with cGVHD

Type of Intervention	Rating
Dependency and Overprotection	
Assess parents for risk of overprotective behavior	CIII
Psychotherapy for parental distress	CIII
Psychotherapy or cognitive behavioral therapy for dependent children to manage low self-esteem, decreased social competence, low school achievement, depression, anxiety, and inability to form close interpersonal relationships	CIII
Cognitive Development	
Pediatric neuropsychological assessment of cognitive function	BII
Evaluation for correctable causes of cognitive dysfunction such as endocrine or metabolic disorders	BIII
Refer to pediatric neuropsychologist for cognitive rehabilitation	CIII

Table 28.8: Recommendations for Managing the Psychosocial Needs of Family Caregivers of Patients with cGVHD

Type of Intervention	Rating
Psychoeducational group programs to provide information, identify resources, and promote problem-solving and coping skills	BIIb
Psychotherapy for caregiver distress	BIIb
Individual teaching of problem-solving and coping skills	BIIb
Combination programs including education, support, psychotherapy, and respite care	BIIb

Table 28.9: Evidence-Based Rating Scale for Recommendations for Managing Psychosocial Issues of cGVHD and Its Treatment [5]

Category	Definition
Strength of the Recommendation	
A	Should always be offered
B	Should generally be offered
C	Evidence for efficacy is insufficient to support a recommendation for or against, or evidence for efficacy might not outweigh adverse consequences or cost of the approach. Optional
D	Moderate evidence for lack of efficacy or for adverse outcome supports a recommendation against use. Should generally not be offered
E	Good evidence for lack of efficacy or for adverse outcome supports a recommendation against use. Should never be offered
Quality of Evidence Supporting the Recommendation	
I	Evidence from > = 1 properly randomized, controlled trial
II	Evidence for > = well-designed clinical trial without randomization, from cohort or case-controlled analytic studies (preferably from >1 center), or from multiple time series or dramatic results from uncontrolled experiments
III	Evidence from opinions of respected authorities based on clinical experience, descriptive
Qualifier for Categories I and II	
A	Evidence derived directly from study(s) in GVHD
B	Evidence derived indirectly from study(s) in analogous or other pertinent disease

CAREGIVER NEEDS

Family caregivers are key resources in the care of patients undergoing HSCT who might otherwise need more expensive inpatient care [102]. Most studies of family caregivers of adult patients undergoing HSCT have only covered the immediate posttransplant period of 3 months or less [103–106]. Those that have studied caregivers for at least 1 year posttransplant have found that while caregivers find positive aspects to their caregiving [17], they continue to experience depression and anxiety at higher levels than patients [107], have impaired relationships with both patients and extended family [107, 108], suffer from negative role changes [17, 68], and yearn for life to return to normal [17]. Because patients with cGVHD are known to experience more negative moods and are often unable to resume normal roles and return to normal activities, it might be expected that caregivers of patients with cGVHD will also experience more negative psychosocial sequelae than caregivers of patients without cGVHD.

TREATMENT OPTIONS IN RESPONSE TO NEEDS

Few studies have been reported that address the treatment of psychosocial needs for patients with cGVHD. There is a slightly larger body of literature investigating interventions for psychosocial problems following HSCT. Most evidence for the treatment of psychosocial problems of patients with cGVHD comes from studies of patients with cancer or other chronic illness. Tables 28.1 to 28.8 contain recommendations for managing psychosocial issues in patients with cGVHD. The strength of the evidence supporting of the recommendations is graded according to the scale in Table 28.9.

REFERENCES

1. Socie G, Stone JV, Wingard, JR. Long-term survival and late deaths after allogeneic bone marrow transplantation. Late Effects Working Committee of the International Bone Marrow Transplant Registry. *N Engl J Med*. 1999;341:14–21.

2. Baker KS, Fraser CJ. Quality of life and recovery after graft-versus-host disease. *Best Pract Res Clin Haem*. 2008;21:333–341.

3. Heinonen H, Volin L, Zevon MA, Uutela A, Barrick C, Ruutu T. Stress among allogeneic bone marrow transplantation patients. *Patient Educ Couns*. 2005;56:62–71.

4. Martin PJ, Weisdorf D, Przepiorka D, et al. National Institutes of Health consensus development project on criteria for clinical trials in chronic graft-versus-host disease: VI. Design of clinical trials working group report. *Biol Blood Marrow Transplant* 2006;12:491–505.

5. Couriel D, Carpenter PA, Cutler C, et al. Ancillary therapy and supportive care of chronic graft-versus-host disease: National Institutes of Health consensus development project on criteria for clinical trials in chronic graft-versus-host disease: V. Ancillary therapy and supportive care working group report. *Biol Blood Marr Trans*. 2006;12:375–396.

6. Fraser CJ, Bhatia S, Ness K, et al. Impact of chronic graft-versus-host disease on the health status of hematopoietic cell transplantation survivors: a report from the Bone Marrow Transplant Survivor Study. *Blood*. 2006;108:2867–2873.

7. Chiodi S, Spinelli S, Ravera G, et al. Quality of life in 244 recipients of allogeneic bone marrow transplantation. *Brit J Haem*. 2000;110:614–619.

8. Duell T, van Lint MT, Ljungman P, et al. Health and functional status of long-term survivors of bone marrow transplantation. *Ann Intern Med*. 1997;126:184–192.

9. Sherman RS, Cooke E, Grant M. Dialogue among survivors of hematopoietic cell transplantation: support-group themes. *J Psychosoc Onc*. 2005;23:1–24.

10. Fraser CJ, Baker KS. The management and outcome of chronic graft-versus-host disease. *Brit J Haem*. 2007;138:131–145.

11. Ferrell B, Grant M, Schmidt GM, et al. The meaning of quality of life for bone marrow transplant survivors. *Canc Nurs*. 1992;15:153–160.

12. Slovacek L, Slovackova B, Jebavy L. Global quality of life in patients who have undergone the hematopoietic stem cell transplantation: finding from transversal and retrospective study. *Exp Oncol*. 2005;27:238–242.

13. Savani BN, Donohue T, Kozanas E, et al. Increased risk of bone loss without fracture risk in long-term survivors after allogeneic stem cell transplantation. *Biol Blood Marrow Transplant*. 2007;13:517–520.

14. Beglinger LJ, Duff K, Van Der Heiden S, et al. Neuropsychological and psychiatric functioning pre- and posthematopoietic stem cell transplantation in adult cancer patients: a preliminary study. *J Int Neuropsychol Soc*. 2007;13:172–177.

15. Jacobs S, Small BJ, Booth-Jones M, Jacobsen PB, Fields KK. Changes in cognitive functioning in the year after hematopoietic stem cell transplantation. *Cancer*. 2007;110:1560–1567.

16. Wingard JR, Curbow B, Baker F, Piantadosi S. Health, functional status, and employment of adult survivors of bone marrow transplantation. *Ann Int Med*. 1991;114:113–118.

17. Boyle D, Blodgett L, Gnesdiloff S, et al. Caregiver quality of life after autologous bone marrow transplantation. *Cancer Nurs*. 2000;23:193–203.

18. Williams LA. Theory of caregiving dynamics. In: Smith MJ, Liehr PR, eds. Middle range theory for nursing. 2nd ed. New York: Springer, 2008:261–276.

19. Lesko LM. Bone marrow transplantation: support of the patient and his/her family. *Support Care Cancer*. 1994;2:35–49.

20. Mishel MH, Braden CJ. Finding meaning: antecedents of uncertainty in illness. *Nurs Res*. 1988;37:98–103, 127.

21. Mishel MH, Sorenson DS. Uncertainty in gynecological cancer: a test of the mediating functions of mastery and coping. *Nurs Res*. 1991;40:167–171.

22. Penrod J. Living with uncertainty: concept advancement. *J Adv Nurs*. 2007;57:658–667.

23. Andrykowski MA. Psychosocial factors in bone marrow transplantation: a review and recommendations for research. *Bone Marrow Transplant*. 1994;13:357–375.

24. Andrykowski MA, Henslee PJ, Barnett RL. Longitudinal assessment of psychosocial functioning of adult survivors of allogeneic bone marrow transplantation. *Bone Marrow Transplant*. 1989;4:505–509.

25. Hengeveld MW, Houtman RB, Zwann FE. Psychological aspects of bone marrow transplantation: a retrospective study of 17 long-term survivors. *Bone Marrow Transplant*. 1988;3:69–75.

26. Syrjala KL, Chapko MK, Vitaliano PP, Cummings C, Sullivan KM. Recovery after allogeneic marrow transplantation: prospective study of predictors of long-term physical and psychosocial functioning. *Bone Marrow Transplant*. 1993;11:319–327.

27. Hirai K, Shiozaki M, Motooka H, et al. Discrimination between worry and anxiety among cancer patients: development of a brief cancer-related worry inventory. *Psychooncology*. 2008;May 6. (Accessed June 27, 2008, at http://www3.interscience.wiley.com/cgi-bin/fulltext/119030481/PDFSTART).

28. Mishel MH, Clayton MF. Theories of uncertainty in illness. In: Smith MJ, Liehr PR, eds. Middle range theory for nursing. 2nd ed. New York: Springer, 2008:55–84.

29. Seligman MEP, Walker EF, Rosenhan DL. Abnormal psychology. 4th ed. New York: W.W. Norton, 2001.

30. Bevans MF, Mitchell SA, Marden S. The symptom experience in the first 100 days following allogeneic hematopoietic stem cell transplantation (HSCT). *Support Care Cancer*. 2008;16: 1243–1254

31. Grant M, Ferrell B, Schmidt GM, Fonbuena P, Niland JC, Forman SJ. Measurement of quality of life in bone marrow transplantation survivors. *Qual Life Res*. 1992;1:375–384.

32. Beanlands HJ, Lipton JH, McCay EA, et al. Self-concept as a "BMT patient," illness intrusiveness, and engulfment in allogeneic bone marrow transplant recipients. *J Psychosom Res*. 2003;55:419–425.

33. Lawrence-Smith G, Sturgeon D. Treating learned helplessness in hospital: a reacquaintance with self-control. *Br J Hosp Med (Lond)*. 2006;67:134–136.

34. Anderson-Hanley C, Sherman ML, Riggs R, Agocha VB, Compas BE. Neuropsychological effects of treatments for adults with cancer: meta-analysis and review of the literature. *J Int Neuropsychol Soc*. 2003;9:967–982.

35. Tannock IF, Ahles TA, Ganz PA, Van Dam FS. Cognitive impairment associated with chemotherapy for cancer: report of a workshop. *J Clin Oncol*. 2004;22:2233–2239.

36. Fann JR, Alfano CM, Roth-Roemer S, Katon WJ, Syrjala KL. Impact of delirium on cognition, distress, and health-related quality of life after hematopoietic stem-cell transplantation. *J Clin Oncol*. 2007;25:1223–1231.

37. Harder H, Cornelissen JJ, Van Gool AR, Duivenvoorden HJ, Eijkenboom WM, van den Bent MJ. Cognitive functioning and quality of life in long-term adult survivors of bone marrow transplantation. *Cancer.* 2002;95:183–192.

38. Hjermstad MJ, Loge JH, Evensen SA, Kvaløy SO, Fayers PM, Kaasa S. The course of anxiety and depression during the first year after allogeneic or autologous stem cell transplantation. *Bone Marrow Transplant.* 1999;24:1219–1228.

39. Syrjala KL, Dikmen S, Langer SL, Roth-Roemer S, Abrams JR. Neuropsychologic changes from before transplantation to 1 year in patients receiving myeloablative allogeneic hematopoietic cell transplant. *Blood.* 2004;104:3386–3392.

40. Chohan R, Vij R, Adkins D, et al. Long-term outcomes of allogeneic stem cell transplant recipients after calcineurin inhibitor-induced neurotoxicity. *Br J Haematol.* 2003;123:110–113.

41. Poppelreuter M, Weis J, Mumm A, Orth HB, Bartsch HH. Rehabilitation of therapy-related cognitive deficits in patients after hematopoietic stem cell transplantation. *Bone Marrow Transplant.* 2008;41:79–90.

42. Andrykowski MA, Schmitt FA, Gregg ME, Brady MJ, Lamb DG, Henslee-Downey PJ. Neuropsychologic impairment in adult bone marrow transplant candidates. *Cancer.* 1992;70:2288–2297.

43. Harder H, Van Gool AR, Cornelissen JJ, et al. Assessment of pre-treatment cognitive performance in adult bone marrow or haematopoietic stem cell transplantation patients: a comparative study. *Eur J Cancer.* 2005;41:1007–1016.

44. Harder H, Duivenvoorden HJ, van Gool AR, Cornelissen JJ, van den Bent MJ. Neurocognitive functions and quality of life in haematological patients receiving haematopoietic stem cell grafts: a one-year follow-up pilot study. *J Clin Exp Neuropsychol.* 2006;28:283–293.

45. Meyers CA, Weitzner M, Byrne K, Valentine A, Champlin RE, Przepiorka D. Evaluation of the neurobehavioral functioning of patients before, during, and after bone marrow transplantation. *J Clin Oncol.* 1994;12:820–826.

46. Harder H, Van Gool AR, Duivenvoorden HJ, et al. Case-referent comparison of cognitive functions in patients receiving haematopoietic stem-cell transplantation for haematological malignancies: two-year follow-up results. *Eur J Cancer.* 2007;43:2052–2059.

47. Meyers CA, Weitzner MA, Valentine AD, Levin VA. Methylphenidate therapy improves cognition, mood, and function of brain tumor patients. *J Clin Oncol.* 1998;16:2522–2527.

48. Sostak P, Padovan CS, Yousry TA, Ledderose G, Kolb HJ, Straube A. Prospective evaluation of neurological complications after allogeneic bone marrow transplantation. *Neurology.* 2003;60:842–848.

49. Andrykowski MA, Henslee PJ, Barnett RL. Longitudinal assessment of psychosocial functioning of adult survivors of allogeneic bone marrow transplantation. *Bone Marrow Transplant.* 1989;4:505–509.

50. Fritzsche K, Struss Y, Stein B, Spahn C. Psychosomatic liaison service in hematological oncology: need for psychotherapeutic interventions and their realization. *Hematol Oncol.* 2003;21:83–89.

51. Khan AG, Irfan M, Shamsi TS, Hussain M. Psychiatric disorders in bone marrow transplant patients. *J Coll Physicians Surg Pak.* 2007;17:98–100.

52. Arora M. Therapy of chronic graft-versus-host disease. *Best Pract Res Clin Haematol.* 2008;21:271–279.

53. Brown ES, Chandler PA. Mood and cognitive changes during systemic corticosteroid therapy. *Prim Care Companion J Clin Psychiatry.* 2001;3:17–21.

54. The Boston Collaborative Drug Surveillance Program. Acute adverse reactions to prednisone in relation to dosage. *Clin Pharmacol Ther.* 1972;13:694–698.

55. Naber D, Sand P, Heigl B. Psychopathological and neuropsychological effects of 8-days' corticosteroid treatment. A prospective study. *Psychoneuroendocrinology.* 1996;21:25–31.

56. Wada K, Yamada N, Suzuki H, Lee Y, Kuroda S. Recurrent cases of corticosteroid-induced mood disorder: clinical characteristics and treatment. *J Clin Psychiatry.* 2000;61:261–267.

57. Levy MR, Fann, JR. The neuropsychiatry of hematopoietic stem cell transplantation. *Eur J Psychiat.* 2006;20:107–128.

58. Hjermstad MJ, Knobel H, Brinch L, et al. A prospective study of health-related quality of life, fatigue, anxiety and depression 3–5 years after stem cell transplantation. *Bone Marrow Transplant.* 2004;34:257–266.

59. DiMartini AF, Trzepacz PT, Daviss SR. Prospective study of FK506 side effects: anxiety or akathisia? *Biol Psychiatry.* 1996;40:407–411.

60. DiMartini A, Pajer K, Trzepacz P, Fung J, Starzl T, Tringali R. Psychiatric morbidity in liver transplant patients. *Transplant Proc.* 1991;23:3179–3180.

61. Fung JJ, Alessiani M, Abu-Elmagd K, et al. Adverse effects associated with the use of FK 506. *Transplant Proc.* 1991;23:3105–3108.

62. Molassiotis A, van den Akker OB, Milligan DW, et al. Quality of life in long-term survivors of marrow transplantation: comparison with a matched group receiving maintenance chemotherapy. *Bone Marrow Transplant.* 1996;17:249–258.

63. Molassiotis A, van den Akker OB, Milligan DW, Boughton BJ. Gonadal function and psychosexual adjustment in male long-term survivors of bone marrow transplantation. *Bone Marrow Transplant.* 1995;16:253–259.

64. Brody EM. The Donald P. Kent Memorial Lecture. Parent care as a normative family stress. *Gerontologist.* 1985;25:19–29.

65. Hirst M. Carer distress: a prospective, population-based study. *Soc Sci Med.* 2005;61:697–708.

66. Hoyert DL, Seltzer MM. Factors related to the well-being and life activities of family caregivers. *Fam Relat.* 1992;41:74–81.

67. George LK, Gwyther LP. Caregiver well-being: a multidimensional examination of family caregivers of demented adults. *Gerontologist.* 1986;26:253–259.

68. Zabora JR, Smith ED, Baker F, Wingard JR, Curbow B. The family: the other side of bone marrow transplantation. *J Psychosoc Oncol.* 1992;10:35–46.

69. Bertero CM. Types and sources of social support for people afflicted with cancer. *Nurs Health Sci.* 2000;2:93–101.

70. Helgeson VS. Social support and quality of life. *Qual Life Res.* 2003;12(Suppl 1):25–31.

71. Cohen S, Wills TA. Stress, social support, and the buffering hypothesis. *Psychol. Bull.* 1985;98:310–357.

72. Lazarus RS, Folkman S. Stress, appraisal, and coping. New York, Springer Publishing Company, 1984.

73. Uchino BN, Cacioppo JT, Kiecolt-Glaser JK. The relationship between social support and physiological processes: a review with emphasis on underlying mechanisms and implications for health. *Psychol Bull.* 1996;119:488–531.

74. Von Ah DM, Kang DH, Carpenter JS. Predictors of cancer-related fatigue in women with breast cancer before, during, and after adjuvant therapy. *Cancer Nurs.* 2008;31:134–144.

75. Jacobsen PB, Sadler IJ, Booth-Jones M, Soety E, Weitzner MA, Fields KK. Predictors of posttraumatic stress disorder

symptomatology following bone marrow transplantation for cancer. *J Consult Clin Psychol.* 2002;70:235–240.

76. Andrykowski MA, Bishop MM, Hahn EA, et al. Long-term health-related quality of life, growth, and spiritual well-being after hematopoietic stem-cell transplantation. *J Clin Oncol.* 2005;23:599–608.

77. Hjermstad M, Holte H, Evensen S, Fayers P, Kaasa S. Do patients who are treated with stem cell transplantation have a health-related quality of life comparable to the general population after 1 year? *Bone Marrow Transplant.* 1999;24:911–918.

78. Syrjala KL, Langer SL, Abrams JR, Storer BE, Martin PJ. Late effects of hematopoietic cell transplantation among 10-year adult survivors compared with case-matched controls. *J Clin Oncol.* 2005;23:6596–6606.

79. Ustun C, Ho G Jr. Eosinophilic fasciitis after allogeneic stem cell transplantation: a case report and review of the literature. *Leuk Lymphoma.* 2004;45:1707–1709.

80. Marks DI, Gale DJ, Vedhara K, Bird JM. A quality of life study in 20 adult long-term survivors of unrelated donor bone marrow transplantation. *Bone Marrow Transplant.* 1999;24:191–195.

81. Humphreys CT, Tallman B, Altmaier EM, Barnette V. Sexual functioning in patients undergoing bone marrow transplantation: a longitudinal study. *Bone Marrow Transplant.* 2007;39: 491–496.

82. Mumma GH, Mashberg D, Lesko LM. Long-term psychosexual adjustment of acute leukemia survivors: impact of marrow transplantation versus conventional chemotherapy. *Gen Hosp Psychiatry.* 1992;14:43–55.

83. Tauchmanovà L, Selleri C, Rosa GD, et al. High prevalence of endocrine dysfunction in long-term survivors after allogeneic bone marrow transplantation for hematologic diseases. *Cancer.* 2002;95:1076–1084.

84. McPhee SJ, Ganong WF. Pathophysiology of disease: an introduction to clinical medicine. 5th ed. New York: Lange Medical Books, 2006.

85. Manne S, DuHamel K, Winkel G, et al. Perceived partner critical and avoidant behaviors as predictors of anxious and depressive symptoms among mothers of children undergoing hemopaietic stem cell transplantation. *J Consult Clin Psychol.* 2003;71:1076–1083.

86. DuHamel KN, Manne S, Nereo N, et al. Cognitive processing among mothers of children undergoing bone marrow/stem cell transplantation. *Psychosom Med.* 2004;66:92–103.

87. Green M, Solnit AJ. Reactions to the threatened loss of a child: a vulnerable child syndrome. Pediatric management of the dying child, part III. *Pediatrics.* 1964;34:58–66.

88. Thomasgard M, Metz WP. Parental overprotection and its relation to perceived child vulnerability. *Am J Orthopsychiatry.* 1997;67:330–335.

89. Thomasgard M. Parental perceptions of child vulnerability, overprotection, and parental psychological characteristics. *Child Psychiatry Hum Dev.* 1998;28:223–240.

90. Thomasgard M, Metz WP. Parent–child relationship disorders: what do the Child Vulnerability Scale and the Parent Protection Scale measure? *Clin Pediatr.* 1999;38:347–356.

91. Thomasgard M, Metz WP. Parental overprotection revisited. *Child Psychiatry Hum Dev.* 1993;24:67–80.

92. Perkins JL, Kunin-Batson AS, Youngren NM, et al. Long-term follow-up of children who underwent hematopoietic cell transplant (HCT) for AML or ALL at less than 3 years of age. *Pediatr Blood Cancer.* 2007;49:958–963.

93. Bolland CM, Krance RA, Heslop HE. Hematopoietic stem cell transplantation in pediatric oncology. In: Pizzo PA, Poplack DG, eds. Principles and practices of pediatric oncology. 5th ed. Philadelphia: Lippincott, Williams & Wilkins, 2006:476–500.

94. Phipps S, Rai SN, Leung WH, Lensing S, Dunavant M. Cognitive and academic consequences of stem-cell transplantation in children. *J Clin Oncol.* 2008;26:2027–2033.

95. Smedler AC, Nilsson C, Bolme P. Total body irradiation: a neuropsychological risk factor in pediatric bone marrow transplant recipients. *Acta Paediatr.* 1995;84:325–330.

96. Arvidson J, Larsson B, Lönnerholm G. A long-term follow-up study of psychosocial functioning after autologous bone marrow transplantation in childhood. *Psychooncology.* 1999;8:123–134.

97. Halberg FE, Wara WM, Weaver KE, et al. Total body irradiation and bone marrow transplantation for immunodeficiency disorders in young children. *Radiother Oncol.* 1990;18 (Suppl 1):114–117.

98. Kaleita TA, Shields WD, Tesler A, Feig SA. Normal neurodevelopment in four young children treated with bone marrow transplantation for acute leukemia or aplastic anemia. *Pediatrics.* 1989;83:753–757.

99. Simms S, Kazak AE, Golomb V, Goldwein J, Bunin N. Cognitive, behavioral, and social outcome in survivors of childhood stem cell transplantation. *J Pediatr Hematol Oncol.* 2002;24:115–119.

100. Phipps S, Dunavant M, Srivastava DK, Bowman L, Mulhern RK. Cognitive and academic functioning in survivors of pediatric bone marrow transplantation. *J Clin Oncol.* 2000;18:1004–1011.

101. Kupst MJ, Penati B, Debban B, et al. Cognitive and psychosocial functioning of pediatric hematopoietic stem cell transplant patients: a prospective longitudinal study. *Bone Marrow Transplant.* 2002;30:609–617.

102. Frey P, Stinson T, Siston A, et al. Lack of caregivers limits use of outpatient hematopoietic stem cell transplant program. *Bone Marrow Transplant.* 2002;30:741–748.

103. Gaston-Johansson F, Lachica EM, Fall-Dickson JM, Kennedy MJ. Psychological distress, fatigue, burden of care, and quality of life in primary caregivers of patients with breast cancer undergoing autologous bone marrow transplantation. *Oncol Nurs Forum.* 2004;31:1161–1169.

104. Donnelly JM, Kornblith AB, Fleishman S, et al. A pilot study of interpersonal psychotherapy by telephone with cancer patients and their partners. *Psychooncology.* 2000;9:44–56.

105. Grimm PM, Zawacki KL, Mock V, Krumm S, Frink BB. Caregiver responses and needs. An ambulatory bone marrow transplant model. *Cancer Pract.* 2000;8:120–128.

106. Williams LA. Whatever it takes: informal caregiving dynamics in blood and marrow transplantation. *Oncol Nurs Forum.* 2007;34:379–387.

107. Langer S, Abrams J, Syrjala K. Caregiver and patient marital satisfaction and affect following hematopoietic stem cell transplantation: a prospective, longitudinal investigation. *Psychooncology.* 2003;12:239–253.

108. Keogh F, O'Riordan J, McNamara C, Duggan C, McCann SR. Psychosocial adaptation of patients and families following bone marrow transplantation: a prospective, longitudinal study. *Bone Marrow Transplant.* 1998;22:905–911.

29

Secondary Malignancies and Other Late Effects

Gérard Socié and H. Joachim Deeg

Large numbers of patients now survive long term following hematopoietic stem cell transplantation (SCT), and late clinical effects of SCT are, thus, of major concern. Chronic graft versus host disease (cGVHD) and the associated immunodeficiency are the primary causes of transplant-related mortality late after allogeneic SCT and contribute directly or indirectly to most late complications. Despite the advent of new treatment modalities the incidence of cGVHD has remained high, related to several changes in clinical SCT practice (1) the expanded use of human leukocyte antigen (HLA) matched unrelated and HLA nonidentical related donors; (2) the increasing use of SCT in older patients; (3) the increasing use of viable donor lymphocyte infusions after SCT to treat relapsed disease or to achieve full donor chimerism after nonmyeloablative transplantation; (4) the increasing use of peripheral blood stem cells instead of bone marrow as a source of stem cells. In addition to cGVHD and its therapy, the major risk factor for late complications after SCT is the use of irradiation in the pretransplant conditioning regimen. The interrelationship between cGVHD, total-body irradiation (TBI), and nonmalignant late effects are summarized in Figures 29.1 and 29.2.

Secondary malignant diseases are of particular clinical concern as more patients survive the early phase after SCT and remain free of their original disease [1, 2].

Nonmalignant late effects are heterogeneous, and although often non–life threatening, they significantly impair the quality of life of long-term survivors [3].

Extensive reviews with references have been published [1, 2], and, thus, only selected references are included in this chapter. Several chapters in this book (late infections, metabolic and endocrine effects, and psycho-social and quality of life issues, pediatric cGVHD) also refer to the relationship between cGVHD and late effect and will not be discussed here. Recommendations for screening for cGVHD, formulated at the National Institute of Health (NIH) sponsored workshop, have recently been published [4].

NONMALIGNANT LATE EFFECTS

Ocular Effects

Kerato-conjunctivitis sicca and cataracts are the two most common late complications affecting the anterior segment of the eye.

Cataract formation, particularly posterior subcapsular cataracts, has long been recognized in recipients of SCT [5, 6]. The two main risk factors for cataract development are exposure to TBI and steroids therapy for cGVHD [5–7]. After single dose TBI almost all patients develop cataracts within 3 to 4 years, and most if not all need surgical repair. The probability of developing cataracts after fractionated TBI is in the range of 30% at 3 years, but may be as high as 80% at 6 to 10 years after SCT [5–7]. In a multivariate analysis, the use of TBI, single as compared to fractionated dose TBI, and the use of steroid treatment for longer than 3 months were associated with a significantly increased risk of cataract development [7]. The radiation effect was dose rate dependent [8, 9]. The largest series to date included a cohort of 1,064 patients and identified as factors independently associated with an increased risk of cataracts; older age (>23 years), higher radiation exposure rate (>4 cGy/min), allogeneic rather than autologous SCT, and steroid administration [10]. Finally, in prospective studies comparing the incidence of cataracts and predisposing risk factors, patients who received cyclophosphamide and TBI (Cy/TBI) had a higher incidence of cataracts than patients treated with busulfan and cyclophosphamide (Bu/Cy) [11]. The only satisfactory treatment for cataract is surgical removal of the lens from the eye to restore transparency of the visual axis. Modern cataract surgery is a low-risk procedure and improves visual acuity in 95% of eyes in the general population; an analysis of results in transplanted patients has yet to be presented.

Kerato-conjunctivitis sicca of the eyes is usually part of a more general syndrome that also includes xerostomia, dryness of the skin, and, in women, vaginitis. All these manifestations are closely related to cGVHD [12–15]. In its most extensive

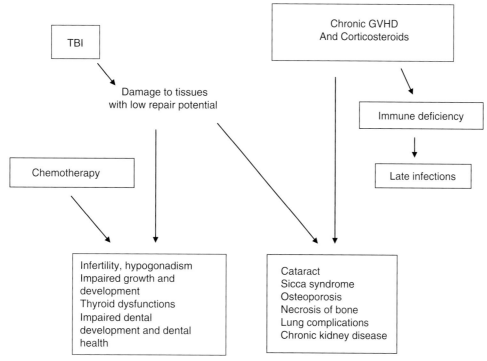

Figure 29.1 Transplant therapy and long-term complications. GVHD, graft versus host disease; TBI, total-body irradiation.

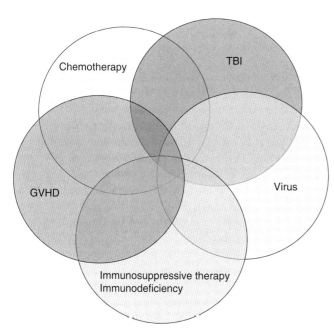

Figure 29.2 Multifactorial etiology of posttransplantation late effects. GVHD, graft versus host disease; TBI, total body irradiation. See Plate 76 in the color plate section.

form the clinical picture may be that of a Sjögren-like syndrome, as described in detail in other chapters of this book.

Pulmonary Effects

Significant late toxicity involving both the airways and the lung parenchyma is observed in at least 15 to 40 of patients after SCT [3, 16–19]. Most studies have been performed in adult patients, and results are still conflicting, because of differences in patient selection and evaluation criteria, limited sample size, and short follow-up. Moreover, the various pulmonary syndromes are not well defined or definable because of overlapping mechanisms and because they represent a continuous spectrum rather than distinct disorders. Sensitivity to cytotoxic agents and irradiation, infections, and immune-mediated lung injury associated with GVHD are the most prominent factors, which contribute to late respiratory complications. Impaired growth of both lungs and chest wall can be additional factors in patients who are transplanted as young children.

Restrictive Lung Disease

Restrictive lung disease is frequently observed 3 to 6 months after SCT in patients conditioned with TBI and receiving an allogeneic SCT, but in most cases it is not symptomatic. Restrictive disease is often stable and, in fact, may resolve, partially or completely, within 2 years of SCT. However, some patients do develop severe late restrictive defects and may eventually die from respiratory failure [16].

Chronic Obstructive Lung Disease

Chronic obstructive pulmonary disease with reduced forced expiratory volume in 1 second (FEV_1)/forced vital capacity (FVC) and FEV_1 develops in up to 20% of long-term survivors after SCT. The pathogenesis is not well understood, but cGVHD, TBI, hypogammaglobulinemia, GVHD prophylaxis with methotrexate, and infections have been described as risk factors [3]. Details are discussed in Chapter 21.

Complications of Bones and Joints

Avascular Necrosis of Bone

The incidence of avascular necrosis of bone (AVN) has been reported at 4% to more than 10%. The mean time from transplant to the diagnosis of AVN is 18 months, and joint pain is usually the first sign [20–24]. The diagnosis is sometimes made early by standard radiographs alone; magnetic resonance imaging is the investigation of choice. The hip joint is affected in more than 80% of cases with bilateral involvement occurring in more than 60% of cases. Other locations described include the knee (10% of patient with AVN), wrist, and ankle. Symptomatic relief of pain and orthopedic measures to decrease the pressure on the affected joints are of value, but most adult patients with advanced damage will require surgery. By 5 years about 80% of patients will have undergone total hip replacement. Short-term results of joint replacement are excellent in more than >85%, but further long-term follow-up is required, particularly in young patients, to determine outcome over an extended life span [25]. Steroid use (both total dose and duration) is the strongest risk factor for AVN [20–24]. Thus, long-term use, even of low dose steroids, should be avoided whenever possible. The second major risk factor is TBI, the highest risks being associated with single doses of 10 Gy or higher and more than 12 Gy in fractionated doses.

Osteoporosis

Hematopoietic SCT can induce bone loss and osteoporosis via the toxic effects of TBI, chemotherapy, iatrogenic hypogonadism and may be compounded by prolonged inactivity of patients after SCT (see reviews in References 26 and 27). Osteopenia and osteoporosis are characterized by a reduced bone mass and increased susceptibility to bone fracture. These conditions are distinguished by the degree of reduction in bone mass and can be quantified on dual energy X-ray absorptiometry (DEXA), a semiquantitative method to assess bone mineral density (BMD), is a validated method used to detect osteoporosis (T-score of equal to or less than –2.5 standard deviations below age-related mean BMD) and osteopenia (T-score of –1.0 to –2.4 standard deviations below age-related mean BMD). Other markers of bone loss include elevated alkaline phosphatase, particularly in women, as well as high C-terminal propeptide. Increased urinary excretion of hydroxyproline can also be used to assess bone loss and response to treatment [28]. The cumulative dose and number of days of glucocorticoid therapy and the number of days of cyclosporine or tacrolimus therapy showed significant associations with loss of bone mass. Nontraumatic fractures occurred in 10% of patients. Using WHO criteria, nearly 50% of patients after SCT have low bone density, a third have osteopenia, and approximately 10% have osteoporosis by 12 to 18 months after SCT.

Few studies on the safety and efficacy of bisphosphonate for prevention of bone loss after HCT have been reported. Results of a randomized study in adult allogeneic HCT recipients showed less bone loss in patients receiving additional pamidronate (60 mg before and 1, 2, 3, 6, and 9 months after HCT) compared to patients receiving 1,000 mg calcium carbonate and 800 IU vitamin D daily, and estrogen (women) or testosterone (men) alone [29]. In a retrospective study of pediatric HCT recipients, treatment with bisphosphonates was well tolerated and was associated with improvement in BMD [30]. Preventive measures of bone loss after HCT are indicated. Many experts recommend the use of antiresorptive treatments (gonadal hormonal replacement or bisphosphonates) in patients with gonadal failure and with cGVHD requiring treatment with glucocorticoid [31]. Physicians and patients should be aware of osteonecrosis of the jaw, a rare but well recognized potentially serious toxicity of bisphosphonate, which is reported more frequently with intravenous formulations [32].

Hormone replacement after HCT should be individualized with the pros and cons discussed carefully with each patient *before initiation of replacement,* and *reassessed at least yearly* if treatment is continued beyond 1 to 3 years after HCT. Increased risk of breast cancer, coronary heart disease (CHD), stroke, and venous thromboembolism was reported in the Women's Health Initiative (WHI) study (nontransplanted women older than 50 years) with continuous combined estrogen-progestin replacement versus placebo, for an average of 5.2 years. Nonetheless, this study also showed a significantly reduced risk of bone fractures and colon cancer [33]. The risk of breast cancer in postmenopausal women on hormone replacement therapy (outside the transplant setting) increases with increasing hormone use, but the impact declines again after cessation of replacement, and is basically no longer detectable by about 5 years [34]. The risk of developing a secondary malignancy begins to rise, starting 5 years after HCT. Whether combined hormone replacement contributes to an increased risk of secondary cancers, in particular, breast cancer after HCT, is difficult to establish. These findings should be considered in the context of other benefits and risks associated with the use of hormone replacement after HCT. The results of the unopposed estrogen versus placebo WHI study (nontransplant postmenopausal women) showed an increase in the risk of stroke, a decrease in the risk of hip fracture, and no effects on CHD incidence or increased risk of breast cancer with an average follow-up of 6.8 years [35]. Thus, considering all available data, the benefit of administration of estrogen combined with progestin (for adult women with a uterus) or estrogen alone (for adult women without a uterus) in young women with gonadal failure after HCT is reasonable, unless other contraindications are present. Hormone replacement should not be administered in patients with a history of cardiovascular disease, hyper coagulation disorders (i.e., venous thrombosis, pulmonary embolism, and stroke), breast cancer, or liver disease

SECONDARY MALIGNANCIES

Secondary malignancies are a known complication of conventional chemotherapy and radiation treatment for patients with a variety of primary cancers. Secondary cancers are now being increasingly recognized as a complication among SCT recipients.

The magnitude of risk of secondary malignancies after SCT has been found to be increased four-fold to 11-fold compared to the general population. The estimated actuarial incidence is reported to be about 3% to 4% at 10 years, increasing to 10% to 12% at 15 years after allogeneic SCT [1, 2, 36–39].

Risk factors for the development of secondary malignancies include exposure to chemotherapy and radiation before transplantation, use of TBI and high-dose chemotherapy used in preparation for SCT, infection with viruses such as *Epstein-Barr virus* (EBV) and *Hepatitis B and C viruses* (HBV and HCV), immunodeficiency after transplant, aggravated by the use of immunosuppressive drugs for prophylaxis and treatment of GVHD, including the use of monoclonal and polyclonal antibodies, HLA nonidentity, and T-cell depletion, the type of transplant (autologous vs. allogeneic), the source of hematopoietic stem cells used, and the primary malignancy. However, assessment of risk factors for all secondary malignancies in aggregate is somewhat artificial because of the heterogeneous nature of the secondary malignancies, with differing clinico-pathological features, distinct pathogenesis, and hence very distinct risk factors associated with their development (reviewed in References 1 and 2).

Currently secondary malignancies after SCT are categorized into three distinct groups: (1) myelodysplasia and acute myeloid leukemia, (2) lymphoma, including lymphoproliferative disorders, and (3) solid tumors. Leukemia and lymphomas develop relatively early in the posttransplant period. Solid cancers, on the other hand, have a longer latency period, and are being observed with increasing frequency as the proportion of long-term surviving patients increase.

Secondary Leukemia after Allogeneic SCT

Secondary leukemia in the setting of allogeneic SCT refers to leukemia of donor cell origin or a *new* leukemia developing in surviving patient cells. Both are extremely rare complications, raising important questions on leukemogenesis. Recently, the Seattle team has suggested that transfer with the donor graft of otherwise silent malignant cells could also be responsible for leukemias arising from donor cells. However, no clear evidence links these secondary leukemias to cGVHD. Nevertheless, with increasing use of older donors (especially for patients receiving reduced intensity conditioning) special attention must be given to the search for hematological abnormalities in the donor and of clear need for donor's surveillance.

The development of new leukemias in patient cells is most likely related to cytotoxic conditioning therapy; there is no evidence to support a role of cGVHD.

Lymphomas

Posttransplant lymphoproliferative disorders (PTLD) are the most common secondary malignancy in the **first year** after allogeneic SCT. Most of these cases are related to compromised immune function and EBV reactivation. The large majority of the PTLD have a B-cell origin, although some T-cell PTLDs

Table 29.1: Site Specific Risk Factors for Secondary Cancers

Risk Factor	Second Cancer
TBI	Melanoma, Thyroid
Limited Field Irradiation	SCC Buccal
T-cell Depletion	Melanoma
chronic GVHD	SCC Buccal and Skin; Thyroid
HCV	Liver
EBV	Lymphoma

EBV, *Epstein-Barr virus*; GVHD, graft versus host disease; HCV, *Hepatitis C virus*; SCC, squamous-cell carcinomas; TBI, total-body irradiation.

have been described [40, 41]. These malignancies are excluded from the present discussion of late effects; they have been extensively been reviewed elsewhere.

Nevertheless, several cases of late-occurring lymphomas have been reported in the literature. It is believed that these late-occurring lymphomas represent an entity that is distinct from the early-occurring B-cell PTLD [42–46]. In a large study of 18,000 SCT recipients, the only risk factor associated with the development of the late-occurring lymphoma was extensive cGVHD.

"Secondary" Hodgkin disease (HD) has also been observed among SCT recipients. SCT recipients followed as part of a large cohort study were at a 6-fold increased risk of developing HD when compared with the general population [47]. Most of the reported cases were of the mixed cellularity subtype, and most of these cases contained the EBV genome. These cases differed from the EBV-associated PTLD by the absence of risk factors commonly associated with EBV-associated PTLD, by a later onset (>2.5 years), and relatively good prognosis. The increased incidence of HD among SCT recipients could possibly be explained by exposure to EBV and overstimulation of cell-mediated immunity, but no clear evidence for a link with cGVHD has been established.

Solid Tumors

Solid tumors have been described after syngeneic, allogeneic, and autologous SCT. The increase in the risk of solid tumors has ranged from 2.1-fold to 2.7-fold when compared to an age- and sex-matched general population [48, 49]. The risk increased with increasing follow-up, and, among those who survived 10 or more years after transplantation, was reported to be 8.3 times as high as expected in the general population. Types of solid tumors reported in excess among SCT recipients, were those typically associated with exposure to radiation therapy, including melanoma, squamous-cell carcinomas (SCC) of the oral cavity and salivary glands, and cancers of the brain, liver, uterine cervix, thyroid, and breast, as well as sarcomas of the bone and connective tissues (Table 29.1). There is a need to follow this cohort of patients long term in order to describe in greater detail the risk of new solid malignancies.

Pathogenesis

Little is known about the pathogenesis of solid tumors. An interaction of cytotoxic therapy, genetic predisposition, viral infection, and GVHD with the resulting antigenic stimulation and the use of immunosuppressive therapy, all appear to play a role in the development of new solid tumors [50, 51].

Radiation-related cancers generally have a long latency period, and the risk of such cancers is particularly high among patients undergoing irradiation at a young age. A large series reported an increased risk of brain and thyroid cancers after TBI given as part of myeloablative conditioning, although most of these patients had also received cranial irradiation before SCT. Both thyroid cancer and brain tumors have been reported after exposure to radiation to the craniospinal axis and the neck when given as part of the conventional therapy for childhood acute lymphoblastic leukemia, HD, and *primary* brain tumors. Similarly, osteogenic sarcoma and other connective tissue tumors have been recognized as secondary malignancies developing after radiation therapy in nontransplanted patients. Those studies indicated a strong dose-response relationship for radiation exposure, in addition to an increased risk with increasing exposure to alkylating chemotherapy agents. The increased risk of thyroid, breast, brain, bone, and soft tissue malignancies seen after SCT appear to be related, at least in part, to cumulative doses of radiation exposure, both as a result of the pretransplant treatment-regimens, and the conditioning regimen used for transplantation.

Immunologic impairment may predispose patients to the development of squamous-cell carcinoma of the buccal cavity and skin, particularly in the context of cGVHD. These tumors have been observed particularly in patients with aplastic anemia conditioned with limited field irradiation or treated with Azathioprine for cGVHD [52]. In immune suppressed patients, oncogenic viruses, such as human papillomaviruses, may contribute to squamous-cell cancers of the skin and buccal mucosa. The observed excess risk of squamous-cell cancers of the buccal cavity and skin in males is unexplained, but may be indicative of an interaction between ionizing radiation, immunodeficiency, and, conceivable factors such as smoking habits or alcohol consumption.

Patients with a family history of early-onset ($<$age 40 years) cancers are at an increased risk for developing secondary cancers, and genetic predisposition is likely to have a substantial impact on the risk of secondary cancers. Studies exploring genetic predisposition and gene-environment interactions have focused thus far on patients exposed to nontransplant conventional therapy for cancer. Future studies are needed in the transplant population to understand how genetic predisposition interacts with myeloablative chemotherapy, TBI, and the attendant posttransplant immunosuppression, thereby leading to secondary solid tumors.

Skin and Mucosal Carcinoma and cGVHD

As already implied above, transplant recipients with cGVHD have an especially high risk of developing SCC of the oral cavity and skin, with rather aggressive behavior being noted for some of these tumors. Among solid organ transplant recipients the frequency of rejection episodes (requiring intensified immunosuppression) and the duration of immunosuppressive therapy strongly correlate with the occurrence of skin cancer. Patients undergoing SCT, in contrast to solid organ recipients, generally receive immunosuppressive therapy only for limited periods of time, unless they develop cGVHD. Thus, prolonged immunosuppression and (persistent) cGVHD are usually linked. A case-control analysis in SCT recipients was designed to quantify the association of GVHD and its therapy with the development of secondary SCC (including those of the oral mucosa) [52]. This case-control study included 183 patients with posttransplant solid cancers (58 SCC, 125 non-SCC) and 501 matched control patients within a cohort of 24,011 patients who received HCT at 215 centers worldwide. Results showed that cGVHD and its therapy were strongly related to the risk of SCC, whereas no such increase in risk was found for non-SCC cancers. Long duration of cGVHD therapy ($p = 0.0001$), the use of Azathioprine, particularly when combined with cyclosporine and steroids ($p = 0.0002$), and the severity of cGVHD ($p = 0.004$) were identified as major risk factors for the development of SCC. Since Azathioprine was used mostly in patients who received prolonged immunosuppressive therapy and had severe cGVHD, the independent effects of these factors could not be evaluated. Consistent with a previous cohort study, there was no evidence that cGVHD or duration of therapy were related to the development of non-SCC solid cancers.

In a separate study the Seattle group evaluated the incidence of and risk factors for basal cell carcinoma (BCC) and SCC in survivors of SCT [53]. Patient-, disease-, treatment-, and toxicity-related factors were analyzed in regards to the risk of BCC and SCC in a retrospective cohort study of 4,810 patients who received allogeneic SCT and who survived for at least 100 days. Among allogeneic SCT recipients, 237 developed at least one skin or mucosal cancer (BCC, n = 158; SCC, n = 95). Among the 95 SCC, 24 occurred on internal mucosal surfaces, such as the tongue, tonsil, vocal cord, esophagus, and genitourinary tract (cervix, vagina, and vulva). Twenty-year cumulative incidence rates of BCC and SCC were 6.5% and 3.4%, respectively. TBI was a significant risk factor for BCC (but not for SCC), most strongly among patients who were younger than 18 years at SCT. Light-skinned patients had an increased risk of BCC. Acute GVHD was associated with increased risk of SCC, and cGVHD with both BCC and SCC. Thus, this analysis suggested that immutable factors, such as age and complexion, have a significant impact on the development of BCC and SCC. However, specific treatment modalities (radiotherapy) and transplant-related complications (GVHD) may modify the risk. These additional risk factors suggest a contribution of immunologic mechanism and DNA and tissue repair in the development of BCC and SCC. Overall these data confirmed previous reports that showed that exposure to ionizing radiation increased the risk of BCC but not SCC.

The major predisposing factor for cGVHD is preceding acute GVHD, that is, a syndrome characterized by alloreactivity and immunodeficiency. The immunodeficiency is further aggravated by the treatment of cGVHD, which may continue over several years. However, cGVHD, which most frequently affects the skin, liver, mouth, and eyes, also shows features of autoimmunity and inflammation. Both aspects are relevant since patients with autoimmune disorders develop malignant tumors more frequently than individuals with apparently normal immunity. Chronic inflammation and scar formation have also been associated with an increased risk of cancer. The interactions between inflammation and immunosuppression are not fully understood, but one might speculate that immunosuppression administered in a milieu of inflammation, as occurs with cGVHD, would interfere with tissue repair and thereby enhance the risk of tumor evolution. The risk would be further heightened when immunosuppressive therapies were given for prolonged periods, as observed in previous investigations in solid organ transplant recipients. If immunosuppression consisted of compounds that are known carcinogens then one would also expect new malignancies in recipients of SCT, which has been reported, in fact, in patients with severe aplastic anemia. In addition it suggests that other components; in particular interactions with agents, such as Cyclosporine (CSP), and the duration of treatment and severity of cGVHD are contributing factors. Reports from the early 1980s suggested that CSP, in many instances given at doses much higher than in use today, contributed to the development of malignancies, in particular posttransplant lymphoproliferative disorders. More recent work suggests that CSP may induce phenotypic changes and enhance invasiveness of nontransformed cells via a TGF β-dependent mechanism. Finally, it should be noted that Mycophenolate mofetil (MMF) (which has largely replaced Azathioprine in the treatment of cGVHD) has a mechanism of action similar to Azathioprine and could, thus, represent a potent risk factor in the future!

Thyroid Carcinoma and cGVHD
While thyroid carcinoma is generally considered a prototype of radiation-induced carcinoma, recent data from the European group strongly suggest that cGVHD may play a role in the genesis of this cancer. We performed a retrospective analysis comparing data obtained by means of a two-step questionnaire from the 166 centers who replied, and data reported to the European Group for Blood and Marrow Transplantation (EBMT) registry on their transplantation activity [54]. During the follow-up period (1985 to 2003), 32 instances of thyroid carcinoma were found within the EBMT cohort of 68,936 patients who received SCT. The standardized incidence ratio of thyroid carcinoma in the transplant population was 3.26, in comparison with the general European population. Multivariate analysis revealed that young age at SCT was the strongest risk factor (relative risk [RR], 24.61 for ages 0 to 10 years; RR, 4.80 for ages 11 to 20 years). Other risk factors were irradiation (RR, 3.44), female sex (RR, 2.79), and cGVHD (RR, 2.94). Nine patients showed no clinical signs of thyroid disease at diagnosis. Total thyroidectomy and iodine ablation was the standard treatment for the majority of patients, and only one patient died because of cancer progression.

Treatment and Prevention
Treatment strategies for patients developing solid tumors after SCT are not well defined [55, 56]. Concerns regarding limited bone marrow reserve and excessive organ toxicity because of prior therapy preclude the use of intensive approaches. Small case series reveal a broad spectrum, that is, favorable outcomes and, hence, a recommendation for an intensive approach as well as aggressive tumor growth and early relapse after standard therapy. A comprehensive study of a large number of patients with second solid tumors will help to determine the nature of these tumors and their outcomes as compared to de novo occurring tumors. Extending the follow-up of SCT recipients to 20 years after transplantation will help clarify the risks of radiation-associated cancers such as breast, lung, and colon cancers. These epithelial cancers typically develop at a median of 15 to 20 years after exposure to radiation and are beginning to emerge among cancer survivor populations treated with conventional therapy. These data indicate that SCT survivors face an increasing risk of solid cancers with time from transplantation and require life-long surveillance. Preventive measures that need to be considered include programs to educate clinicians and survivors about the risk of secondary malignancies, and measures taken to decrease the morbidity associated with secondary malignancies, such as adopting healthy lifestyle choices. Other measures include intervention programs for smoking cessation; periodic and aggressive screening for breast, lung, skin, colorectal, prostate, thyroid, and cervical cancers; chemoprevention for specific cancers; and avoidance of unnecessary exposure to sunlight, especially among patients who have received radiation. By understanding the risk factors for secondary malignancies, and taking measures to avoid them, it may be possible to decrease the incidence of the most devastating delayed consequences in cancer survivors while maintaining high cure rates.

KEY POINTS

Type of posttransplantation late effects
- Nonmalignant late effects
- Malignant late effects
- Health status and social integration
- Quality of life and sexuality
- cGVHD and immune reconstitution

Nonmalignant late effects are heterogeneous in nature and intensity
- Endocrine dysfunction
- Thyroid function
- Gonadal, fertility
- Growth and development
  - Skeletal disorders
  - Ocular problems
- Respiratory tract problems
- Restrictive lung disease
- Obstructive lung disease
  - Salivary function and dental problems

– Liver complication
– Vascular complication

*Any organ or tissue can be the target of late effects after allogeneic stem cell transplantation*Recommendations for solid tumors

- Encourage patients to self-examination
  - Breast
  - Oral cavity
  - Skin
- Avoid high-risk behaviors
  - Smoking
  - Excessive, unprotected skin ultraviolet (UV) exposure
- Life-long clinical assessment in yearly intervals
  - Symptom review and clinical examination
  - Specific screening
- Treatment of cGVHD

Recommendations for skeletal disorders

- Monitoring
  - Clinical symptoms (pain)
  - Dual photon densitometry (osteopenia) at one year and regularly for patients on steroids
  - Magnetic resonance imaging (MRI) in suspicion of AVN
- Patient counseling
  - Regular exercise, compliance of prevention and treatment
- Treatment
  - Osteopenia
    - Vitamin D and calcium supplementation, bisphosphonates
    - Hormonal replacement (estrogens)
- Avascular necrosis of the bone
  - Symptomatic relief of pain
  - Orthopedic measures to decrease the pressure on the affected joints
  - Surgical joint replacement

Recommendations for ocular complications

- Monitoring
  - Ocular clinical symptom evaluation
  - Schirmer's testing
  - Ocular fundus exam
  - Split lamp examination
- Patient counseling
  - Contact lens are discouraged in case of sicca syndrome
- Treatment
  - Cataracts
  - Surgical repair with lens extraction
  - Sicca syndrome
  - Systemic treatment of cGVHD
  - Topical lubricants
  - Caveat topical corticosteroids, cyclosporine

REFERENCES

1. Deeg HJ, Socie G. Malignancies after hematopoietic stem cell transplantation: many questions, some answers. *Blood.* 1998;91(6):1833–1844.
2. Ades L, Guardiola P, Socié G. Second malignancies after allogeneic hematopoietic stem cell transplantation: new insight and current problems. *Blood Rev.* 2002;16(2):135–146.
3. Socie G, Salooja N, Cohen A, et al. Nonmalignant late effects after allogeneic stem cell transplantation. *Blood.* 2003;101(9):3373–3385.
4. Rizzo JD, Wingard JR, Tichelli A, et al. Recommended screening and preventive practices for long-term survivors after hematopoietic cell transplantation: joint recommendations of the European Group for Blood and Marrow Transplantation, the Center for International Blood and Marrow Transplant Research, and the American Society of Blood and Marrow Transplantation. *Biol Blood Marrow Transplant.* 2006;12(2):138–151.
5. Deeg HJ, Flournoy N, Sullivan KM, et al. Cataracts after total body irradiation and marrow transplantation: a sparing effect of dose fractionation. *Int J Radiat Oncol Biol Phys.* 1984;10(7):957–964.
6. Tichelli A, Gratwohl A, Egger T, et al. Cataract formation after bone marrow transplantation. *Ann Intern Med.* 1993;119(12):1175–1180.
7. Benyunes MC, Sullivan KM, Deeg HJ, et al. Cataracts after bone marrow transplantation: long-term follow-up of adults treated with fractionated total body irradiation. *Int J Radiat Oncol Biol Phys.* 1995;32(3):661–670.
8. Belkacemi Y, Ozsahin M, et al. Cataractogenesis after total body irradiation. *Int J Radiat Oncol Biol Phys.* 1996;35(1):53–60.
9. Belkacemi Y, Pene F, et al. Total-body irradiation before bone marrow transplantation for acute leukemia in first or second complete remission. Results and prognostic factors in 326 consecutive patients. *Strahlenther Onkol.* 1998;174(2):92–104.
10. Belkacemi Y, Labopin M, Vernant JP, et al. Cataracts after total body irradiation and bone marrow transplantation in patients with acute leukemia in complete remission: a study of the European Group for Blood and Marrow Transplantation. *Int J.Radiat Oncol Biol Phys.* 1998;41(3):659–668.
11. Socie G, Clift RA, Blaise D, et al. Busulfan plus cyclophosphamide compared with total-body irradiation plus cyclophosphamide before marrow transplantation for myeloid leukemia: long-term follow-up of 4 randomized studies. *Blood.* 2001;98(13):3569–3574.
12. Gratwohl A, Moutsopoulos HM, Chused TM, et al. Sjogren-type syndrome after allogeneic bone-marrow transplantation. *Ann Intern Med.* 1977;87(6):703–706.
13. Janin-Mercier A, Devergie A, Arrago JP, et al. Systemic evaluation of Sjogren-like syndrome after bone marrow transplantation in man. *Transplantation.* 1987;43(5):677–679.
14. Jabs DA, Wingard J, Green WR, et al. The eye in bone marrow transplantation. III. Conjunctival graft-vs-host disease. *Arch Ophthalmol.* 1989;107(9):1343–1348.
15. Tichelli A, Duell T, Weiss M, et al. Late-onset keratoconjunctivitis sicca syndrome after bone marrow transplantation: incidence and risk factors. European Group or Blood and Marrow Transplantation (EBMT) Working Party on Late Effects. *Bone Marrow Transplantation.* 1996;17(6):1105–1111.
16. Crawford SW, Fisher L. Predictive value of pulmonary function tests before marrow transplantation. *Chest.* 1992;101(5):1257–1264.
17. Crawford SW, Pepe M, Lin D, Benedett F, Deeg HJ. Abnormalities of pulmonary function tests after marrow transplantation predict nonrelapse mortality. *Am J Respir Crit Care Med.* 1995;152(2):690–695.
18. Soubani AO, Miller KB, Hassoun PM. Pulmonary complications of bone marrow transplantation 19. *Chest.* 1996;109(4):1066–1077.

19. Cerveri I, Fulgoni P, Giorgiani G, et al. Lung function abnormalities after bone marrow transplantation in children: has the trend recently changed? *Chest.* 2001;120(6):1900–1906.

20. Atkinson K, Cohen M, Biggs J. Avascular necrosis of the femoral head secondary to corticosteroid therapy for graft-versus-host disease after marrow transplantation: effective therapy with hip arthroplasty. *Bone Marrow Transplantation.* 1987;2(4):421–426.

21. Enright H, Haake R, Weisdorf D. Avascular necrosis of bone: a common serious complication of allogeneic bone marrow transplantation. *Am J Med.* 1990;89(6):733–738.

22. Socie G, Selimi F, Sedel A, et al. Avascular necrosis of bone after allogeneic bone marrow transplantation: clinical findings, incidence and risk factors. *Br J Haematol.* 1994;86(3):624–628.

23. Socie G, Cahn JY, Carmelo J, et al. Avascular necrosis of bone after allogeneic bone marrow transplantation: analysis of risk factors for 4388 patients by the Societe Francaise de Greffe de Moelle (SFGM). *Br J Haematol.* 1997;97(4):865–870.

24. Fink JC, Leisenring WM, Sullivan KM, Sherrard DJ, Weiss NS. Avascular necrosis following bone marrow transplantation: a case-control study. *Bone.* 1998;22(1):67–71.

25. Bizot P, Nizard R, Socie G, Gluckman E, Witvoet J, Sedel L. Femoral head osteonecrosis after bone marrow transplantation. *Clin Orthop.* 1998;(357):127–134.

26. Schimmer AD, Minden MD, Keating A. Osteoporosis after blood and marrow transplantation: clinical aspects. *Biol Blood Marrow Transplant.* 2000;6(2A):175–181.

27. Weilbaecher KN. Mechanisms of osteoporosis after hematopoietic cell transplantation. *Biol Blood Marrow Transplant.* 2000;6(2A):165–174.

28. Withold W, Wolf HH, Kollbach S, et al. Monitoring of bone metabolism after bone marrow transplantation by measuring two different markers of bone turnover. *Eur J Clin Chem Clin Biochem.* 1996;34(3):193–197.

29. Kananen K, Volin L, Laitinen K, Alfthan H, Ruutu T, Välimäki MJ. Prevention of bone loss after allogeneic stem cell transplantation by calcium, vitamin D, and sex hormone replacement with or without pamidronate. *J Clin Endocrinol Metab.* 2005;90(7):3877–3885.

30. Carpenter PA, Hoffmeister P, Chesnut III B, et al. Bisphosphonate therapy for reduced bone mineral density in children with chronic graft-versus-host disease. *Biol Blood Marrow Transplant.* 2007;13(6):683–690.

31. Couriel D, Carpenter PA, Cutler C, et al. Ancillary therapy and supportive care of chronic graft-versus-host disease: national institutes of health consensus development project on criteria for clinical trials in chronic Graft-versus-host disease: V. Ancillary Therapy and Supportive Care Working Group Report. *Biol Blood Marrow Transplant.* 2006;12(4):375–396.

32. Mavrokokki T, Cheng A, Stein B, Goss A. Nature and frequency of bisphosphonate-associated osteonecrosis of the jaws in Australia. *J Oral Maxillofac Surg.* 2007;65(3):415–423.

33. Rossouw JE, Anderson GL, Prentice RL, et al. Risks and benefits of estrogen plus progestin in healthy postmenopausal women: principal results From the Women's Health Initiative randomized controlled trial. *JAMA.* 2002;288(3):321–333.

34. Li CI, Malone KE, Porter PL, et al. Relationship between long durations and different regimens of hormone therapy and risk of breast cancer. *JAMA.* 2003;289(24):3254–3263.

35. Anderson GL, Limacher M, Assaf AR, et al. Effects of conjugated equine estrogen in postmenopausal women with hysterectomy: the Women's Health Initiative randomized controlled trial. *JAMA.* 2004;291(14):1701–1712.

36. Witherspoon RP, Fisher LD, Schock G, et al. Secondary cancers after bone marrow transplantation for leukemia or aplastic anemia. *N Engl J Med.* 1989;321(12):784–789.

37. Deeg HJ, Witherspoon RP. Risk factors for the development of secondary malignancies after marrow transplantation. *Hematol Oncol Clin North Am.* 1993;7(2):417–429.

38. Witherspoon RP, Deeg HJ, Storb R. Secondary malignancies after marrow transplantation for leukemia or aplastic anemia. *Transplantation.* 1994;57(10):1413–1418.

39. Socie G. Secondary malignancies. *Curr Opin Hematol.* 1996;3(6):466–470.

40. Cohen JI. Epstein-Barr virus lymphoproliferative disease associated with acquired immunodeficiency. *Medicine (Baltimore).* 1991;70(2):137–160.

41. Curtis RE, Travis LB, Rowlings PA, et al. Risk of lymphoproliferative disorders after bone marrow transplantation: a multi-institutional study. *Blood.* 1999;94(7):2208–2216.

42. Zutter MM, Durnam DM, Hackman RC, et al. Secondary T-cell lymphoproliferation after marrow transplantation. *Am J Clin Pathol.* 1990;94(6):714–721.

43. Verschuur A, Brousse N, Raynal B, et al. Donor B cell lymphoma of the brain after allogeneic bone marrow transplantation for acute myeloid leukemia. *Bone Marrow Transplant.* 1994;14(3):467–470.

44. Schouten HC, Hopman AH, Haesevoets AM, Arenda J-M. Large-cell anaplastic non-Hodgkin's lymphoma originating in donor cells after allogenic bone marrow transplantation. *Br J Haematol.* 1995;91(1):162–166.

45. Meignin V, Devergie A, Brice P, et al. Hodgkin's disease of donor origin after allogeneic bone marrow transplantation for myelogeneous chronic leukemia. *Transplantation.* 1998;65(4):595–597.

46. Rivet J, Moreau D, Daneshpouy M, et al. T-cell lymphoma with eosinophilia of donor origin occurring 12 years after allogeneic bone marrow transplantation for myeloma. *Transplantation.* 2001;72(5):965.

47. Rowlings PA, Curtis RE, Passweg JR, et al. Increased incidence of Hodgkin's disease after allogeneic bone marrow transplantation. *J Clin Oncol.* 1999;17(10):3122–3127.

48. Curtis RE, Rowlings PA, Deeg HJ, et al. Solid cancers after bone marrow transplantation. *N Engl J Med.* 1997;336(13):897–904.

49. Bhatia S, Louie AD, Bhatia R, et al. Solid cancers after bone marrow transplantation. *J Clin Oncol.* 2001;19(2):464–471.

50. Socie G, Scieux C, Gluckman E, et al. Squamous cell carcinomas after allogeneic bone marrow transplantation for aplastic anemia: further evidence of a multistep process. *Transplantation.* 66(5):667–670.

51. Daneshpouy M, Socie G, Clavel C, et al. Human papillomavirus infection and anogenital condyloma in bone marrow transplant recipients. *Transplantation.* 71(1):167–169.

52. Curtis RE, Metayer C, Rizzo JD, et al. Impact of chronic GVHD therapy on the development of squamous-cell cancers after hematopoietic stem-cell transplantation: an international case-control study. *Blood.* 2005;105(10):3802–3811.

53. Leisenring W, Friedman DL, Flowers MED, Schwartz JL, Deeg HJ. Nonmelanoma skin and mucosal cancers after hematopoietic cell transplantation. *J Clin Oncol*. 2006;24(7):1119–1126.

54. Cohen A, Rovelli A, Van Lint MT, et al. Risk for secondary thyroid carcinoma after hematopoietic stem-cell transplantation: an EBMT Late Effects Working Party Study. *J Clin Oncol*. 2007;25(17):2449–2454.

55. Socie G, Henry-Amar M, Devergie A, et al. Poor clinical outcome of patients developing malignant solid tumors after bone marrow transplantation for severe aplastic anemia. *Leuk Lymphoma*. 1992;7(5–6):419–423.

56. Favre-Schmuziger G, Hofer S, Passweg J, et al. Treatment of solid tumors following allogeneic bone marrow transplantation. *Bone Marrow Transplant*. 2000;25(8):895–898.

30

Health-Related Quality of Life (HRQOL) in Chronic Graft versus Host Disease

Sandra A. Mitchell and Bryce B. Reeve

INTRODUCTION AND BACKGROUND

General studies of the late effects in survivors of allogeneic hematopoietic stem cell transplantation (HSCT) suggest that chronic graft versus host disease (cGVHD) has deleterious consequences for physical, mental, and social aspects of functioning and for health-related quality of life (HRQOL) [1, 2]. These studies' findings imply that following allogeneic HSCT, cGVHD negatively affects physical function, domestic and vocational role function, marital, family and social interaction, and psychosocial recovery, and may be associated with a number of bothersome symptoms including fatigue, depression, pain, bowel changes, and dyspareunia [3–5]. Systematic prospective, longitudinal evaluation of HRQOL using standardized measures is needed, of new treatment approaches and to gain a better understanding of the overall impact of cGVHD on general physical and mental health, functioning, symptom burden, and well-being, and to gauge the effectiveness of new treatment approaches. Over the past several years, both the National Institutes of Health/National Cancer Institute and the U.S. Food and Drug Administration have been increasingly interested in understanding how patient-reported outcomes (PROs) (symptoms, functional performance and quality of life) should be incorporated as enpoints into trials of new therapies [6–9], and how PROs can be used to evaluate therapeutic response in cGVHD [10]. A recent Institute of Medicine report noted that studies of interventions to alleviate symptoms and improve quality of life and function in cancer survivors were urgently needed [11], and achieving quality of life for cancer survivors has been identified as a priority by the American Society of Clinical Oncology, the Oncology Nursing Society and the National Cancer Institute [12–14].

We begin by exploring theoretical aspects of HRQOL as a multidimensional construct, examining the significance of HRQOL for transplant survivors with cGVHD and briefly reviewing what we know about the impact of cGVHD on HRQOL (to include symptoms, functional status, and general well-being). The application of this construct as an outcome measure in clinical trials of new therapies for cGVHD, including

a critical appraisal of available measures and methods and considerations in the use of systematic HRQOL assessments in clinical practice with long-term survivors of allogeneic HSCT with cGVHD are discussed. We conclude by analyzing future directions for integrating HRQOL evaluation into practice and research.

DEFINING HRQOL

Health-related quality of life (HRQOL) is a global construct that has evolved in response to the need to evaluate the patient's overall sense of well-being and how it relates to disease and treatment. Beliefs, expectations, and experiences of the individual influence their assessment of their HRQOL, and thus the individual should be considered as the best source to evaluate their HRQOL. This has been affirmed by the World Health Organization in their definition of quality of life as "an individual's perception of their position in life, in the context of the culture and values systems in their life, and in relation to their goals, expectations, standards and concerns" [15]. The term HRQOL limits the focus to the effects of health, illness and treatment on quality of life, and excludes aspects of quality of life that are not related to health, such as political freedom or transportation.

Quality of life has been conceptualized in a number of different ways in the literature, including references to the ability to lead a normal life, to lead a socially useful life (e.g., through social and vocational roles), and to achieve one's life goals, and to experience happiness and satisfaction with life. One researcher has defined quality of life as the difference or the gap, between a person's hopes and expectations and their present life experiences. Essential to the concept of HRQOL is the notion that the meaning of one's current situation is essential: two individuals may have exactly the same objective state of health but they may perceive their HRQOL quite differently.

Though there is no universally agreed upon definition, there is consensus in the literature that HRQOL is a multidimensional construct, that it includes the broad domains of emotional, physical, functional, social, financial, and spiritual

Table 30.1: Selected Items that Measure Symptoms or Functional Status

Lee[†] cGVHD Symptom Scale [31]	MOS-SF-36[†] Physical Function Subscale [32]
How bothered have you been by any of the following symptoms within the past month:	*Does your health now limit you in these activities:*
■ Abnormal skin color	■ Lifting or carrying groceries
■ Itchy skin	■ Climbing one flight of stiars
■ Dry eyes	■ Bending, kneeling, or stooping
■ Ulcers in the mouth	■ Walking several blocks
■ Frequent cough	■ Bathing or dressing yourself
■ Difficulty swallowing solid foods	
■ Joint or muscle aches	
■ Limited joint movement	
■ Muscle cramps	
■ Weak muscles	

[†] *Note*: These items reflect only a sample of items from this scale.

well-being; that the individual is the best judge of his or her own HRQOL; and that quality of life is dynamic and changes over time [16–24]. Studies that operationalize (measure) quality of life differently may have distinct findings even for the same patient population, and the definition of the construct of HRQOL should be selected to fit the study purpose and patient population and will guide the selection of HRQOL measures.

A number of authors have argued that many of our current approaches to measuring HRQOL actually measure the related concepts of health status, symptoms, or functional status [25, 26]; or that they measure the variables that influence quality of life (e.g., mood, physical function) rather than quality of life itself [24]. Conceptual ambiguity in the field of HRQOL research has resulted in a tendency to use the same terms to mean different things, and thus it has been difficult to compare findings across studies and to translate knowledge into clinical practice. For the purposes of this chapter, we define HRQOL as a multidimensional construct that encompasses health status, symptoms, and aspects of physical, emotional, social, and spiritual functioning and well-being, together with overall life satisfaction, happiness, and sense of purpose and fulfillment, at a point in time when health, illness, and treatment conditions are relevant [18].

DISTINGUISHING HRQOL FROM SYMPTOMS AND FUNCTIONAL STATUS

An important issue in HRQOL measurement is distinguishing among symptoms, functional status, and the domains of HRQOL [27–29]. HRQOL measures may include questions about common disease- or treatment-related symptoms, and about functional status and daily activities; however, it is important to note that the three concepts are distinct. HRQOL measures are often used in tandem with measures of functional status and symptoms so that the relationship among these constructs can be assessed. Table 30.1 gives examples of symptoms and functional status items [30, 31].

Symptoms are experienced deviations from an individual's perception of his or her normal, healthy state of being, and may be conceptualized as multidimensional in nature with aspects that include perception, character, frequency/persistence, intensity, distress, and interference with function [32–34]. Whether symptoms should be scaled for intensity, frequency, interference, or all of these dimensions remains a topic of continued debate in the literature [35–37]. Measurement of the degree of distress or bother [38, 39] associated with individual symptoms acknowledges not only the presence of a symptom, but also encompasses simultaneously its severity, persistence, and interference. For example, skin itching may be rated as mild in severity, but may be experienced as extremely bothersome or distressing either because it persists throughout the day or because it interferes with social or vocational functioning. Symptom burden may be considered the collective representation of the features and impact of bothersome symptoms, as reported from the patient's perspective [40, 41]. Both theory and research [33, 42, 43] suggest that the experience of multiple bothersome symptoms either sequentially or concurrently has an exponential rather than multiplicative impact on symptom burden.

Cella [44] has described several possible relationships between symptom intensity, symptom duration and HRQOL that may be observed, and his analysis underscores the importance of distinguishing these constructs. For example, the relationship between symptom intensity and HRQOL may be linear (that is, as symptoms increase or decrease, HRQOL increases or decreases) or the relationship may be moderated by symptom intensity (i.e., HRQOL is affected by a symptom only once a given level of symptom severity is reached or only until a plateau in the decline of HRQOL is reached). The relationship between symptom duration and HRQOL can also vary across time and clinical circumstances, for example: (1) a decline in quality of life can occur once a symptom is experienced and quality of life remains low; (2) with persistence of a symptom there is adaptation with the result that there is a diminished effect of the symptom on quality of life; and (3) an individual becomes increasingly bothered by a persistent symptom over time, and the long duration of the symptom initiates a decline in quality of life. Thus, the relationship between symptoms and HRQOL may vary both within and across patients as disease status changes and as multiple symptoms occur.

Functional status is another concept that is related to, but distinct from according to the Functional Outcomes Model, postulated by Leidy [45] and recently extended by Stull, Leidy, Jones, and Stahl [46], functional status comprises an individual or population's ability to undertake activities designed to meet basic needs, fulfill life roles, and maintain health and well-being. It is conceptually distinct from symptoms and from quality of life. Functional status has four dimensions: capacity, performance, reserve, and capacity utilization. Functional capacity, reflecting the maximum possible level of function is distinct from functional performance [45]. Individuals choose to function at a level that reflects their greatest physical and psychological comfort. Functional performance is defined as the physical, psychological, social, occupational, and spiritual activities that individuals do in the normal course of their lives to meet basic needs, fulfill usual roles, and maintain their health and well-being. The term functional reserve refers to the difference between functional capacity and performance. Functional reserve is the latent functional ability that can be called upon in time of perceived need. It is a dynamic construct and is defined relative to capacity and performance. Individuals with different functional capacities can still perform an activity at the same level, the difference being the amount of functional reserve utilized to achieve a given level of performance, and therefore the ease with which an activity is performed. Encroachment upon functional reserve may be expressed through the development of symptoms, for example, fatigue, weakness, pain, or dyspnea [47]. Leidy's framework also posits that individuals who have diminishing functional capacity can continue to sustain functional performance through higher capacity utilization.

CONCEPTUAL MODELS OF HRQOL FOR APPLICATION TO LONG-TERM TRANSPLANT SURVIVORS WITH CGVHD

A number of models have been proposed to explain the domains of HRQOL and to depict relationships among the domains. Three models with potential application to understanding and measuring HRQOL in long-term survivors of HSCT, with who are experiencing cGVHD, are depicted in Figures 30.1 through 30.3. The conceptual models for HRQOL developed by Ferrans et al. (Figure 30.1) and by Ferrell et al. (Figure 30.2) were developed independently although they are quite similar in terms of the HRQOL domains identified. Both models were developed and further validated on the basis of qualitative data, including interviews with HSCT recipients and survivors of HSCT [48, 49].

Ferrans [47] has recently revised a model of HRQOL originally proposed by Wilson and Cleary [50]. Figure 30.3 depicts

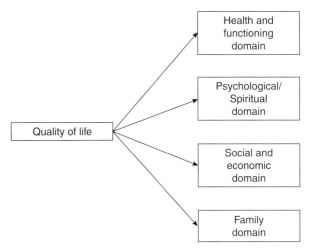

Figure 30.1 Ferrans conceptual model for quality of life.
Ferrans CE. Development of a quality of life index for patients with cancer. *Oncol Nurs Forum*, 17;1990:17. Used with permission.

relationships among the elements of the revised Wilson and Cleary model of HRQOL. Since it is also critical to understand the complex factors that may contribute to overall HRQOL individual and environmental, characteristics of the environment and the individual, as well as biological and physiological variables that influence symptoms, functional status HRQOL are also portrayed. As you move from left to right, the model progresses from the cellular level, to the level of the individual, to the societal level.

More recently, investigators in the field of HRQOL outcomes evaluation have drawn a conceptual distinction between measures/items that assess the *status* of a particular aspect of HRQOL (e.g., how much fatigue do you have) versus a measure/item that asks the respondent to make an *evaluation* of that state (e.g., how satisfied are you with your current level of fatigue) [18]. This distinction is important because some HRQOL measures are composed predominantly of status questions while evaluation questions comprise the majority of items in other measures. Answers to these two types of questions (status and evaluation) must be interpreted quite differently and may explain why there has been variability observed in the predictors of HRQOL both within and across populations. A distinction should also be made between indicators of HRQOL (e.g., what is quality of life, what refers to quality of life?) and determinants of HRQOL (i.e., what contributes to or influences quality of life) [24].

CONSIDERATIONS IN SELECTING A MEASURE OF HRQOL, SYMPTOMS OR FUNCTIONAL STATUS IN CGVHD

There are a wide range of potential measures of HRQOL from which to choose. As a starting point, Salek offers a compendium summarizing available measures and psychometric data, though this text has not been updated for 10 years. PROQOLID is an Internet resource describing more than

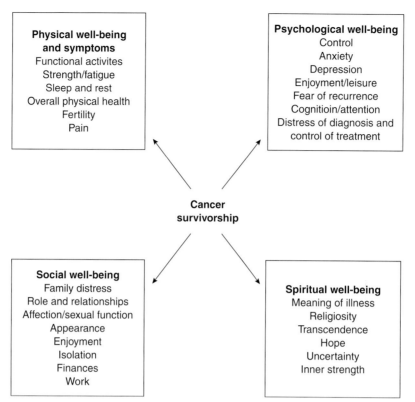

Figure 30.2 Quality of life model applied to cancer survivors.
Quality of Life in Long-Term Cancer Survivors by BR Ferrell, K.H. Dow, S. Leigh, J.Ly, & P. Gulasekaram. 1995, *Oncol Nurs Forum*, 22, p. 916. Used with permission.

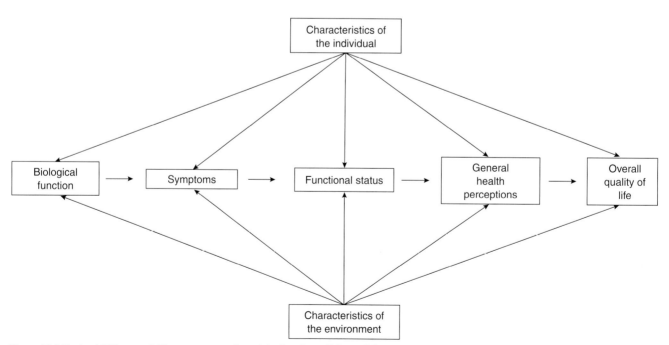

Figure 30.3 Revised Wilson and Cleary conceptual model of quality of life model.
Conceptual Model of Health-Related Quality of Life; C.E. Ferrans, J.J. Zerwic, JE Wilbur & J.L Larson, 2005; *J Nurs Scholarsh*, 37 (4), p. 338. Used with permission.

600 available measures of symptoms, functional status, and HRQOL, offering details concerning the psychometric properties of the instruments and access to translated instruments, user manuals, and the contacts necessary to secure licensing agreements.

A number of factors should be considered in the final selection of an instrument to measure HRQOL, symptoms, or functional status [54]. No one measure is ideal for all situations, and evidence for the pyschometric properties of a measure should be evaluated with respect to the population within which the measure was tested. When selecting a measure of HRQOL, researchers and clinicians have a number of decision points. A wide array of valid and reliable measures is currently available to capture HRQOL, functional status, and symptom assessments at varying levels of specificity, and none has been identified as a gold standard. Pearce, Sanson-Fisher, and Campbell have recently published a review of the existing scales to measure HRQOL in cancer survivors, and identified nine measures developed specifically to measure HRQOL in this population, though none fully met all of the authors' rigorous psychometric standards [51].

HRQOL measures can be distinguished as generic versus disease-specific. Generic instruments (such as the MOS-SF-36 or the Sickness Impact Profile) produce scores for all domains of HRQOL, whereas disease-specific instruments (such as the Lee cGVHD Symptom Scale) focus on concerns specific to illness or treatment. Generic measures offer the advantage of comparisons with the general population and can be used across disease or treatment group [52]. However, generic measures tend to be broad, and may therefore be so general that they fail to address the issues of greatest concern. On the other hand, while disease-specific measures tend to have greater face validity, and may be more responsive to change, they may overlook critical aspects of HRQOL. There is general agreement that both generic and condition-specific instruments should be used.

HRQOL measures should be valid (measure what they say they measure), reliable (capable of producing the same results in the same patient group when assessed repeatedly) and sensitive or responsive to changes. Measures offered in multiple languages should also have available evidence of their linguistic and cultural equivalence. Frost et al. have recently proposed guidelines for establishing sufficient evidence of the reliability and validity of patient-reported outcome measures, including measures of HRQOL [53]. Other considerations in selecting an HRQOL measure include barriers to access and use the measure (e.g., permission to use, costs), whether the measure has floor or ceiling effects in specific populations, the method of administration (self-administered, telephone survey, or in-person interview), the clarity and number of questions, the ease of scoring, the availability of the measure in languages other than English, and in cognitively impaired or pediatric populations whether proxy-ratings of HRQOL using the measure have been shown to be valid and reliable [54]. Population characteristics such as disease and treatment type, age, performance status, and illness burden may affect completion rates

and will shape decisions about whether a measure of overall HRQOL or a more specific measure (e.g., of symptom burden or functional status) is most appropriate. In the context of selecting an HRQOL measure for research, the study hypothesis and conceptual framework for measurement also greatly influence the choice of a measure [55], that is, whether global well-being or specific domains of symptoms or functional status are thought to be relevant outcomes in assessing benefit or are likely to change with intervention.

Generic instruments, such as the SF-36 and the Functional Assessment of Chronic Illness Therapy (FACIT) battery of HRQOL measures, provide the opportunity to compare study findings to relevant norms and to identify minimally important clinical differences. This information may be particularly valuable to the clinician who is screening populations or to the researcher interested in addressing specific hypotheses. The dimension(s) of HRQOL of greatest interest and one's purpose(s) in measuring these outcomes should also be clearly identified and used to guide rational selection from among the available measures.

The only available cGVHD-specific HRQOL measure is the Lee cGVHD Symptom Scale, though a cGVHD-specific module for the MD Anderson Symptom Inventory is undergoing preliminary psychometric and feasibility testing (personal communication, L. Williams, June 30, 2008). The Lee cGVHD Symptom scale assesses the degree to which respondents are bothered by each of the 30 symptoms that are common in cGVHD. Participants are asked to frame their responses around the degree of bother experienced in the past month. Responses are captured on a five-point Likert scale ("no symptoms or not bothered at all," "slightly bothered," "moderately bothered," "bothered quite a bit," or "extremely bothered"). The measure provides seven subscales (energy, skin, nutrition, muscles/joints, breathing, psychosocial, eye/mouth) and items are summed to produce a summary score of cGVHD-specific symptom distress. Test–retest reliability for the overall tool was modest ($r = 0.64$), as one would expect with a summative symptom inventory, since symptoms fluctuate from day to day [30]. However, individual symptom subscales that clinically tend to have greater consistently, such as ocular symptoms ($r = 0.93$) and mouth symptoms ($r = 0.87$), had stronger test-retest reliability. Internal consistency reliability assessed using Cronbach's alpha was $\alpha = 0.90$ for the overall score. Discriminant validity was supported by the low correlations between selected subscale scores on the cGVHD symptom scale and unrelated domains of the SF-36 and FACT-BMT. Convergent validity was supported by the fact that the energy subscale correlated most closely with physical domains on the SF-36 and FACT-BMT, whereas, the psychological subscale correlated best with scores for emotional function on the FACT-BMT and mental health on the SF-36 [30]. The Lee cGVHD Symptom Scale takes approximately 5 minutes to complete.

Overall, little is known about the psychometric properties of measures of symptoms, functional status and HRQOL in patients with cGVHD, and studies to explore the reliability and validity of the measures of symptoms, functional status, and

Table 30.2: Patient-Reported Outcome Measures Recommended for Evaluating Therapeutic Response in Adults with Chronic GVHD

Instrument*	Lee Chronic GVHD Symptom Scale	Human Activity Profile (HAP)	Medical Outcomes Study Short Form-36 (MOS-SF-36)	Functional Assessment of Cancer Therapy-Bone Marrow Transplant (FACT-BMT)
Outcome Measured	Chronic GVHD-specific symptom bother	Functional performance and activity limitations	Self-reported general health status	Health-related quality of life
Content Domains	30 symptoms common in cGVHD Seven subscales (energy, skin, nutrition, lung, psychosocial, eye and mouth) and items are summed to produce a summary score of chronic GVHD-specific symptom bother	94 oxygen-demanding activities of daily living. The activities are arranged in a hierarchical fashion beginning with getting in and out of bed and progressing through more physically demanding activities and ending with running or jogging 3 miles in 30 minutes or less	The 36 items evaluate: physical functioning, physical role functioning, emotional role functioning, social functioning, bodily pain, mental health, vitality, and general health	FACT-G has four domains: Physical Well-Being, Social Well-Being, Emotional Well-Being, and Functional Well-Being. BMT Module: 18 areas of concern specific to hematopoietic stem cell transplant recipients
Number of Items	30	94	36	45 Items (27 for FACT-G and 18 for BMT module)
Response Frame	Degree of symptom bother experienced within the past month.	The last time they had an opportunity to perform the activity independently	Past four weeks; a single item asks about health in comparison to one year ago	Within the past seven days
Languages Available	English, Spanish translation has been used and developed.	English	English, Spanish, and more than 50 other languages	English, Spanish, and more than 20 other languages
Advantages/ Disadvantages	Chronic GvHD-specific, brief, strong face validity and thorough preliminary psychometric evaluation.	Ceiling and floor effects are limited, ease of questionnaire administration and scoring. Values for healthy age-matched samples available for adjusted activity score	Reliability, validity and sensitivity to change extensively supported. Extensively used in clinical trials	Reliability, validity and sensitivity to change extensively supported. Extensively used in clinical trials
Time Required to Complete Questionnaire	5 minutes	7 minutes	7 minutes	5–10 minutes
Procurement/Costs	No costs. Contact: sjlee@fhcrc.org	No costs. Contact: ddaughto@unmc.edu	Needs an annual license to use. Visit: sf-36.org	Scoring and interpretation manuals have a nominal cost, visit: facit.org

* The recommendation to use these instruments as a response measure in cGVHD does not imply permission for their use in clinical trials. Investigator teams wishing to collect these data should follow the procedure established by the organizations that hold copyright for each instrument.

HRQOL identified in the recently proposed cGVHD response criteria (see Table 30.2) [10] are urgently needed. Results from one analysis suggest that the trial outcome index (TOI) of the functional assessment of cancer therapy-bone marrow transplantation module (FACT-BMT) may be more sensitive to the occurrence of cGVHD compared to the Medical Outcomes Study Short Form-12 (an abbreviated version of the SF-36) [56].

MORBIDITY AND MORTALITY BURDEN OF cGVHD

Chronic GVHD is a chronic, multisystem alloimmune late complication of allogeneic HSCT. Occurring in between 33% and 80% of patients who survive 150 days after allogeneic transplant, it is a major cause of late mortality, significant morbidity and impairments in HRQOL. While the precise pathogenesis of cGVHD remains elusive, the attack on host tissues is initially mediated by donor T cells recognizing antigens expressed on normal tissues, and likely also involves immune dysregulation of donor derived lymphocyte clones secondary to thymic atrophy, lymphocyte depletion, and loss of thymic epithelial secretory function [57].

The incidence of cGVHD varies depending on the age of the stem cell recipient, gender mismatch between recipient and donor, the degree of HLA disparity, the use of unmanipulated or T-cell-depleted stem cell sources, the use of donor lymphocyte infusions, and a history of prior acute GVHD [58, 59]. With the increased use of donor lymphocyte infusions, and a reduction in early posttransplant mortality there has been a resultant increase in the number of long-term survivors and with this, it may be anticipated that the incidence of cGVHD will rise [60, 61].

Clinically, cGVHD is characterized by multisystem disease manifestations, which frequently mimic the clinical features of autoimmune diseases. The manifestations include skin changes (lichenoid and sclerodermatous skin changes, erythematous rash, skin ulcers, changes in pigmentation, loss of accessory structures like hair, dystrophic nails), ocular dryness, grittiness and pain, sicca symptoms, abdominal cramping, esophageal dysmotility, weight loss, hepatic dysfunction, obstructive lung disease, joint contractures, myositis, polyserositis, immunodeficiency (including hypogammaglobulinemia and functional asplenia), and the development of autoantibodies including antinuclear antibody, antierythrocyte antibodies, and antiplatelet antibodies [62, 63]. Among those who survive 2 or more years following allogeneic HSCT, cGVHD is a leading cause of nonrelapse mortality and a major predictor of serious morbidity [64–67]. Studies examining late effects following allogeneic HSCT suggest that patients with cGVHD requiring immunosuppressive therapy 2 years after transplant are at a particularly high risk for nonrelapse death, primarily from infectious complications [68]. The range of clinical manifestations and the consequences of cGVHD for health status, quality of life, symptoms, and functional status are summarized in Figure 30.4.

IMPACT OF cGVHD ON HRQOL, SYMPTOMS AND FUNCTIONAL STATUS

In recent years HRQOL has become a common concern in healthcare, and it has been the focus of considerable research in oncology [69, 70] and following HSCT [22, 71–74]. Although there are no published reports that directly and systematically characterize HRQOL, symptoms or functional status in samples comprised exclusively of patients with cGVHD, general studies of HRQOL following allogeneic HSCT provide clues to the possible impact of cGVHD on these specific dimensions as well as the impact on overall health and well-being.

A number of studies have shown that the presence of extensive cGVHD is a consistent predictor of impaired quality of life [1, 3, 56, 75–81], although interestingly, one study noted that continued immunosuppressive therapy does not itself seem to have a negative influence on HRQOL [1]. Moreover, studies comparing transplant survivors with and without cGVHD suggest that those survivors with cGVHD experience significantly more fatigue, depression, pain, bowel changes, and dsypareunia [1, 4, 82]. Relative to those transplant survivors without cGVHD, physical, sexual, and social functioning is also noted to be lower [80, 82]. Transplant survivors with more severe cGVHD also have impaired physical and psychosocial recovery both at 1 year after transplant [4, 80], and over the longer term [5, 77]. In a study of health outcomes following allogeneic HSCT for chronic myeloid leukemia, cGVHD was the strongest risk factor for the development of several significant medical late effects such as hypothyroidism, osteoporosis, and was also a predictor for inferior overall health and mental health, as well as functional impairment, activity limitations, and pain [3]. Another key finding of this study was the fact that those with resolved cGVHD had HRQOL, functional and health status outcomes comparable to those with no history of cGVHD.

The literature suggests that a variety of clinical and treatment-related variables influence symptoms, functional status, and HRQOL in HSCT survivors with cGVHD including age, gender, cGVHD severity, intensity of immunosuppression, the time elapsed since cGVHD was diagnosed, and comorbidity. In prior studies of survivors of hematopoietic stem cell transplantation, inferior HRQOL has been associated with the occurrence of cGVHD [1, 3, 75–77, 79, 81, 83], the presence of more physical symptoms [84], lower levels of physical functioning [85–87], and a greater number of comorbid conditions and late effects of high-dose chemoradiotherapy, such as hypothyroidism, liver dysfunction, osteoporosis or relapse [77]. Research also suggests that gender differentially influences posttransplant quality of life, with males reporting poorer quality of life [85]. While some studies suggest that older age at transplantation may predict impaired overall HRQOL [88], other studies have failed to find a relationship between older age at transplant and impairments in HRQOL during survivorship following the procedure [89].

Across several studies, more extensive cGVHD had a consistent negative association with HRQOL [2, 3, 80, 90] although

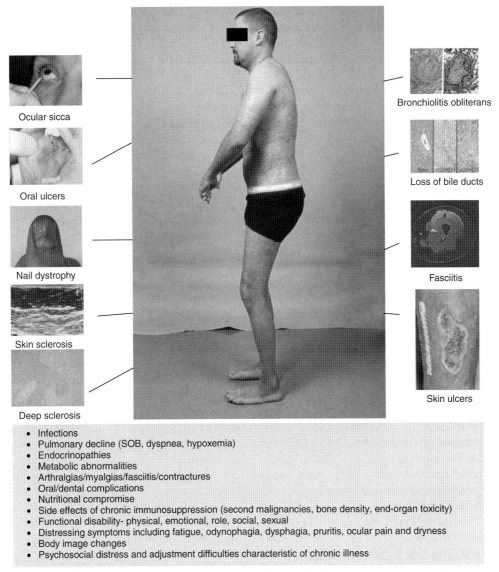

- Ocular sicca
- Oral ulcers
- Nail dystrophy
- Skin sclerosis
- Deep sclerosis
- Bronchiolitis obliterans
- Loss of bile ducts
- Fasciitis
- Skin ulcers

- Infections
- Pulmonary decline (SOB, dyspnea, hypoxemia)
- Endocrinopathies
- Metabolic abnormalities
- Arthralgias/myalgias/fasciitis/contractures
- Oral/dental complications
- Nutritional compromise
- Side effects of chronic immunosuppression (second malignancies, bone density, end-organ toxicity)
- Functional disability- physical, emotional, role, social, sexual
- Distressing symptoms including fatigue, odynophagia, dysphagia, pruritis, ocular pain and dryness
- Body image changes
- Psychosocial distress and adjustment difficulties characteristic of chronic illness

Figure 30.4 Clinical manifestations of cGVHD and its effects on health status, symptoms, functional status and quality of life. See Plate 77 in the color plate section.

in one study, the simple presence or absence of immunosuppressive therapy did not predict HRQOL outcomes [1]. There is also some evidence to suggest that the length of time that has elapsed since the cGVHD diagnosis influences symptom burden and psychological distress. Heinonen et al. (2005) observed a general improvement in the prevalence and severity of distressing symptoms across the first 5 years of recovery following allogeneic HSCT. Other studies indicate, however, that symptoms such as moderate to severe fatigue, skin dryness, pain, joint stiffness, weakness, tremor, eye symptoms, dyspnea, cognitive dysfunction, and problems with sleep, all symptoms that are consistent with cGVHD and its treatment, remain prominent difficulties for HSCT survivors over the long term [2, 3, 77, 82, 91].

Making inferences about HRQOL in cGVHD from the post-HSCT literature is challenging in part because there is heterogeneity in the samples (ages, preparative regimen intensities, mixed autologous, and allogeneic recipients), measures,

data analytic approaches, length of follow-up, and timing of HRQOL assessment relative to the transplant. The literature is also difficult to interpret because psychological aspects of HRQOL, such as anxiety, depression, and limitations in social or vocational functioning, can result from or be intensified by HSCT and cGVHD. All of these aspects may influence an individual's reporting of HRQOL and this heterogeneity together with issues of response shift [92], the absence of data to guide determination of the minimally important clinical difference (MICD) in this population [93], and the magnitude of intra-individual variation in HRQOL reports across time [94] makes it extremely difficult to draw definitive conclusions. The impact of cGVHD on HRQOL can only be distinguished from the more general effects of HSCT using prospective, longitudinal designs that follow patients from the time of transplant, characterize changes in cGVHD severity and intensity of immunosuppression over time, and utilize samples sizes that permit stratification and statistical control of covariates such as baseline psychological symptoms.

Selected Issues in Measuring and Interpreting HRQOL Outcomes

Timing of Outcome Assessment

When and how often to assess HRQOL outcomes is determined by a multitude of considerations including the research hypotheses, the measurement conceptual model, and clinical utility [95]. The rate at which the concept of interest is likely to vary within an individual and its expected rate of change given the natural history of the disease or following an intervention also influence decisions about the timing of outcome assessment. It is often desirable to time HRQOL assessments to coincide with monitoring intervals for other clinical events (e.g., cGVHD response measurements). These considerations must be balanced by issues of respondent burden, researcher time and effort, the need to have consistency in the timing of HRQOL across treatment arms, the measure's established sensitivity to change, and the data analytic challenges associated with multiple time points of assessment.

Response Shift

Response shift is the change in scores that may occur over time as respondents adjust their expectations on the basis of changes in their health status or circumstances [96, 97]. This change may be an adjustment in the respondent's internal standards of measurement (i.e., *recalibration*), a change in the respondent's values (i.e., *reprioritization*), or a redefinition of the construct by the respondent (i.e., *reconceptualization*) [98]. Another explanation of response shift is that individuals readjust their evaluation of their status to maintain hope or according to what they perceive should be normal [99, 100]. In some situations, response shift can lead to HRQOL scores that are difficult to accurately interpret. For example, an intervention aimed at increasing adolescent cancer survivors' confidence in engaging in physically challenging activities actually resulted in a decrease in global QOL ratings [101]. The researchers hypothesized that response shift occurred as a result of the intervention, and caused participants to reconsider their current life quality given the change in perceived accessibility of physical activities and make a downward comparison. Response shift is often observed in longitudinal studies or repeated measures over time, and may account for HRQOL scores that paradoxically increase, decrease or are unchanged.

Health Status Versus Preference-Based Assessment

Work in HRQOL measurement has originated from two different approaches: health status assessment and health value/preference/utility assessment. Health status assessment describes a person's functioning or satisfaction with functioning in one or more domains (e.g., physical, emotional, social). In contrast, preference-based HRQOL measures assess the value or desirability of a health state against an external metric such as the trade-offs the individual is willing to make to improve their health, balancing the amount of time they would spend in their current health state versus taking a "gamble" or chance of having sudden death (or another undesired health state), or improvement to perfect health. A utility is thus assigned to their current health state that reflects their preference for this health state compared to the undesired health state and perfect health. Various approaches to eliciting preferences exist, including visual analogue scales, standard gamble, and time trade-off [102]. For example, with the standard gamble, suppose we wish to assign a preference score to the overall state of health for a patient recovering from a stem cell transplant. The respondent is offered a hypothetical choice between remaining in their current state of health for a specified period of time (say 1 year), versus taking a gamble. In the gamble they are offered a probability (say 20% probability) of spending that same year in perfect health or the probability of immediate death (or some other undesired health state). The probability is varied until the respondent is unable to decide between remaining in their current health state and taking the lottery. With poorer current health state, a respondent will accept even gambles that have a comparatively low probability of achieving perfect health. Though preference-based approaches to HRQOL measurement have generally had more limited application in oncology than health assessment approaches, the health utilities index (HUI) has been used in survivors of childhood cancer [103] and a recent report describes efforts to develop utilities for health states assessed in cancer patients using the Functional Assessment of Cancer-General (FACT-G) [104]. Preference-based approaches to HRQOL may not be suitable to elicit HRQOL assessments from proxy respondents [105] and may post interpretive challenges for both patients and investigators.

Minimally Important Clinical Difference

An important advance in HRQOL research has been the concept of the minimally important difference (MID). The MID is defined as the smallest difference in score on a measure that the patient perceives as beneficial, and some have extended this definition to include differences that would mandate a change in the patient's management [106, 107]. Synonymous terms include the minimally important clinical difference (MICD), clinically significant difference, and minimum clinically important difference. Differences in scores smaller than the MICD are considered clinically unimportant, even if statistical significance is reached. Though various recommendations for MICD with the SF-36 have been proposed for the thresholds of MICD from the normative value of 50 [31], a general consensus of an MICD of 5 points for each of the SF-36 domain scales and 3 points for the physical component summary (PCS) and mental component summary (MCS) scores exists in the literature [107, 108]. In the design and reporting of HRQOL data, MICD estimates can be used to develop hypotheses and for power analyses, and are extremely useful in interpreting study results, although more studies are needed to identify MCIDs in cancer populations.

TECHNOLOGICAL ADVANCES OPTIMIZE THE EVALUATION OF HRQOL OUTCOMES

Electronic technology has been developed that allows data concerning HRQOL, functional status and self-report of symptoms to be gathered using touch-screen computers, interactive voice response systems, telephone monitoring, or Internet-based surveys, thus eliminating several steps associated with completion of paper and pencil questionnaires. A growing number of instruments have been adapted for and evaluated in a web-based format [109]. Feasibility testing indicates that these measures are generally well-accepted by patients and that technology increases the ease, cost-effectiveness, and efficiency of survey administration and may decrease missing data [110–113]. A recent report describes the feasibility and outcomes associated with use of an innovative web-based system for very frequent HRQOL and symptom self-assessment following HSCT [114]. Advances in the development of item banks and computerized adaptive testing (CAT) continue at a rapid pace [115], and the National Institutes of Health's PROMIS (Patient-Reported Outcomes Measurement Information System; www.NIHpromis.org) offers improved precision and efficiency with which HRQOL outcomes are measured, reduced respondent burden, and enhanced comparability of health outcome measures [116, 117].

CONCLUSIONS AND DIRECTIONS FOR PRACTICE AND RESEARCH

HRQOL data can provide information to guide clinical decision making on several levels. It can help clinicians in decision making by informing them about the impact of specific treatments on patient outcomes, and identifying and prioritizing the treatment of problems that have a significant impact on symptoms, functional status, and HRQOL. It can also be used to improve communication between clinicians and patients, and to help patients in making decisions about more than one treatment option. Lastly, information about HRQOL outcomes can be used to shape health care policy and inform decisions by governmental institutions and pharmaceutical industry.

Despite fulfilling some of these objectives, the application of HRQOL in clinical care and research is an evolving field, and it has had some challenges. First, there is a need to reach consensus within the field to standardize the definitions of HRQOL, and the domains that make up HRQOL, to reduce the ambiguity and confusion among researchers that limits the theoretical or practice value of findings [118]. Second, with no agreed upon single measures of HRQOL, numerous HRQOL measures exist that limit the ability to contrast results across multiple studies using different HRQOL measures. Projects like the PROMIS offer an attractive solution to this issue by building HRQOL item banks from existing measures and linking all items on to a common metric to allow any set of measures

formed from the bank to be compared or combined together. Third, response burden is a constant concern when assessing HRQOL in ill or older adult populations. While single item HRQOL measures are simple to use and interpret, they may lack content validity and be imprecise [119] except perhaps for screening [120]. Last, better effort needs to be taken to improve the interpretability of HRQOL scores for patients, clinicians, and policymakers. Martin urges that consideration be given to including graphical analysis in addition to statistical analysis, and that there be attention to parsimony and plainness when interpreting and reporting HRQOL outcomes [121]. The availability of psychometrically sound and decision-relevant HRQOL measures will enhance our capacity to improve care delivery by identifying the most efficacious interventions and translating these research findings into useful information for decision-making [122].

REFERENCES

1. Chiodi S, Spinelli S, Ravera G, et al. Quality of life in 244 recipients of allogeneic bone marrow transplantation. *Br J Haematol.* 2000;110(3):614–619.
2. Sutherland HJ, Fyles GM, Adams G, et al. Quality of life following bone marrow transplantation: A comparison of patient reports with population norms. *Bone Marrow Transplantation.* 1997;19(11):1129–1136.
3. Baker KS, Gurney JG, Ness KK, et al. Late effects in survivors of chronic myeloid leukemia treated with hematopoietic cell transplantation: Results from the Bone Marrow Transplant Survivor Study. *Blood.* Sep 15 2004;104(6):1898–1906.
4. Syrjala KL, Langer S, Abrams J, Storer B, Martin P. Physical and mental recovery after hematopoietic stem cell transplantation. *Discovery Medicine.* Oct 2004;4(23):263–269.
5. Syrjala KL, Langer SL, Abrams JR, et al. Recovery and long-term function after hematopoietic cell transplantation for leukemia or lymphoma. *J Am Med Assoc.* 2004;291(19):2335–2343.
6. Acquadro C, Berzon R, Dubois D, et al. Incorporating the patient's perspective into drug development and communication: An ad hoc task force report of the Patient-Reported Outcomes (PRO) Harmonization Group meeting at the Food and Drug Administration, February 16, 2001. *Value Health.* Sep-Oct 2003;6(5):522–531.
7. Revicki DA, Osoba D, Fairclough D, et al. Recommendations on health-related quality of life research to support labeling and promotional claims in the United States. *Qual Life Res.* 2000;9(8):887.
8. Minasian LM, O'Mara A. Introduction. *J Natl Cancer Inst Monogr.* 2007(37):1–2.
9. Ganz PA, Goodwin PJ. Health-related quality of life measurement in symptom management trials. *J Natl Cancer Inst Monogr.* 2007(37):47–52.
10. Pavletic SZ, Martin P, Lee SJ, et al. Measuring therapeutic response in chronic graft-versus-host disease: National Institutes of Health Consensus Development Project on Criteria for Clinical Trials in Chronic Graft-versus-Host Disease: IV. Response Criteria Working Group report. *Biol Blood Marrow Transplant.* Mar 2006;12(3):252–266.

11. IOM. *From cancer patient to survivor: Lost in transition.* Washington DC: National Academies Press; 2006.

12. Berry DL. *Oncology Nursing Society 2005–2009 Research Agenda.* Pittsburgh: Oncology Nursing Society; 2007.

13. NCI. *Report of the President's Cancer Panel Living beyond cancer: Finding a new balance.* Bethesda, MD: National Cancer Institute; 2004.

14. Outcomes of cancer treatment for technology assessment and cancer treatment guidelines. American Society of Clinical Oncology. *J Clin Oncol.* Feb 1996;14(2):671–679.

15. The World Health Organization Quality of Life assessment (WHOQOL): Position paper from the World Health Organization. *Soc Sci Med.* Nov 1995;41(10):1403–1409.

16. Bloom JR, Kang SH, Petersen DM, Stewart SL. Quality of life in long-term cancer survivors. In: Feuerstein M, ed. *Handbook of cancer survivorship.* New York: Springer Publishing; 2007: 43–65.

17. Buchanan DR, O'Mara AM, Kelaghan JW, Minasian LM. Quality-of-life assessment in the symptom management trials of the National Cancer Institute-supported Community Clinical Oncology Program. *J Clin Oncol.* Jan 20 2005;23(3):591–598.

18. Ferrans CE. Definitions and conceptual models of quality of life. In: Lipscomb J, Gotay, CC, Snyder, C, eds. *Outcomes assessment in cancer: measures, methods, and applications.* Cambridge: Cambridge University Press. 2005;14–30.

19. King CR, Ferrell BR, Grant M, Sakurai C. Nurses' perceptions of the meaning of quality of life for bone marrow transplant survivors. *Cancer Nurs.* Apr 1995;18(2):118–129.

20. Haas BK. A multidisciplinary concept analysis of quality of life. *West J Nurs Res.* Dec 1999;21(6):728–742.

21. Ferrans CE. Development of a conceptual model of quality of life. *Sch Inq Nurs Pract.* Fall 1996;10(3):293–304.

22. Hacker ED. Quantitative measurement of quality of life in adult patients undergoing bone marrow transplant or peripheral blood stem cell transplant: A decade in review. *Oncology Nursing Forum.* 2003;30(4):613–629.

23. King CR. Advances in how clinical nurses can evaluate and improve quality of life for individuals with cancer. *Oncology Nursing Forum.* 2006;33(Suppl 1):5–12.

24. Moons P, Budts W, De Geest S. Critique on the conceptualisation of quality of life: A review and evaluation of different conceptual approaches. *Int J Nurs Stud.* Sep 2006;43(7):891–901.

25. Anderson KL, Burckhardt CS. Conceptualization and measurement of quality of life as an outcome variable for health care intervention and research. *J Adv Nurs.* Feb 1999; 29(2):298–306.

26. Moons P. Why call it health-related quality of life when you mean perceived health status? *Eur J Cardiovasc Nurs.* Dec 2004;3(4):275–277.

27. Ferrans CE. Differences in what quality-of-life instruments measure. *J Natl Cancer Inst Monogr.* 2007(37):22–26.

28. Sousa KH, Williamson A. Symptom status and health-related quality of life: Clinical relevance. *J Adv Nurs.* Jun 2003;42(6):571–577.

29. Moinpour CM, Donaldson GW, Redman MW. Do general dimensions of quality of life add clinical value to symptom data? *J Natl Cancer Inst Monogr.* 2007;(37):31–38.

30. Lee S, Cook EF, Soiffer R, Antin JH. Development and validation of a scale to measure symptoms of chronic graft-versus-host disease. *Biol Blood Marrow Transplant.* 2002;8(8):444–452.

31. Ware JE, Jr., Kosinski M, Bjorner JB, Turner-Bowker DM, Gandek B, Maruish ME. *User's manual for the SF-36v2 health survey.* 2nd ed. Lincoln, RI: QualityMetric Incorporated; 2007.

32. Finlayson TL, Moyer CA, Sonnad SS. Assessing symptoms, disease severity, and quality of life in the clinical context: A theoretical framework. *Am J Manag Care.* May 2004; 10(5):336–344.

33. Lenz ER, Pugh LC. The theory of unpleasant symptoms. In: Smith MJ, Liehr PR, eds. *Middle range theory for nursing.* New York: Springer Publishing Company, Inc.; 2003:69–90.

34. Posey AD. Symptom perception: A concept exploration. *Nurs Forum.* Jul–Sep 2006;41(3):113–124.

35. Chang CH, Cella D, Clarke S, Heinemann AW, Von Roenn JH, Harvey R. Should symptoms be scaled for intensity, frequency, or both? *Palliat Support Care.* Mar 2003;1(1): 51–60.

36. Tishelman C, Degner LF, Rudman A, et al. Symptoms in patients with lung carcinoma: Distinguishing distress from intensity. *Cancer.* Nov 1 2005;104(9):2013–2021.

37. Wu AW, Dave NB, Diener-West M, Sorensen S, Huang IC, Revicki DA. Measuring validity of self-reported symptoms among people with HIV. *AIDS Care.* Oct 2004; 16(7):876–881.

38. Goodell TT, Nail LM. Operationalizing symptom distress in adults with cancer: A literature synthesis. *Oncol Nurs Forum.* Mar 2005;32(2):E42–47.

39. Lacasse C, Beck SL. Clinical Assessment of Symptom Clusters. *Sem Oncol Nurs.* 2007;23(2):106–112.

40. Cleeland C. Symptom burden: Multiple symptoms and their impact as patient-reported outcomes. *J Natl Cancer Inst Monogr.* 2007;37:16–21.

41. Gapstur RL. Symptom burden: A concept analysis and implications for oncology nurses. *Oncol Nurs Forum.* May 2007;34(3):673–680.

42. Barsevick AM, Whitmer K, Nail LM, Beck SL, Dudley WN. Symptom cluster research: Conceptual, design, measurement, and analysis issues. *J Pain Symptom Manage.* Jan 2006;31(1): 85–95.

43. Beck SL. Symptom clusters: Impediments and suggestions for solutions. *J Natl Cancer Inst Monogr.* 2004(32):137–138.

44. Cella DF. Quality of life: Concepts and definition. *J Pain Symptom Manage.* Apr 1994;9(3):186–192.

45. Leidy NK. Functional status and the forward progress of merry-go-rounds: Toward a coherent analytical framework. *Nurs Res.* 1994;43(4):196–202.

46. Stull DE, Leidy NK, Jones PW, Stahl E. Measuring functional performance in patients with COPD: A discussion of patient-reported outcome measures. *Curr Med Res Opin.* Nov 2007;23(11):2655–2665.

47. Ferrans CE, Zerwic JJ, Wilbur JE, Larson JL. Conceptual model of health-related quality of life. *J Nurs Scholarsh.* 2005;37(4):336–342.

48. Belec RH. Quality of life: Perceptions of long-term survivors of bone marrow transplantation. *Oncol Nurs Forum.* Jan–Feb 1992;19(1):31–37.

49. Ferrell B, Grant M, Schmidt GM, et al. The meaning of quality of life for bone marrow transplant survivors. Part 1. The impact of bone marrow transplant on quality of life. *Cancer Nurs.* Jun 1992;15(3):153–160.

50. Wilson IB, Cleary PD. Linking clinical variables with health-related quality of life. A conceptual model of patient outcomes. *JAMA*. Jan 4 1995;273(1):59–65.

51. Pearce NJ, Sanson-Fisher R, Campbell HS. Measuring quality of life in cancer survivors: A methodological review of existing scales. *Psychooncology*. Oct 31 2007.

52. Coons SJ, Rao S, Keininger DL, Hays RD. A comparative review of generic quality-of-life instruments. *PharmacoEconomics*. 2000;17(1):13–35.

53. Frost MH, Reeve BB, Liepa AM, Stauffer JW, Hays RD. What is sufficient evidence for the reliability and validity of patient-reported outcome measures? *Value Health*. Nov-Dec 2007;10(Suppl 2):S94–S105.

54. Scientific Advisory Committee of the Medical Outcomes Trust. Assessing health status and quality of life instruments: Attributes and review criteria. *Quality of Life Research*, 2002; 11:193–205.

55. Rothman ML, Beltran P, Cappelleri JC, Lipscomb J, Teschendorf B. Patient-reported outcomes: Conceptual issues. *Value Health*. Nov-Dec 2007;10(Suppl 2):S66–75.

56. Lee SJ, Kim HT, Ho VT, et al. Quality of life associated with acute and chronic graft-versus-host disease. *Bone Marrow Transplantation*. Aug 2006;38(4):305–310.

57. Horwitz ME, Sullivan KM. Chronic graft-versus-host disease. *Blood Reviews*. Jan 2006;20(1):15–27.

58. Pavletic SZ, Smith LM, Bishop MR, et al. Prognostic factors of chronic graft-versus-host disease after allogeneic blood stem-cell transplantation. *Am J Hematol*. Apr 2005;78(4):265–274.

59. Remberger M, Kumlien G, Aschan J, et al. Risk factors for moderate-to-severe chronic graft-versus-host disease after allogeneic hematopoietic stem cell transplantation. *Biol Blood Marrow Transplant*. 2002;8(12):674–682.

60. Lee SJ. New approaches for preventing and treating chronic graft-versus-host disease. *Blood*. Jun 1 2005;105(11):4200–4206.

61. Sala-Torra O, Martin PJ, Storer B, et al. Serious acute or chronic graft-versus-host disease after hematopoietic cell transplantation: A comparison of myeloablative and nonmyeloablative conditioning regimens. *Bone Marrow Transplant*. May 2008;41(10):887–893.

62. Cutler C, Giri S, Jeyapalan S, Paniagua D, Viswanathan A, Antin JH. Acute and chronic graft-versus-host disease after allogeneic peripheral-blood stem-cell and bone marrow transplantation: a meta-analysis.[see comment]. *Journal of Clinical Oncology*. Aug 15 2001;19(16):3685–3691.

63. Lee S. New approaches for preventing and treating chronic graft-versus-host disease. *Blood*. Jun 1 2005;105(11):4200–4206.

64. Vogelsang GB, Lee L, Bensen-Kennedy DM. Pathogenesis and treatment of graft-versus-host disease after bone marrow transplant. *Annu Rev Med*. 2003;54:29–52.

65. Duell T, van Lint MT, Ljungman P, et al. Health and functional status of long-term survivors of bone marrow transplantation. EBMT Working Party on Late Effects and EULEP Study Group on Late Effects. European Group for Blood and Marrow Transplantation. *Ann Intern Med*. Feb 1 1997;126(3):184–192.

66. Singhal S, Powles R, Treleaven J, Kulkarni S, Horton C, Mehta J. Long-term outcome of adult acute leukemia patients who are alive and well two years after allogeneic bone marrow transplantation from an HLA-identical sibling. *Leuk Lymphoma*. Jul 1999;34(3–4):287–294.

67. Socie G, Stone JV, Wingard JR, et al. Long-term survival and late deaths after allogeneic bone marrow transplantation. Late Effects Working Committee of the International Bone Marrow Transplant Registry. *N Engl J Med*. Jul 1 1999;341(1):14–21.

68. Singhal S, Mehta J. Reimmunization after blood or marrow stem cell transplantation. *Bone Marrow Transplantation*. 1999;23(7):637–646.

69. Lipscomb, J., Gottay, C. C., Snyder, C. (Eds) *Outcomes assessment in cancer: Measures, methods, and applications*. Cambridge University Press, 2004.

70. Bottomley A, Aaronson NK. International perspective on health-related quality-of-life research in cancer clinical trials: The European Organisation for Research and Treatment of Cancer experience. *J Clin Oncol*. Nov 10 2007;25(32):5082–5086.

71. Prieto JM, Atala J, Blanch J, et al. Psychometric study of quality of life instruments used during hospitalization for stem cell transplantation. *J Psychosom Res*. Aug 2004;57(2):201–211.

72. Tsimicalis A, Stinson J, Stevens B. Quality of life of children following bone marrow transplantation: Critical review of the research literature. *Eur J Oncol Nurs*. Sep 2005;9(3):218–238.

73. Baker KS, Fraser CJ. Quality of life and recovery after graft-versus-host disease. *Best Pract Res Clin Haematol*. Jun 2008;21(2):333–341.

74. Mosher CE, Redd WH, Rini CM, Burkhalter JE, Duhamel KN. Physical, psychological, and social sequelae following hematopoietic stem cell transplantation: A review of the literature. *Psychooncology*. Aug 1 2008.

75. Baker F, Wingard JR, Curbow B, et al. Quality of life of bone marrow transplant long-term survivors. *Bone Marrow Transplant*. May 1994;13(5):589–596.

76. Bush NE, Haberman M, Donaldson G, Sullivan KM. Quality of life of 125 adults surviving 6–18 years after bone marrow transplantation. *Soc Sci Med*. 1995;40(4):479–490.

77. Kiss TL, Abdolell M, Jamal N, Minden MD, Lipton JH, Messner HA. Long-term medical outcomes and quality-of-life assessment of patients with chronic myeloid leukemia followed at least 10 years after allogeneic bone marrow transplantation. *J Clin Oncol*. 2002;20(9):2334–2343.

78. Molassiotis A, Morris PJ. Quality of life in patients with chronic myeloid leukemia after unrelated donor bone marrow transplantation. *Cancer Nurs*. Oct 1999;22(5):340–349.

79. Socie G, Mary JY, Esperou H, et al. Health and functional status of adult recipients 1 year after allogeneic haematopoietic stem cell transplantation. *Br J Haematol*. 2001;113(1):194–201.

80. Syrjala KL, Chapko MK, Vitaliano PP, Cummings C, Sullivan KM. Recovery after allogeneic marrow transplantation: Prospective study of predictors of long-term physical and psychosocial functioning. *Bone Marrow Transplantation*. 1993;11(4):319–327.

81. Yano K, Kanie T, Okamoto S, et al. Quality of life in adult patients after stem cell transplantation. *Int J Hematol*. Apr 2000;71(3):283–289.

82. Worel N, Biener D, Kalhs P, et al. Long-term outcome and quality of life of patients who are alive and in complete remission more than two years after allogeneic and syngeneic stem cell transplantation. *Bone Marrow Transplantation*. 2002;30(9):619–626.

83. Molassiotis A. A correlational evaluation of tiredness and lack of energy in survivors of haematological malignancies. *Eur J Cancer Care (Engl)*. Mar 1999;8(1):19–25.

84. Molassiotis A, Boughton BJ, Burgoyne T, van den Akker OB. Comparison of the overall quality of life in 50 long-term survivors of autologous and allogeneic bone marrow transplantation. *J Adv Nurs*. 1995;22(3):509–516.

85. Heinonen H, Volin L, Zevon MA, Uutela A, Barrick C, Ruutu T. Stress among allogeneic bone marrow transplantation patients. *Patient Education and Counseling.* 2005;56(1):62–71.

86. Kopp M, Holzner B, Meraner V, et al. Quality of life in adult hematopoietic cell transplant patients at least 5 yr after treatment: A comparison with healthy controls. *Eur J Haematol.* Apr 2005;74(4):304–308.

87. Prieto JM, Saez R, Carreras E, et al. Physical and psychosocial functioning of 117 survivors of bone marrow transplantation. *Bone Marrow Transplant.* Jun 1996;17(6):1133–1142.

88. Andrykowski MA, Henslee PJ, Farrall MG. Physical and psychosocial functioning of adult survivors of allogeneic bone marrow transplantation. *Bone Marrow Transplantation.* 1989;4(1):75–81.

89. Redaelli A, Stephens JM, Brandt S, Botteman MF, Pashos CL. Short- and long-term effects of acute myeloid leukemia on patient health-related quality of life. *Cancer Treat Rev.* Feb 2004;30(1):103–117.

90. Andrykowski MA, Greiner CB, Altmaier EM, et al. Quality of life following bone marrow transplantation: Findings from a multicentre study. *Br J Cancer.* 1995;71(6):1322–1329.

91. Rusiewicz A, DuHamel KN, Burkhalter J, et al. Psychological distress in long-term survivors of hematopoietic stem cell transplantation. *Psychooncology.* Apr 2008;17(4):329–337.

92. Tierney DK, Facione N, Padilla G, Dodd M. Response shift: A theoretical exploration of quality of life following hematopoietic cell transplantation. *Cancer Nurs.* Mar-Apr 2007;30(2):125–138.

93. Osoba D. The clinical value and meaning of health-related quality-of-life outcomes in oncology. In: Lipscomb J, Gotay, CC, Snyder, C, eds. *Outcomes assessment in cancer: measures, methods, and applications.* Cambridge: Cambridge University Press; 2005:386–405.

94. Donaldson GW, Moinpour CM. Individual differences in quality-of-life treatment response. *Med Care.* Jun 2002;40(Suppl 6):III39–53.

95. Sprangers MA, Moinpour CM, Moynihan TJ, Patrick DL, Revicki DA. Assessing meaningful change in quality of life over time: A users' guide for clinicians. *Mayo Clin Proc.* Jun 2002;77(6):561–571.

96. Schwartz C, Andresen E, Nosek M, Krahn G. Response shift theory: Important implications for measuring quality of life in people with disability. *Arch Phys Med Rehabil.* Apr 2007;88(4):529–536.

97. Schwartz CE, Rapkin BD. Reconsidering the psychometrics of quality of life assessment in light of response shift and appraisal. *Health Qual Life Outcomes.* Mar 23 2004;2:16.

98. Visser MRM, Oort FJ, Sprangers MAG. Methods to detect response shift in quality of life data: A convergent validity study. *Quality of Life Research.* 2005;14(3):629–639.

99. Varricchio CG. Measurement issues in quality-of-life assessments. *Oncol Nurs Forum.* Jan 2006;33(Suppl 1):13–21.

100. Westerman MJ, Hak T, Sprangers MA, Groen HJ, van der Wal G, The AM. Listen to their answers! Response behaviour in the measurement of physical and role functioning. *Qual Life Res.* Apr 4 2008; 17(4):549–558.

101. Schwartz CE, Feinberg RG, Jilinskaia E, Applegate JC. An evaluation of a psychosocial intervention for survivors of childhood cancer: Paradoxical effects of response shift over time. *Psychooncology.* Jul-Aug 1999;8(4):344–354.

102. Feeny DH. The roles for preference-based measures in support of cancer research and policy. In: Lipscomb J, Gotay CC, Snyder C, eds. *Outcomes assessment in cancer: Measures, methods and applications.* New York: Cambridge University Press; 2005:69–92.

103. Grant J, Cranston A, Horsman J, et al. Health status and health-related quality of life in adolescent survivors of cancer in childhood. *J Adolesc Health.* May 2006;38(5):504–510.

104. Dobrez D, Cella D, Pickard AS, Lai JS, Nickolov A. Estimation of patient preference-based utility weights from the functional assessment of cancer therapy – general. *Value Health.* Jul-Aug 2007;10(4):266–272.

105. Furlong W, Barr RD. Commentary on Cox CL, Lensing S, Rai SN et al. Proxy assessment of quality of life in pediatric clinical trials: Application of the Health Utilities Index 3. *Qual Life Res* 2005; 14: 1045–1056. *Qual Life Res.* Sep 2006;15(7):1291–1293; discussion 1295–1296.

106. Revicki D, Hays RD, Cella D, Sloan J. Recommended methods for determining responsiveness and minimally important differences for patient-reported outcomes. *J Clin Epidemiol.* Feb 2008;61(2):102–109.

107. Bjorner JB, Wallenstein GV, Martin MC, et al. Interpreting score differences in the SF-36 Vitality scale: Using clinical conditions and functional outcomes to define the minimally important difference. *Curr Med Res Opin.* Apr 2007;23(4):731–739.

108. Norman GR, Sloan JA, Wyrwich KW. Interpretation of changes in health-related quality of life: The remarkable universality of half a standard deviation. *Med Care.* May 2003;41(5):582–592.

109. Jones JB, Snyder CF, Wu AW. Issues in the design of Internet-based systems for collecting patient-reported outcomes. *Qual Life Res.* Oct 2007;16(8):1407–1417.

110. Lind L, Karlsson D. A system for symptom assessment in advanced palliative home healthcare using digital pens. *Med Inform Internet Med.* Sep–Dec 2004;29(3–4):199–210.

111. Berry DL, Trigg LJ, Lober WB, et al. Computerized symptom and quality-of-life assessment for patients with cancer part I: Development and pilot testing. *Oncol Nurs Forum.* Sep 2004;31(5):E75–83.

112. Mullen KH, Berry DL, Zierler BK. Computerized symptom and quality-of-life assessment for patients with cancer part II: Acceptability and usability. *Oncol Nurs Forum.* Sep 2004;31(5):E84–89.

113. Carpenter JS, Rawl S, Porter J, et al. Oncology outpatient and provider responses to a computerized symptom assessment system. *Oncol Nurs Forum.* Jul 2008;35(4):661–669.

114. Bush N, Donaldson G, Moinpour C, et al. Development, feasibility and compliance of a web-based system for very frequent QOL and symptom home self-assessment after hematopoietic stem cell transplantation. *Qual Life Res.* Feb 2005;14(1):77–93.

115. Garcia SF, Cella D, Clauser SB, et al. Standardizing patient-reported outcomes assessment in cancer clinical trials: A patient-reported outcomes measurement information system initiative. *J Clin Oncol.* Nov 10 2007;25(32):5106–5112.

116. Cella D, Yount S, Rothrock N, et al. PROMIS Cooperative Group. *Med Care.* 2007 May;45(5 Suppl 1):S3–S11.

117. Rose M, Bjorner JB, Becker J, Fries JF, Ware JE. Evaluation of a preliminary physical function item bank supported the expected advantages of the Patient-Reported Outcomes

Measurement Information System (PROMIS). *J Clin Epidemiol.* Jan 2008;61(1):17–33.

118. McHorney CA, Cook KF. The ten Ds of health outcomes measurement for the twenty-first century. In: Lipscomb J, Gotay, CC, Snyder, C, eds. *Outcomes Assessment in Cancer: Measures, methods, and applications.* Cambridge: Cambridge University Press; 2005:590–609.

119. McHorney CA. Generic health measurement: Past accomplishments and a measurement paradigm for the 21st century. *Ann Intern Med.* Oct 15 1997;127(8 Pt 2):743–750.

120. Butt Z, Wagner LI, Beaumont JL, et al. Use of a single-item screening tool to detect clinically significant fatigue, pain, distress, and anorexia in ambulatory cancer practice. *J Pain Symptom Manage.* Jan 2008;35(1):20–30.

121. Martin P. Seattle Symposium on Cancer Research Outcomes: Commentary on the papers by Donaldson and Moinpour and by Osoba. *Med Care.* Jun 2002;40(Suppl 6):III54–55.

122. Lipscomb, J., Donaldson, M. S. Hiatt, R. A. (2007). Cancer outcomes research and the arenas of application. *JNCI Monographs*, 33, 1–7

PART IV: SPECIAL CONSIDERATIONS IN CHRONIC GVHD

31

Design of Clinical Trials Testing Treatment for Chronic Graft versus Host Disease

Paul J. Martin, Donna Przepiorka, and Stephanie J. Lee

INTRODUCTION

Approximately 4,000 patients have allogeneic hematopoietic cell transplantation (HCT) annually throughout the world, and 40% to 60% of those who survive beyond the first 3 months develop chronic graft versus host disease (GVHD). Even though nearly 1,500 people develop chronic GVHD each year, no drugs have been approved for its treatment. New therapies are needed, since chronic GVHD has major adverse effects on long-term morbidity and late nonrelapse mortality after allogeneic HCT. The complexity of chronic GVHD, however, has made it difficult to design, conduct, and analyze clinical trials involving these patients, even when promising treatment options are available.

The National Institutes of Health Consensus Development Project on Criteria for Clinical Trials in Chronic Graft-Versus-Host Disease clarified organized and codified a number of issues in this disease that are vital for successful drug development, and material in this chapter draws heavily from those recommendations [1]. For design of a successful clinical trial in this complex disorder, three critically important questions must be considered (1) who will be enrolled in the trial, (2) how will subjects be treated, and (3) how will results be evaluated? The following sections address the selection of participants, treatment methods, data collection, primary and secondary endpoints, biostatistical considerations, and overall assessment of safety and efficacy, as applied to clinical trials of treatments for chronic GVHD.

SELECTION OF PARTICIPANTS

General Considerations

The prestudy evaluation is critical to defining the patient population of the clinical trial. The diagnosis of chronic GVHD should be established according to accepted criteria [2]. Whenever feasible, the diagnosis of chronic GVHD should be confirmed by tissue biopsy and the extent of visible disease documented by photography before treatment is initiated in these trials [3]. Prestudy evaluations should also survey clinical and laboratory parameters that may affect outcome, account for the probable risk-benefit ratio to individual participants, and provide a baseline that will allow results to be interpreted. Information from well-documented baseline evaluations can be used not only to confirm eligibility for enrollment but also for discovery of previously unidentified prognostic factors.

Patients with chronic GVHD have heterogeneous clinical manifestations, which makes it difficult to accrue a seemingly homogeneous cohort in any study. Inclusion and exclusion criteria must balance the need for a representative selection of subjects (arguing that a large proportion of people with chronic GVHD should be eligible) versus the need for clear interpretation (arguing that the study population should be as homogeneous as possible). In general, phase III trials should be more inclusive, whereas phase II trials may need to be more restrictive in order to facilitate the use of early and intermediate endpoints. Inclusion of children is encouraged in both phase II and phase III studies and may require assessments of additional endpoints, such as growth and development, which are relevant to this population. Studies limited to enrollment of children may also be feasible through the participation of pediatric-oriented cooperative groups. In treatment trials, inclusion criteria depend primarily on whether the population of interest has newly diagnosed chronic GVHD requiring "primary" therapy or more advanced chronic GVHD that has already not improved or has recurred after primary therapy, thus requiring "secondary" treatment. Criteria for secondary treatment should be clearly delineated in the protocol, for example, when primary therapy has failed as indicated by progression of chronic GVHD signs and symptoms during therapy. In some circumstances, secondary therapy may also be instituted for persistent steroid-dependent chronic GVHD. Steroid-intolerant patients with steroid-responsive chronic GVHD could also be enrolled in clinical trials of secondary therapy, provided that steroid intolerance is strictly defined. Inclusion of steroid-intolerant

Acknowledgments: The authors gratefully acknowledge the contributions of many colleagues who participated in the National Institutes of Health Consensus Development Project on Criteria for Clinical Trials in Chronic Graft-Versus-Host Disease. The conclusions in this article have not been formally disseminated by the Food and Drug Administration and should not be construed to represent any Agency determination or policy.

patients would not pose a problem when the primary endpoint is safety, but stratification may be needed in a randomized trial where the primary endpoint is efficacy, since the response rate among steroid-intolerant patients could be higher than among those with steroid-refractory or steroid-dependent chronic GVHD.

Recognition of overlap syndromes where chronic GVHD occurs together with manifestations typical of acute GVHD has increased recently. Inclusion of patients with such overlap syndromes may complicate the interpretation of phase II trials because the response of individual organs may depend on whether acute or chronic GVHD is predominant. Such patients might still be included in phase III trials where resolution of GVHD, discontinuation of therapy, or survival is a component of the primary endpoint. Stratification would be needed in order to account for different expected outcomes according to the presence or absence of acute GVHD, and unambiguous response criteria would be required for phase II trials where shorter-term clinical response is the primary endpoint.

A key issue for clinical trials testing secondary therapy is whether and how to limit enrollment of patients with far advanced chronic GVHD that has produced irreversible organ damage. Even if the study intervention inhibits disease activity, efficacy might not be evident if most of the clinical manifestations represent irreversible damage that accumulated during the prior course of the disease. Patients with such far advanced chronic GVHD can probably best contribute to studies where the primary endpoint is related to safety and tolerance. Patients with irreversible damage as the only manifestation of chronic GVHD should be excluded from trials designed to measure improvement in chronic GVHD, although it may be appropriate to include these patients in studies where the primary endpoint is survival, prevention of chronic GVHD progression, palliation of disease manifestations that are ordinarily considered irreversible (e.g., through the use of antifibrotic medications), or reduction in the dose of steroid treatment. Patients with both reversible and irreversible manifestations of chronic GVHD can be enrolled in trials with endpoints related to clinical improvement, as long as the protocol gives clear guidance on how previously established irreversible damage is assessed. Organs or sites affected by irreversible damage could be excluded for purposes of evaluating improvement, but they should be included for purposes of evaluating possible progression of the disease. Clinical trials for secondary treatment of chronic GVHD could benefit enormously from the availability of markers distinguishing active disease from irreversible organ damage.

Exclusion Criteria

In clinical trials of treatment for chronic GVHD, exclusion criteria generally address the presence of (1) uncontrolled infection at the time of enrollment, (2) contraindications to administration of the study intervention or known inability of the patient to tolerate the study intervention, and (3) complications such as recurrent or progressive malignancy that might affect the study

endpoints or temper the effort to control chronic GVHD. Other typical exclusion criteria include pregnancy or breast-feeding, an unwillingness to comply with any critical components of study treatment or response evaluation, or short duration of anticipated survival due to other comorbidities.

Considerations for Drug Development

Conventionally, new agents have been tested for safety and for initial assessment of efficacy among patients with steroid-refractory GVHD, under the premise that only patients at very high risk of poor outcomes should be subjected to the unknown risks of a new agent. This approach, however, poses several practical problems.

If the phase II experience in patients with steroid-refractory GVHD is encouraging, a pivotal phase III controlled study may be necessary as a formal demonstration of efficacy. Because response may be easier to assess in patients with newly diagnosed chronic GVHD lacking extensive organ damage, a pivotal phase III study is likely to enroll patients with newly diagnosed GVHD, where a new agent could be tested as an "add-on" to "standard" first-line therapy. However, if the phase II data were generated in a steroid-refractory population, there may be no data on safety and efficacy in newly diagnosed patients to support study planning. Options include forging ahead with the phase III study based on extrapolations from the phase II study or conducting a separate phase II study in patients with newly diagnosed chronic GVHD before undertaking a phase III study.

Defining the control treatment in a phase III study for chronic GVHD poses a major challenge. Documentation of the new agent's superiority over standard therapy is difficult, since no one treatment is accepted as standard of care in patients with steroid-refractory chronic GVHD. Furthermore, placebo-controlled trials are unappealing for patients who have clinically significant symptoms. Approaches that offer all patients some chance of benefit from participation in the study, such as crossover designs, may improve enrollment, but criteria for changing therapy need to be explicit and unambiguous.

TREATMENT METHODS

Management and Evaluation of Chronic GVHD

The level of guidance regarding the management of chronic GVHD in protocols should consider the balance between physician autonomy necessary for optimal patient care, the expertise of the treating physicians, and the consistency required to allow study interpretation. In general, the more prescribed the treatment approach, the more likely it is to conflict with local practice, thereby causing study deviations. Endpoint assessment is another area where expertise varies. Specific training toward study goals and proper procedures for all study personnel should be considered an important tool to ensure quality and consistency in conduct of the study.

Administration of Study Medications and Other Interventions

Protocols for treatment of chronic GVHD must provide appropriate guidelines for administration of the study medication or intervention, including the initial dosage, monitoring of drug concentrations in the blood, any reductions in dose or frequency of administration indicated because of toxicity, and any tapering of doses or frequency of administration at the end of treatment. Use of other medications or interventions could potentially affect drug levels, the course of chronic GVHD, or manifestations of organ dysfunction. If such drugs are allowed, details of their use should be recorded in the case-report forms.

Administration of Glucocorticoids

Standard steroid therapy currently represents a well-established mainstay of initial treatment for chronic GVHD. Protocols should provide guidelines for tapering of glucocorticoid doses and should specify daily or alternate day administration. The guidelines should indicate the appropriate starting dose and any adjustments in glucocorticoids doses, depending on toxicity and changes in GVHD severity. Tapering of steroid doses prompted by clinical improvement, however, could mask the full benefit of an effective investigational agent, while continued administration of high-dose steroids could mask the absence of benefit from an ineffective investigational agent. A fixed starting dose and taper schedule may be appropriate for clinical trials where administration of glucocorticoids is an integral component of the intervention being tested and for trials to evaluate short-term efficacy of a new regimen. In longer-term trials, however, adherence to a fixed schedule is likely to be impossible because of variation among subjects in persistence of chronic GVHD and tolerability of glucocorticoid-related side effects.

Ancillary Therapy and Supportive Care

Protocols should provide guidelines for prevention of opportunistic infection in patients with chronic GVHD [4]. Protocols should also acknowledge that organ or site-specific therapies are an important component of symptom management in patients with chronic GVHD [4]. Allowable site-specific therapies should be specified in the protocol, and the therapies used for patients should be recorded in the case report forms.

DATA COLLECTION

Timing of Data Collection

Calendar-driven data collection (e.g., every 3 or 6 months) is strongly recommended for clinical trials of treatment for chronic GVHD. Insufficiently frequent assessment could overlook differences in time to response between study arms, while too frequent assessments might make it difficult to detect changes from one evaluation to the next and would unnecessarily add to the resource burden of the study. Calendar-driven data collection should be supplemented by event-driven collection of GVHD-related data at the time of treatment success or treatment failure. Collection of adverse event data should also be event-driven. Note that these recommendations apply only to collection of research data. The frequency of clinical visits is determined by medical need.

Either longitudinal or time-to-event analysis can be accommodated by calendar-driven data collection, although careful planning would be required if treatment involves cycles of different length between the study arms. For GVHD therapy trials, we strongly favor real-time collection of prespecified data from physicians and patients during clinic visits. This approach ensures the capture of detailed and directed information that may be necessary to document response assessments [5].

Case-Report Forms

Investigators are often tempted to collect any and all data elements that might possibly be used in an analysis. Overcollection of data adds to the burden of participation experienced not only by physicians but also by subjects. Excessive data collection can compromise enthusiasm for the trial and increase the probability that critical data elements will be missed or that inappropriate analysis could occur. Conversely, elimination of unnecessary data collection facilitates the conduct of clinical trials.

Standardized case-report forms should be used, with the level of detail determined by the study goals. Data collected retrospectively from medical charts intended for clinical care lack details needed to assess the results of clinical trials. Instead, a checklist form can be used routinely for assessment and documentation of chronic GVHD manifestations during clinic visits and subsequently made part of the medical record. Consistent template-driven documentation at an appropriate level of detail through the real-time use of standard assessment forms enables comparisons with previous assessments or with the patient's baseline condition. If time points for assessment are standardized, then data for all patients in each study arm can be easily aggregated for analysis. The information from case-report forms of this design can effectively describe not only the initial onset and final resolution of chronic GVHD but also its severity across time.

Case-report forms for the baseline assessment of chronic GVHD should collect information regarding eligibility for enrollment in the trial, manifestations that indicate prognosis, and the severity of manifestations in each organ or site potentially affected by the disease [6]. Previously recognized prognostic indicators at the onset of chronic GVHD include performance status, lichen planus-like versus sclerotic skin lesions, percent body surface affected by rash, diarrhea, weight loss >10%, oral involvement, platelet count, total bilirubin, progressive onset from prior acute GVHD versus onset without prior acute GVHD or after resolution of prior acute GVHD, and type and dose of previously administered immunosuppressive medications [6, 7].

At each subsequent calendar-driven assessment point, the dose and schedule of the investigational agent should be recorded together with the reasons for any dose reduction, and the assessment of severity should be repeated together with any other necessary endpoint information specified by the study design. Drug diaries can be used to identify the maximum, minimum, or average dose of the investigational agent during intervals between assessment points. The amount of concomitant immunosuppressive medications, ancillary therapies, and supportive care (e.g., physical therapy, massage, punctal plugs) should also be recorded. In trials where the blood levels of an investigational medication are not monitored and adjusted as part of the study, it may also be useful to record the administration of specific concomitant medications that might affect the concentration of investigational agents in the blood. All concomitant medications must be recorded in studies to be submitted for regulatory review.

Patient-Reported Outcomes

Information in the case-report form can include quality of life or functional assessments as reported by patients. Collection of patient-reported data should use instruments that have been validated in patients with chronic GVHD. Established methods of instrument administration and scoring should be used, whenever such instruments and methods are available. Each instrument should define clinically meaningful differences that qualify as improvement or worsening between two assessments based on statistical considerations or clinical perceptions. Results should report both population changes and the percentage of patients with clinically meaningful difference in self-reported outcomes before and after treatment. We encourage the development of instruments to capture parent or self-reported data from pediatric patients. The Lee symptom scale [8] has been validated among patients with chronic GHVD. Other more general instruments such as the SF-36, FACT-BMT, CHRI, HAP, or ASK have been used in a variety of clinical trials but have not been validated specifically for assessment of outcomes among patients with chronic GVHD [5].

Adverse Events and Serious Adverse events

The protocol document should specify a safety-monitoring plan that includes definitions of adverse events (AEs) and serious adverse events (SAEs) in accordance with 21 CFR 312.21(a), taking into consideration the study design, known and potential risks of the investigational product, the patient population under study, and any regulatory or sponsor requirements. Although all AEs are of interest in phase I and phase II studies, complications related to HCT raise the background of expected and unrelated events, thereby confounding safety analyses in early-phase trials. In large randomized trials that are not intended for regulatory review, it would be pragmatic to define the relevant AEs that require tracking, thereby minimizing undue burden on study personnel and potentially improving the quality of the data, as long as patient safety is not jeopardized by less complete reporting of AEs. Reporting of all AEs is generally necessary in trials intended for regulatory

review. Regardless of whether a study is intended for regulatory review, the protocol should specify the scope and time requirements for reporting and reviewing AEs in order to protect the integrity of the study and safety of participants [9].

Considerations for Multi-institutional Studies

The numbers of patients with chronic GVHD in any single institution are generally not sufficient for studies intended to establish safety and efficacy for investigational products within a reasonable time frame. Studies that enroll patients at several institutions are more likely to meet accrual targets and provide the necessary data to analyze outcomes in a robust manner. Multicenter studies are complicated, however, by the divergent standards that evolved based on local experience. Uniform training of individuals who assess patients, follow protocol-mandated procedures, examine histopathology, perform chronic GVHD grading, and assess clinical trial endpoints may improve compliance and reproducibility. Likewise, centralized review of histopathology, clinical grading, and response assessments may improve reproducibility and uniformity among institutions. These quality enhancements add greatly to the costs of conducting clinical trials.

PRIMARY AND SECONDARY ENDPOINTS
Selection of Endpoints

The choice of specific primary and secondary endpoints will be influenced by regulatory needs, the intervention's mechanism of action, study phase, indication (prevention, primary treatment, or secondary treatment), and by the presence or absence of blinding. Potential primary and secondary endpoints include physician-assessed response (complete response, partial response, stable disease, or no response, progression); patient-reported outcomes; time to GVHD progression; transplant-related mortality; disease-free survival; overall survival; survival to resolution of chronic GVHD; and survival to permanent discontinuation of immunosuppressive treatment (Table 31.1). GVHD response and patient-reported outcomes could be applied globally or to specific organs, depending on the nature of the intervention and the organs or sites affected by the disease.

Valid primary and secondary endpoints of chronic GVHD treatment studies should focus on the clinical benefits of central importance to patients: survival free of the underlying disease, freedom from chronic GVHD manifestations, treatment and complications, and improvement in symptoms, function, and quality of life. Intermediate endpoints that reflect the degree of chronic GVHD activity, such as physician assessment, biochemical tests, and biomarkers [10] are important only to the extent that they may predict or confirm one of the patient-experienced outcomes [11, 12]. Since chronic GVHD typically has a prolonged clinical course, extended follow-up is strongly encouraged to ensure that responses are durable. The minimum duration of response required to designate treatment as "successful" will vary according to trial design and endpoint. Requirements for

Table 31.1: Summary of Recommendations [1]

Who will be enrolled?
- Inclusion and exclusion criteria should encompass as many people with chronic GVHD as possible without compromising the ability to interpret results of the study
- Baseline evaluations should document the need for therapy, identify prognostic characteristics, and specifically characterize the condition of subjects at the time of enrollment, so that results of therapy can be interpreted

How will participants be treated?
- Within reason, the study protocol should specify or provide guidance regarding the dosing and dose adjustment of all immunosuppressive medications, including the study drug. Reasons for deviations should be noted in case-report forms

How will results be evaluated?
- Case-report forms should be calendar-driven by the protocol to provide assessment of chronic GVHD and adverse events at regular intervals. Patient-reported measures should be incorporated whenever feasible. Standardized and clinically validated measures should be used
- Primary and secondary endpoints should be selected for their ability to demonstrate clinical benefit, which can be an improvement in the way a patient feels or functions or a prolongation of survival. Endpoints should account for competing outcomes such as death or recurrent malignancy. Composite endpoints may be required in some specific protocols
- Biostatistical analysis should incorporate considerations of competing events and concomitant therapy, appropriate power calculations, interim analyses, sensitivity analysis and missing measurements

GVHD, graft versus host disease.

durability of response should be prespecified in the definition of endpoints. Where applicable, criteria for failure of primary therapy and failure of secondary treatment should be defined.

From a clinical point of view, three concurrent elements idealize "success" in the management of chronic GVHD (1) resolution of reversible disease manifestations, (2) withdrawal of all immunosuppressive medications, and (3) subsequent long-term survival without recurrent malignancy. None of the endpoints listed in Table 31.2 completely embodies all three elements. Relapse-free survival to permanent discontinuation of immunosuppressive treatment comes closest to this ideal, since this endpoint amounts to cure of chronic GVHD. This endpoint is better suited to phase III trials than phase II trials, since previous studies have shown that the median duration of immunosuppressive treatment for chronic GVHD exceeds 2 years [7].

Disease Activity versus Damage

The distinction between disease *activity* and *damage* plays a critical role in the clinical management of chronic GVHD and interpretation of response. Disease *activity* can cause manifestations that would be expected to resolve after pathogenic

immunological mechanisms are controlled. Examples include an erythematous rash, oral erythema and lichenoid changes, diarrhea, transaminase elevations, and eosinophilia (Table 31.3). Sometimes disease activity leads to fibrosis such as sclerotic skin changes, fasciitis, and contractures. If progression of these manifestations can be halted by treatment, resolution may occur very slowly during a period of months to years through a prolonged process of tissue remodeling. Disease *damage* leads to manifestations that are generally considered to be irreversible since tissue destruction has occurred. Examples include ocular and oral sicca, bronchiolitis obliterans, and vitiligo. At best, an arrest of disease activity would be expected to halt progression of these manifestations. Measurement of response in clinical trials should account for differences in the expected rates of improvement between inflammatory and fibrotic manifestations of chronic GVHD. Under rare circumstances, an arrest of previously progressive damage could be considered as therapeutic benefit, even if the intervention does not provide functional improvement.

Response as an Endpoint

Most phase II studies have relied on GVHD response as the primary endpoint. While "response" is easily recognized in clinical practice, documentation of response for purposes of clinical trials is much more difficult. Scales for measurement of response have not yet been validated, and as noted above, perceived response may depend on the inflammatory or fibrotic nature of disease manifestations. Changes in ancillary treatment and supportive care may enhance or mask symptoms. Response assessments are subject to bias, particularly in open-label, single-arm studies.

Complete response, strictly defined partial response, and validated early surrogate markers of success or failure are highly appropriate endpoints for phase II studies. Results for these endpoints can be assessed within the first several months after enrollment and are not greatly affected by subsequent management or other competing late events such as recurrent malignancy. Outcomes with wider scope such as permanent resolution of chronic GVHD or survival are highly appropriate endpoints for pivotal phase III studies, but statistical methods must account for concomitant treatment and competing events such as death or recurrent malignancy during immunosuppressive treatment. Since chronic GVHD may decrease the risk of recurrent malignancy while increasing the risk of other causes of death, composite endpoints that account for trade-offs between these two competing risks are most appropriate. Stratification may help ensure that competing risks are balanced between arms.

Supporting Information from Physician and Patient Participants

Physician behavior and patient self-reports can provide additional information about responses. For physicians, changes in the dose of immunosuppressive medications and addition of new medications likely reflect the clinical impression of response. Patients can be queried about quality of life or

Table 31.2: Potential Primary and Secondary Endpoints for Chronic GVHD Treatment Trials

Endpoint*	Interpretation	Time to Endpoint	Biostatistical Notes
GVHD response	Response to treatment according to organ-specific or summary measures	Short	Scales for measurement of response have not yet been validated. Results may be affected by changes in ancillary treatment and supportive care. Endpoint is subject to bias, and has greater validity in blinded trials. Most appropriate as a primary endpoint in phase II studies and possibly in selected phase III studies
Patient-reported outcomes	Self-assessed morbidity caused by chronic GVHD or treatment	Short	Missing data and informative censoring are major problems. Few sensitive instruments are available. Results may be affected by changes in ancillary treatment and supportive care. Endpoint is subject to bias, and has greater validity in blinded trials. Best used as a secondary endpoint
Transplant-related mortality	Death before recurrence or progression of malignancy	Long	Endpoint measures failure rather than success. Also known as "chronic GVHD-specific mortality" in the literature. Best used as a secondary endpoint
Relapse-free survival	Survival without recurrent malignancy	Long	Objective endpoint, but not specific to chronic GVHD. Best used as a secondary endpoint
Overall survival	Survival	Long	Objective endpoint, ultimate gold standard, but may not be specific to chronic GVHD. Best used as a secondary endpoint
Relapse-free survival to resolution of GVHD†	Complete response	Long	Endpoint must account for continued immunosuppressive treatment. Best used as a primary endpoint in phase III studies
Relapse-free survival to permanent discontinuation of immunosuppressive treatment†	Cure	Long	Best used as a primary endpoint in phase III studies

* Endpoint probabilities can be estimated as cumulative incidence or as proportions of success or failure at a specified time point with complete follow-up. Cumulative incidence estimates can be influenced by the frequency of competing risks. Endpoint rates (i.e., hazards) can be estimated and compared by Cox regression.
† Secondary treatment is considered to be an indication of failure.
GVHD, graft versus host disease.

Table 31.3: Time to Onset of Response, According to Pathophysiology of Disease Manifestations

Pathophysiology	Onset of Response	Manifestations
Inflammation	Weeks	Cutaneous erythema Oral manifestations Diarrhea Abnormal liver function
Fibrosis	Months	Cutaneous sclerosis Fasciitis Panniculitis
Destruction	Not seen	Oral and ocular sicca Bronchiolitis obliterans Vitiligo

symptom scales, and they can report changes in performance and function with the use of standardized questionnaires. Physician behavior and "patient-reported outcomes" may be more sensitive to subtle differences in disease activity, but they each involve subjective assessments with uncertain reliability and probable susceptibility to bias, especially in open-label studies. In blinded trials, however, these assessments may be used to support other more objective response criteria.

BIOSTATISTICAL CONSIDERATIONS

Prevention Trials

In some situations, a clinical trial may be designed to prevent severe chronic GVHD, for example through alterations in the nature or source of the graft. Because of competing risks (e.g., death and recurrent malignancy before the onset of chronic GVHD), cumulative incidence estimates, rather than Kaplan-Meier methods, should be used to evaluate the proportion of patients who develop chronic GVHD. Since patients can develop chronic GVHD only if they are engrafted with donor cells and survive for some minimal time, usually 80 to 100 days, after HCT, cumulative incidence curves should be calculated from the onset of the prevention intervention, which may vary according to the design of the study. Death without prior chronic GVHD should always be treated as a competing risk. Events that may influence the speed with which immunosuppressive medications are withdrawn, such as disease progression or decreasing donor chimerism, may or may not be considered competing events since they may indirectly affect onset of chronic GVHD.

Treatment Trials

Primary and secondary endpoints in chronic GVHD treatment trials require careful statistical consideration, as summarized in Table 31.2. In all cases, endpoints, timing of assessments, and statistical methods should be prespecified. Kaplan-Meier estimates can be used to evaluate survival, and cumulative incidence estimates can be considered for evaluation of other simple and composite endpoints, depending on the type of treatment and the length of follow-up. All trials should be adequately powered to evaluate a prespecified statistical hypothesis regarding the primary endpoint, and the statistical hypothesis should address a clinically meaningful benefit. Sample size calculations should address potential study dropouts. Large imbalances for risk factors that might affect outcome can be prevented by appropriate stratification for balance. In trials that enroll a large number of subjects, stratification is generally not necessary because the likelihood of a significant imbalance in risk factors between arms is low. The risk of an imbalance is higher in trials that enroll smaller numbers of subjects. Techniques for biased adaptive randomization may be able to prevent an imbalance in the distribution of multiple risk factors between arms.

Late phase studies should have Data and Safety-Monitoring Boards (DSMBs), particularly if they involve multiple institutions. Scheduled interim analyses may be necessary to evaluate not only efficacy but also toxicity and futility, a need illustrated by three trials that tested the use of thalidomide to prevent or treat chronic GVHD [13–15]. DSMBs may be appropriate for phase II studies testing agents with insufficiently characterized safety profiles that might jeopardize the safety of subjects or for studies that involve particularly vulnerable populations such as children.

The conduct and interpretation of clinical trials for treatment of chronic GVHD would be greatly enhanced by development of biostatistical methods that could account for baseline prognostic characteristics and for changes in both the severity of disease manifestations and the overall intensity of immunosuppressive treatment. Crossover designs may be biostatistically robust if failure is required before patients crossover (in reality, these are extended access trials) or if treatment remains blinded before and after crossover. On the other hand, crossover designs can confound the assessment of longer-term outcomes such as survival and cannot be used in studies testing an investigational agent added to another treatment.

Post hoc analyses should demonstrate that a favorable difference in outcome does not reflect imbalance in the distribution of baseline risk factors among arms of the study. Analyses should also evaluate whether the intervention has reduced the overall level of systemic immunosuppression and the amount of topical therapy. If this is not the case, then a secondary analysis should be carried out in order to correct for possible confounding effects of ancillary treatment and supportive care on the primary endpoint. Finally, favorable results for the primary endpoint should be supported by favorable or neutral results for secondary efficacy endpoints and by the absence of side effects that outweigh the benefits demonstrated by the efficacy endpoints. These analyses should be prespecified in the protocol.

Handling of Missing Data

Missing data hamper the evaluation of patient-reported outcomes and other endpoints. Imputation has been used as a technique to deal with missing data for patient-reported outcomes. Missing data can also affect the assessment of response when the study arms have different dropout rates, resulting in informative censoring. Protocols should specify how missing data will be treated, and sample size estimates should make allowances for dropout and informative censoring, when necessary. Sensitivity testing under worst-case assumptions for missing data can be used to ensure robust results.

STUDIES INTENDED FOR REGULATORY REVIEW

The ultimate goal of the drug development pathway is to define content in the product label. Thus, additional considerations of clinical trial design, eligibility criteria, details of treatment, endpoint choice, and study conduct are required in preparing trials intended for licensing review. The characteristics of adequate and well-controlled studies needed for regulatory approval in the United States are summarized in 21 CFR 314.126(b). These characteristics include (1) a clear statement of the objectives and methods of analysis, with an implicit emphasis on prospective design; (2) a valid comparison with a control to provide a quantitative assessment of effect; (3) a method of selection of subjects that provides adequate assurance that they have the disease being studied; (4) a method to avoid bias in the assignment of subjects to treatment and controls groups; (5) adequate measures to minimize bias on the part of subjects, observers, and analysts of the data; (6) well-defined and reliable methods to assess subjects' response; and (7) an analysis that is adequate to assess the effects of the treatment. In the United States, sponsors and investigators should consider requesting a Special Protocol Assessment from the Food and Drug Administration (FDA) before beginning a clinical trial intended to support a licensing application [16].

FDA can approve a new drug application (NDA) or a new indication only after determining that the drug meets the statutory standards for safety and effectiveness, among other requirements. FDA may refuse to approve an application if there is insufficient information about a drug to determine whether it is safe for use under the conditions prescribed or if there is a lack of substantial evidence that the drug will have its purported effect on the defined population under the conditions of use prescribed.

Assessment of efficacy involves the measurement of an outcome variable that reflects clinical benefit, together with an evaluation of the statistical robustness and reproducibility of the trial results. Endpoints should be selected to provide evidence of meaningful clinical benefit for patients. Tools and instruments used to capture endpoint information must be well characterized and validated. Clear definitions of failure and success must be provided.

Endpoints of limited scope and subjective endpoints that are not supported by objective measurements may be highly appropriate for the assessment of some interventions. For example, stabilization of pulmonary function tests might be appropriate in the evaluation of an inhalational agent for treatment of bronchiolitis obliterans in patients who previously showed consistent deterioration before enrollment in the study. As another example, trials to evaluate a steroid-sparing agent could have a reduction in glucocorticoid-related side effects as the primary endpoint.

CHALLENGES FOR THE FUTURE

Improvements in clinical trial design can facilitate advances in the treatment of chronic GVHD only if drugs or devices previously approved for other indications or new therapeutic agents currently under development have activity against physiologic pathways leading to development or progression of the disease. Current understanding of the pathophysiology leading to chronic GVHD is limited, but deeper insight could come from nonclinical models and from studies of other diseases that result in similar clinical manifestations, such as scleroderma and Sjogren's syndrome. A more sophisticated understanding of the pathogenesis of chronic GVHD, combined with the availability of agents directed at specific targets in pathways leading to development of the disease, could lead to improvements in outcomes for patients after allogeneic HCT.

Further effort is needed to overcome a variety of barriers to successful completion of clinical trials in patients with chronic GVHD. Enrollment rates in clinical trials can be extremely rapid in studies where a novel and potentially effective investigational agent is available only through participation in a clinical trial. Enrollment rates are predictably much slower in clinical trials with products that are readily available as a result of approval for another indication. Physicians who believe that a product is inadequately effective for chronic GVHD on the basis of personal experience, case reports, or limited phase II studies have little clinical motivation to enroll patients, while those who believe that a product is effective can prescribe it at their own discretion, thereby avoiding the burdens and restrictions imposed by participating in the trial. Enrollment will be slow, unless physicians can set aside such personal beliefs in order to improve the quality of evidence regarding the efficacy of products for treatment of chronic GVHD. Enrollment can potentially be improved by designs that leave the smallest possible "footprint" on clinical practice and by ensuring that reimbursement for costs is commensurate with the amount of work required for the study.

Clinical trials in patients with chronic GVHD have been hampered by the absence of validated scales based on objective measurements that can be used to assess response and outcome after treatment. Many clinical trials have used "clinical improvement," partial response, or complete response as endpoints, often at unspecified times after enrollment. As a more rigorous endpoint, some trials have used time to discontinuation of all immunosuppressive treatment as an indicator of cure, but ascertainment of this endpoint requires lengthy follow-up. Progress in the field would be helped greatly by development of a validated shorter-term endpoint that could be used in future early-phase clinical trials to evaluate new approaches for treatment of chronic GVHD, such as determining the optimal biological dose for a drug that has little or no toxicity. Such endpoints would make it much easier to evaluate the merits of new approaches for treatment of chronic GVHD by shortening the time needed to assess outcomes and to identify promising new approaches. So far, nearly all treatment studies of chronic GVHD have been conducted with the use of agents that have been approved for other indications. Academic investigators have found it very difficult to attract the interest of industry partners, because chronic GVHD is an orphan indication with no established template for an approval path at the FDA. Successful identification of validated short-term endpoints could create future opportunities to test novel agents that have not already been approved for other indications.

REFERENCES

1. Martin PJ, Weisdorf DW, Przepiorka D, et al. National Institutes of Health consensus development project on criteria for clinical trials in chronic graft-versus-host disease: VI. Design of Clinical Trials Working Group report. *Biol Blood and Marrow Transplant.* 2006;12:491–505.
2. Filipovich AH, Weisdorf D, Pavletic, et al. National Institutes of Health consensus development project on criteria for clinical trials in chronic graft-versus-host disease: I. Diagnosis and Staging Working Group report. *Biol Blood and Marrow Transplant.* 2005;11:945–955.
3. Shulman HM, Kleiner D, Lee SJ, et al. Histopathologic diagnosis of chronic graft-versus-host disease: National Institutes of Health consensus development project on criteria for clinical trials in chronic graft-versus-host disease: II. Pathology Working Group report. *Biol Blood and Marrow Transplant.* 2006;12:31–47.
4. Couriel D, Carpenter P, Cutler C, et al. Ancillary Therapy and Supportive Care of chronic graft-versus-host disease: National Institutes of Health consensus development project on criteria for clinical trials in chronic graft-versus-host disease: V. Ancillary Therapy and Supportive Care Working Group report. *Biol Blood and Marrow Transplant.* 2006;12:375–396.
5. Pavletic SZ, Martin P, Lee SJ, et al. Measuring therapeutic response in chronic graft-versus-host disease: National Institutes

of Health consensus development project on criteria for clinical trials in chronic graft-versus-host disease: VI. Response Criteria Working Group report. *Biol Blood and Marrow Transplant.* 2006;12:252–266.

6. Lee SJ, Vogelsang GB, Flowers MED. Chronic graft-versus-host disease. *Biol Blood and Marrow Transplant.* 2003;9:215–233.

7. Stewart BL, Storer B, Storek J, et al. Duration of immunosuppressive treatment for chronic graft-versus-host disease. *Blood.* 2004;104:3501–3506.

8. Lee S, Cook EF, Soiffer R, et al. Development and validation of a scale to measure symptoms of chronic graft-versus-host disease. *Biol Blood and Marrow Transplant.* 2002;8:444–452.

9. International Conference on Harmonization. Guidelines for Good Clinical Practice. Geneva, Switzerland: International Conference on Harmonization; May 1, 1996.

10. Schultz, KR, Miklos DB, Fowler D, et al. Toward biomarkers for chronic graft-versus-host disease: National Institutes of Health consensus development project on criteria for clinical trials in chronic graft-versus-host disease: III. Biomarker Working Group report. *Biol Blood and Marrow Transplant.* 2006;12:126–137.

11. Wittes RE. Antineoplastic agents and FDA regulations: square pegs for round holes? *Cancer Treatment Reports.* 1987;71: 795–806.

12. Anonymous. Outcomes of cancer treatment for technology assessment and cancer treatment guidelines. American Society of Clinical Oncology. *Journal of Clinical Oncology.* 1996;14: 671–679.

13. Chao NJ, Parker PM, Niland JC, et al. Paradoxical effect of thalidomide prophylaxis on chronic graft-vs.-host disease. *Biol Blood Marrow Transplant.* 1996;2:86–92.

14. Koc S, Leisenring W, Flowers ME, et al. Thalidomide for treatment of patients with chronic graft-versus-host disease. *Blood.* 2000;96:3995–3996.

15. Arora M, Wagner JE, Davies SM, et al. Randomized clinical trial of thalidomide, cyclosporine, and prednisone versus cyclosporine and prednisone as initial therapy for chronic graft-versus-host disease. *Biol Blood Marrow Transplant.* 2001;7:265–273.

16. *Food and Drug Administration.* Guidance for Industry: Special Protocol Assessment. May, 2002.

32

SPECTRUM OF CHRONIC GRAFT VERSUS HOST DISEASE IN UNIQUE CLINICAL SITUATIONS

The Role of Stem-Cell Source Including Cord Blood Stem Cells, Reduced-Intensity Conditioning, and Donor Leukocyte Infusions

Mohamad Mohty, Juliet N. Barker, and Claudio Anasetti

INTRODUCTION

Several risk factors were found to be associated with the incidence and severity of chronic graft versus host disease (cGVHD) after allogeneic stem-cell transplantation (allo-SCT). The most important factor is likely to be the development of significant acute GVHD; but other classical risk factors including older age, a female donor (especially to a male patient), or some diagnoses such as chronic myeloid leukemia (CML) or aplastic anemia, were also reported. Some unique clinical situations such as the use of mismatched or unrelated donors (URDs) may be also associated with a higher risk of cGVHD, likely because of an increased reactivity between donor immune effectors and host cells. In the last decade, exploring cGVHD has also gained in importance, as more transplant centers are increasingly using allogeneic granulocyte colony-stimulating factor (G-CSF)-mobilized peripheral blood stem cells (PBSC). The latter has been associated with an increased incidence of cGVHD in most studies of human leukocyte antigen (HLA)-matched sibling transplantation. More recently, the use of the so-called reduced intensity or nonmyeloablative conditioning (RIC) regimens with or without systematic donor leukocyte infusion (DLI) also showed that cGVHD is still a major limitation. Similarly, the natural history of cGVHD appears to be modified after cord blood transplantation, and will need to be closely monitored. The aim of this chapter is to address the clinical, biological, and therapeutic features of cGVHD in the specific context of the above-mentioned unique clinical situations.

IMPACT OF STEM-CELL SOURCE ON cGVHD: BONE MARROW VERSUS PERIPHERAL BLOOD STEM CELLS

In the past decade, the availability of recombinant human G-CSF for hematopoietic stem-cell (HSC) mobilization represented a major advance in the field of allo-SCT. G-CSF-mobilized PBSCs have emerged as an attractive alternative to bone marrow (BM) as stem-cell source. In 1994 and 1995, the first large series of allo-SCT using PBSCs from G-CSF-mobilized donors were reported [1–8], and the use of allogeneic PBSCs as stem-cell source has since rapidly grown in this setting [9]. All prospective randomized trials comparing allogeneic PBSCs to BM could confirm that the use of PBSCs is associated with faster hematological recovery [10]. However, the use of PBSCs for allo-SCT is still not universally accepted. This is in part due to unresolved concerns about the long-term effects of growth factor treatment in healthy volunteers [11] and uncertainty about whether this stem-cell source is associated with more acute and cGVHD.

Nine prospective randomized controlled trials enrolling 1,111 patients with various hematologic malignancies comparing HLA-matched, related allogeneic unmanipulated PBSC transplantation with BM transplantation have been performed and published thus far [10]. Using an individual patient data meta-analysis including data from these nine randomized trials, there is a highly significant increase in the odds of developing of both extensive stage and overall (any stage) cGVHD in patients receiving allogeneic PBSCs. At 3 years, 47% and

68% of patients treated with PBSCs developed extensive or any stage cGHVD versus 31% and 52%, after BM, respectively. At 5 years, the corresponding figures for PBSC versus BM were 51% versus 35% for extensive stage cGVHD, and 73% versus 56% for any stage, respectively. However, in these randomized trials, allo-SCT using PBSCs was, overall, associated with a statistically significant improvement in disease-free survival (DFS) over allo-SCT using BM (59% vs. 53% at 3 years and 54% vs. 47% at 5 years, respectively). This difference was more pronounced in patients with more advanced disease (mainly acute leukemia and CML; 41% vs. 27% at 3 years; and 32% vs. 21% at 5 years) than in patients with early disease, likely due to a decrease in relapse in both late-stage and early-stage disease patients, while transplant-related mortality (TRM) was not different [10].

These findings slightly differed from those of another meta-analysis showing that the risk of relapse after PBSC transplantation may be lower than after BM transplantation, without reaching a statistical significance [12]. In addition, long-term results obtained from 141 PBSC and 272 BM recipients reported to the International Bone Marrow Transplant Registry and the European Group for Blood and Marrow Transplantation, showed that cGVHD was more frequent after PBSC compared to BM transplantation, yet relapse rates were similar in both groups. DFS rates were higher after PBSC than BM transplantation for patients with advanced CML (33% vs. 25%) but lower for those in first chronic phase (41% vs. 61%) due to higher rates of late TRM. On the other hand, overall survival and DFS were similar after PBSC and BM transplantation for early and advanced acute leukemia [13].

In terms of clinical presentation and therapeutic features, the French randomized trial was able to assess in detail the cGVHD organ-specific involvement and long-term immunosuppressive treatments. Among patients receiving PBSCs, recurrence of cGVHD following cessation of all immunosuppressive therapy is statistically more significant in comparison to BM recipients. Moreover, systemic immunosuppressive therapy had to be restarted rather shortly after initial cessation (median time, 3.8 months), and a highly significant proportion of PBSC recipients needed a second-line immunosuppressive regimen, as compared to BM. From the functional point of view, time to reach a Karnofsky performance status score of 90% (symptomatic but able to perform normal activity) tended to be higher in the PBSC group. This altered quality of survival could also be measured by the higher number of days of inpatient hospitalization experienced by cGVHD patients from the PBSC group, following day 100 after transplantation. The most relevant clinical features encountered in patients developing cGVHD after allo-SCT with PBSC were also assessed. Based on the type of cutaneous lesions, there was no significant difference in the number of patients with lichenoid lesions between PBSC and BM recipients. However, there was a trend, to more sclerodermatous cGVHD in PBSC recipients, suggesting more generalized cGVHD cutaneous manifestations associated with the use of allogeneic PBSCs. Oral and vaginal involvements did not appear to be significantly different after

PBSC transplantation. However, a higher incidence of ocular symptoms is usually seen in PBSC recipients. While there is no difference between PBSC and BM allo-SCT in terms of incidence of hepatic involvement, a longer time to normalization of hepatic abnormalities, especially serum bilirubin, was observed in the PBSC group. Other severe organ involvement (pulmonary symptoms, musculoskeletal and gastrointestinal tract) was only seen in the PBSC group. When assessed in terms of number of organs involved, cGVHD patients who had received PBSCs had a significantly higher number of organs involved (usually more than three organs involved) [14].

From the biological standpoint, we observed that at all time points after day 100 following transplantation, and during the first 3 years of follow-up, the mean absolute peripheral blood lymphocyte counts were higher among PBSC recipients compared with BM recipients [14], suggesting that more circulating alloreactive T lymphocytes derived from the donor may mediate, at least in part, more frequent and more severe cGVHD. Compared with BM, PBSC grafts contain 10-fold higher number of T cells, higher number of monocytes [15], skewed distribution of dendritic cells [16], and the absence of mesenchymal stem cells [17]. Another prominent feature of PBSC grafts is the significantly higher content of CD34+ stem cells, which not only participate in engraftment, but also have an immunogenic role [18–21]. With this background, several investigators tested the hypothesis whether there was a correlation between the cellular composition of the graft, especially CD34+ cell dose, and the risk of cGVHD, and other transplant-related events. Different studies demonstrated that an increased CD34+, but not CD3+, cell dose was significantly associated with an increased incidence of cGVHD, especially in its clinical extensive form after PBSC transplantation. Patients receiving the highest CD34+ cell dose (usually in excess of $8 > 10^6/$Kg) are likely to have a higher risk of developing extensive cGVHD [22–24]. Moreover, in patients surviving relapse-free beyond day 100 and evaluable for cGVHD, a "high" CD34+ cell dose had a negative impact on overall survival and DFS because of an increased cGVHD-related mortality [23], suggesting that allogeneic PBSC and BM do not appear to be simply interchangeable sources of hematopoietic grafts, and well-established dogma in the allogeneic BM transplantation setting need yet to be established in the PBSC setting.

At present, little is known to explain this surprising association between CD34+ cell dose and the risk of detrimental cGVHD after PBSC transplantation. Study of the different differentiation pathways and lymphoid and dendritic cell repopulation potential of G-CSF mobilized CD34+ PBSC may bring insights to elucidate the pathophysiology underlying the association between CD34+ cell dose and cGVHD.

Since extensive or severe cGVHD can adversely affect quality of life, the systematic use of allogeneic PBSCs (especially in patients with less advanced diseases) should be weighed to the higher risk of disease recurrence with BM against long-term consequences of cGVHD that is usually a good marker of an efficient immune graft-versus-leukemia effect. Nevertheless, it is important to note that these findings apply only to matched sibling fully myeloablative allo-SCT, and may not be completely valid in the context of RIC allo-SCT or alternative donor strategies.

CHRONIC GVHD AFTER REDUCED-INTENSITY CONDITIONING REGIMENS AND DONOR LEUKOCYTE INFUSIONS

Allo-SCT procedures are currently undergoing a profound evolution. The spectra of patients and diseases for which this approach is now considered have increased considerably over the past years. Despite the development of new potent drugs, outcome remains poor for a large proportion of patients. Also, given the peak age incidence of hematologic malignancies (usually median age >60), the vast majority of patients are excluded from high-dose chemotherapy, thereby precluding access to standard allo-SCT for those in need. On this background, several groups have launched RIC allo-SCT programs dedicated to patient not eligible for standard myeloablative allo-SCT. Indeed, the immune reactions between donor-derived immunocompetent T lymphocytes and host-type tumor cells have been well established to be the major antitumor agent in allo-SCT (graft-vs.-tumor effect; GVT). Therefore, non-myeloablative or RIC regimens development aimed to obtain minimal procedure-related toxicity, while securing engraftment to harness the GVT effect. One major advantage of RIC transplantation is the possibility of modulating immune reactivity by achieving a transient mixed chimeric state without rejection. Full donor chimerism could be later restored by a DLI, to provide optimal GVT reactivity. The RIC approach has been rapidly adopted worldwide and shown to be feasible in several disease settings, with the added benefit of expanding the transplant option to patients' categories who are ineligible for fully myeloablative allo-SCT. Several thousands of RIC transplants have been reported thus far. Unfortunately, most of the studies reported on small heterogeneous groups of patients, with respect to disease status. Also, the indications for RIC allo-SCT with respect to the patients' disease risk status and eligibility for RIC allo-SCT are not clearly delineated. In addition, few data are available to weigh the risk of TRM and morbidity versus risk of disease relapse. The comparison between different RIC allo-SCT series often blurs these distinctions. In general, the median age was within the fifth decade, although some were in the sixth and seventh decades. In addition to the heterogeneous demographic and disease features, complexity in data interpretation is illustrated by the use of different RIC and GVHD prophylaxis regimens. In these studies, the RIC regimen usually included a purine analog (mainly fludarabine) administered with or without low-dose irradiation and antibodies such as alemtuzumab or antithymocyte globulin (ATG). Donor origin is also variable with studies mixing data from related and URDs. The source of stem cells investigated in RIC allo-SCT includes most commonly PBSCs, which may contribute to a higher incidence of cGVHD. Some of the trials also included an alkylating agent such as melphalan or busulfan. Of note, TRM was generally relatively low, in the 5% to 25% range, although some trials reported a rate as high as 66% in cases of advanced disease [25, 26].

Conclusions related to the incidence or severity of cGVHD are very difficult to draw from these studies, and it is not clear that RIC transplants reduce the risk of cGVHD, though in theory, reduction of the "inflammatory" component of the conditioning as in RIC regimens may lead to the reduction of the rate and/or severity of acute GVHD and cGVHD. However, such hypothesis is yet to be proven, at least in clinical practice, where cGVHD remains a matter of concern after RIC allo-SCT. Older recipient age and its corollary of altered immune functions is a further confounding factor in this setting. Moreover, the distinction between acute and chronic forms of GVHD seems to be blurred after RIC allo-SCT, with clinically "acute" forms occurring much later than usual, or clinically "chronic" forms occurring very early, raising questions about the need for continuous immunosuppression and its corollary of long-term infectious complications. Table 32.1 summarizes the incidence of cGVHD in some large comparative studies between RIC and standard allo-SCT. A delay in the median time to onset of acute GVHD after RIC allo-SCT could translate into delayed onset of cGVHD features. In patients receiving fludarabine and low-dose total body irradiation (TBI), Mielcarek et al. [27] demonstrated that patients undergoing RIC allo-SCT had a delayed initiation of corticosteroid treatment for any GVHD symptoms, suggesting a delayed onset of cGVHD in this group. The frequent use of prolonged mycophenolate mofetil rather than the classical short-term methotrexate in RIC allo-SCT may have accounted for this delay. In another multicenter study where both RIC and conventional allo-SCT patients received comparable GVHD prophylaxis, median times to the onset of acute and cGVHD were significantly delayed in the RIC group, without a statistically significant difference in the incidence of cGVHD among RIC transplantation patients compared to myeloablative conditioning regimen [28]. The delayed time to onset of cGVHD in the RIC setting is likely a reflection of the state of mixed chimerism in these patients. In our own experience using fludarabine, busulfan, and ATG-based RIC regimen, the cumulative incidence of extensive cGVHD did not exceed 26% at 2 years, with ATG as part of the RIC and the choice of the stem-cell source (BM vs. PBSC) providing a powerful tool to modulate both acute and cGVHD incidence [32].

In terms of cGVHD features, Busca et al. [33] did not report any difference between patients after RIC or conventional conditioning in either the stage of cGVHD (limited or extensive), the type of onset, or extent of organ involvement. However, patients receiving RIC regimens are more likely to have refractory or steroid-dependent cGVHD requiring second-line treatments [29, 32, 34] although, the possibility of discontinuation of systemic immunosuppressive therapy was either comparable to conventional allo-SCT [33] or significantly higher [27].

Despite relatively wider use, data on the application of DLI following RIC allo-SCT and its correlation with cGVHD remain limited. The largest experience published by Peggs et al. [35] showed that both acute and cGVHD were very common

Table 32.1: Selected Comparative Studies Assessing cGVHD after Reduced-Intensity Conditioning versus Myeloablative Conventional Allo-SCT (Only Studies with >50 Patients are Included)

Author [references]	N	Type of Conditioning	Donor Type	GVHD Prophylaxis	cGVHD Incidence	Follow-Up (median)	Comment
Mielcarek [27]	RIC: 44 MAC: 52	RIC: Flu-low TBI MAC: Cy-TBI, Bu-Cy, Flu-Bu	MRD, MUD	CSA-MMF CSA-MMF or MTX	RIC: 73% MAC: 71%	~12 m.	Delayed initiation of corticosteroid treatment for cGVHD after RIC
Couriel [29]	RIC: 63 MAC: 74	RIC: Flu-Cy, other MAC: Bu-Cy, Flu-Mel	MRD	Tac-MTX Long MTX	RIC: 14% MAC: 40%	20 m.	Higher rate of relapsing cGVHD with MAC
Perez-Simon [28]	RIC: 150 MAC: 88	RIC: Flu-Mel, Flu-Bu MAC: Bu-Cy, Cy-TBI	MRD	CSA-MTX Short MTX	RIC: 71% MAC: 63%	13 m.	Higher incidence of limited, but not extensive cGVHD in RIC patients
Kim [30]	RIC: 63 MAC: 41	RIC: Flu-Bu + other MAC: TBI or Bu-Cy-based	MRD	RIC: CSA-MTX or MMF MAC: CSA-MTX	RIC: 57% MAC: 72%	13 m.	
Aoudjhane [31]	RIC: 315 MAC: 407	RIC: Flu-Bu, Flu-low TBI MAC: various	MRD	RIC: CSA-MTX or MMF MAC: CSA-MTX	RIC: 48% MAC: 56%	14 m.	In multivariate analysis, the risk of cGVHD was lower after RIC

Bu, busulfan; CSA, cyclosporine A; cGVHD, chronic graft versus host disease; Cy, cyclophosphamide; Flu, fludarabine; long, day 1, 3, 6, and 11 methotrexate; m., months; MAC, myeloablative conditioning; Mel, melphalan; MMF, mycophenolate mofetil; MRD, matched related donor; MTX, methotrexate; MUD, matched unrelated donor; N, number of patients; ref, reference; RIC, reduced-intensity conditioning; Short, day 1, 3 and 6 methotrexate; Tac, tacrolimus; TBI, total body irradiation.

after RIC allo-SCT, occurred at lower T-cell doses, and were more severe in the URD cohort. Moreover, conversion from mixed to full donor chimerism occurred in the majority of patients. Presence of mixed chimerism in the granulocyte lineage at the time of DLI did not predict for chimerism response or GVHD. DLIs and subsequent GVHD allowed achieving disease responses mainly in indolent lymphoid malignancies. Nonetheless, it remains unclear whether this type of approach is suitable for patients with other malignancies. Overall, the timing and dosage of DLI that can be administered with relative safety remain poorly defined, especially in the RIC setting where the persistence of host antigen presenting cells could have an impact on the development of GVHD, limiting its application.

In terms of risk factors of GVHD, the impact of donor HLA matching is likely to be comparable between the RIC allo-SCT setting and the standard myeloablative setting. Indeed, the clinical importance of donor matching for classical class I HLA-A, -B and -C and class II HLA-DR and -DQ alleles and antigens has been widely demonstrated [36] and now serves as the gold standard for donor selection worldwide [37]. Historically, the associations of HLA matching and clinical outcome were defined in patients receiving the classical sources of stem cells (BM replete with T cells, T-cell depleted BM, or PBSC) following standard myeloablative conditioning regimens. Ho et al. were among the first to describe the detrimental effects of

donor HLA disparity following RIC allo-SCT [38]. In a retrospective analysis of 111 patients who underwent RIC allo-SCT from URDs, of whom 78 were 10/10 matched at HLA-A, B, C, DRB1, DQB1 and 33 were mismatched at one or more HLA-C antigen/allele (24 HLA-C only; nine HLA-C + other locus mismatch). HLA-C disparity did not impair engraftment. Overall survival at 2 years was 30% in HLA-C-mismatched and 51% in 10/10-matched patients ($p = 0.008$). In Cox regression, HLA-C mismatch was an independent predictor of death. Also, treatment-related mortality was higher in the HLA-C-mismatched group [38]. In particular, HLA-C disparity can provoke graft versus host allorecognition after RIC allo-SCT, increasing the risk of clinically severe acute GVHD and its corollary cGVHD, lowering overall survival. However, participation of HLA-C in graft-versus-leukemia effects is suggested by the association of lower disease recurrence with transplantation from HLA-C mismatched donors.

The impact of CD34+ stem-cell dose on the incidence of cGVHD is less well defined in the setting of RIC allo-SCT. The Spanish retrospective analysis found that the CD34+ cell dose significantly influenced the development of cGVHD, only among patients receiving more than percentile 75 of CD34+ cells versus those receiving p75 or fewer cells [39]. However, other studies of RIC allo-SCT from related donors found no correlation between CD34+ cell dose and incidence of cGVHD [40–42]. Heterogeneous post-transplant immunosuppression

Table 32.2: Incidence of Chronic GVHD after UCBT

Author	Year	N	Age (years)	(%)	Comments
UCB Bank, Registry or Multicenter					
Rubinstein [47]	1998	562	82% < 18	25	Generally limited, rarely a cause of death, did not correlate with HLA-mismatch
Laughlin [49]	2001	68	31 (17–58)	38	11/12 patients had limited disease
Gluckman [50]	2006	925 (malignancy)	11 (0.1–56)	29	Increased incidence if low cell dose or 3–4 antigen HLA-mismatch
		279 (nonmalignant)	3 (0.25–10)	24	Increased incidence if 3–4 antigen HLA-mismatch
Single Center					
Wagner 48]	2002	102	7 (0.2–56)	9	All extensive diagnosed at a median of 5 months
Wall [51]	2005	32	1.6 (0.5–3.9)	26	
Barker [44]	2005	23	24 (13–53)	23	All extensive
Kernan [52]	2006	316	4.6 (0.1–18)	21	
Brunstein [53]	2007	110	51 (17–69)	23	No factor was predictive
Ballen [54]	2007	21	49 (24–63)	31	2/5 with extensive and 3/5 with limited disease

cGVHD, chronic graft versus host disease; HLA, human leukocyte antigen; N, number of patients; UCB, umbilical cord blood; UCBT, umbilical cord blood transplantation.

regimens with or without prior T-cell depletion may account for these different findings.

In summary, it appears that although RIC regimens do not appear to decrease the incidence of cGVHD, the natural history of the disease is modified. However, one should bear in mind that poor standardization and reproducibility of the diagnostic criteria for cGVHD and the gradation of disease severity complicate comparison between studies. The use of the consensus document elaborated by the Working Group of the NIH Consensus Development Project [43], will likely help standardizing the criteria for diagnosis of cGVHD, and providing uniformity in describing the extent and prognosis of disease in the RIC setting.

CHRONIC GVHD AFTER UMBILICAL CORD BLOOD TRANSPLANTATION

Umbilical cord blood (UCB) is increasingly being used as an alternative HSC source with the advantage of rapid availability and less stringent requirement for HLA-match. While early experience with UCB transplantation (UCBT) was associated with poor engraftment and high TRM in recipients of low UCB cell dose, more recent data has been associated with much improved survival [44] making UCBT an increasingly attractive alternative for some patients. From the earliest experience of UCBT a less than expected incidence of acute GVHD has been observed given the degree of HLA disparity [45–48]. Most UCB grafts that have been transplanted to date have been

either 5/6 or 4/6 HLA-A,B antigen and DRB1 allele matched to the recipient. However, at high-resolution typing the degree of HLA-mismatch to the recipient is considerable. For example, the median patient-recipient HLA-match of 72 UCB units transplanted at Memorial Sloan-Kettering Cancer Center has been 5/10 (unpublished data). The exact reasons for the relatively low incidence of GVHD are unknown but likely result from the functional immaturity of the infused lymphocytes including decreased cytotoxicity, an altered cytokine profile, decreased HLA expression and increased regulatory T cells and are under investigation.

The incidence of cGVHD has also been lower than expected but is less well described especially in adults. To date, both single institution and registry studies have revealed a relatively low incidence of cGVHD after almost exclusively HLA-mismatched UCBT that has ranged between 9% and 38% (Table 32.2). However, these studies have varied in their reporting of whether the cGVHD is limited or extensive and whether HLA-mismatch has any influence on the incidence of this complication. For these reasons the comparison of how the cGVHD after UCBT compares to that after the transplantation of adult sources of allogeneic HSC should be considered as preliminary. However, while no randomized studies of URD HSC and UCB transplantation have been performed to date, a number of retrospective studies have compared the outcomes of UCBT and URD transplants including the incidence of cGVHD (Table 32.3). For example, Eapen et al. have reported the outcomes of children ≤ 16 years transplanted for the treatment of leukemia or myelodysplasia with HSC from either 8/8 allele

Table 32.3: Comparison of Chronic GVHD after UCBT and URD or Sibling Donor Transplants

Author	Year	N	Donor	HLA – Match (%)	cGVHD Incidence	Comment
Pediatric Series						
Rocha [55]	2001	99	UCBT	8 match	25% (1–17)	(1) N engrafted survivors after day 100 with cGVHD: UCBT 12%; URD 43%; T-URD 11% (2) UCBT HR 0.24 (95%CI: 0.01–0.66), p = 0.002
		262	URD	82 match	46% (37–53)	
		180	T-URD	57 match	12% (6–17)	
Eapen [56]	2007	503	UCBT	7 match*	82/466 = 18%	(1) *Criteria for "match" were A, B antigen, DRB1 allele for UCB but A, B, C, DRB1 alleles for URD recipients (2) cGVHD incidence was similar in UCB and matched URD transplant recipients (3) cGVHD rates were similar in matched and mismatched UCBT recipients
		282	URD	41 match*	Matched URD: 37/ 116 = 32% Mismatched URD: 66/166 = 40%	
Adult Series						
Takahashi [57]	2004	68	UCBT	0 match	13/54 = 24% extensive	UCBT HR 0.60 (0.28–1.28) p = 0.18
		45	URD	87 match	14/35 = 40% extensive	
Laughlin [58]	2004	150	UCBT	0 match	33% extensive	Although UCBT recipients had a higher incidence of cGVHD overall as compared to matched URD BMT recipients (HR 1.62; 95%CI 1.08–2.42, p = 0.02), UCBT recipients had the least extensive cGVHD (p = 0.03)
		450	URD	82 match	URD match: 52% extensive URD mismatch: 71% extensive	
Rocha [59]	2004	98	UCBT	6 match	30%	Multivariate analysis cGVHD risk was not different between the 2 groups. RR for UCBT recipients: 0.64 (0.37–1.1), p = 0.11
		584	URD	100 match	46%	
Takahashi [60]	2007	100	UCBT	0 match	28% extensive	UCBT HR (extensive cGVHD) 0.49 (95%CI: 0.29–0.85), p = 0.01
		71	Sib	76 match	55% extensive	

BMT, bone marrow transplantation; cGVHD, chronic graft versus host disease; CI, confidence interval; HLA, human leukocyte antigen; HR, hazards ratio; M, HLA-match; MM, HLA-mismatch; N, number of patients; RR, relative risk; sib, sibling T-URD, unrelated donor with T-cell depletion; UCBT, umbilical cord blood transplantation; URD, unrelated donor.

matched URD BM (n = 116), mismatched marrow (n = 166), or 4–6/6 A,B antigen, DRB1 allele matched single unit UCB grafts (n = 503) after a myeloablative preparative regimen [56]. This study has the distinction of the only analysis that has compared UCBT with the transplantation of the current gold standard of 8/8 HLA-A, B, C, DRB1 allele matched URD BM. These authors reported incidences of cGVHD of 18% in UCB, 32% in HLA-matched, and 40% in HLA-mismatched URD transplant recipients, respectively, with no significant difference in the cGVHD incidence in UCBT recipients and allele matched marrow. Further, there was no difference in the incidence of cGVHD after 6/6 HLA-matched and 1 and 2 antigen mismatched UCBT in this study.

Laughlin et al. reported that 35/69 (51%) of adult single unit UCBT recipients, 86/243 (35%) of 6/6 HLA-matched URD transplant recipients, and 17/43 (40%) of HLA-mismatched URD transplant recipients developed cGVHD [58]. While this suggested a higher rate of cGVHD among UCBT recipients as compared to that of HLA-matched marrow, among those

patients with cGVHD the proportion with extensive disease was lower among UCBT recipients than those receiving URD marrow with rates of 33% in UCB, 52% in matched BM, and 71% in mismatched marrow, respectively. Rocha et al. performed a similar analysis in adult UCBT and HLA-matched URD marrow transplant recipients in Europe [61]. In this study the 2-year cGVHD incidence was 30% in UCBT and 46% in URD adult transplant recipients (p = 0.07). Interestingly, Takahashi and colleagues have reported that the incidence of extensive cGVHD after UCBT (n = 100) of 28% was significantly less than that of 55% in 71 HLA-identical related donor transplant recipients in Japan [60]. This study suggests for the first time that UCB may have advantages over even sibling donor HSC from the standpoint of cGVHD. The lower incidence of cGVHD after UCBT was further confirmed in a large Japanese multicentre study which investigated the clinical features of cGVHD in 1,072 Japanese patients with hematologic malignancies who received a transplant through the Japan Cord Blood Bank Network. The cumulative incidence of cGVHD 2 years after UCBT was 28%. Multivariate analysis identified risk factors of cGVHD: higher patient body weight, higher number of mismatched antigens for GVHD direction, myeloablative preparative regimen, use of mycophenolate mofetil in GVHD prophylaxis, and development of grades II to IV acute GVHD. Most importantly, this study suggested that cGVHD after UCBT is associated with improved survival, perhaps due to an immune graft-versus-malignancy effect, since development of cGVHD was favorably associated with both overall survival and event-free survival [62].

Beyond the incidence of cGVHD after UCBT, the pattern and severity of organ involvement and its response to therapy have yet to be fully explored. The first effort to address this issue has been performed by Arora et al. [63] In this study 123 patients with cGVHD after URD transplantation were compared to 47 patients with cGVHD after UCBT. URD transplant recipients were significantly younger (median age 25 vs. 39 years, $p = 0.002$), and the grafts were mostly 6/6 HLA-matched (67% as compared to 10% in the UCBT recipients, $p < 0.001$). Fifty-three percent of URD recipients received cyclosporine-A (CSA) and methotrexate GVHD prophylaxis with 33% receiving T-cell depletion whereas 64% of UCBT recipients received CSA and mycophenolate mofetil prophylaxis with 34% receiving CSA and corticosteroids. Interestingly, there was no difference in the incidence of preceding acute GVHD in these cGVHD patients, the time to cGVHD onset, or the organ involvement with cGVHD in the two groups. However, UCBT recipients were more frequently responsive (complete or partial remission) to treatment [48% URD vs. 74% UCB at 2 months ($p = 0.005$); 49% vs. 78% at 6 months ($p = 0.001$); and 51% vs. 72% at 1 year ($p = 0.003$)], respectively. In addition, TRM after the diagnosis of cGVHD was higher after URD transplantation with a 1-year post-cGVHD TRM of 27% (95%CI: 19%–35%) after URD versus 11% (95%CI: 2%–22%) after UCBT ($p = 0.055$). In both groups, thrombocytopenia and no response to therapy at 2 months were independently associated with increased mortality whereas a progressive onset of cGVHD was only a significant predictor of increased mortality in the URD group. Also, URD transplant recipients were significantly more likely to have the poor prognostic factor of platelet count less than 100,000 at the onset of cGVHD (URD 54% and UCB 23%, $p = 0.003$). These data suggest that cGVHD following UCBT is more responsive to therapy and is associated with lower TRM. It is possible that the findings in favor of UCBT may have even been more striking if it were not for the fact that 121 of 123 URD recipients in this study received BM as the HSC source rather than PBSC.

In summary, while cGVHD does occur after UCBT current data suggests that (1) the incidence is less than expected based on the degree of HLA disparity of the UCB grafts; (2) the incidence of extensive disease is either comparable or lower than that of matched URD marrow transplantation; and (3) that cGVHD after UCBT may be more responsive to treatment and associated with a lower TRM than seen after URD transplantation. Much remains to be understood concerning the natural history, pattern, and severity of organ involvement

of the cGVHD after UCBT, the role of HLA-match, the ideal prophylaxis and therapy for this disease, whether there is any association between cGVHD and protection against relapse, and the comparison with URD PBSC. However, it is likely that once the limitation of engraftment after UCBT can be reliably resolved, with strategies such as double unit UCBT, for example, the potential benefit of a reduced risk for severe extensive cGVHD, particularly as compared to the transplantation of mismatched URD HSC, may make UCB an attractive HSC source for many patients. This is particularly relevant given the increased cGVHD that has been seen after the transplantation of PBSC from volunteer donors (especially in the setting of mismatch) and the resultant adverse impact on the quality of life for these patients.

REFERENCES

1. Tanaka J, Imamura M, Zhu X, et al. Potential benefit of recombinant human granulocyte colony-stimulating factor-mobilized peripheral blood stem cells for allogeneic transplantation. *Blood.* 1994;84:3595–3596.

2. Korbling M, Przepiorka D, Huh YO, et al. Allogeneic blood stem cell transplantation for refractory leukemia and lymphoma: potential advantage of blood over marrow allografts. *Blood.* 1995;85:1659–1665.

3. Korbling M, Przepiorka D, Gajewski J, Champlin RE, Chan KW. With first successful allogeneic transplantations of apheresis-derived hematopoietic progenitor cells reported, can the recruitment of volunteer matched, unrelated stem cell donors be expanded substantially? *Blood.* 1995;86:1235.

4. Korbling M, Huh YO, Durett A, et al. Allogeneic blood stem cell transplantation: peripheralization and yield of donor-derived primitive hematopoietic progenitor cells (CD34+ Thy-1dim) and lymphoid subsets, and possible predictors of engraftment and graft-versus-host disease. *Blood.* 1995;86:2842–2848.

5. Bensinger WI, Weaver CH, Appelbaum FR, et al. Transplantation of allogeneic peripheral blood stem cells mobilized by recombinant human granulocyte colony-stimulating factor. *Blood.* 1995;85:1655–1658.

6. Schmitz N, Dreger P, Suttorp M, et al. Primary transplantation of allogeneic peripheral blood progenitor cells mobilized by filgrastim (granulocyte colony-stimulating factor). *Blood.* 1995;85:1666–1672.

7. Russell JA, Luider J, Weaver M, et al. Collection of progenitor cells for allogeneic transplantation from peripheral blood of normal donors. *Bone Marrow Transplant.* 1995;15:111–115.

8. Azevedo WM, Aranha FJ, Gouvea JV, et al. Allogeneic transplantation with blood stem cells mobilized by rhG-CSF for hematological malignancies. *Bone Marrow Transplant.* 1995;16:647–653.

9. Gratwohl A, Baldomero H, Frauendorfer K, Urbano-Ispizua A, Niederwieser D. Results of the EBMT activity survey 2005 on haematopoietic stem cell transplantation: focus on increasing use of unrelated donors. *Bone Marrow Transplant.* 2007;39:71–87.

10. Stem Cell Trialists' Collaborative Group. Allogeneic peripheral blood stem-cell compared with bone marrow transplantation in the management of hematologic malignancies: an individual patient data meta-analysis of nine randomized trials. *J Clin Oncol.* 2005;23:5074–5087.

11. Bennett CL, Evens AM, Andritsos LA, et al. Haematological malignancies developing in previously healthy individuals who received haematopoietic growth factors: report from the Research on Adverse Drug Events and Reports (RADAR) project. Br J Haematol. 2006;135:642–650.

12. Cutler C, Giri S, Jeyapalan S, Paniagua D, Viswanathan A, Antin JH. Acute and chronic graft-versus-host disease after allogeneic peripheral-blood stem-cell and bone marrow transplantation: a meta-analysis. J Clin Oncol. 2001;19:3685–3691.

13. Schmitz N, Eapen M, Horowitz MM, et al. Long-term outcome of patients given transplants of mobilized blood or bone marrow: A report from the International Bone Marrow Transplant Registry and the European Group for Blood and Marrow Transplantation. Blood. 2006;108:4288–4290.

14. Mohty M, Kuentz M, Michallet M, et al. Chronic graft versus host disease after allogeneic blood stem cell transplantation: long term results of a randomized study. Blood. 2002;100:3128–3134.

15. Blaise D, Kuentz M, Fortanier C, et al. Randomized trial of bone marrow versus lenograstim-primed blood cell allogeneic transplantation in patients with early-stage leukemia: a report from the Societe Francaise de Greffe de Moelle. J Clin Oncol. 2000;18:537–546.

16. Arpinati M, Green CL, Heimfeld S, Heuser JE, Anasetti C. Granulocyte-colony stimulating factor mobilizes T helper 2-inducing dendritic cells. Blood. 2000;95:2484–2490.

17. Bacigalupo A, Francesco F, Brinch L, Van Lint MT. Bone marrow or peripheral blood as a source of stem cells for allogeneic transplants. Curr Opin Hematol. 2000;7:343–347.

18. Ryncarz RE, Anasetti C. Expression of CD86 on human marrow CD34(+) cells identifies immunocompetent committed precursors of macrophages and dendritic cells. Blood. 1998;91:3892–3900.

19. Rondelli D, Lemoli RM, Ratta M, et al. Rapid induction of CD40 on a subset of granulocyte colony-stimulating factor-mobilized CD34(+) blood cells identifies myeloid committed progenitors and permits selection of nonimmunogenic CD40(-) progenitor cells. Blood. 1999;94:2293–2300.

20. Rondelli D, Anasetti C, Fortuna A, et al. T cell alloreactivity induced by normal G-CSF-mobilized CD34⁺ blood cells. Bone Marrow Transplant. 1998;21:1183–1191.

21. van Rhee F, Jiang YZ, Vigue F, et al. Human G-CSF-mobilized CD34-positive peripheral blood progenitor cells can stimulate allogeneic T-cell responses: implications for graft rejection in mismatched transplantation. Br J Haematol. 1999;105:1014–1024.

22. Zaucha JM, Gooley T, Bensinger WI, et al. CD34 cell dose in granulocyte colony-stimulating factor-mobilized peripheral blood mononuclear cell grafts affects engraftment kinetics and development of extensive chronic graft-versus-host disease after human leukocyte antigen-identical sibling transplantation. Blood. 2001;98:3221–3227.

23. Mohty M, Bilger K, Jourdan E, et al. Higher doses of CD34⁺ peripheral blood stem cells are associated with increased mortality from chronic graft-versus-host disease after allogeneic HLA-identical sibling transplantation. Leukemia. 2003;17:869–875.

24. Sohn SK, Kim JG, Kim DH, Lee NY, Suh JS, Lee KB. Impact of transplanted CD34⁺ cell dose in allogeneic unmanipulated peripheral blood stem cell transplantation. Bone Marrow Transplant. 2003;31:967–972.

25. Mohty M, Nagler A, Killmann NM. Reduced-intensity conditioning allogeneic stem cell transplantation: hype, reality or time for a rethink? Leukemia. 2006;20:1653–1654.

26. Blaise D, Vey N, Faucher C, Mohty M. Current status of reduced-intensity-conditioning allogeneic stem cell transplantation for acute myeloid leukemia. Haematologica. 2007;92:533–541.

27. Mielcarek M, Martin PJ, Leisenring W, et al. Graft-versus-host disease after nonmyeloablative versus conventional hematopoietic stem cell transplantation. Blood. 2003;102:756–762.

28. Perez-Simon JA, Diez-Campelo M, Martino R, et al. Influence of the intensity of the conditioning regimen on the characteristics of acute and chronic graft-versus-host disease after allogeneic transplantation. Br J Haematol. 2005;130:394–403.

29. Couriel DR, Saliba RM, Giralt S, et al. Acute and chronic graft-versus-host disease after ablative and nonmyeloablative conditioning for allogeneic hematopoietic transplantation. Biol Blood Marrow Transplant. 2004;10:178–185.

30. Kim DH, Sohn SK, Baek JH, et al. Retrospective multicenter study of allogeneic peripheral blood stem cell transplantation followed by reduced-intensity conditioning or conventional myeloablative regimen. Acta Haematol. 2005;113:220–227.

31. Aoudjhane M, Labopin M, Gorin NC, et al. Comparative outcome of reduced intensity and myeloablative conditioning regimen in HLA identical sibling allogeneic haematopoietic stem cell transplantation for patients older than 50 years of age with acute myeloblastic leukaemia: a retrospective survey from the Acute Leukemia Working Party (ALWP) of the European group for Blood and Marrow Transplantation (EBMT). Leukemia. 2005;19:2304–2312.

32. Mohty M, Bay JO, Faucher C, et al. Graft-versus-host disease following allogeneic transplantation from HLA-identical sibling with antithymocyte globulin-based reduced-intensity preparative regimen. Blood. 2003;102:470–476.

33. Busca A, Rendine S, Locatelli F, et al. Chronic graft-versus-host disease after reduced-intensity stem cell transplantation versus conventional hematopoietic stem cell transplantation. Hematology. 2005;10:1–10.

34. de Lavallade H, Mohty M, Faucher C, Furst S, El-Cheikh J, Blaise D. Low-dose methotrexate as salvage therapy for refractory graft-versus-host disease after reduced-intensity conditioning allogeneic stem cell transplantation. Haematologica. 2006;91:1438–1440.

35. Peggs KS, Thomson K, Hart DP, et al. Dose-escalated donor lymphocyte infusions following reduced intensity transplantation: toxicity, chimerism, and disease responses. Blood. 2004;103:1548–1556.

36. Flomenberg N, Baxter-Lowe LA, Confer D, et al. Impact of HLA class I and class II high-resolution matching on outcomes of unrelated donor bone marrow transplantation: HLA-C mismatching is associated with a strong adverse effect on transplantation outcome. Blood. 2004;104:1923–1930.

37. Hurley CK, Setterholm M, Lau M, et al. Hematopoietic stem cell donor registry strategies for assigning search determinants and matching relationships. Bone Marrow Transplant. 2004;33:443–450.

38. Ho VT, Kim HT, Liney D, et al. HLA-C mismatch is associated with inferior survival after unrelated donor non-myeloablative hematopoietic stem cell transplantation. Bone Marrow Transplant. 2006;37:845–850.

39. Perez-Simon JA, Diez-Campelo M, Martino R, et al. Impact of CD34⁺ cell dose on the outcome of patients undergoing reduced-intensity-conditioning allogeneic peripheral blood stem cell transplantation. Blood. 2003;102:1108–1113.

40. Mohty M, Bagattini S, Chabannon C, et al. CD8⁺ T cell dose affects development of acute graft-vs-host disease following

reduced-intensity conditioning allogeneic peripheral blood stem cell transplantation. *Exp Hematol.* 2004;32:1097–1102.

41. Panse JP, Heimfeld S, Guthrie KA, et al. Allogeneic peripheral blood stem cell graft composition affects early T-cell chimerism and later clinical outcomes after non-myeloablative conditioning. *Br J Haematol.* 2005;128:659–667.

42. Baron F, Maris MB, Storer BE, et al. High doses of transplanted CD34+ cells are associated with rapid T-cell engraftment and lessened risk of graft rejection, but not more graft-versus-host disease after nonmyeloablative conditioning and unrelated hematopoietic cell transplantation. *Leukemia.* 2005;19:822–828.

43. Filipovich AH, Weisdorf D, Pavletic S, et al. National Institutes of Health consensus development project on criteria for clinical trials in chronic graft-versus-host disease: I. Diagnosis and staging working group report. *Biol Blood Marrow Transplant.* 2005;11:945–956.

44. Barker JN, Weisdorf DJ, DeFor TE, et al. Transplantation of 2 partially HLA-matched umbilical cord blood units to enhance engraftment in adults with hematologic malignancy. *Blood.* 2005;105:1343–1347.

45. Kurtzberg J, Laughlin M, Graham ML, et al. Placental blood as a source of hematopoietic stem cells for transplantation into unrelated recipients. *N Engl J Med.* 1996;335:157–166.

46. Gluckman E, Rocha V, Boyer-Chammard A, et al. Outcome of cord-blood transplantation from related and unrelated donors. Eurocord Transplant Group and the European Blood and Marrow Transplantation Group. *N Engl J Med.* 1997;337:373–381.

47. Rubinstein P, Carrier C, Scaradavou A, et al. Outcomes among 562 recipients of placental-blood transplants from unrelated donors. *N Engl J Med.* 1998;339:1565–1577.

48. Wagner JE, Barker JN, DeFor TE, et al. Transplantation of unrelated donor umbilical cord blood in 102 patients with malignant and nonmalignant diseases: influence of CD34 cell dose and HLA disparity on treatment-related mortality and survival. *Blood.* 2002;100:1611–1618.

49. Laughlin MJ, Barker J, Bambach B, et al. Hematopoietic engraftment and survival in adult recipients of umbilical-cord blood from unrelated donors. *N Engl J Med.* 2001;344:1815–1822.

50. Gluckman E, Rocha V. Donor selection for unrelated cord blood transplants. *Curr Opin Immunol.* 2006;18:565–570.

51. Wall DA, Carter SL, Kernan NA, et al. Busulfan/melphalan/antithymocyte globulin followed by unrelated donor cord blood transplantation for treatment of infant leukemia and leukemia in young children: the Cord Blood Transplantation study (COBLT) experience. *Biol Blood Marrow Transplant.* 2005;11:637–646.

52. Martin PL, Carter SL, Kernan NA, et al. Results of the cord blood transplantation study (COBLT): outcomes of unrelated donor umbilical cord blood transplantation in pediatric patients with lysosomal and peroxisomal storage diseases. *Biol Blood Marrow Transplant.* 2006;12:184–194.

53. Brunstein CG, Barker JN, Weisdorf DJ, et al. Umbilical cord blood transplantation after nonmyeloablative conditioning: impact on transplantation outcomes in 110 adults with hematologic disease. *Blood.* 2007;110:3064–3070.

54. Ballen KK, Spitzer TR, Yeap BY, et al. Double unrelated reduced-intensity umbilical cord blood transplantation in adults. *Biol Blood Marrow Transplant.* 2007;13:82–89.

55. Rocha V, Cornish J, Sievers EL, et al. Comparison of outcomes of unrelated bone marrow and umbilical cord blood transplants in children with acute leukemia. *Blood.* 2001;97:2962–2971.

56. Eapen M, Rubinstein P, Zhang MJ, et al. Outcomes of transplantation of unrelated donor umbilical cord blood and bone marrow in children with acute leukaemia: a comparison study. *Lancet.* 2007;369:1947–1954.

57. Takahashi S, Iseki T, Ooi J, et al. Single-institute comparative analysis of unrelated bone marrow transplantation and cord blood transplantation for adult patients with hematologic malignancies. *Blood.* 2004;104:3813–3820.

58. Laughlin MJ, Eapen M, Rubinstein P, et al. Outcomes after transplantation of cord blood or bone marrow from unrelated donors in adults with leukemia. *N Engl J Med.* 2004;351:2265–2275.

59. Rocha V, Labopin M, Sanz G, et al. Transplants of umbilical-cord blood or bone marrow from unrelated donors in adults with acute leukemia. *N Engl J Med.* 2004;351:2276–2285.

60. Takahashi S, Ooi J, Tomonari A, et al. Comparative single-institute analysis of cord blood transplantation from unrelated donors with bone marrow or peripheral blood stem-cell transplants from related donors in adult patients with hematologic malignancies after myeloablative conditioning regimen. *Blood.* 2007;109:1322–1330.

61. Rocha V, Labopin M, Sanz G, et al. Transplants of umbilical-cord blood or bone marrow from unrelated donors in adults with acute leukemia. *N Engl J Med.* 2004;351:2276–2285.

62. Narimatsu H, Miyakoshi S, Yamaguchi T, et al. Chronic graft-versus-host disease following umbilical cord blood transplantation: retrospective survey involving 1072 patients in Japan. *Blood.* 2008 Sep 15;112(6):2579–2582. Epub 2008 Jun 16.

63. Arora M, Nagaraj S, Wagner JE, et al. Chronic graft-versus-host disease (cGVHD) following unrelated donor hematopoietic stem cell transplantation (HSCT): higher response rate in recipients of unrelated donor (URD) umbilical cord blood (UCB). *Biol Blood Marrow Transplant.* 2007;13:1145–1152.

33

Pediatric Chronic Graft versus Host Disease

Kristin Baird, Alan S. Wayne, and David A. Jacobsohn

INTRODUCTION

Allogeneic Transplantation in Pediatrics

Allogeneic hematopoietic stem cell transplantation (allo-HSCT) is curative for many pediatric diseases. Most children transplanted for cancer, severe combined immunodeficiency syndrome [1], aplastic anemia [2], sickle cell anemia [3], thalassemia [4], and certain metabolic disorders [5] are expected to survive. This has led to an ever-increasing population of long-term survivors. Recent studies demonstrate the major impact that late effects have on the individual survivors and society as a whole [6, 7].

Chronic Graft versus Host Disease

Chronic graft versus host disease (cGVHD) is the most significant nonrelapse cause of morbidity and mortality following stem cell transplantation (SCT) for malignancies [8]. Although the rates of cGVHD are lower in children than adults [9–11], the incidence of cGVHD in children has increased in association with the use of peripheral blood and unrelated donors [8, 12–16]. The manifestations and mechanisms of cGVHD in children and adults appear similar, although the natural history and response to therapy are different. cGVHD and its current treatments have a spectrum of deleterious effects on normal growth and organ development in children. In addition, the impact of prolonged immunosuppression is of particular concern in childhood, a critical time of immunologic development in response to common infections and immunizations.

Data and research focused on cGVHD in pediatrics are limited. Most studies are small and are often grouped into larger adult series. In comparison to adults, relatively small numbers of children and adolescents undergo transplantation. Furthermore, pediatric patients are commonly referred to pediatric transplant centers and subsequently return to a home treatment center, where the consequences of transplant may not be systematically studied. Treating and preventing the secondary effects of allo-HSCT remain critical adjuncts to the care of children with life-threatening illnesses requiring transplantation; however, the treatment and prevention of cGVHD need to be approached with consideration of graft-versus-leukemia (GVL) effects, which have benefit in the setting of transplantation for certain malignancies [13].

INCIDENCE OF cGVHD IN PEDIATRICS

The incidence of cGVHD is lower in children than adults. Analysis of data from the International Bone Marrow Transplant Registry (IBMTR) published in 2000, shows a 15% 3-year cumulative incidence of cGVHD in 2,052 children receiving human leukocyte antigen (HLA)-matched sibling bone marrow transplants (BMTs). All of these patients received a myeloablative preparative regimen and approximately one-third received total body irradiation (TBI). Two-thirds of the patients had malignant disease and most received cyclosporine (CSA)-based GVHD prophylaxis. Factors that were associated with lower rates of cGVHD were younger age, nonmalignant disease, and the use of methotrexate (MTX) with CSA for GVHD prophylaxis [17].

Zecca et al. conducted a retrospective analysis of 696 consecutive pediatric patients that underwent transplant in Italy between 1991 and 1999. The indication for transplant was malignancy in two-thirds, the majority of patients received bone marrow (BM) as the stem cell source and two-thirds had HLA-matched sibling donors. The incidence of cGVHD was 25%, with 16% categorized as limited and 9% as extensive and a median time to diagnosis of 116 days posttransplantation. The factors most highly associated with cGVHD included patient age >15 years, donor age >5 years, female donor into a male recipient, the use of TBI, malignant disease as indication for transplant, and previous grade II to IV acute GVHD (aGVHD). aGVHD had the highest relative risk (RR = 2.14) for the development of cGVHD. Cord blood was associated with lower incidence of cGVHD in comparison to BM or PBSCs (p = 0.0073). cGVHD was associated with a lower relapse rate in patients with acute lymphoblastic leukemia (ALL). The 6-year disease-free survival (DFS) was 68% in malignant diseases in the presence of cGVHD and 54% in the absence of

Table 33.1: Unrelated Donor Bone Marrow Transplantation: Pediatric Series

Patients (n)	Probability of Myeloid Engraftment (%)	aGVHD Grades II–IV	cGVHD	cGVHD Comments	Reference
UD (88)	100	83% matched 98% MM	60% matched 69% MM	37% extensive	Balduzzi 1995 [18]
MUD (17)	83	63%	54%	38% extensive	Davies BJH 1997 [19a]
MUD (50)	93	49% matched 67% MM	50% matched 55% MM	Lower relapse rates in patients with cGVHD	Davies JCO 1997 [19b]
MUD (28)		64%	57%	20% extensive	Saarinen-Pihkala 2001 [24]
MRD (37)		38%	26%	13% extensive	
MUD (363)	98	47%	39%	Female donor into female recipient = significantly higher rates. Lower relapse rates in patients with cGVHD	Bunin 2002 [20]
MUD (88)	98	85%	58%	47% extensive	Woolfrey 2002 [23]
MUD* (66[†])	97	40% matched 42% 1 MM 37% 2–3 MM	20% matched 34% 1 MM 40% 2–3 MM	10% extensive 14% extensive 20% extensive	Giebel 2003 [22]
MUD (23)	100	48%	46%	13% extensive	Talano 2006 [21]

Notes: MM, mismatched; MRD, matched related donor; MUD, matched unrelated donor; *n*, number; RD, related donor; TRM, transplant related mortality; UD, unrelated donor.
* High-resolution typing (10 allelle); [†] 4 received peripheral blood stem cells (PBSC).

cGVHD ($p = 0.0013$). cGVHD did not correlate with DFS in nonmalignant diseases [13].

STEM CELL SOURCE

Unrelated Donors

Pediatric patients appear to tolerate alternative donor transplants (matched unrelated and mismatched related) better than adults. Studies of unrelated donor BMT in the pediatric population during the 1980s through the early 1990s report high incidences of cGVHD (50%–69%) [18, 19]. More recent studies, however, suggest a decreasing incidence of cGVHD (39%–46%) (Table 33.1) [20, 21]. A joint Polish and Italian study prospectively evaluated 63 children transplanted from unrelated donors selected by high-resolution typing of both HLA class I and class II loci. They observed low incidences of severe aGVHD, cGVHD, and graft failure, with rates comparable to those seen in children transplanted from HLA-identical siblings [22].

In 2002, investigators in Seattle published results on unrelated donor marrow transplantation for children with ALL. All patients ($n = 88$) received the same conditioning regimen with cyclophosphamide and TBI and most received CSA with MTX for GVHD prophylaxis. Fifty-six patients had an HLA-matched donor and 32 had a single antigen mismatch. Of those patients surviving past day 80, 47% developed extensive cGVHD and limited cGVHD was observed in 11% [23].

A population-based study from seven Nordic centers of 65 pediatric transplant patients who underwent BMT for ALL from either matched sibling donors ($n = 37$) or unrelated donors ($n = 28$) was published in 2001. GVHD prophylaxis in the matched sibling group consisted of CSA in all and MTX in 67% of patients. GVHD prophylaxis in the unrelated donor group consisted of CSA and MTX with 64% receiving antithymocyte globulin (ATG) and 11% also having T-cell depletion. cGVHD was significantly higher in the unrelated group (57% vs. 26%; $p = 0.05$). The treatment-related mortality (TRM), event free survival (EFS), and overall survival (OS) were not significantly different; however, patients with sibling donors had higher relapse rate and earlier time to relapse [24].

Peripheral Blood Stem Cells

BM remains the predominant stem cell source employed in pediatric transplantation. However, alternative sources have been utilized with increasing frequency. As in the adult setting, the use of granulocyte colony-stimulating factor (G-CSF) mobilized PBSC has increased in pediatrics [12, 25]. Studies in adults have demonstrated a higher incidence of cGVHD or refractory cGVHD when using PBSC versus BM [26–28]. In adults, this approach has been associated with decreased TRM and decreased relapse rates in leukemia patients despite an increased incidence of cGVHD [29]. In children, however, data are less clear (Table 33.2). A retrospective IBMTR study in pediatrics reported poorer survival with PBSC transplants

Table 33.2: Peripheral Blood Stem Cell Transplantation: Pediatric Series

Patients (n)	Probability of Myeloid Engraftment (%)	aGVHD Grades II–IV (%)	cGVHD (%)	cGVHD Comments	Reference
MRD PBSC (58)	98	16	64	43% extensive cGVHD	Watanabe 2000 [32]
MRD PBSC (25)	100	62	29	cGVHD 17% at day 100, 21% at 1 year	Benito 2001 [33]
MRD PBSC (143)	97	27	33	Grade and organ involvement same in BM versus PBSC	Eapen 2004 [12]
MRD BM (630)	96	28	19		
MRD PBSC (90)	94	25	64	Extensive skin cGVHD associated with decreased DFS	Diaz 2005 [30]
MUD PBSC (38)	97	62	65	50% extensive in PBSC	Meisel 2007 [31]
MUD BM (23)	96	55	59	26% extensive in BM	

aGVHD, acute graft versus host disease; BM, bone marrow; cGVHD, chronic graft versus host disease; DFS, disease-free survival; MRD, matched related donor; MUD, matched unrelated donor; n, number; PBSC, peripheral blood stem cell.

in comparison to BM despite similar rates of relapse. Patients in this study had similar rates of aGVHD, but rates of cGVHD were higher with a RR of 1.85 in the PBSC group [12]. A recent Spanish study of 90 children who underwent PBSC transplants reported a high cumulative incidence of cGVHD (64%). However, those with cGVHD had improved DFS with lower relapse rates and similar TRM. In multivariate analysis several variables had a negative impact on DFS: the presence of extensive skin involvement (RR = 16.22), thrombocytopenia (RR = 43.65), and a Lansky Performance Status score <80 (RR = 9.25). Despite higher DFS in those with cGVHD (65% vs. 49%), there were several deaths attributed to cGVHD and infectious complications [30]. More recently, Meisel et al. retrospectively analyzed the outcome of 23 BM and 38 PBSC transplants. They reported more rapid engraftment in the PBSC recipients, but no significant differences in TRM, aGVHD, cGVHD, OS, or relapse-free survival (RFS) [31]. This is one of the few studies not to observe an increase in cGVHD with PBSC versus BM. This might be related to the fact that these were unrelated donors with high median age (38–41 years), and the cGVHD incidence was high in both groups (PBSC 65% vs. BM 59%). However, there was a trend toward more extensive cGVHD in the PBSC group (50% vs. 26%) [31]. Thus, despite the lack of randomized studies in children, it appears that the risk of cGVHD with PBSC is higher than BM [32, 33].

Umbilical Cord Blood

There is significant interest in cord blood as a source of stem cells in light of the relative toxicities, costs, donor risks, and delays associated with obtaining marrow or PBSC from unrelated donors. Because of the relatively limited stem cell doses in umbilical cord blood units, this source has been most frequently utilized in pediatric patients. Results are promising with high engraftment rates (>80%) and low incidence of acute and chronic GVHD, which allows for a greater degree of HLA-mismatch (Table 33.3) [13, 17, 34–40].

In 1998, Rubinstein et al. reported the outcomes for 562 umbilical cord blood (UCB) recipients (460 patients < 18 years of age). Severe aGVHD (grade III or IV) occurred in 23% and cGVHD in 25% of those who survived for 6 months or more. cGVHD was generally limited and contributed to death in only three patients. cGVHD occurred in 80% of those with severe aGVHD, as compared to 18% of those without ($p < 0.001$). The incidence of cGVHD did not correlate with the extent of HLA disparity or other variables. The rate of relapse among recipients with leukemia was 9% within the first 100 days, 17% within 6 months, and 26% by 1 year. Relapse risk was associated with the severity of GVHD, type of leukemia (acute myeloid leukemia [AML] = highest risk), and advanced stage of disease [41].

A recent IBMTR publication reported a 6% 3-year cumulative incidence of cGVHD in 113 children who received matched sibling umbilical cell blood transplantation (UCBT). Patients whose indication for HSCT was a nonmalignant diagnosis had even lower rates of cGVHD [17]. The Eurocord registry reviewed 99 UCBT transplants and observed a 12% 2-year incidence of cGVHD. Half of these patients had one or more HLA antigen mismatch(es). The indication for transplant was leukemia for all of the patients, although preparative regimens and GVHD prophylaxis were variable. HLA-matched unrelated BM recipients (n = 262) had a 46% cumulative incidence of cGVHD and recipients of T-cell depleted HLA-matched unrelated BM (n = 180) had an 11% incidence of cGVHD [42].

In 2007, Eapen et al. reported the outcome of 501 unrelated UCBT in patients <16 years of age. They found a 9% risk of aGVHD and an 18% risk of cGVHD. In addition, they found similar rates of cGVHD for matched and 1- and 2- antigen mismatched UCB donors [40]. These findings were further supported by a recent comprehensive review evaluating the impact of HLA matching on GVHD incidence in UCBT. Although they identified a trend suggesting an impact of matching on risk of severe grade III to IV aGVHD, there was no impact of degree of matching on cGVHD [43]. There is also a suggestion

Table 33.3: Cord Blood Transplantation: Pediatric Series

Patients (n)	Probability of Myeloid Engraftment (%)	aGVHD Grades II–IV (%)	cGVHD	cGVHD Comments	Reference
Sibling (44)	85	3	6	All limited	Wagner 1995 [34]
UD (562)	91	45	25	cGVHD generally limited	Rubinstein 1998 [41]
Sibling (113)	85	14	6	15% cGVHD with BMT	Rocha 2000 [17]
UD (99)	80	35	12	46% UD BMT 11% T-deplete UD BMT	Rocha 2001 [42]
UD (30)	89	37.2	0	cGVHD evaluation only followed for 1 year	Thomson 2000 [35]
UD (44)	82	44	28	Rates of GVHD did not differ with degree of MM	Yu 2001 [36]
UD (102)	88	39	9	Relapse rates unaffected by acute or cGVHD	Wagner 2002 [38]
UD (501)	76–85	39	18	cGVHD rates similar for matched and 1- and 2- antigen MM UCB	Eapen 2007 [40]

aGVHD, acute graft versus host disease; BMT, bone marrow transplant; cGVHD, chronic graft versus host disease; MM, mismatch; N, number; UCB, umbilical cord blood; UD, unrelated donor.

that cGVHD in unrelated UCBT is more responsive to therapy than recipients of unrelated BMT [44].

PREPARATIVE REGIMEN

Reduced Intensity Conditioning Regimens in Pediatrics

Another trend in transplantation is the use of nonmyeloablative or reduced intensity transplant (RIT) preparative regimen with the goal of decreasing both short- and long-term toxicities. Trials suggest no increase in the incidence of GVHD in comparison to standard myeloablative regimens, although other toxicities are markedly reduced. The approach has been studied in the setting of acquired severe aplastic anemia [45] and combined immunodeficiency syndromes [46]. Pilot studies in pediatric cancer patients establishing the feasibility of this approach have recently been initiated [47]. Although acute transplant-related toxicity has been low and early engraftment rates high, several studies have shown a high incidence of subsequent graft failure, particularly in patients with nonmalignant disease [48–51].

One study utilizing a preparative regimen consisting of busulfan, fludarabine, and ATG was closed secondary to a high rate of graft failure (21%) in patients with nonmalignant disorders. Despite these findings, the authors found the regimen to be well tolerated with 89% OS and 2-year 74% EFS [51]. Slavin et al. reported nine patients ≤20 years of age who received fludarabine, busulfan, and ATG followed by matched sibling allografts for leukemia and nonmalignant disorders. cGVHD developed in 4/9 patients [52]. At Children's Memorial Hospital in Chicago there is a growing experience with the same regimen. Of 13 patients transplanted for nonmalignant disorders,

8 survived past day 100 with complete donor chimerism and were evaluable for cGVHD. Of these, three had extensive cGVHD [50]. In order to minimize cGVHD in young patients with chronic granulomatous disease, Horwitz et al. followed a preparative regimen of fludarabine, cyclophosphamide, and ATG with T-cell-depleted grafts followed shortly by donor lymphocyte infusion (DLI). Of the six patients under the age of 21 years, two had graft failure and one died. Of the remaining three patients only one patient developed limited cGVHD [53]. Additional clinical trials are needed to determine whether long-term toxicities and rates of cGVHD are diminished with reduced intensity conditioning in children.

PATHOBIOLOGY

Despite growing research into the pathobiology of cGVHD, there are limited data specific to pediatrics. Although the scientific basis for this is not completely understood, studies consistently show that lower donor or recipient age reduces the incidence of cGVHD. These differences have been hypothesized to be due in part to a lower exposure of young donors and recipients to infections. Prior donor or recipient cytomegalovirus (CMV) infection has been associated with higher rates of cGVHD [54, 55]. Murine models suggest that age may influence antigen-presenting cell (APC) function, and APCs from older recipients are more effective at inducing aGVHD [56]. In addition, CD4+ T-lymphocyte regeneration following intensive chemotherapy exposure is directly related to thymic function and therefore to recipient age. Mackall et al. observed an inverse relationship between patient age and CD4+ lymphocyte counts after high-dose chemotherapy in children, adolescents, and young adults with cancer. In addition, CD4 count recovery was directly correlated to the appearance of CD45RA + CD4$^+$ T lymphocytes, and there was a higher proportion of this population of cells in patients exhibiting thymic enlargement [57].

As previously discussed, one of the clearest demonstrations of the impact of donor age is the lower rate of cGVHD seen with UCB transplants. Overall, UCB has an immature T-cell phenotype with increased numbers of naïve T cells that are shifted toward a Th2 phenotype [58]. As part of this Th2 shift, neonatal CD8$^+$ T cells require exogenous IL-4 to develop into Tc2 cells and upon activation with anti-CD3/B7, cord blood CD8$^+$ T cells coexpress CD4, CCR5, and CXCR4. When compared to adult peripheral blood, UCB shows decreased expression of certain cell surface markers, cytokine secretion, and T-cell activation. The decreased ability of UCB T cells to activate is associated with a physical linkage of CD26, a T-cell activation antigen, with CD45RA outside lipid rafts. This in turn may lead to impaired immune responses and decreased incidence of cGVHD in UCBT [59].

It is likely that the Th2 bias of UCB cells is due to antigen presentation at priming and not due to intrinsic T cell defects. UCB dendritic cells are characteristically immature and inefficient in antigen presentation [60, 61]. Although monocytes derived from adult peripheral blood and from UCB have equally immature phenotypes, UCB dendritic cells appear to have attenuated activation in response to inflammatory stimulation and are therefore intrinsically biased against a Th1 response [54].

Although UCB B cells have low expression of HLA class II and high levels of empty HLA-DR molecules, they are able to elicit a mixed lymphoid reaction similar to adult B cells [62]. However, when compared to adult B cells, UCB B cells are less sensitive to the costimulatory effects of IL-2 and have lower surface expression of CD62L and CCR7, suggesting they may have possible homing defects [55]. Overall, the decreased incidence of cGVHD seen with UCB transplantation is likely due to diminished T-cell activation and decreased antigen presentation by dendritic cells and B cells, ultimately resulting in increased T-cell tolerance.

The Children's Oncology Group (COG) recently published an analysis of peripheral blood biomarkers in 52 newly diagnosed children with extensive cGVHD. The patients had been enrolled on a COG phase III cGVHD therapeutic trial and peripheral blood samples were evaluated for 13 known or suspected biomarkers. Patient samples were compared with 28 time-matched controls with no cGVHD. Soluble B cell-activating factor (BAFF), anti-dsDNA antibody, soluble IL-2 receptor alpha, and soluble CD13 were elevated in early-onset cGVHD in comparison to controls. Furthermore, sBAFF and anti-dsDNA were elevated in late-onset cGVHD. In combination, the four biomarkers had both high specificity (84%) and sensitivity (100%) for the diagnosis of cGVHD. Levels of sBAFF and sCD13 were higher in patients with hepatic cGVHD, whereas anti-dsDNA levels were higher in patients with joint, sclerodermatous, and ocular involvement. Elevated sBAFF was significantly associated with lichenoid skin rash and joint involvement, elevated IL-6 and monocyte chemoattractant protein-1 (MCP-1) with joint manifestations, and

elevated anticardiolipin antibody with ocular involvement. No association was found with gastrointestinal (GI), pulmonary, or musculoskeletal cGVHD [63]. Biomarkers have the potential to help predict the risk of developing cGVHD, improving classification, and directing cGVHD research and treatment. Further investigation and large study validation are required.

MANIFESTATIONS

Manifestations of cGVHD are discussed at length throughout this book. In this chapter we highlight those features that have been studied specifically in children, or where there are relevant pediatric caveats.

The Impact of Staging and Grading on Survival

Thrombocytopenia, progressive onset, extensive skin involvement, GI involvement, and low Karnofsky performance status at diagnosis of cGVHD are associated with decreased survival [64–66]. A Johns Hopkins study evaluated both adults and children; however, there were not sufficient numbers of pediatric patients to examine these groups separately [66]. Nonetheless, there appeared to be no effect of age on the entire model suggesting the same parameters would apply to pediatrics.

CLINICAL MANIFESTATIONS

Cutaneous

Cutaneous manifestations of cGVHD in children are similar to those found in adults. Specific pediatric recommendations are listed in Text Boxes 33.1 and 33.2.

Musculoskeletal

In general, musculoskeletal involvement of cGVHD in children is the same as in adults and can result in myositis, fasciitis, muscle weakness, cramping, and pain. The Children's Hospital of Philadelphia reviewed their experience with 14 patients with orthopedic complications of cGVHD. All patients had positive skin biopsies and several patients had positive biopsies showing chronic inflammation or lymphocytic infiltrates in muscle (n = 5), joint capsules (n = 3), fascia (n = 4), nerve (n = 1), and fat (n = 1). All patients were treated with CSA and prednisone, as well as physical and occupational therapy. Most patients did well and by self-report had high-level functioning. Three patients underwent surgical procedures, which involved joint capsular releases for contractures. In all cases, contractures recurred within 6 months [67]. Thus, medical management with physical and occupational therapy is recommended. Other commonly encountered orthopedic complications include osteoporosis and avascular necrosis [68, 69]. These are overwhelmingly the result of corticosteroid therapy for cGVHD. Careful follow-up with bone density studies and use of vitamin D and calcium supplementation in conjunction with biphosphonates in select patients is recommended. (Text Box 33.3)

Text Box 33.1 Cutaneous*

- When estimating body surface area involved, the classic "rule of nines" does not apply to children.

Adults		Children	
Anatomic Structure	Surface Area (%)	Anatomic Structure	Surface Area (%)
Head and neck	9	Head and neck	18
Anterior torso	18	Anterior torso	18
Posterior torso	18	Posterior torso	18
Each leg	18	Each leg	13.5
Each arm	9	Each arm	9
Genitalia/perineum	1	Genitalia/perineum	1

- Children are at increased risk of systemic effects from topical steroids because of a greater skin surface area to body weight ratio.
- Middle to upper strength topical steroids use should be limited.
- The use of topical steroids under occlusive dressings should be avoided.
- The use of potent steroids on the face of young children, or on any site in infants less than 1 year of age, should be avoided.

Text Box 33.2 Vulvovaginal*

- Vulvovaginal GVHD should be considered in post-pubertal females. Although rare, vulvovaginal GVHD has been observed in prepubertal females.
- Examination by a pediatric gynecologic practitioner is recommended when evaluating vulvovaginal GVHD.

Text Box 33.3 Musculoskeletal*

- Children with sclerotic skin changes, range of motion (ROM) measurements should be obtained. Although there are no established norms for ROM below the age of 4 years, individual response or progression may be captured.
- The definition of reduced bone mineral density in children uses age and sex- normalized standard-deviation scores (Z-scores) rather than T-scores. A Z-score of <−2.0 is below the standard deviation of normal for age and should be considered concerning. In the appropriate clinical context of a chronically ill child, in particular on corticosteroids, concern for osteopenia with an approximate Z-score of <−1.5 and osteoporosis is a Z-score <−2.5 is warranted. The incorrect application of T-scores to children may lead to misdiagnosis and inappropriate treatment.
- The use of bisphosphonates in children is limited, and most experience is with pamidronate, where definitive dosing has not been established.

Eyes

There appear to be no unique pediatric manifestations of ocular cGVHD. It is important to follow patients closely with serial Schirmer's tests to assess degree of wetting and to intervene early at the onset of ocular involvement even prior to the evolution of symptoms. Schirmer's test without anesthesia is not recommended for children under 9 years old. The procedure may be difficult to perform in younger children and consultation with an ophthalmologist with specific expertise in cGVHD may be needed for objective scoring in these children (Text Box 33.4) [70].

Text Box 33.4 Ocular*

- Regular surveillance for keratoconjunctivitis sicca is necessary through regular examination and Schirmer's testing (every 3 months). Patients should see an ophthalmologist at least once annually.
- Schirmer's testing can typically be done both with and without anesthesia in children above the age of 9 years. However, many young children can only perform the study with topical anesthetic, or will have difficulty complying at all.
- In patients <40 years of age, 15 mm of wetting in a nonanesthetized eye and 10 mm of wetting in an anesthetized eye are normal.
- When found early, ocular sicca generally responds to local measures in conjunction with systemic immunosuppression.

Mouth

In general, children with isolated oral cGVHD can be treated with corticosteroid rinses. Responses to topical therapy are varied and many patients require systemic treatment. No treatment has been shown to have significant benefit over another and some may lead to increased rates of oral squamous cell carcinoma [71]. Secondary infections with viruses (especially herpes simplex) and yeasts are frequent; therefore, using a local antifungal preparation in combination with topical steroids is recommended. The largest single-center series of oral cGVHD in pediatric patients included 49 patients seen at a multidisciplinary pediatric HSCT clinic at the Dana-Farber Cancer Institute. Subjective and objective assessments of mucosal, salivary gland, and sclerotic pathology were performed. Oral mucosal involvement was identified in nearly half (45%) of patients; however, only 8% of patients reported mouth pain and all patients reported being able to eat well. The most common manifestation was erythema (42%), followed by reticular (36%) and ulcerative (21%) lesions. Ten percent reported dry mouth, although no patients reported difficulty swallowing. Forty-five percent of patients required specific therapy for oral mucosal cGVHD despite being treated with at least one systemic immunomodulatory agent.

Salivary gland and sclerotic disease were rarely observed (Text Box 33.5) [72].

Text Box 33.5 Oral*

▪ Oral manifestations in children generally respond well to dexamethasone rinses.

▪ Avoid the use of high potency steroids in very young child because of the potential for greater systemic effects.

▪ Parents' assistance may be necessary to aid children with topical oral therapies in order improve pediatric compliance.

Gastrointestinal tract

Children with cGVHD may have varied GI complaints consisting of nausea, anorexia, abdominal pain, cramping, or diarrhea. While these symptoms may be related to cGVHD, more often they are attributable to other causes including acute GVHD, infection, dysmotility, lactose intolerance, pancreatic insufficiency, or drug-related side effects [64]. As many of these problems are easily remedied, full evaluation of symptoms, including upper and lower endoscopy, is important [73].

Weight loss and reduced body mass index remain critical issues in children with multiorgan cGVHD. Maintaining adequate nutrition is essential and careful evaluation of growth (and head circumference in infants) is required. In adult patients with cGVHD, low body mass index (BMI) is a predictor for mortality. The group at Children's Memorial Hospital performed a retrospective study on 18 children with extensive cGVHD. They found that patients with multiorgan involvement had a mean maximal decrease in BMI of 20.9% and most dropped below 10th percentile in expected weight-for-age. This change in BMI indicated both a significant decrease in weight and often a plateau in stature. In contrast, patients with one organ system involved had a mean maximal decrease in BMI of 5% and did not fall below 10th percentile for weight. The authors concluded that weight loss and malnutrition are clinically significant issues in children with multisystem cGVHD and that weight loss is likely another systemic manifestation of cGVHD that may contribute to increased mortality in this group [74].

Liver

Hepatic cGVHD is typically manifested by bile duct destruction and bridging fibrosis resulting in obstructive jaundice [75]. Patients will show elevated alkaline phosphatase, gamma-glutamyl transferase (GGT), and direct serum bilirubin. While cholestasic hepatic cGVHD is the classic manifestation of liver involvement, hepatitic cGVHD is being identified more often, with some patients presenting with isolated elevations of serum alanine aminotransferase (ALT) and aspartate aminotransferase (AST) [76, 77]. First

described in adult patients, recently this hepatitic pattern has been reported in a case series of six pediatric patients. The underlying diagnosis, pretransplant conditioning, and GVHD prophylaxis varied for these patients and PBSCs were used in four. Hepatic GVHD was detected between days 149 and 310 posttransplant. Two patients had prior aGVHD involving the skin and/or GI tract and only two patients had cGVHD preceding the diagnosis of hepatic GVHD. On histologic review, no patients had significant duct loss and only one had significant lymphocytic infiltration of the bile ducts. Bile duct epithelial damage and significant portal/periportal inflammation were present in all and lobular necro-inflammation was seen in five patients. Five patients improved with immunosuppression and one died with progressive GVHD. The authors concluded that the clinical and histologic patterns of hepatitic cGVHD are similar to that described in adults [78].

Evaluation of a child with suspected liver cGVHD must include viral studies for hepatitis A, B, C, and *Epstein-Barr virus* (EBV), *Cytomegalovirus* (CMV), *Varicella zoster virus* (VZV), and adenovirus to exclude infection as a cofactor or cause for hepatic dysfunction. Also, drug toxicity (e.g., fluconazole, calcineurin inhibitors) can cause elevations of bilirubin and hepatic transaminases. Liver biopsy is required to confirm the diagnosis, particularly important for those patients with no other signs or symptoms of cGVHD.

Respiratory Tract

A serious life-threatening manifestation of cGVHD is lung involvement in the form of bronchiolitis obliterans (BO), which develops in 5% to 20% of patients after allo-HSCT [79]. In a retrospective study from Minnesota of 2,859 SCT recipients, the overall 3-year incidence of BO was 3% and their 5-year survival was 10%. While not a strictly pediatric study, there was a large number of pediatric patients included (median age, 24.7 years; range, 0.1–67.4 years) [80].

Patients with early BO may be asymptomatic but typically present with cough, wheezing, or dyspnea on exertion [81, 82]. Pulmonary function studies (PFTs) may show decreased forced expiratory volume in 1 second /full volume capacity (FEV_1/FVC) ratio (0.7) and FEV_1 < 75% predicted and rapid declines are commonly seen thereafter. PFTs in children must be interpreted with caution. The predicted norms are based on healthy age-matched controls and vary with normal growth. Care must be taken to follow not only percent predicted values but also absolute values over time, as pediatric patients post-HSCT may not continue on the normal growth curves for height and weight. Also patients having received TBI or chest wall irradiation may not have proportional chest wall growth. Other clinical diagnoses can be associated with these findings, therefore an extensive work-up is recommended. Evaluation should include high-resolution computer-assisted tomography (CT) scan of the chest (inspiratory and expiratory phase) to evaluate for characteristic air trapping and bronchiolar cuffing. In younger children, CT scanning in the inspiratory and expiratory phase may not be possible, and for the very young (<5 years of age) sedation may be required. Bronchoalveolar lavage to evaluate for possible concurrent infection and aggressive therapy of such is essential. Biopsy may be needed for definitive diagnosis. However, this is commonly avoided due to the risks of the procedure, in which case the term Bronchiolitis Obliterans Syndrome (BOS) is applied. Pneumothorax, pneumomediastinum, and subcutaneous emphysema are rare and often represent advanced disease (Text Box 33.6).

Text Box 33.6 Pulmonary*

■ Formal pulmonary function testing (PFT) including spirometry, lung volumes, and diffusing capacity can be difficult to measure in children <7 years of age. However, some highly compliant children perform PFTs with proper coaching. In those unable to comply, negative plethysmography can be used.

■ PFT values must be carefully evaluated in pediatric patients, and actual measured values be followed because predicted normal values vary with age, weight, and height. Therefore, percent predicted values might spuriously show serial decrease over time without substantive decline in absolute values, particularly in patients posttransplant who may not have normal growth for age because of chronic illness, steroid use, or TBI.

Hematopoietic System

Thrombocytopenia is the most common hematopoietic manifestation of cGVHD, though any cytopenia may been seen. Cytopenias may result from stromal damage, but antibody mediated autoimmune neutropenia [83], anemia [84], and thrombocytopenia [85] have also been reported. It is important to eliminate drug toxicity, infection, graft failure, or disease relapse as the underlying cause. A number of studies (mostly in adults) have shown that thrombocytopenia at the time of cGVHD diagnosis confers a poor prognosis [86, 64], although thrombocytopenia may be a poor prognostic factor independent of GVHD [87]. Eosinophilia is also frequently seen in children and can precede the development of overt cGVHD [88].

Immune System

The immune system of children with cGVHD may be severely compromised from effects of the underlying disease as well as its therapy, and infection is the leading cause of death in patients with active cGVHD. Patients with cGVHD have reduced numbers and function of lymphocytes putting them at high risk for fungal, viral, and bacterial infections. In addition, patients with barrier breakdown due to mucosal involvement (skin, oral, or GI) are at increased risk for infections [89–91]. Patients may be functionally asplenic, evidenced by persistence of Howell-Jolly bodies and a higher incidence of pneumococcal sepsis [92, 93]. Functional asplenia can persist despite resolution of other manifestations of cGVHD; therefore,

lifelong prophylaxis against encapsulated organisms is recommended. Patients should also receive prophylaxis against Pneumocystis until complete resolution of cGVHD and for at least 6 months after discontinuation of immunosuppressive therapy. Centers for Disease Control and Prevention (CDC) recommendations for infection prophylaxis are available online (http://www.cdc.gov/mmwr/preview/mmwrhtml/rr4910a1.htm). Supplemental intravenous immunoglobulin (IVIG) replacement should be provided for individuals with the combination of severe hypogammaglobunemia, (IgG <400 mg/dl) and recurrent infections. Patients at risk for CMV should be monitored closely with CMV polymerase chain reaction (PCR) or antigenemia. Patients receiving steroid rinses for oral GVHD are at high risk for local Candidal infections and topical antifungal prophylaxis (e.g., nystatin swishes or clotrimazole troches) should be used. Consideration should also be given to antifungal and antiviral prophylaxis, although this is dependent on individual patient risk factors and the intensity of the therapy they are receiving.

Children with cGVHD should be closely monitored, aggressively evaluated, and rapidly treated for possible infection. Treatment should include organism-specific antimicrobial agents and empiric broad-spectrum antibacterial coverage for fever or other signs of serious infection [94]. Vaccinations should be delayed until there is no active cGVHD and immunosuppressive therapy has been discontinued. All patients should receive posttransplant immunizations according to CDC recommendations (http://www.cdc.gov/mmwr/preview/mmwrhtml/rr4910a1.htm) (Text Box 33.7) [95].

Text Box 33.7 Immunity*

■ Recovery of immune function after HSCT is variable and depends on the interaction of several factors including stem cell source, GVHD, and immunosuppression.

■ (Re)vaccination schedules are variable and relying on a generalized schedule for immunization is not practical. Children undergoing HSCT have often missed routine childhood immunizations, therefore a review of patient-specific immunization history is indicated. For general reference see Chapter 25 and for up-to-date guidelines, visit the Centers for Disease Control and Prevention (CDC) website, http://www.cdc.gov/mmwr/preview/mmwrhtml/rr4910a1.htm.

■ Heptavalent conjugated pneumococcal vaccine is recommended at 12 and 14 months after HCT for patients less than or equal to 5 years of age. Children between 2 and 5 years of age should receive one dose of the 23-valent pneumococcal vaccine 2 months after the last dose of the heptavalent conjugated vaccine.

■ Varicella-Zoster Vaccine should be only given if patients are immunocompetent at 24 months (not on immune suppression and with no GVHD for 6 months). If patients were previously vaccinated, revaccinate. If patients were never vaccinated with positive serology, do not vaccinate. If patients were never vaccinated with negative serology, vaccinate. Pediatric patients aged 12 months to 12 years receive a single dose; patients aged ≥13 years should receive two doses, 4–8 weeks apart.

PREVENTION

Despite the many effective methods to prevent aGVHD, there has been limited success in regard to cGHVD. Techniques such as depletion of donor T cells have been investigated in the prevention of GVHD. Despite lower rates of aGVHD, T-cell depletion increases the risk of graft rejection, mixed chimerism, and relapse [96]. Reported rates of clinically extensive cGVHD also remain high after matched unrelated donor transplants despite T-cell depletion [24, 96–99]. Several preventative agents, such as CSA and MTX, have been given in varied prophylactic regimens and do not appear to significantly impact the development of cGVHD [100].

ATG is widely used before HSCT with HLA-matched unrelated donors or mismatched relatives to prevent both graft rejection and GVHD. The addition of ATG has resulted in low rates of GVHD after pediatric mismatched cord blood transplant similar to matched unrelated BM transplants [101]. Notably, many UCB transplant regimens include ATG suggesting a possible contribution of this agent to diminished GVHD after UCBT. Despite encouraging results, however, ATG may negatively impact immune reconstitution [102].

TREATMENT

The approach to treatment of cGVHD in pediatrics is mostly extrapolated from experience in adults. While there is no proven "standard therapy," prednisone and CSA are commonly employed as frontline therapy. One alternate-day regimen improved survival in high-risk patients with thrombocytopenia and extensive skin involvement [86]. Patients should be evaluated for response to treatment and monitored for side effects of therapy at a minimum of every 3 months (Table 33.4). Therapy should be continued for at least 3 months after maximal response and weaned with careful monitoring for recurrent cGVHD. Investigators at Johns Hopkins observed that 90% of patients who ultimately respond to therapy show signs of response by 3 months [103].

SALVAGE REGIMENS

Sirolimus

Sirolimus (Rapamycin) is a macrocyclic triene antibiotic with immunosuppressive, antifungal, and antitumor properties that inhibits signal transduction and cell cycle progression after binding to FKBP12 [104]. Sirolimus has been shown to have activity in the prevention and treatment of aGVHD [105–108] and is now being studied in the chronic setting. Several recent studies show good overall response rates (63%–93%) in cGVHD [107–109]. No studies to date have been performed on a pediatric population and dosing and pharmacokinetics (PK) remain incompletely defined and are usually based on data from solid organ transplant populations.

Mycophenolate Mofetil

Mycophenolate mofetil (MMF) is an antimetabolite used as an alternative immunosuppressant that inhibits the proliferation of T and B lymphocytes and is currently in use for aGVHD prophylaxis. At Johns Hopkins, a retrospective review of 26 patients with refractory cGVHD treated with MMF combined with tacrolimus showed this steroid-sparing combination was well tolerated, and nearly half the patients showed an objective response [110]. A retrospective study from City of Hope National Medical Center evaluated any patient (age ranges 2.5–55 years) receiving MMF as part of their treatment regimen over a 2-year period ($n = 34$). MMF was added to standard CSA, tacrolimus, and/or prednisone as either salvage ($n = 24$) or first-line ($n = 10$) therapy. Nine (90%) of 10 patients receiving MMF as first-line and 18 (75%) of 24 receiving it as second-line therapy responded. Of the patients, 12 (35%) had complete response (CR), 15 (44%) had a partial response (PR), 5 (15%) had stable disease (SD), and only 2 (6%) had progressive GVHD (PD). Out of the 30 patients initially receiving steroids, 73% were able to decrease steroid dosing with a median decrease of 50%. Few patients had to discontinue MMF because of side effects to treatment [111].

MMF has been evaluated in several pediatric trials. Italian investigators studied the safety and efficacy of MMF as salvage therapy for cGVHD in 15 children following HSCT. Patients were 3 to 16 years of age and had received grafts from HLA-compatible siblings ($n = 8$), partially matched related donors ($n = 2$), or matched unrelated donors ($n = 5$). Each had developed extensive cGVHD that was previously unresponsive to standard immunosuppressive therapy. Patients were treated with MMF at doses of 15 to 40 mg/kg/day in combination with other concurrent immunosuppressive therapy. The overall response rate was 60%, with 13% having a CR, 33% having a combined CR and PR in varied organs, 13% with a PR, and 27% with PD. When analyzed by organ system, the best responses were with GI tract (60% of CRs), mouth (33% of CRs), or skin involvement (43% of CRs) excluding sclerotic manifestations. For those who responded to MMF, 45% tolerated a significant reduction of steroids and 27% were able to discontinue steroids completely [112]. Investigators in Seattle reported a very promising CR rate of 65% in 26 pediatric patients who had previously progressed on prednisone and CSA. MMF was added to their regimen. For complete resolution, MMF therapy needed to be continued for up to 3 years in several cases. The drug was remarkably well tolerated with only transient leucopenia reported in one patient [113]. Thus, MMF may have efficacy in cGVHD although it may take several months for effects to be seen.

Pentostatin

Pentostatin is a nucleoside analog that irreversibly inhibits adenosine deaminase causing profound immunosuppression [114, 115]. An early case review of five patients treated with pentostatin

Table 33.4: Guidelines for Evaluations at Least 5 Years Following Transplantation

Examination	Baseline Evaluation	Every 1–3 Months	Every 6 Months	Annual
History and Physical				
Complete history & physical	X	X		
Height	X	X		
Weight	X	X		
Skin exam	X	X		
Nutritional assessment	X	X		
Tanner evaluation	X		X	
Developmental evaluation	X		X	
Functional and quality-of-life assessment	X			X
Laboratory Evaluation				
Complete blood counts	X	X		
Complete chemistries	X	X		
Immunoglobulin levels	X	X		
Lipid profile	X		X	
Iron indices	X		X	
Endocrinologic function	X		X	
Nutritional assessment	X		X	
Evaluations				
Schirmer's evaluation	X		X[††]	
Pulmonary function tests	X		X[††]	
Bone densitometry	X			X
ECHO or MUGA	X			X
ECG	X			X
Consultations				
Physiatry or PT evaluation for ROM	X	X[*]		
Ophthalmology	X			X[†]
Dental evaluation	X		X	
Gynecologist (as indicated)	X			

ECG, electrocardiogram; ECHO, echocardiogram; MUGA scan, multi gated acquisition scan; PT, physical therapy; ROM, range of motion.

[*] Patients with fasciitis or sclerotic manifestations; [†]more frequent evaluations for patients with organ involvement.

[††] Patients may require more or less frequent evaluations depending on individual disease manifestations.

for cGVHD at Johns Hopkins reported significant response in all patients [116]. These observations lead to an open-label phase II study of pentostatin for patients with steroid refractory cGVHD dosed at 4 mg/m² intravenously every 2 weeks for 12 doses. Therapy was continued as long as benefit was documented, and corticosteroid taper was initiated after three doses of pentostatin. Fifty-eight heavily pretreated adult and pediatric patients (5–64 years) were enrolled: 32 (55%) had an objective response; however, when stratified for age, younger patients (< 33 years) had a better response rate (77%) in comparison to older individuals (37.5%). Infection was the most significant toxicity, with 11 (20%) grade III to IV infectious events. Overall survival at 1 and 2 years was 78% and 70% respectively, with cGVHD with or without infection accounting for the majority of deaths [117].

Hydroxychloroquine

Hydroxychloroquine (HCQ) is a lysosomotropic 4-aminoquinoline antimalarial drug that has been used to effectively treat autoimmune disorders [118, 119]. A phase II trial in children and adults studied the addition of HCQ to patients with steroid-resistant or -dependent cGVHD. Forty patients were treated with HCQ 800 mg (12 mg/kg) per day. Of 32 evaluable patients (20 children, 12 adults), 17 had objective responses (3 CR, 14 PR). Of note, all patients with documented response tolerated at least a 50% wean in their steroid dosing. No hematologic, hepatic, renal, or retinal toxicity was observed. Adults and children had similar response rates [120].

Thalidomide

Thalidomide is an agent that initially showed promise with response rates of 20% to 30% in high-risk patients [121]. Unfortunately, side effects (particularly sedation, constipation, neutropenia, and neurologic toxicity) are often intolerable and the drug has fallen out of favor. In addition, thalidomide has been reported to cause a significant flare of skin manifestations in some patients [122]. Two reports of thalidomide use in pediatrics suggest that this drug has activity in steroid refractory cGVHD and may be better tolerated by children [123, 124].

Anticytokine Therapy and Monoclonal Antibodies

Various monoclonal antibodies and anticytokine therapies are being explored in the treatment of cGVHD, in hopes of bringing such targeted therapies with more favorable side effect profiles to this patient population.

Patients with cGVHD commonly exhibit B-cell dysfunction manifested by autoantibodies. Thus, rituximab an anti-CD20 monoclonal antibody, has been investigated as a treatment for cGVHD. Cutler et al. evaluated 21 patients who were treated with 38 cycles of rituximab in a phase I/II study. Rituximab was well tolerated and toxicity was limited to infectious events. A clinical response rate of 70% was reported, although limited to patients with cutaneous and musculoskeletal manifestations [125]. Other monoclonal antibodies, such as infliximab and etanercept (anti TNF-α) and daclizumab (anti IL2R-α), are also being explored in cGVHD, often based on initial experience with aGVHD [126]. Etanercept is a recombinant human soluble tumor necrosis factor alpha (TNF-α) receptor fusion protein that inhibits TNF-α, a major mediator in the pathogenesis of GVHD. Investigators in Italy evaluated the safety and efficacy of etanercept in 21 patients with steroid refractory aGVHD ($n = 13$) and cGVHD ($n = 8$). Overall, 52% responded to treatment with etanercept, including five patients (62%) with cGVHD, with one CR and four PRs. Clinical responses were seen most commonly in patients with refractory gut aGVHD. CMV reactivation was commonly encountered [127]. A small pediatric case series of three patients with idiopathic pulmonary syndrome after HSCT treated with etanercept in combination with other immunosuppressive agents revealed promising results [128].

Extracorporeal Photopheresis

Extracorporeal Photopheresis (ECP) involves the infusion of autologous peripheral blood mononuclear cells collected by apheresis, incubated with the photoactivatable drug 8-methoxypsoralen (8-MOP) and UVA irradiation. Phase I and II data suggest that ECP is an effective treatment for both acute and chronic GVHD. In a review of early studies, Greinix et al. published the results of 11 reports involving a total of 151 patients. Response rates ranged from 40% to 81% [129]. Importantly, it was noted that adverse reactions to ECP were uncommon. Newer studies show similar response rates of up to 61% to 71% particularly of skin, liver, eye, and oral manifestations including those patients with steroid refractory disease [130–133]. Studies using ECP for GVHD are primarily in adults, but there have been several trials that have either included or exclusively enrolled children. Children appear to show similar overall response rates (60%–75%) but may have more CRs than adults [134].

The treatment of children in these trials is sporadic and most trials restrict enrollment to individuals weighing more than 30 to 40 kg. One European study evaluated the use of ECP in 44 pediatric patients with acute and chronic GVHD. This study enrolled children with weights as low as 10 kg and therapy was delivered with minimal side effects. Hypotension was seen in approximately 50% of patients, but this was mild and did not require discontinuation of treatment. An overall response rate of 59% was reported, and 44% of patients were able to discontinue all other immunosuppression and another 29% to reduce immunosuppression [134]. One out of 77 developed GI bleeding, which has been previously reported [132–135]. Salvaneschi et al. treated 35 children with steroid refractory acute and chronic GVHD. Eighteen of these had extensive cGVHD with a 78% response rate and 67% were able to taper steroids. ECP was safe and well tolerated [136]. Despite the encouraging results of this treatment modality, ECP in children has limitations associated with small patient size, including the inability to tolerate significant fluid shifts and difficulty with venous access, which may be prohibitive with current technologies.

TOXICITY AND LATE EFFECTS

Cancer remains the leading indication for SCT in pediatrics and SCT contributes to 5-year cancer survival rates that now exceed 80%. With improvements in posttransplant DFS rates, acute and long-term toxicities have assumed an ever-increasing impact on organ function, quality of life, and overall survival [6]. As these children reach adulthood with chronic, life-altering posttransplant complications, the implications for both the individual survivors and society is substantial. While progress toward developing less toxic therapies continues, such as non-myeloablative SCT [14], treating and preventing secondary effects remain a critical adjunct to the care of children requiring transplantation. Special considerations include the effects of conditioning regimens on the growing child, for example, decrease in linear growth, infertility, endocrinopathies, and neurocognitive dysfunction [27, 137–139]. In addition, the toxicity profiles of cGVHD and its treatment are substantial. This is particularly important during critical periods of normal growth and development. Thus the treatment of cGVHD in pediatrics must include consideration for possible impact on growth, nutrition, organ function and development, psychosocial functioning, and the development of normal immunity. cGVHD and its treatment can inhibit growth. Children may experience catch-up growth if growth plates remain open after cGVHD is controlled and immunosuppression tapered; however, their full predicted height may not be reached. The consequences of long-term corticosteroid use in children are well described, and deleterious effects on growth and bone density may develop even after discontinuation of therapy [140, 141].

Investigators at St. Jude Children's Research Hospital recently published a large prospective cohort study to evaluate the incidence and risk factors for late sequelae in pediatric HSCT survivors. All patients underwent comprehensive surveillance tests and were followed for at least 3 years after HSCT. With a median follow-up of 9 years, 135 of the 155 participants (87%) were found to have late sequelae. The majority had multiple chronic health conditions (12%: 1, 46%: 2–4, and 30%: 5–9). Risk factors for increasing number of late effects included young age at the time of HSCT, female sex, high radiation dose, and history of cGVHD. The cumulative incidence at 10 years for common late events was as follows: osteonecrosis 13.8%, chronic renal insufficiency 26.8%, hypothyroidism 45.1%, growth hormone deficiency 31.2%, female hypogonadism 57.4%, osteopenia 47.7%, cataracts 43.4%, pulmonary dysfunction 63.2%, and male hypogonadism 20.3% [142]. This study emphasizes the high incidence and varied late effects of patients with cGVHD. Close follow-up evaluation and treatment for these chronic conditions is imperative.

Another recent prospective study focused on risk factors and clinical outcome of pulmonary and cardiac late effects following HSCT. Investigators evaluated the cardiac and lung function of 162 pediatric patients prior to HSCT and then annually for 5 years. The 5-year cumulative incidence of lung and cardiac impairment was 35% and 26%, respectively. cGVHD was the major risk factor for reduced lung function while TBI alone and together with pretransplant anthracyclines were the most significant risk factors for cardiac dysfunction. This study demonstrated that deterioration of pulmonary and cardiac function after HSCT was often asymptomatic, emphasizing the need for lifelong monitoring [143].

SUPPORTIVE CARE

Age-based, multidisciplinary, ancillary supportive care is essential to the optimal management of cGVHD in the pediatric patient [94]. As in adults, local care with the use of topical therapies is strongly encouraged to minimize toxicities of systemic therapy. Unfortunately, pediatric specific studies are lacking and most recommendations reflect extrapolation from adult studies [94]. Skin care should include topical moisturizers, antipruritic agents, and strict photoprotection as well as close surveillance for cutaneous malignancy. Maintenance of good oral and dental hygiene, routine dental cleaning, and endocarditis prophylaxis are recommended. The oropharynx should also be carefully screened for malignancy. Ocular care consists of photoprotection, regular evaluation for infection, cataract formation, and increased intraocular pressure. Regional care may include artificial tears, ocular ointments, punctal occlusion, humidified environment, occlusive eye wear, moisture chamber eyeglasses, or gas-permeable scleral contact

lenses. Response to GI manifestations may include dietary modification, enzyme supplementation for malabsorption, gastroesophageal reflux management, esophageal dilatation, and ursodeoxycholic acid for hyperbilirubenemia. Pulmonary support requires infection surveillance, *Pneumocystis jirovecii* prophylaxis, and treatment of gastroesophageal reflux. Patients with pulmonary cGVHD may benefit from inhaled corticosteroids, bronchodilators, supplementary oxygen, and pulmonary rehabilitation. Consideration of lung transplantation is given to the rare appropriate candidate with severe BO.

Patients should be monitored closely for neurologic and psychologic dysfunction. Individuals may benefit from treatment for depression, pain, or neuropathic syndromes with tricyclic antidepressants, selective serotonin reuptake inhibitors, or anticonvulsants. Regular monitoring for early signs of musculoskeletal manifestations (e.g., decreased range of motion) and early intervention with physical therapy, occupational therapy, and splinting of contractures may help preserve range of motion in involved joints. Bone densitometry and calcium and 25-OH vitamin levels should be monitored and treatment should include calcium and vitamin D supplements, and, in selected patients, bisphosphonates [144].

CONCLUSIONS

There are substantial challenges to advancing research and care of children with cGVHD, including specific obstacles to conducting research in pediatric populations. Certain measurements or evaluations may be difficult or impossible to perform on young children (e.g., Schirmer's test). In addition, tools may lack age-specific norms (e.g., PFTs and ROM for children <4 years old). It may be difficult to obtain Institutional Review Board (IRB) approval for potentially toxic therapies, and studies in adults commonly must be completed before pediatric trials are approved. Nontherapeutic research evaluations that do not offer direct benefit to the patient (e.g., invasive biologic studies) may not be ethically appropriate in children. Finally, it may be difficult to accrue adequate numbers of pediatric subjects with the cGVHD manifestations targeted by a given study. It is critical that clinical trials be designed to include pediatric patients with accrual goals of sufficient numbers to produce statistically significant conclusions. In addition, such trials should integrate biologic studies whenever possible in order to maximize discovery and advances in pediatric cGVHD.

*Text Boxes: Considerations for pediatric patients are based on recommendations of the NIH Consensus Development Project on Criteria for Clinical Trials in cGVHD [94].

REFERENCES

1. Notarangelo LD, Forino C, Mazzolari E. Stem cell transplantation in primary immunodeficiencies. *Curr Opin Allergy Clin Immunol.* 2006;6:443–448.

2. Kennedy-Nasser AA, Leung KS, Mahajan A, et al. Comparable outcomes of matched-related and alternative donor stem cell transplantation for pediatric severe aplastic anemia. *Biol Blood Marrow Transplant.* 2006;12:1277–1284.

3. Walters MC. Stem cell therapy for sickle cell disease: transplantation and gene therapy. *Hematology Am Soc Hematol Educ Program.* 2005;66–73.

4. Gaziev J, Lucarelli G. Stem cell transplantation for thalassaemia. *Reprod Biomed Online.* 2005;10:111–115.

5. Peters C, Steward CG. Hematopoietic cell transplantation for inherited metabolic diseases: an overview of outcomes and practice guidelines. *Bone Marrow Transplant.* 2003;31:229–239.

6. Oeffinger KC, Mertens AC, Sklar CA, et al. Chronic health conditions in adult survivors of childhood cancer. *N Engl J Med.* 2006;355:1572–1582.

7. Hewitt M, Rowland JH, Yancik R. Cancer survivors in the United States: age, health, and disability. *J Gerontol A Biol Sci Med Sci.* 2003;58:82–91.

8. Higman MA, Vogelsang GB. Chronic graft versus host disease. *Br J Haematol.* 2004;125:435–454.

9. Storb R, Prentice RL, Sullivan KM, et al. Predictive factors in chronic graft-versus-host disease in patients with aplastic anemia treated by marrow transplantation from HLA-identical siblings. *Ann Intern Med.* 1983;98:461–466.

10. Atkinson K, Horowitz MM, Gale RP, et al. Risk factors for chronic graft-versus-host disease after HLA-identical sibling bone marrow transplantation. *Blood.* 1990;75:2459–2464.

11. Ochs LA, Miller WJ, Filipovich AH, et al. Predictive factors for chronic graft-versus-host disease after histocompatible sibling donor bone marrow transplantation. *Bone Marrow Transplant.* 1994;13:455–460.

12. Eapen M, Horowitz MM, Klein JP, et al. Higher mortality after allogeneic peripheral-blood transplantation compared with bone marrow in children and adolescents: the Histocompatibility and Alternate Stem Cell Source Working Committee of the International Bone Marrow Transplant Registry. *J Clin Oncol.* 2004;22:4872–4880.

13. Zecca M, Prete A, Rondelli R, et al. Chronic graft-versus-host disease in children: incidence, risk factors, and impact on outcome. *Blood.* 2002;100:1192–1200.

14. Busca A, Rendine S, Locatelli F, et al. Chronic graft-versus-host disease after reduced-intensity stem cell transplantation versus conventional hematopoietic stem cell transplantation. *Hematology.* 2005;10:1–10.

15. Lee SJ, Vogelsang G, Flowers ME. Chronic graft-versus-host disease. *Biol Blood Marrow Transplant.* 2003;9:215–233.

16. Akpek G, Chinratanalab W, Lee LA, et al. Gastrointestinal involvement in chronic graft-versus-host disease: a clinicopathologic study. *Biol Blood Marrow Transplant.* 2003;9:46–51.

17. Rocha V, Wagner JE, Jr., Sobocinski KA, et al. Graft-versus-host disease in children who have received a cord-blood or bone marrow transplant from an HLA-identical sibling. Eurocord and International Bone Marrow Transplant Registry Working Committee on Alternative Donor and Stem Cell Sources. *N Engl J Med.* 2000;342:1846–1854.

18. Balduzzi A, Gooley T, Anasetti C, et al. Unrelated donor marrow transplantation in children. *Blood.* 1995;86:3247–3256.

19a. Davies SM, Wagner JE, Defor T, et al. Unrelated donor bone marrow transplantation for children and adolescents with aplastic anaemia or myelodysplasia. *Br J Haematol.* 1997;96:749–756.

19b. Davies SM, Wagner JE, Shu A, et al. Unrelated donor bone marrow transplantation for children with acute leukemia. *J Clin Oncol.* 1997;15(2):557-565.

20. Bunin N, Carston M, Wall D, et al. Unrelated marrow transplantation for children with acute lymphoblastic leukemia in second remission. *Blood.* 2002;99:3151–3157.

21. Talano JM, Casper JT, Camitta BM, et al. Alternative donor bone marrow transplant for children with Philadelphia chromosome ALL. *Bone Marrow Transplant.* 2006;37:135–141.

22. Giebel S, Giorgiani G, Martinetti M, et al. Low incidence of severe acute graft-versus-host disease in children given haematopoietic stem cell transplantation from unrelated donors prospectively matched for HLA class I and II alleles with high-resolution molecular typing. *Bone Marrow Transplant.* 2003;31:987–993.

23. Woolfrey AE, Anasetti C, Storer B, et al. Factors associated with outcome after unrelated marrow transplantation for treatment of acute lymphoblastic leukemia in children. *Blood.* 2002;99:2002–2008.

24. Saarinen-Pihkala UM, Gustafsson G, Ringden O, et al. No disadvantage in outcome of using matched unrelated donors as compared with matched sibling donors for bone marrow transplantation in children with acute lymphoblastic leukemia in second remission. *J Clin Oncol.* 2001;19:3406–3414.

25. Grupp SA, Frangoul H, Wall D, et al. Use of G-CSF in matched sibling donor pediatric allogeneic transplantation: a consensus statement from the Children's Oncology Group (COG) Transplant Discipline Committee and Pediatric Blood and Marrow Transplant Consortium (PBMTC) Executive Committee. *Pediatr Blood Cancer.* 2006;46:414–421.

26. Cutler C, Antin JH. Peripheral blood stem cells for allogeneic transplantation: a review. *Stem Cells.* 2001;19:108–117.

27. Cutler C, Giri S, Jeyapalan S, et al. Acute and chronic graft-versus-host disease after allogeneic peripheral-blood stem-cell and bone marrow transplantation: a meta-analysis. *J Clin Oncol.* 2001;19:3685–3691.

28. Flowers ME, Parker PM, Johnston LJ, et al. Comparison of chronic graft-versus-host disease after transplantation of peripheral blood stem cells versus bone marrow in allogeneic recipients: long-term follow-up of a randomized trial. *Blood.* 2002;100:415–419.

29. Champlin RE, Schmitz N, Horowitz MM, et al. Blood stem cells compared with bone marrow as a source of hematopoietic cells for allogeneic transplantation. IBMTR Histocompatibility and Stem Cell Sources Working Committee and the European Group for Blood and Marrow Transplantation (EBMT). *Blood.* 2000;95:3702–3709.

30. Diaz MA, Gonzalez-Vicent M, Gonzalez ME, et al. Long term outcome of allogeneic PBSC transplantation in pediatric patients with hematological malignancies: a report of the Spanish Working Party for Blood and Marrow Transplantation in Children (GETMON) and the Spanish Group for Allogeneic Peripheral Blood Transplantation (GETH). *Bone Marrow Transplant.* 2005;36:781–785.

31. Meisel R, Laws HJ, Balzer S, et al. Comparable long-term survival after bone marrow versus peripheral blood progenitor cell transplantation from matched unrelated donors in children with hematologic malignancies. *Biol Blood Marrow Transplant.* 2007;13:1338–1345.

32. Watanabe T, Kajiume T, Abe T, et al. Allogeneic peripheral blood stem cell transplantation in children with hematologic malignancies from HLA-matched siblings. *Med Pediatr Oncol.* 2000;34:171–176.

33. Benito AI, Gonzalez-Vicent M, Garcia F, et al. Allogeneic peripheral blood stem cell transplantation (PBSCT) from HLA-identical sibling donors in children with hematological diseases: a single center pilot study. *Bone Marrow Transplant.* 2001;28:537–543.

34. Wagner JE, Kernan NA, Steinbuch M, et al. Allogeneic sibling umbilical-cord-blood transplantation in children with malignant and non-malignant disease. *Lancet.* 1995;346:214–219.

35. Thomson BG, Robertson KA, Gowan D, et al. Analysis of engraftment, graft-versus-host disease, and immune recovery following unrelated donor cord blood transplantation. *Blood.* 2000;96:2703–2711.

36. Yu LC, Wall DA, Sandler E, et al. Unrelated cord blood transplant experience by the pediatric blood and marrow transplant consortium. *Pediatr Hematol Oncol.* 2001; 18:235–245.

37. Gluckman E, Rocha V, Chevret S. Results of unrelated umbilical cord blood hematopoietic stem cell transplantation. *Rev Clin Exp Hematol.* 2001;5:87–99.

38. Wagner JE, Barker JN, DeFor TE, et al. Transplantation of unrelated donor umbilical cord blood in 102 patients with malignant and nonmalignant diseases: influence of CD34 cell dose and HLA disparity on treatment-related mortality and survival. *Blood.* 2002;100:1611–1618.

39. Barker JN. Who should get cord blood transplants? *Biol Blood Marrow Transplant.* 2007;13 (Suppl 1):78–82.

40. Eapen M, Rubinstein P, Zhang MJ, et al. Outcomes of transplantation of unrelated donor umbilical cord blood and bone marrow in children with acute leukaemia: a comparison study. *Lancet.* 2007;369:1947–1954.

41. Rubinstein P, Carrier C, Scaradavou A, et al. Outcomes among 562 recipients of placental-blood transplants from unrelated donors. *N Engl J Med.* 1998;339:1565–1577.

42. Rocha V, Cornish J, Sievers EL, et al. Comparison of outcomes of unrelated bone marrow and umbilical cord blood transplants in children with acute leukemia. *Blood.* 2001;97: 2962–2971.

43. Kamani N, Spellman S, Hurley CK, et al. State of the art review: HLA matching and outcome of unrelated donor umbilical cord blood transplants. *Biol Blood Marrow Transplant.* 2008; 14:1–6.

44. Arora M, Nagaraj S, Wagner JE, et al. Chronic graft-versus-host disease (cGVHD) following unrelated donor hematopoietic stem cell transplantation (HSCT): higher response rate in recipients of unrelated donor (URD) umbilical cord blood (UCB). *Biol Blood Marrow Transplant.* 2007;13: 1145–1152.

45. Storb R, Weiden PL, Sullivan KM, et al. Second marrow transplants in patients with aplastic anemia rejecting the first graft: use of a conditioning regimen including cyclophosphamide and antithymocyte globulin. *Blood.* 1987;70:116–121.

46. Buckley JD, Lampkin BC, Nesbit ME, et al. Remission induction in children with acute non-lymphocytic leukemia using cytosine arabinoside and doxorubicin or daunorubicin: a report from the Childrens Cancer Study Group. *Med Pediatr Oncol.* 1989;17:382–390.

47. Kletzel M, Jacobsohn D, Tse W, et al. Reduced intensity transplants (RIT) in pediatrics: a review. *Pediatr Transplant.* 2005;9 (Suppl 7):63–70.

48. Iannone R, Casella JF, Fuchs EJ, et al. Results of minimally toxic nonmyeloablative transplantation in patients with sickle cell anemia and beta-thalassemia. *Biol Blood Marrow Transplant.* 2003;9:519–528.

49. Del Toro G, Satwani P, Harrison L, et al. A pilot study of reduced intensity conditioning and allogeneic stem cell transplantation from unrelated cord blood and matched family donors in children and adolescent recipients. *Bone Marrow Transplant.* 2004;33:613–622.

50. Jacobsohn DA, Duerst R, Tse W, et al. Reduced intensity haemopoietic stem-cell transplantation for treatment of non-malignant diseases in children. *Lancet.* 2004;364: 156–162.

51. Horn B, Baxter-Lowe LA, Englert L, et al. Reduced intensity conditioning using intravenous busulfan, fludarabine and rabbit ATG for children with nonmalignant disorders and CML. *Bone Marrow Transplant.* 2006;37:263–269.

52. Slavin S, Nagler A, Naparstek E, et al. Nonmyeloablative stem cell transplantation and cell therapy as an alternative to conventional bone marrow transplantation with lethal cytoreduction for the treatment of malignant and nonmalignant hematologic diseases. *Blood.* 1998;91:756–763.

53. Horwitz ME, Barrett AJ, Brown MR, et al. Treatment of chronic granulomatous disease with nonmyeloablative conditioning and a T-cell-depleted hematopoietic allograft. *N Engl J Med.* 2001;344:881–888.

54. Langrish CL, Buddle JC, Thrasher AJ, et al. Neonatal dendritic cells are intrinsically biased against Th-1 immune responses. *Clin Exp Immunol.* 2002;128:118–123.

55. Tasker L, Marshall-Clarke S. Functional responses of human neonatal B lymphocytes to antigen receptor cross-linking and CpG DNA. *Clin Exp Immunol.* 2003;134:409–419.

56. Ordemann R, Hutchinson R, Friedman J, et al. Enhanced allostimulatory activity of host antigen-presenting cells in old mice intensifies acute graft-versus-host disease. *J Clin Invest.* 2002;109:1249–1256.

57. Mackall CL, Fleisher TA, Brown MR, et al. Age, thymopoiesis, and CD4+ T-lymphocyte regeneration after intensive chemotherapy. *N Engl J Med.* 1995;332:143–149.

58. Delespesse G, Yang LP, Ohshima Y, et al. Maturation of human neonatal CD4+ and CD8+ T lymphocytes into Th1/Th2 effectors. *Vaccine.* 1998;16:1415–1419.

59. Kobayashi S, Ohnuma K, Uchiyama M, et al. Association of CD26 with CD45RA outside lipid rafts attenuates cord blood T-cell activation. *Blood.* 2004;103:1002–1010.

60. Hunt DW, Huppertz HI, Jiang HJ, et al. Studies of human cord blood dendritic cells: evidence for functional immaturity. *Blood.* 1994;84:4333–4343.

61. Sorg RV, Kogler G, Wernet P. Identification of cord blood dendritic cells as an immature CD11c- population. *Blood.* 1999;93:2302–2307.

62. Garban F, Ericson M, Roucard C, et al. Detection of empty HLA class II molecules on cord blood B cells. *Blood.* 1996;87: 3970–3976.

63. Fujii H, Cuvelier G, She K, et al. Biomarkers in newly diagnosed pediatric extensive chronic graft-versus-host disease: a report from the Children's Oncology Group. *Blood.* 2008 Mar 15;111(6): 3276–85.

64. Akpek G, Zahurak ML, Piantadosi S, et al. Development of a prognostic model for grading chronic graft-versus-host disease. *Blood*. 2001;97:1219–1226.

65. Lee S, Cook EF, Soiffer R, et al. Development and validation of a scale to measure symptoms of chronic graft-versus-host disease. *Biol Blood Marrow Transplant*. 2002;8:444–452.

66. Akpek G, Lee SJ, Flowers ME, et al. Performance of a new clinical grading system for chronic graft-versus-host disease: a multicenter study. *Blood*. 2003;102:802–809.

67. Beredjiklian PK, Drummond DS, Dormans JP, et al. Orthopaedic manifestations of chronic graft-versus-host disease. *J Pediatr Orthop*. 1998;18:572–575.

68. Stern JM, Chesnut CH, 3rd, Bruemmer B, et al. Bone density loss during treatment of chronic GVHD. *Bone Marrow Transplant*. 1996;17:395–400.

69. Tauchmanova L, De Rosa G, Serio B, et al. Avascular necrosis in long-term survivors after allogeneic or autologous stem cell transplantation: a single center experience and a review. *Cancer*. 2003;97:2453–2461.

70. Pavletic SZ, Martin P, Lee SJ, et al. Measuring Therapeutic Response in Chronic Graft-versus-Host Disease: National Institutes of Health Consensus Development Project on Criteria for Clinical Trials in Chronic Graft-versus-Host Disease: IV. Response Criteria Working Group Report. *Biol Blood Marrow Transplant*. 2006;12:252–266.

71. Imanguli MM, Pavletic SZ, Guadagnini JP, et al. Chronic graft versus host disease of oral mucosa: review of available therapies. *Oral Surg Oral Med Oral Pathol Oral Radiol Endod*. 2006;101:175–183.

72. Treister NS, Woo SB, O'Holleran EW, et al. Oral chronic graft-versus-host disease in pediatric patients after hematopoietic stem cell transplantation. *Biol Blood Marrow Transplant*. 2005;11:721–731.

73. Jacobsohn DA, Montross S, Anders V, et al. Clinical importance of confirming or excluding the diagnosis of chronic graft-versus-host disease. *Bone Marrow Transplant*. 2001;28:1047–1051.

74. Browning B, Thormann K, Seshadri R, et al. Weight loss and reduced body mass index: a critical issue in children with multiorgan chronic graft-versus-host disease. *Bone Marrow Transplant*. 2006;37:527–533.

75. Shulman HM, Sharma P, Amos D, et al. A coded histologic study of hepatic graft-versus-host disease after human bone marrow transplantation. *Hepatology*. 1988;8:463–470.

76. Strasser SI, Shulman HM, Flowers ME, et al. Chronic graft-versus-host disease of the liver: presentation as an acute hepatitis. *Hepatology*. 2000;32:1265–1271.

77. Akpek G, Boitnott JK, Lee LA, et al. Hepatitic variant of graft-versus-host disease after donor lymphocyte infusion. *Blood*. 2002;100:3903 3907.

78. Melin-Aldana H, Thormann K, Duerst R, et al. Hepatitic pattern of graft versus host disease in children. *Pediatr Blood Cancer*. 2007;49:727–730.

79. Afessa B, Litzow MR, Tefferi A. Bronchiolitis obliterans and other late onset non-infectious pulmonary complications in hematopoietic stem cell transplantation. *Bone Marrow Transplant*. 2001;28:425–434.

80. Dudek AZ, Mahaseth H, DeFor TE, et al. Bronchiolitis obliterans in chronic graft-versus-host disease: analysis of risk factors and treatment outcomes. *Biol Blood Marrow Transplant*. 2003;9:657–666.

81. Ratanatharathorn V, Ayash L, Lazarus HM, et al. Chronic graft-versus-host disease: clinical manifestation and therapy. *Bone Marrow Transplant*. 2001;28:121–129.

82. Filipovich AH, Weisdorf D, Pavletic S, et al. National Institutes of Health consensus development project on criteria for clinical trials in chronic graft-versus-host disease: I. Diagnosis and staging working group report. *Biol Blood Marrow Transplant*. 2005;11:945–956.

83. Khouri IF, Ippoliti C, Gajewski J, et al. Neutropenias following allogeneic bone marrow transplantation: response to therapy with high-dose intravenous immunoglobulin. *Am J Hematol*. 1996;52:313–315.

84. Au WY, Lo CM, Hawkins BR, et al. Evans' syndrome complicating chronic graft versus host disease after cadaveric liver transplantation. *Transplantation*. 2001;72:527–528.

85. Tomonari A, Tojo A, Lseki T, et al. Severe autoimmune thrombocytopenia after allogeneic bone marrow transplantation for aplastic anemia. *Int J Hematol*. 2001;74:228–232.

86. Sullivan KM, Witherspoon RP, Storb R, et al. Prednisone and azathioprine compared with prednisone and placebo for treatment of chronic graft-v-host disease: prognostic influence of prolonged thrombocytopenia after allogeneic marrow transplantation. *Blood*. 1988;72:546–554.

87. Nevo S, Enger C, Hartley E, et al. Acute bleeding and thrombocytopenia after bone marrow transplantation. *Bone Marrow Transplant*. 2001;27:65–72.

88. Jacobsohn DA, Schechter T, Seshadri R, et al. Eosinophilia correlates with the presence or development of chronic graft-versus-host disease in children. *Transplantation*. 2004;77:1096–1100.

89. Siadak M, Sullivan KM. The management of chronic graft-versus-host disease. *Blood Rev*. 1994;8:154–160.

90. Storek J, Witherspoon RP, Webb D, et al. Lack of B cells precursors in marrow transplant recipients with chronic graft-versus-host disease. *Am J Hematol*. 1996;52:82–89.

91. Maury S, Mary JY, Rabian C, et al. Prolonged immune deficiency following allogeneic stem cell transplantation: risk factors and complications in adult patients. *Br J Haematol*. 2001;115:630–641.

92. Rege K, Mehta J, Treleaven J, et al. Fatal pneumococcal infections following allogeneic bone marrow transplant. *Bone Marrow Transplant*. 1994;14:903–906.

93. Kulkarni S, Powles R, Treleaven J, et al. Chronic graft versus host disease is associated with long-term risk for pneumococcal infections in recipients of bone marrow transplants. *Blood*. 2000;95:3683–3686.

94. Couriel D, Carpenter PA, Cutler C, et al. Ancillary therapy and supportive care of chronic graft-versus-host disease: national institutes of health consensus development project on criteria for clinical trials in chronic Graft-versus-host disease: V. Ancillary Therapy and Supportive Care Working Group Report. *Biol Blood Marrow Transplant*. 2006;12:375–396.

95. Vogelsang GB. How I treat chronic graft-versus-host disease. *Blood*. 2001;97:1196–1201.

96. Green A, Clarke E, Hunt L, et al. Children with acute lymphoblastic leukemia who receive T-cell-depleted HLA mismatched marrow allografts from unrelated donors have an increased incidence of primary graft failure but a similar overall transplant outcome. *Blood*. 1999;94:2236–2246.

97. Oakhill A, Pamphilon DH, Potter MN, et al. Unrelated donor bone marrow transplantation for children with relapsed acute

lymphoblastic leukaemia in second complete remission. *Br J Haematol.* 1996;94:574–578.

98. Fleming DR, Henslee-Downey PJ, Romond EH, et al. Allogeneic bone marrow transplantation with T cell-depleted partially matched related donors for advanced acute lymphoblastic leukemia in children and adults: a comparative matched cohort study. *Bone Marrow Transplant.* 1996;17: 917–922.

99. Bunin N, Saunders F, Leahey A, et al. Alternative donor bone marrow transplantation for children with juvenile myelomonocytic leukemia. *J Pediatr Hematol Oncol.* 1999; 21:479–485.

100. Horwitz ME, Sullivan KM. Chronic graft-versus-host disease. *Blood Rev.* 2006;20:15–27.

101. Wall DA, Carter SL, Kernan NA, et al. Busulfan/melphalan/antithymocyte globulin followed by unrelated donor cord blood transplantation for treatment of infant leukemia and leukemia in young children: the Cord Blood Transplantation study (COBLT) experience. *Biol Blood Marrow Transplant.* 2005;11:637–646.

102. Duval M, Pedron B, Rohrlich P, et al. Immune reconstitution after haematopoietic transplantation with two different doses of pre-graft antithymocyte globulin. *Bone Marrow Transplant.* 2002;30:421–426.

103. Wingard JR, Piantadosi S, Vogelsang GB, et al. Predictors of death from chronic graft-versus-host disease after bone marrow transplantation. *Blood.* 1989;74:1428–1435.

104. Sehgal SN. Rapamune (Sirolimus, rapamycin): an overview and mechanism of action. *Ther Drug Monit.* 1995;17:660–665.

105. Benito AI, Furlong T, Martin PJ, et al. Sirolimus (rapamycin) for the treatment of steroid-refractory acute graft-versus-host disease. *Transplantation.* 2001;72:1924–1929.

106. Cutler C, Antin JH. Sirolimus for GVHD prophylaxis in allogeneic stem cell transplantation. *Bone Marrow Transplant.* 2004;34:471–476.

107. Couriel DR, Saliba R, Escalon MP, et al. Sirolimus in combination with tacrolimus and corticosteroids for the treatment of resistant chronic graft-versus-host disease. *Br J Haematol.* 2005;130:409–417.

108. Johnston LJ, Brown J, Shizuru JA, et al. Rapamycin (sirolimus) for treatment of chronic graft-versus-host disease. *Biol Blood Marrow Transplant.* 2005;11:47–55.

109. Jurado M, Vallejo C, Perez-Simon JA, et al. Sirolimus as part of immunosuppressive therapy for refractory chronic graft-versus-host disease. *Biol Blood Marrow Transplant.* 2007;13: 701–706.

110. Mookerjee B, Altomonte V, Vogelsang G. Salvage therapy for refractory chronic graft-versus-host disease with mycophenolate mofetil and tacrolimus. *Bone Marrow Transplant.* 1999;24:517–520.

111. Lopez F, Parker P, Nademanee A, et al. Efficacy of mycophenolate mofetil in the treatment of chronic graft-versus-host disease. *Biol Blood Marrow Transplant.* 2005;11:307–313.

112. Busca A, Saroglia EM, Lanino E, et al. Mycophenolate mofetil (MMF) as therapy for refractory chronic GVHD (cGVHD) in children receiving bone marrow transplantation. *Bone Marrow Transplant.* 2000;25:1067–1071.

113. Yusuf U SJ, Stephan V. Mycophenolate Mofetil (MMF) as salvage treatment for steroid-refractory chronic graft-versus-host-disease (GVHD) in children [abstract]. *Blood.* 2001;98:398a.

114. Giblett ER, Anderson JE, Cohen F, et al. Adenosine-deaminase deficiency in two patients with severely impaired cellular immunity. *Lancet.* 1972;2:1067–1069.

115. Saven A, Piro L. Newer purine analogues for the treatment of hairy-cell leukemia. *N Engl J Med.* 1994;330:691–697.

116. Goldberg JD, Jacobsohn DA, Margolis J, et al. Pentostatin for the treatment of chronic graft-versus-host disease in children. *J Pediatr Hematol Oncol.* 2003;25:584–588.

117. Jacobsohn DA, Chen AR, Zahurak M, et al. Phase II study of pentostatin in patients with corticosteroid-refractory chronic graft-versus-host disease. *J Clin Oncol.* 2007;25: 4255–4261.

118. Mackenzie AH. Antimalarial drugs for rheumatoid arthritis. *Am J Med.* 1983;75:48–58.

119. Olson NY, Lindsley CB. Adjunctive use of hydroxychloroquine in childhood dermatomyositis. *J Rheumatol.* 1989;16: 1545–1547.

120. Gilman AL, Chan KW, Mogul A, et al. Hydroxychloroquine for the treatment of chronic graft-versus-host disease. *Biol Blood Marrow Transplant.* 2000;6:327–334.

121. Vogelsang GB, Farmer ER, Hess AD, et al. Thalidomide for the treatment of chronic graft-versus-host disease. *N Engl J Med.* 1992;326:1055–1058.

122. Schlossberg H, Klumpp T, Sabol P, et al. Severe cutaneous ulceration following treatment with thalidomide for GVHD. *Bone Marrow Transplant.* 2001;27:229–230.

123. Cole CH, Rogers PC, Pritchard S, et al. Thalidomide in the management of chronic graft-versus-host disease in children following bone marrow transplantation. *Bone Marrow Transplant.* 1994;14:937–942.

124. Rovelli A, Arrigo C, Nesi F, et al. The role of thalidomide in the treatment of refractory chronic graft-versus-host disease following bone marrow transplantation in children. *Bone Marrow Transplant.* 1998;21:577–581.

125. Cutler C, Miklos D, Kim HT, et al. Rituximab for steroid-refractory chronic graft-vs.-host disease. *Blood.* 2006.

126. Srinivasan R, Chakrabarti S, Walsh T, et al. Improved survival in steroid-refractory acute graft versus host disease after nonmyeloablative allogeneic transplantation using a daclizumab-based strategy with comprehensive infection prophylaxis. *Br J Haematol.* 2004;124:777–786.

127. Busca A, Locatelli F, Marmont F, et al. Recombinant human soluble tumor necrosis factor receptor fusion protein as treatment for steroid refractory graft-versus-host disease following allogeneic hematopoietic stem cell transplantation. *Am J Hematol.* 2007;82:45–52.

128. Yanik G, Hellerstedt B, Custer J, et al. Etanercept (Enbrel) administration for idiopathic pneumonia syndrome after allogeneic hematopoietic stem cell transplantation. *Biol Blood Marrow Transplant.* 2002;8:395–400.

129. Greinix HT, Volc-Platzer B, Knobler RM. Extracorporeal photochemotherapy in the treatment of severe graft-versus-host disease. *Leuk Lymphoma.* 2000;36:425–434.

130. Couriel D, Hosing C, Saliba R, et al. Extracorporeal photopheresis for acute and chronic graft-versus-host disease: does it work? *Biol Blood Marrow Transplant.* 2006;12: 37–40.

131. Couriel DR, Hosing C, Saliba R, et al. Extracorporeal photochemotherapy for the treatment of steroid-resistant chronic GVHD. *Blood.* 2006;107:3074–3080.

132. Foss FM, DiVenuti GM, Chin K, et al. Prospective study of extracorporeal photopheresis in steroid-refractory or steroid-resistant extensive chronic graft-versus-host disease: analysis of response and survival incorporating prognostic factors. *Bone Marrow Transplant.* 2005;35:1187–1193.

133. Rubegni P, Cuccia A, Sbano P, et al. Role of extracorporeal photochemotherapy in patients with refractory chronic graft-versus-host disease. *Br J Haematol.* 2005;130:271–275.

134. Messina C, Locatelli F, Lanino E, et al. Extracorporeal photochemotherapy for paediatric patients with graft-versus-host disease after haematopoietic stem cell transplantation. *Br J Haematol.* 2003;122:118–127.

135. Dall'Amico R, Livi U, Milano A, et al. Extracorporeal photochemotherapy as adjuvant treatment of heart transplant recipients with recurrent rejection. *Transplantation.* 1995;60: 45–49.

136. Salvaneschi L, Perotti C, Zecca M, et al. Extracorporeal photochemotherapy for treatment of acute and chronic GVHD in childhood. *Transfusion.* 2001;41:1299–1305.

137. Brougham MF, Wallace WH. Subfertility in children and young people treated for solid and haematological malignancies. *Br J Haematol.* 2005;131:143–155.

138. Phipps S, Dunavant M, Srivastava DK, et al. Cognitive and academic functioning in survivors of pediatric bone marrow transplantation. *J Clin Oncol.* 2000;18:1004–1011.

139. Woolfrey AE, Gooley TA, Sievers EL, et al. Bone marrow transplantation for children less than 2 years of age with acute myelogenous leukemia or myelodysplastic syndrome. *Blood.* 1998;92:3546–3556.

140. Falcini F, Taccetti G, Trapani S, et al. Growth retardation in juvenile chronic arthritis patients treated with steroids. *Clin Exp Rheumatol.* 1991;9 (Suppl 6):37–40.

141. Lai HC, FitzSimmons SC, Allen DB, et al. Risk of persistent growth impairment after alternate-day prednisone treatment in children with cystic fibrosis. *N Engl J Med.* 2000;342: 851–859.

142. Leung W, Ahn H, Rose SR, et al. A prospective cohort study of late sequelae of pediatric allogeneic hematopoietic stem cell transplantation. *Medicine (Baltimore).* 2007;86:215–224.

143. Uderzo C, Pillon M, Corti P, et al. Impact of cumulative anthracycline dose, preparative regimen and chronic graft-versus-host disease on pulmonary and cardiac function in children 5 years after allogeneic hematopoietic stem cell transplantation: a prospective evaluation on behalf of the EBMT Pediatric Diseases and Late Effects Working Parties. *Bone Marrow Transplant.* 2007;39:667–675.

144. Carpenter PA, Hoffmeister P, Chesnut CH, et al. Bisphosphonate therapy for reduced bone mineral density in children with chronic graft-versus-host disease. *Biol Blood Marrow Transplant.* 2007 Jun;13(6):683–90.

34

Principles of Interdisciplinary Practice in the Care of Patients with Chronic Graft versus Host Disease

Viki Anders, Carina Moravec, and Sandra A. Mitchell

INTRODUCTION

Patients with chronic graft versus host disease (cGVHD) experience a variety of health needs that result directly from the physical, functional, and psychosocial effects of the disease, are produced as side effects of immunosuppressive treatments, or derive from the late treatment effects of high-dose therapy and hematopoietic stem cell transplantation (HSCT). The achieving optimal outcomes for patients with cGVHD requires the coordinated efforts of an interdisciplinary team delivering a comprehensive range of clinical services in both community-based and specialty care settings. The services must be designed to promptly detect, effectively mitigate, and, where possible, prevent these sequelae. This chapter focuses on the principles of interdisciplinary practice in the care of patients with cGVHD. The chapter examines seven fundamental elements for successful interdisciplinary practice in cGVHD. These elements address (1) the composition, functioning, leadership, and coordination of the team, (2) the organizational service delivery model, (3) communication and collaboration, (4) eliminating barriers to access to needed services, (5) the development of standards of care, standard operating procedures, and evidence-based guidelines, (6) involvement of patient and family, and (7) coordination and continuity of care between specialty care centers and community. Case vignettes illustrate the application of the principles of interdisciplinary care and analyze the features of interdisciplinary team functioning that contribute to optimal clinical outcomes in HSCT survivors with cGVHD and the family members and communities who are caring for them.

THE NEED FOR INTERDISCIPLINARY PRACTICE TO OPTIMIZE OUTCOMES IN PATIENTS WITH cGVHD

There is a growing recognition that a patient-centered interdisciplinary approach to the delivery of health care is fundamental to achieving optimal patient outcomes [1, 2], particularly for those patients experiencing a multisystem illness such as cGVHD [3]. No one health care profession has all the knowledge needed to provide total patient-centered care because the needs of patients with cGVHD are both multidimensional and complex. The challenges of meeting these needs are magnified by the fact that other conditions such as infection, late effects of treatment, and comorbidities may mimic the heterogeneous manifestations of cGVHD and by the fact that there is a wide range of potential treatment approaches without a clear standard of therapy. Moreover, treatment and follow-up must often be coordinated across a variety of settings and perhaps across geographical distance. A further challenge is that many health care professionals in oncology lack knowledge of the late effects of treatment including cGVHD. Furthermore, the health care system has done little to address reimbursement constraints for the delivery of survivorship care, particularly for those survivors coping with late effects of treatment such as cGVHD. Within this context, optimizing the quality and cost-effectiveness of care and ensuring accountability for outcomes presents a significant challenge that can only be met through effective interdisciplinary practice. Interdisciplinary practice is also essential to health care organizational effectiveness and has the potential to reduce professional burnout [4].

INTERDISCIPLINARY PRACTICE – DEFINING FEATURES AND DETERMINANTS OF SUCCESS

Interdisciplinary practice is defined as "a partnership between a team of health professionals and a client in a participatory, collaborative, and coordinated approach to shared decision making around health issues [5]." This definition is noteworthy for its emphasis on coordination and collaboration, and for its inclusion of patients and families as active participants. The term *interdisciplinary* emphasizes collective decision making and action, while the term *multidisciplinary* may imply a shared focus, but individual decision making and parallel action [6, 7]. The interdisciplinary approach is ideal for the management of the complex problems associated with cGVHD.

Collaboration in teams is the process by which interdependent professionals act collectively to meet patient care needs. Determinants of successful collaboration in health care teams include interpersonal relationships within the team, conditions within the organization, and the organization's environment [8].

Interpersonal relationships among team members based on a willingness to collaborate, and the existence of mutual trust, respect, and communication are fundamental to inter-disciplinary collaboration. Moreover, since the collaborative process is voluntary, both a commitment to the spirit of collaboration and to a process of engagement and negotiation are essential [9]. Building trust requires confidence in one's own abilities as well as trust in the ability of others, and it requires time, effort, and patience. Mutual respect implies knowledge and appreciation that the contributions of each member of the team are interdependent and complementary. At both an individual and organizational level, successful collaboration occurs only when competition is minimized and disparities in power equalized. Both competition and inequality of power erode trust and mutual respect.

Martin-Rodriguez et al. suggest that communication has been shown to be a determinant of collaboration for at least three reasons [8]. First, communication is required for team members to exchange information about how their work contributes to clinical outcomes and team objectives. Second efficient communication also allows constructive negotiations with other professionals [9]. Lastly communication is the mechanism by which other components of collaboration such as mutual respect and trust are fostered.

Conditions within an organization that encourage inter-disciplinary collaboration include an organizational structure that is decentralized, egalitarian, and adaptable, as opposed to hierarchical, authoritarian and rigid [4, 10]. An organizational philosophy that values participation, openness, risk taking and interdependence is also essential [11].

In terms of the organizational environment, collaborative practice benefits from an availability of time to interact and spaces to meet. Collaboration requires venues that allow collaborators to share information, develop interpersonal relationships through informal interaction, and address team issues. Studies suggest that sharing space and working in physical proximity reduces professional territoriality, and may facilitate collaboration, especially when conflicts arise [12, 13]. Collaboration also requires mechanisms for coordinated action and communication [14]. The availability of practice standards, policies, interdisciplinary protocols, shared documentation tools, and regular formal meetings involving all team professionals are fundamental to supporting interprofessional collaboration [9, 15, 16].

Element 1: Composition, Coordination, and Leadership of the Interdisciplinary cGVHD Team

The care of patients with cGVHD requires an interdisciplinary team, with a full therapeutic range, together with referral links and an approach to care that strengthens community capacity to meet the diverse needs of HSCT survivors and their families coping with late effects of treatment. Regardless of whether the model of care is a specialty referral practice for cGVHD within a tertiary care center, a clinic designed to provide long-term follow-up of HSCT survivors, or an HSCT clinic that cares for transplant recipients across the trajectory from initial evaluation to long-term follow-up, the management of cGVHD requires the expertise of multiple disciplines. The core team includes the transplant physicians, nurses, advance practice nurses, the community oncologist and/ or internist, the patient, and the patient's family members and/or caregivers. This core team depends on many other disciplines to assist with the diagnosis and treatment of the patient with cGVHD, depending on the individual patient's needs. These disciplines, together with the core team, are shown in Table 34.1. A referral network with these specialties is vital to ensure prompt access to these disciplines when the need arises.

With such a diverse team, mechanisms for team leadership, coordination, and communication are essential. Nurse coordinators, outpatient clinic nurses, and the advanced practice nurse (APN) have fundamental responsibilities in the coordination and leadership of the interdisciplinary team [17]. The nurse is ideally suited to perform intake activities, coordinate team functions, support collaborative working links between team members and develop the systems to ensure that all patients with cGVHD have access to relevant services. With advanced skills in physical examination, differential diagnosis, and treatment, the APN possesses an ideal skill set for the pivotal role of conducting a comprehensive evaluation of the patient with cGVHD, integrating the perspectives of all team members, summarizing the interdisciplinary plan of care in a single document, and communicating the plan to patients, families, and community-based clinicians. With so many different providers involved, the patient and family must be made aware that ongoing collaboration and communication is occurring between members of the interdisciplinary team, if they are to feel that their care is coordinated and not fragmented. Team leadership by a physician and APN can promote the achievement of both day-to-day and strategic leadership functions, including measuring and evaluating outcomes, promoting team communication, coordination, and problem solving, ensuring prompt enrollment of patients onto clinical trials, and sharing in the development of structure standards, procedures, and care protocols that improve clinical and operational outcomes.

In developing a service delivery model, a consistent core team of professionals dedicated to working together to address the needs of patients with cGVHD is indispensable. Consistency in core and ancillary team members promotes the development of expertise in the evaluation and management of cGVHD and in optimizing communication, collaboration, coordination, and joint problem solving [4]. Though not always achievable, a central location to which the consultants travel for patient evaluation is helpful, particularly when a series of consultations is required. Many patients with cGVHD have limited physical capacity for traveling to multiple office locations. In addition the time spent in clinic waiting rooms may also

Table 34.1: Disciplines/Specialties Required in the Care of Patients with cGVHD

Core Team Members	Additional Specialty Services
Hematopoietic Stem Cell Transplantation	Dermatology
■ Physicians	Gastroenterology
■ Nurses	Pulmonology
■ Advanced practice nurses	Ophthalmology
	Oral medicine/dentistry
Community oncologist and/or internist	Pathology
Patient and family	Physical and occupational therapy
	Pain and symptom management
	Psychosocial support
	Infectious diseases
	Gynecology
	Endocrinology
	Hepatology
	Radiology
	Pharmacology
	Otolaryngology
	Neurology
	Psychiatry
	Cardiology
	Speech and language pathology
	Vocational rehabilitation

expose cGVHD patients to infectious risks. If a central location for evaluation cannot be established, referral mechanisms that ensure prompt access are crucial. The consultant must be provided with, or have access to, the necessary records, imaging studies and reports, a summary of the patient's medical history, and the reason for the consultation.

Geographical issues often present barriers to access for patients with cGVHD. Preferred consultants may have offices distant to the cancer center. Moreover, patients with cGVHD often receive care in their home communities by clinicians who have limited exposure to the problems associated with cGVHD. Systems should be established for periodic evaluation of HSCT survivors with active cGVHD by an interdisciplinary team with a focus in cGVHD. Not only does this ensure comprehensive periodic evaluation by a team with expertise in cGVHD, it also serves to strengthen collaborative links between the community and specialty health care providers, ensuring more timely access to specialty care when necessary and fostering community-based expertise in the care of patients with cGVHD.

Element 2: Service Delivery Models for HSCT Survivors with cGVHD

An explicit model to guide the delivery of services to patients with cGVHD can be helpful in designing roles and methods for the delivery of care and in specifying and interpreting the indicators of clinical, operational, and economic effectiveness and quality. Three potential models that may be relevant to patients with cGVHD can be identified from a review of the literature, though none has yet been tested in this patient population.

Chronic Care Model

The Chronic Care Model (CCM) provides a framework for the delivery of chronic disease management interventions within primary health care. The three key elements of the CCM include (1) support of patient self-management through patient education and motivational counseling; (2) the delivery of coordinated care through interdisciplinary teams, emphasizing the role of the nurse case managers and the contribution of advanced practice nursing roles; and (3) clinical information systems to support health care providers in the delivery of evidence-based interventions and adherence to guidelines [18]. Aspects of the CCM that are particularly relevant to the care of patients with cGVHD include the important role of nurses in the coordination and delivery of interdisciplinary care, and nurses' efforts to educate and counsel patients to enhance self-management. The CCM also underscores the importance of developing evidence-based guidelines for cGVHD management to support clinical decision making.

Disease Management Model

Disease management programs are designed to provide an organized method for managing patients with chronic disease and to provide resources for patients that promote better understanding and self-management of their conditions. Disease management is a system of coordinated interventions and communications delivered to populations that have significant self-care needs. It provides access to a spectrum of health care professionals and ensures comprehensive, coordinated care. Important aspects of this model include communication and shared decision making among the patient – lay caregiver – provider triad and a family-focused approach to care.

Elements of a classic disease management support system that may be particularly helpful in the management of patients with cGVHD include 24/7 phone access for consultation, the services of a patient navigator, respite care/home health care, regular review of medication profiles by a pharmacist, access to educational programs and psychosocial support, automated telephone reminder systems, and periodic follow-up phone calls [19].

Clinical outcomes of disease management that are particularly relevant to cGVHD include functional status, incidence of infections, nutritional status, and the optimal management of comorbidities such as renal dysfunction, osteoporosis, and endocrinopathies. Beneficial effects on psychological distress, quality of life, adherence to therapy, and caregiver burden are also relevant outcomes of disease management [19]. Cost-effectiveness of this model in terms of reduction in hospitalization and length of stay, and efficient sourcing and delivery of services can be evaluated.

A strength of the disease management model is its emphasis on developing patients' knowledge, skills, and motivation for effective self-management [20]. This aspect is particularly relevant to patients experiencing cGVHD, since adherence to a treatment regimen, self-management of distressing symptoms, and active participation in measures to prevent functional decline [21] are fundamental to achieving best outcomes.

Survivorship Care Model

Since cGVHD is a prevalent and significant late effect of treatment in this subset of cancer survivors, survivorship care models can provide valuable guidance in the delivery of services to this patient population. Our expanding knowledge that cancer survivors are at risk for physical and psychosocial late effects of treatment has provided an impetus to offer cancer survivors tailored follow-up that emphasizes risk-adapted monitoring and management of late effects [17, 22]. Elements of that follow-up include education, counseling, and health promotion for survivors and their families to promote risk reduction through healthy behaviors, support and advocacy to address psychosocial issues, and targeted surveillance and management of groups of survivors at particular risk for specific complications.

A three-level risk-adapted model for the delivery of survivorship services has recently been proposed by Eiser et al. (2007) [23] and Wallace et al. (2001) [24]. In this model, long-term follow-up proceeds by one of three methods (1) telephone, (2) through nurse or primary-care-led clinics, or (3) through a medically supervised late effects clinic. A similar model could be adapted to cGVHD where patients with no or clinically limited cGVHD are followed distantly with some education and support for early detection of complications, while those with resolving cGVHD receive most of their care from primary care providers with periodic input from the cGVHD specialty program. Those individuals with active cGVHD, and those on intensive immunosuppression, receive most of their care through a cGVHD specialty program, transitioning back to level II when their cGVHD is under improved control.

These three models share a number of features including an emphasis on coordination of care; patient and family education, support and empowerment; and the importance of self-management. The models also underscore the principles of interdisciplinary practice outlined below including communication and the involvement of patient and family. Descriptive and comparative analyses of the strengths and limitations of each of the models for the development, implementation, and evaluation of service delivery in cGVHD is an important area for future study.

CASE STUDY 34.1: THREE INTERDISCIPLINARY CARE MODELS IN cGVHD

A 34-year-old who is 2 years status post unrelated donor HSCT for treatment of non-Hodgkins lymphoma (NHL) has cGVHD involving his skin, eyes, and mouth that has been unresponsive to high-dose prednisone, tacrolimus, and mycophenolate. Recently, he has been responding to treatment with sirolimus. However, he also experienced a fever, productive cough, and mild shortness of breath over the past weekend, and after discussing his symptoms with the on-call transplant physician at the tertiary care center, he was hospitalized in his home community for a course of intravenous antibiotics for the treatment of pneumonia. He is seen regularly at the tertiary care center by oral medicine for management of oral ulcerations and xerostomia, by gastroenterology for management of dysphagia and weight loss, and by ophthalmology for management of severe ocular sicca. He lives more than 600 miles from the transplant center, and visits monthly for cGVHD evaluation including the above specialists, as needed. At a recent visit, he was referred to orthopedics for their recommendations regarding the timing of hip replacement surgery for management of avascular necrosis. Consistent with the CCM, he receives much of his care through his primary health care providers and he and his wife have received extensive teaching by nurses to enhance self-management. He has a nurse case manager at the transplant center who facilitates the coordination of his referrals, and integrates communication between the transplant center and the community clinicians. Aspects of the disease management model include the telephone access for specialty provider consultation, and periodic telephone calls from the transplant case manager. Monthly consultation with a pharmacist who is familiar with the various immunosuppressive agents helps to support self-management. This case also illustrates aspects of the survivorship care model in that in addition to cGVHD, potential late effects such as infection and avascular necrosis also receive evaluation and management.

Element 3: Communication and Collaboration

Effective communication is fundamental to the delivery of interdisciplinary care. Both formal and informal communication must occur among providers in the process of developing and implementing a plan of care. Informal communication occurs during day-to-day interactions, while a formal team meeting convened at a regular time provides an opportunity for the whole team to review findings, share diagnostic impressions, refine a collective plan of care, and coordinate responsibilities for implementing the plan. Communication with patients and families and with community providers about the results of cGVHD evaluations and the plan for ongoing management is another key aspect of interdisciplinary care. Communication must be timely, tailored to preferences, and should contain the information necessary to promote accurate understanding and facilitate necessary action. Communication to other providers and to patients can occur via detailed progress notes, personal communication by telephone, or brief summaries provided by fax or e-mail. Applications of advances in technology including video conferencing, digital images, and other telehealth strategies in the care of HSCT survivors are undergoing development and preliminary evaluation [25–27]. Results suggest that these strategies can play an important role in reducing access barriers for HSCT survivors, including those with cGVHD, and may improve clinical outcomes, reduce cost, and improve patient satisfaction and adherence. Continued development and testing of these strategies is indicated to improve communication with patients and families, and to explore their application in strengthening collaboration with community care providers.

CASE STUDY 34.2: COMMUNICATION

PL is a 32 year old gentleman with a long history of steroid refractory skin and oral cGVHD. Two months after immunosuppression was discontinued, he developed severe abdominal pain and diarrhea. Stool cultures were negative. Prior to initiating treatment with corticosteroids, his local physician contacted the transplant center and arranged for a consultation with the cGVHD team. He was referred to a gastroenterologist familiar with GVHD. An abdominal CT showed an extremely small pancreas, and laboratory studies were consistent with pancreatic enzyme deficiency. He was placed on pancreatic enzyme replacement with resolution of his symptoms.

Providing quality care within an interdisciplinary team also requires team members to develop and sustain partnerships and collaboration. Partnership is a team-based approach to achieving a stated goal. Collaboration is the process of working together within the negotiated framework to achieve the goal of the partnership. In collaboration, values are shared, respect is mutual, and power is shared equally [15]. O'Neill and Krauel suggest that the building blocks of an effective partnership include a shared agenda and mutually beneficial goals, with each partner bringing assets to the partnership, and demonstrating accountability to each other [28]. Respect for each partner's time commitments, tact, and mutual trust are also essential [29, 30].

Baggs defines six critical elements for effective collaborative practice: trust, cooperation, assertiveness, shared decision making, communication, and coordination [31]. At the center of interdisciplinary collaborative practice models are two tenets: (1) patient needs are the foremost priority in the provision of care, and (2) patients require the expertise and skills of different types of providers simultaneously during each encounter or hospital admission [32]. Collaboration requires development of relationships, building trust, and establishing an atmosphere of candor in communication. Barriers to collaboration include competition, territoriality, defensiveness, withholding information, unpredictable or inconsistent behaviors, lack of follow-through, devaluing contributions, intentions or integrity of others, and a lack of mutuality in resolving challenges and disappointments [15, 33].

There is a certain amount of duplication and role overlap that may occur among members of the health care team, and this can result in territorial behaviors within the team members. Territoriality causes the focus on the patient to be displaced and the professionals' role, knowledge base, or authority becomes the focal point. Collaboration provides opportunities for members of the team to develop a shared purpose, recognize divergent and complementary skills and contributions, and promote effective communication [15]. Paradoxically, territoriality may be increased by efforts to artificially define which role components or intervention approaches are the exclusive responsibility or expertise of any one role or one discipline. Establishing

credibility is often a matter of time, patience, and the development of mutual respect, which evolves as team members share common patient-related experiences. Though successful professional collaboration requires effort, it ultimately enhances continuity and reduces care fragmentation [34, 35].

CASE STUDY 34.3: COLLABORATION

WW is a 30-year-old man who had a myeloablative PBSC transplant. Shortly after tapering off immunosuppressants for GVHD, he developed bronchitis. Despite supportive treatment, the dry cough did not resolve and he developed dyspnea on exertion, followed by progression in skin, mouth, and ocular GVHD. A pulmonary consult was requested and bronchiolitits obliterans was confirmed by pulmonary function tests (PFTs), and high-resolution chest CT. Corticosteroids, tacrolimus, inhalers, and antibiotics were added. He had close follow-up with the pulmonary team. Nurses gave him instructions on energy conservation and contacted his home health agency for supplemental oxygen. Respiratory technicians repeated PFTs and walking oximetry frequently. They helped him titrate supplemental oxygen to his symptoms. He enrolled in a pulmonary rehabilitation program that helped him increase muscle strength and manage dyspnea and fatigue. He became depressed on the higher doses of prednisone and was referred to psychiatry for evaluation. Prescribed antidepressants resulted in improved in his mood. Although he has been unable to return to his labor job, he is receiving job retraining through a local vocational retraining program.

Element 4: Access to the Full Range of Disciplines and Therapies

Several barriers can arise in the long-term management of the patient with cGVHD that may limit access to the full range of disciplines and therapies. These barriers include (1) geographic barriers encountered when care for a complex disease entity must be delivered by multiple providers in many different sites, (2) limited access to clinical trials, and (3) barriers created by lack of insurance coverage and by a system of reimbursement that does not align incentives for all involved.

The fact that cGVHD often occurs once the patient has returned to their home community can present geographic barriers to accessing health care professionals with expertise and interest in cGVHD. Though much of the care required by survivors with cGVHD can be effectively delivered by clinicians who are generalists, effective management of cGVHD requires periodic access to providers with specific expertise in the manifestations of cGVHD. Such access is particularly essential for patients with a new diagnosis of cGVHD, those with refractory manifestations, those patients with serious adverse effects of treatment (e.g., life-threatening infection, severe myodystrophy), and for those who demonstrate high-risk features and poor prognostic signs.

Patients with cGVHD also encounter barriers to clinical trial participation and these barriers not only affect the quality of care they receive, but also contribute to inertia in the development of new therapeutic options. Barriers to participation in clinical trials arise due to lack of knowledge about available trials, difficulty in traveling to study sites, and a lack of third-party payment for trial-associated care. Though some states require third-party payers to reimburse for care provided in a clinical trial, these state mandates are not universal, and the language of some of the legislation specifies payment for the costs associated with the treatment of cancer, not necessarily the treatment of late effects such as cGVHD. Patients who elect to participate in trials may incur out-of-pocket expenses for travel and accommodation. For patients with cGVHD who may not have been able to work for several months due to the transplant and acute posttransplant recovery, funds may be unavailable to cover such out-of-pocket expenses.

Survivors of allogeneic HSCT experiencing cGVHD may have lost insurance coverage due to unemployment or may have reached lifetime reimbursement caps that further erode coverage for necessary services. Particular reimbursement challenges include (1) coverage for preventive rehabilitation services to limit the development of functional decline and for frequent dental visits, (2) timely authorizations for referral to specialty consultants, and (3) payment for care by providers with cGVHD-specific expertise (including providers with expertise in the delivery of extracorporeal photopheresis) but who are "out of network."

CASE STUDY 34.4: FULL ACCESS TO RANGE OF DISCIPLINES AND THERAPIES

TC is a 35 year old mother of five, who underwent a matched unrelated transplant 15 months ago. She lives two hours from her transplant center. She has chronic lichenoid GVHD that evolved into sclerotic manifestations with extensive skin scarring and decreased range of motion. Her history is also significant for fungal pneumonia and she is being treated with voriconazole. The patient was eligible for a clinical trial at the transplant center. However in order to enroll, she would need to return to the transplant center twice a week for 6 months. Although the social worker identified some resources, with five children and limited funds she decided to be treated locally. Close follow-up between community providers and the transplant center was maintained. Unfortunately, the patient's prescription coverage reached the annual maximum and she had to pay all subsequent prescription costs out-of-pocket. Two months later she was admitted with acute respiratory failure and progressive fungal pneumonia. At the time of admission, she reported that she had discontinued voriconazole one month earlier because of its expense. This case demonstrates how geographic barriers, limited access to clinical trials, and limitations with insurance coverage present significant challenges for patients and their clinicians and how those challenges may contribute to adverse clinical outcomes.

Element 5: Standards of Care and Evidence-Based Guidelines

Standards of care, standardized screening and assessment instruments, and evidence-based guidelines contribute to effective interdisciplinary care by reducing practice variation and promoting a consistent level of service delivery [4]. Such standards and guidelines also enhance communication with community providers and contribute to continuity of care. Articulation of standards also contributes to identifying,

prioritizing, measuring, and analyzing indicators of service quality and clinical outcomes [36]. Unfortunately, few evidence-based guidelines or systematic reviews published are available to guide the management of allogeneic HSCT survivors with cGVHD. Individual centers and Hutchinson Cancer Research Center and organizations as the National Marrow Donor Program (NMDP) have developed expert consensus guidelines for long-term follow-up of allogeneic HSCT survivors and for the evaluation of survivors with cGVHD. Evidence-based guidelines for the care of allogeneic HSCT survivors [37], and for evidence-based supportive care of the patient with cGVHD are also beginning to be published [21]. While some existing survivorship care guidelines are relevant to allogeneic HSCT survivors with cGVHD, there is an urgent need to evaluate their applicability and to develop guidelines that address unique aspects of cGVHD survivorship care, such as management of obliterative bronchiolitis, prevention/management of osteoporosis, prophylaxis of infection, and standards for the evaluation and management of symptoms such as peripheral neuropathy, myopathy, fatigue, and mood disturbance. Patient and family education standards and informational brochures and other resources for self-care in cGVHD would also support interdisciplinary practice and contribute to improved clinical outcomes.

Confirmation of the diagnosis of cGVHD is one essential standard of care. A recent case report by Bolanos-Meade et al. underscores the importance of histological confirmation of GVHD [38]. They report the case of a 48-year-old white male who developed a generalized maculopapular pruritic rash, attributed to GVHD. He had no other manifestations of GVHD. A skin biopsy was obtained and immunosuppression was started for presumed GVHD. Ultimately, the biopsy revealed findings consistent with Grover's disease. No histopathologic changes of GVHD were observed. Immunosuppression was discontinued and the rash subsequently resolved. This case illustrates the importance of the inclusion of pathologists with expertise in, the histological diagnosis of GVHD on the interdisciplinary team. Slides, and tissue blocks and photographs can be sent to the transplant center for review if the patient cannot return for evaluation by transplant clinicians.

Element 6: Involvement of Patient and Family

Throughout this chapter we have emphasized the importance of including the patient, family members, and informal caregivers in the management of cGVHD. Patient and caregiver education regarding the manifestations of cGVHD is crucial both to empower the patient and family for effective self-management and because many patients are cared for by clinicians who may be unfamiliar with the diverse manifestations of cGVHD. Education also provides patients and their family and friends who care for them the knowledge and skills to understand, manage, and live well with cGVHD and its symptoms and sequelae, to work effectively with their health care team, and to navigate the health care system to find the resources and supports that they need.

Skin: Red skin, red bumps on skin, increased dryness, loss of hair, decreased ability to sweat, lightening, darkening or thickening of skin, blisters or any other changes in the appearance of your skin

Mouth: Sores, white areas, thickening, sensitivity to spicy foods, toothpaste, citrus, carbonated soft drinks increased dryness

Eyes: Increased dryness or grittiness, pink eye, discharge

Gastrointestinal: Diarrhea, stomach cramping, weight loss, yellow tint in white of eyes

Muscles: Diminished movement in joints, weakness

Lungs: Shortness of breath, especially with exercise, cough

Dates: Transplant: _____
 DLI:_____ _____ _____
To reach your GVHD Nurse Practitioner: _____
please call _____
To reach the Attending Physician on Call: _____

Figure 34.1 Reportable signs and symptoms of cGVHD.

CASE STUDY 34.5: INVOLVEMENT OF PATIENT AND CAREGIVERS

EF is a 40 year old male who received a haploidentical bone marrow transplant. He developed lichenoid chronic GVHD of the skin that responded well to corticosteroids plus tacrolimus, thus immunosuppression was tapered off. Because of work obligations, he cancelled his last clinic visit, where he would have received information about various cGVHD manifestations, reportable signs and symptoms, and contact information for the cGVHD clinic (see Figure 34.1). When he returned to the GVHD clinic two years later, he was being treated with diuretics for lower extremity edema. On exam, he was found to have hide-bound sclerotic changes in the lower legs and feet, and contractures involving his wrists, shoulders and ankles, affecting activities of daily living. He had no pigmentary or body hair distribution changes, contributing to the late diagnosis of cGVHD progression. Systemic immunosuppression was added and he was referred to physical and occupational therapy.

Element 7: Coordination and Continuity of Care Between Specialty Center and Community

Moving across the illness trajectory, patients with cGVHD typically experience several transitions in care, including transitions in care settings as well as care providers. These transitions create shifts in the roles and responsibilities of care providers, patients, and their informal caregivers, and whenever such changes occur, the possibility for discontinuity exists.

Continuity of care is of paramount importance in achieving quality care for individuals with a multifaceted condition such as cGVHD. Patients with cGVHD require an extended period of contact with a specialized and complex health care system. Achieving integration across settings and among members of the interdisciplinary team, specialty consultants, and supportive services is a challenge.

Shortell offers a parsimonious definition of continuity of care as the "extent to which services are received as a coordinated uninterrupted succession of events consistent with the needs of the patient" [39]. Continuity of care involves patient, lay caregivers, and health care providers working together to provide a coordinated, comprehensive continuum that meets the needs of patients, provides for transitions between settings, results in improved clinical outcomes, and promotes a cost-effective use of health care resources. Two different dimensions of continuity should be distinguished (1) continuity of plan, that is, the means by which separate episodes of care are joined and structured, and (2) longitudinality, which is a relationship between a patient and a regular source of care that lasts over time [40, 41]. Many clinical approaches to strengthening continuity of care, such as primary provider and case management models, emphasize longitudinality. Discharge planning models, interdisciplinary planning teams, formalized communication and referral mechanisms between providers, integrated documentation tools, and case management plans across settings are examples of models that emphasize continuity of plan.

Barriers to continuity of care include a sense of threat regarding the involvement of health care providers outside one's own institution, together with interagency and interprofessional competition and territoriality. Lack of knowledge regarding the services of other disciplines and resources is compounded when there is a hesitancy or resistance to collaborate. Suboptimal communication between providers and health care settings is magnified by the fact that health records are not easily shared among agencies and providers. Reimbursement issues also affect the range, intensity, duration, and location of services that are available to a patient, at the expense of both quality and continuity of care [42].

Continuity of care aims to achieve and maintain the maximum level of patient multidimensional functioning within the limits imposed by disease, while simultaneously promoting physical and psychospiritual comfort, facilitating transitions between settings and caregivers, and optimizing the use of health care resources [43]. Seven essential elements of continuity of care are listed in Table 34.2. An interdisciplinary approach to care that acknowledges the whole person, including the family, and addresses the highly technical and often complex problems of patients with cGVHD is essential and should be accessible throughout the illness continuum. Though team composition and leadership may shift over time, mutual respect and recognition of each provider's unique contribution are fundamental characteristics of an interdisciplinary approach. Case conferences, shared documentation tools, and interdisciplinary care standards can be effective strategies to facilitate communication and collaboration. A comprehensive, systematic assessment of patient and family needs contributes to continuity of care. Once the needs for care are identified, three key questions should be posed to promote goal setting, teaching, and resource coordination (1) What activities are to be performed to maintain or enhance individual and family functioning? (2) Who will perform these activities and who is the designated alternate?

Table 34.2: Essential Elements of Continuity of Care

Interdisciplinary approach to care
Comprehensive assessment of patient and family needs and
  strengths
Patient and family education and involvement in decision making
Measurable goals and a documented plan for care
Identification and coordination of supplemental resources
Integration of care through each transition
Evaluation

Adapted with permission from: Mitchell-Beddar & Aikin
(1994). Continuity of care. *Seminars in Oncology Nursing*, 10 (4),
p. 254–263.

and (3) what health teaching, referrals, and/or equipment and supplies are required?

Since successful continuity of care requires active participation of patients and families, another required element of continuity of care is patient and family education and involvement in decision making. The identification of measurable goals, development of the plan together with the patient and family, and coordination of supplemental resources (such as home nursing care, laboratory services, medications, rehabilitation, and respite care) are also essential.

Lastly, care must be integrated through each transition in care settings or care providers. An area that can cause particular difficulties for the patient with cGVHD and their caregivers is the transfer of specific medical procedures and technology into the community [44, 45]. It is essential to determine whether the community setting has the necessary educational, procedural, financial, and material supports to effectively transfer the technology into the community. Careful exploration of these issues, together with referral to agencies well in advance of the transition of care, provision of copies of clinic procedures and protocols, and/or an opportunity to observe the care procedure, are essential to assure a smooth transition in care.

Health care team interventions to promote continuity of care also include efforts to help the patient and family verbalize feelings of fear, vulnerability, and helplessness, build trust and confidence in new caregiving personnel, and develop realistic problem solving and contingency planning. Outcome indicators of continuity of care include optimal patient functioning (including physical, psychological, and social function), patient comfort, and patient and family satisfaction [46].

CASE STUDY 34.6: INTERDISCIPLINARY INTEGRATION AND CONTINUITY OF CARE

BF is a 22 year old young man who received a matched unrelated bone marrow transplant. Two months after the transplant he was tapering his immunosuppressive medications and had no evidence of active GVHD but was still on substantial doses of corticosteroids. Prior to discharge to his local oncologist he and his mother attended a discharge class that reviewed important signs and symptoms to report to the transplant team.

His physician received a packet of information that included medical records, written information regarding chronic GVHD, infections and other long-term effects of transplant as well as contact information for the transplant center. Less than a week after discharge he was admitted to a local hospital with fever, diarrhea and elevated liver function tests. Diagnostic imaging showed multiple nodules in his brain and lungs, suspicious for fungal infection. Voriconazole was added. When the local oncologist contacted the transplant center, he noted that the patient's clinical status had improved on voriconazole but he was reluctant to taper steroids because of on-going active GVHD. When the patient was seen in the GVHD clinic after discharge from the hospital, it was concluded that the patient's GVHD was quiescent, thus, a rapid taper of the steroids was initiated. Follow up appointments with the local oncologist as well as the transplant attending were made.

CONCLUSIONS AND DIRECTIONS FOR FUTURE RESEARCH

Several future directions in basic and for translational research, education, and health policy are suggested by this review of interdisciplinary care of the patient with cGVHD. Although interdisciplinary management has been shown to improve outcomes in selected clinical situations, there is an urgent need for demonstration projects testing innovative strategies for the delivery of interdisciplinary care to HSCT survivors with cGVHD. Telehealth methods have shown preliminary evidence that they are feasible, and that they improve clinical and fiscal outcomes as well as patient satisfaction [25]. Such methods and other innovations to improve the interdisciplinary care of cGVHD patients deserve development and evaluation. There is also an immediate need for evidence-based guidelines to direct the diagnosis and management of patients with cGVHD. The recent consensus development process to develop and disseminate guidelines for diagnosis and staging [47] and for evaluation of therapeutic response [48] could be applied to the development of additional evidence-based guidelines addressing specific symptoms and syndromes in cGVHD.

Health care professional education should continue to strengthen the value of collaboration, enhance communication skills, and expand awareness of the importance of involving community providers in the delivery of specialty care. Patients and families also need information to understand the importance of keeping lines of communication open between their community providers and the transplant center by continuing to visit their community providers for regular evaluations. Efforts to build community capacity and expertise in the management of cGVHD are essential. cGVHD is a persistent and pervasive late complication that occurs in up to 80% [49] of allogeneic HSCT survivors. Access to information and consultative support from the specialty center helps community providers fulfill their important role in care delivery. Lastly, a variety of health policy reforms are required to address the needs of HSCT survivors with cGVHD to receive adequate coverage for needed interdisciplinary services, and to fund programs and strategies that address access barriers created by geographic distance and to improve access to clinical trials.

REFERENCES

1. Gittell JH, Fairfield KM, Bierbaum B, et al. Impact of relational coordination on quality of care, postoperative pain and functioning, and length of stay: a nine-hospital study of surgical patients. *Med Care.* 2002;38:807–819.

2. Unutzer J, Katon W, Callahan CM, et al. Collaborative care management of late-life depression in the primary care setting: a randomized controlled trial. *JAMA.* 2002;288:2836–2845.

3. Shlomchik WD, Lee SJ, Couriel D, et al. Transplantation's greatest challenges: advances in chronic graft-versus-host disease. *Biol Blood Marrow Transplant.* 2007;13:2–10.

4. Drinka TJK, Clark PG. *Health care teamwork: Interdisciplinary practice and teaching.* Westport, Auburn House, 2000.

5. Orchard CA, Curran V, Kabene S. Creating a culture for interdisciplinary collaborative professional practice. *Med Educ Online.* 2005;10:1–13.

6. McCallin A. Interdisciplinary practice–a matter of teamwork: an integrated literature review. *J Clin Nurs.* 2001;10:419–428.

7. Sorrells-Jones J. The challenge of making it real: interdisciplinary practice in a "seamless" organization. *Nurs Adm Q.* 1997; 21:20–30.

8. San Martin-Rodriguez L, Beaulieu MD, D'Amour D, et al. The determinants of successful collaboration: a review of theoretical and empirical studies. *J Interprof Care.* 2005; (Suppl 19)1:132–147.

9. Henneman EA, Lee JL, Cohen JI. Collaboration: a concept analysis. *J Adv Nurs.* 1995;21:103–109.

10. D'Amour D, Ferrada-Videla M, San Martin Rodriguez L, et al. The conceptual basis for interprofessional collaboration: core concepts and theoretical frameworks. *J Interprof Care.* 2005;(Suppl 19)1:116–131.

11. Stichler JF. Professional interdependence: the art of collaboration. *Adv Pract Nurs Q.* 1995;1:53–61.

12. Baggs JG, Schmitt MH. Nurses' and resident physicians' perceptions of the process of collaboration in an MICU. *Res Nurs Health.* 1997;20:71–80.

13. Lindeke LL, Block DE. Maintaining professional integrity in the midst of interdisciplinary collaboration. *Nurs Outlook.* 1998;46:213–218.

14. Cabello CC. A collaborative approach to integrating outpatient and inpatient transplantation services. *Outcomes Manag.* 2002;6:67–72.

15. Hanson CM, Spross JA. Collaboration. In: Hamric A, Spross J, Hanson C, eds. *Advanced nursing practice: An integrative approach.* Philadelphia, W.B. Saunders, 1998:229–248.

16. Warren ML, Houston S, Luquire R. Collaborative practice teams: from multidisciplinary to interdisciplinary. *Outcomes Manag Nurs Pract.* 1998;2:95–98.

17. Carlson CA, Hobbie WL, Brogna M, et al. A multidisciplinary model of care for childhood cancer survivors with complex medical needs. *J Pediatr Oncol Nurs.* 2008;25:7–13.

18. Bodenheimer T, Wagner EH, Grumbach K. Improving primary care for patients with chronic illness. *JAMA.* 2002;288: 1775–1779.

19. Pickard AS, Hung SY, McKoy JM, et al. Opportunities for disease state management in prostate cancer. *Dis Manag.* 2005;8:235–244.

20. Linden A, Butterworth SW, Roberts N. Disease management interventions II: what else is in the black box? *Dis Manag.* 2006;9:73–85.

21. Couriel D, Carpenter PA, Cutler C, et al. Ancillary therapy and supportive care of chronic graft-versus-host disease: national institutes of health consensus development project on criteria for clinical trials in chronic graft-versus-host disease: V. Ancillary therapy and supportive care working group report. *Biol Blood Marrow Transplant.* 2006;12:375–396.

22. Friedman DL, Freyer DR, Levitt GA. Models of care for survivors of childhood cancer. *Pediatr Blood Cancer.* 2006;46:159–168.

23. Eiser C, Absolom K, Greenfield D, et al. Follow-up after childhood cancer: evaluation of a three-level model. *Eur J Cancer.* 2006;42:3186–3190.

24. Wallace W, Blacklay A, Eiser C, et al. Developing strategies for long-term follow up of survivors of childhood cancer. *BMJ.* 2001;323:271–274.

25. Wright J, Purdy B, McGonigle S. E-Clinic: an innovative approach to complex symptom management for allogenic blood and stem cell transplant patients. *Canadian Oncology Nurs J.* 2007;17:187–192.

26. Bensink M, Wootton R, Irving H, et al. Investigating the cost-effectiveness of videotelephone based support for newly diagnosed paediatric oncology patients and their families: design of a randomised controlled trial. *BMC Health Serv Res.* 2007;7:38.

27. Guihot A, Becquemin MH, Couderc LJ, et al. Telemetric monitoring of pulmonary function after allogeneic hematopoietic stem cell transplantation. *Transplantation.* 2007;83:554–560.

28. O'Neil E, Krauel P. Building transformational partnerships in nursing. *J Prof Nurs.* 2004;20:295–299.

29. Plowfield LA, Wheeler EC, Raymond JE. Time, tact, talent, and trust: essential ingredients of effective academic-community partnerships. *Nurs Educ Perspect.* 2005;26:217–220.

30. Reina ML, Reina DS, Rushton CH. Trust: The foundation for team collaboration and healthy work environments. *AACN Adv Crit Care.* 2007;18:103–108.

31. Baggs JG. Development of an instrument to measure collaboration and satisfaction about care decisions. *J Adv Nurs.* 1994;20:176–182.

32. King KB, Parinello KA, Baggs JG. Collaboration and advanced practice nursing. In Hickey JV, Ouimette RM, Venegoni SL, eds. *Advanced practice nursing: Changing roles and clinical applications.* Philadelphia, Lippincott, 1995:146–162.

33. Reina ML, Reina DS, Rushton CH. Trust: the foundation for team collaboration and healthy work environments. *AACN Adv Crit Care.* 2007;18:103–108.

34. King KB, Baggs JG. Collaboration. The essence of the acute care nurse practitioner practice. In: Kleinpell RM, Piano MR, eds. *Practice issues for the acute care nurse practitioner.* New York, Springer Publishing Company, 1998:67–78

35. Zwarenstein M, Bryant W. Interventions to promote collaboration between nurses and doctors., Cochrane Database of Systematic Reviews, 2000.

36. LeMaistre CF, Loberiza FR, Jr. What is quality in a transplant program? *Biol Blood Marrow Transplant.* 2005;11:241–246.

37. Rizzo JD, Wingard JR, Tichelli A, et al. Recommended screening and preventive practices for long-term survivors after hematopoietic cell transplantation: joint recommendations of the European Group for Blood and Marrow Transplantation, Center for International Blood and Marrow Transplant Research, and the American Society for Blood and Marrow Transplantation (EBMT/CIBMTR/ASBMT). *Bone Marrow Transplant.* 2006;37:249–261.

38. Bolanos-Meade J, Anders V, Wisell J, et al. Grover's Disease after Bone Marrow Transplantation. *Biol Blood Marrow Transplant.* 2007;13:1116–1117.

39. Shortell SM. Continuity of medical care: conceptualization and measurement. *Med Care.* 1976;14:377–391.

40. Rogers J, Curtis P. The concept and measurement of continuity in primary care. *Am J Public Health.* 1980;70:122–127.

41. Starfield B. Continuous confusion? *Am J Public Health.* 1980;70:117–119.

42. Harris MF, Zwar NA. Care of patients with chronic disease: the challenge for general practice. *Med J Aust.* 2007;187:104–107.

43. Buckwalter K. Exploring the process of discharge planning: Application to the construct of health. In: McLelland E, Kelly K, Buckwalter K, eds. *Continuity of care: Advancing the concept of discharge planning.* New York, Grune & Stratton, 1985: 5–10.

44. McMillan SC, Small BJ, Weitzner M, et al. Impact of coping skills intervention with family caregivers of hospice patients with cancer: a randomized clinical trial. *Cancer.* 2006;106: 214–222.

45. Winkler MF, Ross VM, Piamjariyakul U, et al. Technology dependence in home care: impact on patients and their family caregivers. *Nutr Clin Pract.* 2006;21:544–556.

46. McKeehan K, Coulton C. A systems approach to program development for continuity of care in hospitals. In: McLelland E, Kelly K, Buckwalter K, eds. *Continuity of care: Advancing the concept of discharge planning.* New York, Grune & Stratton, 1985:79–92.

47. Filipovich AH, Weisdorf D, Pavletic S, et al. National Institutes of Health consensus development project on criteria for clinical trials in chronic graft-versus-host disease: I. Diagnosis and staging working group report. *Biol Blood Marrow Transplant.* 2005;11:945–956.

48. Pavletic SZ, Martin P, Lee SJ, et al. Measuring therapeutic response in chronic graft-versus-host disease: National Institutes of Health consensus Development Project on Criteria for Clinical Trials in Chronic Graft-versus-Host Disease: IV. Response Criteria Working Group report. *Biol Blood Marrow Transplant.* 2006;12:252–266.

49. Flowers ME, Parker PM, Johnson LJ, et al. Comparison of chronic graft versus host disease after transplantation of peripheral blood stem cells versus bone marrow in allogeneic recipients: long-term follow-up of a randomized trial. *Blood.* 2002;100:415–419.

35

PATIENT ADVOCACY, EDUCATION AND PSYCHOSOCIAL SUPPORT

Kathleen M. Castro, Susan Stewart, Myra J. Jacobs, and Paula Kim

Many patients consider chronic graft versus host disease (cGVHD) to be worse than the disease for which they receive the transplant. Patients suffering from cGVHD and their caregivers need information and support services that target their specific needs. This is particularly important for patients who may feel isolated in a community that has little experience with cGHVD and for those who live far from their transplant center. Educating patients about services available from the transplant center itself, as well as resources available in the community, can help the patient and their family cope with this trying disease.

The Story of E.F.

I handle the shock of my diagnosis – chronic lymphocytic leukemia (CLL) – during a routine annual physical. I am told not to worry, many people live forty years with this disease. I decide to believe in that prophecy whole heartedly and go on with my life. I am the senior executive of a major worldwide health care research and development company. I travel around the world. I am an in charge, high energy person with two young children and a busy husband and a nanny holding the reigns on the household. Nothing can hold me back. I tell no one of my diagnosis, a career killer for sure.

Four years postdiagnosis, the fatigue and sinus infections become more and more debilitating, and I find myself with my head on my desk wondering why I cannot get through the day. I opt for a chemotherapeutic regimen that is producing great results in patients with CLL. After a full month of treatment, experiencing every major side effect possible, it doesn't work. My once indolent cancer has reared itself into an aggressive defiant cancer. My physician says the only chance left for me is a stem cell transplant.

I read everything I can on the subject and muster up my can do attitude as I await a donor match. I write my goodbye letters to each of my sons, now ages 11 and 14, and save them on my computer, just in case I fail this too. My support system is in full swing, but my husband is let go from his job two days before I enter the hospital. He has missed too many days of work.

The transplant appears to be a success. I am told that things are going so well I will be back on my feet in a year. I believe this and think about re-starting my career. Financially, we figure we can continue living our usual lifestyle for a year, until I am ready to

work again. My husband is still in a daze and trying to figure out what to do. How can he commit to a new job when his wife is having a HSCT? Can't be done.

I get aGVHD, skin rash over 100% of my body, welts, pustules, itching and burning beyond belief. I am exhausted and mortified by the way I look. We try several skin creams and add anti-itch drugs and steroids to my growing regimen of immunosuppressant and prophylactic antibiotics and antivirals. The aGVHD finally comes under control. It becomes a full time job just managing my drug regimens. I create an excel spreadsheet just to keep track of the doses and side effects.

At 120 days post-transplant, my CLL is less than 1% in my marrow. Amazing! I still feel like I was rolled over by a Mack truck to get to this point. My aGVHD has moved on to cGVHD, and I am told I should be thrilled because cGVHD will knock down the CLL in my bone marrow.

So I am now two years post-transplant and find that I have a new chronic disease: chronic graft versus host disease. I am not back on my feet one year later as promised, not even close. My cGVHD flairs are debilitating. I am taking over 52 pills a day, four mouth treatments, and high dose steroids. The fatigue is unbearable at times and I find that the impact on my quality of life is terrible. Depression sets in. My wonderful support network has all gone back to their own lives by now.

I realize the hard way that the myriad of symptoms and long term complications of cGVHD are clearly in their infancy. I knew the transplant was experimental, and now I am again a pioneer, fumbling my way trying to understand and treat this complex disease. I wish I had been informed before the transplant that the recovery could be one year or it could be several years. It certainly would not have changed my decision on the transplant, but it would have dramatically changed how we handled our finances. The drug co-pays alone exceed $14,000 a year. Our house is up for sale, we cannot afford to live there any more.

So the challenge I face now is how to have some semblance of a quality life until we conquer this disease. When not raging from steroids, I try to explain to my family what is going on with me and ask for their patience and support. They are skeptical and don't really get it. I feel very isolated and alone, still limited in my excursions, no crowded places, no concerts or school functions, no airplanes or hotels, no swimming in the lake.

I'm three years post-HSCT. I have been hospitalized several times and am in pain and on morphine most of the year. I had

---

396

eight parallel ribs in my chest simultaneously fracture from the constant steroid bombardment. We have gone through the agonizingly slow process of weaning off the steroids several times. The weight gain and adipose tissue formation in the form of humps on my neck and chest, breast enlargement and girth are almost too much to bear. I still do not recognize my moon face in the mirror even though I have had it for years now. This total body deformation is just horrible to go through.

I tried a month of Rituxan as an alternative to steroids to deal with the skin problems. At the end of my fourth week infusion, I went into respiratory distress. Pulmonary function tests were down below 50% and just getting dressed was a major ordeal. I'm back on steroids. Breathing returned to normal in about a week.

My joint deterioration totally destroyed what little quality of life I have had. I have fallen over twelve times this year – one of my ankles just gives out for no apparent reason. My thumbs and wrists are so weak I cannot open the gas cap on my car or cut a tomato with a knife. I use a cane to walk.

The cGVHD has attacked every mucosal membrane in my body. I have plugs in my tear ducts and use numerous eye drops all day. My eyesight is deteriorating and I see double when my eyes are very dry. I tried the new contact lenses for cGVHD – what an amazing relief to wear them. They also cleared my vision to almost 20/20. However, my insurance will not cover the $8,000 cost. Until we sell our house, I will have to wait for relief for my eyes.

So here I am weaning off the steroids again, waiting for the next event to happen. I am still on 52 pills a day, plus the mouth treatments. In the meantime, I try to come to grips with my new normal and all the hopes and dreams I now know are unlikely to ever happen. I need a new plan. I volunteer my time when I can to help support patients and their families. People tell me I am invaluable to them. However, I am unreliable due to cGVHD flares that can last a few days to a few weeks. I accept the challenge of navigating this new maze in treating the complexities of cGVHD. Ultimately it is manageable, though not an easy path. I need continued support during the long term ups and downs of cGVHD, from both my medical team and my family. The number of specialists required for cGVHD is significant: endocrinologist, gastroenterologist, psychiatrist, pulmonologist, dermatologist, surgeons, the list goes on. It requires coordination from my doctor to find the specialist who is interested in cGVHD and will see patients on a timely basis (during the flare). This is easier said than done. There are few experienced specialists in cGVHD. I am living as strong as I can, but the road is a bumpy one.

Despite advancements in the treatment of cGVHD, many patients still face overwhelming challenges and a poorer than expected quality of life. Worel et al. [1] found 73% of patients reporting good to very good quality of life within 5 years of hematopoietic stem cell transplant (HSCT). However, patients who experienced cGVHD demonstrated significant physical, role, and social impairment. Only 60% of the cGVHD group were able to return to work. Ness et al. [2] studied childhood cancer survivors treated with HSCT and found these survivors were at increased risk for performance limitations that restricted participation in routine daily activities and interpersonal relationships. The physical performance limitations were most common in young adult HSCT survivors who had a major medical condition, cGVHD, or both.

Isolation, mood swings due to medications to control the disease, uncertainty about the course of the disease, and physical changes associated with cGVHD challenge patients and caregivers alike. Few people have heard of cGVHD and, thus, have little appreciation for the struggle those with the diagnosis face. Not only do patients feel isolated emotionally, but they may find that the local health care teams caring for them post-transplant have little experience in handling this disease.

"The treatment for cGVHD made me so sick, it was worse than the transplant. Only now, I had to work on top of it. I thought it would never get better and that I had traded one disease for another. Friends, family and co-workers had never heard of cGVHD. No one understood."

THE IMPACT OF cGVHD

Patients and their loved ones facing a life-threatening disease and the prospect of an allogeneic HSCT approach the treatment with both fear and confusion. The acute needs associated with a HSCT – finding a suitable donor, surviving the treatment, and getting the disease into remission dominate most patients' attention. Though physicians discuss long-term complications such as cGHVD with patients pretransplant, few patients appreciate the life-altering consequences this disease can cause because their immediate focus is on getting through the transplant itself.

When cGVHD persists for several months or years, the impact on both the patient's physical and emotional well-being is significant. Coping with a long-term disease that has no clear course or promise of resolution can strain relationships, finances, and emotional health [3].

The Blood & Marrow Transplant Information Network (BMT InfoNet), an information and peer support network for families facing the prospect of a HSCT [4], invited subscribers to Blood & Marrow Transplant Newsletter [5] and those visiting BMT InfoNet's web site to take a survey in 2007. The 252 survey respondents, 77% of whom had active cGHVD at the time they responded, describe the impact cGVHD has on a patient and support network.

When asked whether cGVHD had interfered with the patient's ability to resume normal activities after transplant, 73% responded "yes." Fatigue was frequently cited as the limiting factor. Other factors that frequently interfere with the resumption of normal activities cited by survivors include ongoing diarrhea, suppressed immune system, shortness of breath, muscle loss, difficulty with dry eyes, and the need to limit exposure to the sun.

The lifestyle changes brought on by cGVHD are not limited to the patient. More than half of those responding to the survey said that cGVHD has interfered with the ability of the patient's family members to engage in normal activities. Many cited inability to enjoy family activities in the sun, lack of sexual desire, shifting family responsibilities from patient to others, and limited ability to socialize with others due to the patient's immunocompromised state as major limiting factors.

Sixty-three percent of respondents reported sadness or depression as a result of cGVHD, and 46% said that family members experienced symptoms as well. Half reported financial problems as a result of cGHVD, and one-third reported marital problems. These survey results demonstrate the continued physical and psychosocial needs of this patient population and their caregivers and offer insight into the various educational needs and supportive care measures that can be provided to this population.

Andrykowski et al. [6] found that patients post-HSCT reported poorer physical, psychological, and social functioning when compared to healthy controls. Recognition of the physical and psychosocial late effects has been accompanied by the realization that for many HSCT survivors, they no longer have their underlying disease but do not have their health restored. Interestingly, this same group of patients also reported increased psychological and interpersonal growth that continued years post-transplantation. Partners and spouses of HSCT patients report more fatigue, depression, and cognitive dysfunction post-transplantation than healthy controls [7]. Partners also report less social support, dyadic satisfaction and spiritual well-being, and more loneliness than HSCT survivors [7].

PATIENT AND RESEARCH ADVOCACY

Navigating and understanding the health care system poses challenges for healthy people. For people diagnosed with disease, the challenges are even greater. Therapies are more complex; patients are living longer with disease and have more treatment options than before. When diagnosed with a potentially life-threatening or chronically debilitating disease, a patient and his/her support network face the immediate needs of making treatment decisions, dealing with side and after affects of such treatments, and hoping the treatment is effective. It is also important for them to maintain a good quality of life. And most importantly, they hope that the disease will not recur.

Effectively dealing with and managing a patient's care along the continuum of their disease is enhanced when the patient, the physician, and the health care team establish a relationship that includes information exchange and methods to ensure that the patient understands the information and feels comfortable with the overall treatment plan. By creating this relationship and providing this information, the patient and their support network become a more informed partner in their care.

The Institute of Medicine Committee (IOM) Report on Psychosocial Services to Cancer Patients/Families in a Community Setting [8] recommends that patient education and advocacy organizations educate patients and their families to expect and request care that meets their psychosocial needs as well as their physical needs.

A critical responsibility of transplant professionals includes providing information about different types of advocacy organizations and the characteristics and benefits of each. Assisting a patient to identify and access appropriate resources empowers the patient and the support network to seek the services that meet their psychosocial, and treatment-related needs.

An advocate is one who speaks or acts on behalf of people, issues, ideas and causes. Each patient may be their own and most effective advocate, along with caregivers, family, friends, and patient advocacy organizations. Self-advocacy occurs when an individual patient or their caregivers speak up personally about their individual care [9]. Each patient should be encouraged to be active in their care, treatment, and decision making. Beyond self-advocacy, a patient advocate can be anyone acting on behalf of a patient to assist the patient to obtain and understand needed information and services, whether from health care professionals, nonprofit advocacy organizations, public or private agencies and companies, or resources such as the Internet. Research advocacy is different from patient advocacy in that it seeks to raise awareness and focus attention on research needs and issues, and it can complement patient advocacy and public policy efforts.

Nonprofit advocacy organizations provide another means of advocacy by providing general and disease-specific services and programs. Many advocacy groups and their leadership take on increasingly important public awareness and shared roles in the continuing advancement of science, influencing public policy and working to bring about change that benefits patients and their support systems.

Nonprofit advocacy organizations and their grassroot volunteers sponsor and host awareness activities and other education events that bring communities together, and spotlight their message in the public arena. These activities are ideal to enhance interactions between health professionals and advocacy groups, strengthening their relationships and improving their understanding of one another.

A nonprofit or not for profit organization (NPO) is a broad term that refers to an organization generally with a stated mission or objective to support and engage in activities of public and private interest. It is intended to function without individual shareholders or owners, but rather with stakeholders, who are generally comprised of all volunteer or volunteer and paid staff. There are numerous legal elements that determine nonprofit status and tax exempt status as designated by the U.S. Internal Revenue Service (IRS). It is advised to exercise due diligence as you determine which advocacy and NPOs you will rely on when providing NPO supplied information to patients, or supporting or affiliating with any NPO so that you have a thorough understanding of the organization. Examples of due diligence include awareness of organization mission, programs, and objectives; and a review of NPO tax returns, (the most common being the IRS Form 990) to keep abreast of an organization's financial status, type of IRS designation, sources of financial support, and allocation of funds. Internal Revenue Service 501(c) 3 is the common designation most people have heard about. However, as with any government regulations, one should understand the implications and parameters

Table 35.1: Nonprofit Advocacy Resource Organizations

BoardSource	www.boardsource.org
Charity Navigator	www.charitynavigator.org
Guidestar	www.guidestar.org
Internal Revenue Service Charities and Non Profits section	http://www.irs.gov/charities/index.html
Wikipedia page for NonProfit	http://en.wikipedia.org/wiki/Non_profit

of other public and private designations when working with NPOs. Resources to understand more about NPOs and how they operate can be found in Table 35.1.

Research advocates can help facilitate cross-community relationships and interactions to accelerate scientific progress of any organization involved in biomedical research, all of which ultimately benefits the patient community. Research and public policy advocacy efforts were extremely effective in advancing research in a number of diseases such as Acquired Immune Deficiency Syndrome (AIDS) and breast cancer in the 1970s and 1980s, and prostate and pancreatic cancer during the 1990s, 2000, and beyond. The HIV/AIDS advocacy organizations were successful in advocating for an expedited drug approval process via the U.S. Food and Drug Administration. These advocacy efforts have also benefited cancer and HSCT patients [10]. The cGVHD community historically lacks a strong unified nonprofit presence in public policy and research focused advocacy as most of the community's attention has been devoted to patient focused services and programs. Even when combined with other forms of GVHD, such as acute GVHD, the patient population numbers remain relatively small, making it difficult when trying to mobilize grassroots and others for action-driven public policy and research advocacy. The physical ways with which cGVHD manifests may also impact mobilization, as the patient population is not limited to one area of medicine and practice.

There are a limited number of patient advocacy and nonprofit resources with a strong interest or focus on cGVHD. Transplant professionals are encouraged to collaborate with qualified advocates and organizations while working to assist medical professionals with information development and dissemination inside and outside of the cGVHD community [11]. Constant vigilance on the part of advocacy organizations, transplant professionals, and cGVHD patients will assure the strides made today are not forgotten tomorrow [10].

Advocacy may be accomplished in a variety of ways, through patient and caregiver education, professional education, community awareness, research advocacy, and public policy. Advocating for patients and family members, assisting them in finding a support network that can help identify emerging therapies and providing them with professional counseling and peer support will aid them to better cope with this challenging disease.

EDUCATION

Because the morbidity and mortality associated with HSCT has decreased, we now have more people living with chronic illness post-transplantation such as cGVHD. It is now generally accepted that patients should be fully informed about health-related matters and should be involved in and accepting responsibility for their health care [12]. Patients have more access to information than ever before and have more responsibility in directing and managing their own health care [12, 13]. The goal of patient education is to support autonomous patient decision making while developing patient competence, confidence, and self-trust in their ability to carry out health behaviors consistent with their medical and psychosocial needs [14]. cGVHD varies widely in its presentation, treatment regimens, and response. Because of this variability, patient-centered treatment plans are an effective method of meeting the outcomes set by both the patient and health care team. These teams should empower patients and their caregivers to advocate for themselves by becoming educated regarding cGVHD and understanding the resources available for education.

Although more than half of the BMT InfoNet survey respondents felt they had sufficient information about cGHVD, 46% said they did not (personal communication, BMT InfoNet, April 2008). When presented with an array of potential options for obtaining information about cGVHD, the following were cited as the sources of information respondents would most likely utilize: (1) a cGVHD Web site, (2) print newsletter, and (3) local meetings with medical experts to discuss cGVHD.

However, providing education and psychosocial support to both patients and their caregivers post-HSCT is challenging. Barriers to these services may include distance from transplant experts, patient fatigue, resumption of normal activities and /or lack of time, financial constraints, lack of transportation, and weak social support [8].

Transplant professionals can help overcome these barriers by delivering information and emotional support to survivors diagnosed with cGVHD beyond routine office visits. Partnering with, or referring patients to, an advocacy organization can enhance patients' ability to cope with their disease. Partnerships might include co-sponsorship and implementation of support programs, such as telephone support groups, teleconferences, webcasts, or town hall meetings on cGVHD or simply a referral to an advocacy organization with print resources about cGVHD that may help patients better understand their disease and treatment options.

Although patient education material regarding cGVHD is limited compared to information for other diseases such as cancer, many excellent resources are available for patients and for advocacy organizations. The National Marrow Donor Program (NMDP) has developed long-term survivor guidelines that specifically discuss follow-up and screening for cGVHD [15]. These guidelines may be used by patients, caregivers, and health care providers. The BMT InfoNet cited above and The National Bone Marrow Transplant Link (nbmtLINK) were founded to specifically support HSCT patients and family members. These organizations provided patient and family education using a variety of methods (DVD, videos, webcasts) in addition to printed materials [16, 17]. Disease-based organizations, such as The Leukemia & Lymphoma Society also offer teleconferences or print materials of interest to patients and health care professionals dealing with cGVHD [18]. Professional societies, such as American Society for Blood and Marrow Transplantation provide information for transplant professionals that advocate for standardized approaches to caring for cGVHD patients through the use of consensus guidelines [19].

Health care providers may find that patients and their caregivers prefer print material provided to them by these organizations as opposed to finding resources on their own [20]. Table 35.2 provides a number of advocacy and professional organizations that assist patient and caregivers with cGVHD and also provide avenues for health care provider education and public policy. While these organizations are not a substitute for medical advice and care provided by health care professionals, they can assist in the education of patients about the disease, and provide sorely needed psychosocial support in the form of support groups, webcasts, symposia, and written educational materials.

The context in which patients consume health information has changed dramatically with the advent of the Internet, advances in telemedicine, and changes in media health coverage and advertising. In 2005, a Harris poll found 71% of people use the Internet for health-related information [21]. Approximately, 39% of cancer patients use the Internet directly and another 15% to 20% of cancer patients use the Internet "indirectly" through family and friends [22]. This has a large impact on the knowledge of patients, how they interact with their health care team, and how these interactions may change the patient–physician relationship. Patients and family members use the Internet for information because of its convenience, accessibility, anonymity, potential for interactivity, social support, and ability to tailor information to a person's own needs [23, 24]. People who use the Internet for health and cancer information are more likely to be female, under the age of 65, have an income over $50,000, have some college education, and have a current or prior diagnosis or family member with a diagnosis of cancer [25, 26]. Rutten et al. [24] also found Hispanics were less likely than other racial groups to use the Internet for cancer information. This may be related to a host of factors including income status previously mentioned, reading levels of cancer web sites and lack of information available in Spanish.

Hesse et al. [27] provided nationally representative estimates of health-related use of the Internet, level of trust in information sources, and preferences for cancer information sources. They found the majority of patients seeking cancer information preferred to go to their physicians first, with the Internet being the second most dominant source of information. Consistent with other cited literature, patients older than 65 were 10 times more likely to go to health care providers than the Internet, whereas patients under the under the age of 65

were equally split between using health care providers or the Internet as sources of cancer information. Respondents had the highest level of trust in cancer information received from physicians while Internet information trust was divided, one-fourth expressing a lot of trust and one-fourth expressing no trust in this information source. Younger age and female sex respondents had more trust in Internet information.

As more patients and their support networks turn to the Internet for information, it is important for health professionals to be educated on how to evaluate Internet sites. Eysenbach et al. (2003) performed a systematic review of health information available on the World Wide Web and found a need for operational definitions of quality criteria. Information may be extremely varied and overwhelming. The Health on the Net (HON)[28] Foundation was formed in 1995 to guide consumers and care providers in finding accurate and reliable information on the Internet. The HON has a code of conduct that outlines what one should look for when evaluating health information on an Internet site [13, 28]. The National Cancer Institute also offers guidelines for consumers and health care providers to use when determining whether health information on an Internet site is reliable [29]. Table 35.3 provides a summary of what to look for in a site using the criteria from both of these organizations. Transplant team members and health care professionals working with cGVHD patients may use the Internet frequently to gain information for themselves. Providers should be aware of how to critique this information and evaluate how it pertains to their population. Helft et al. [30] surveyed American Society of Clinical Oncology (ASCO) members and found that while the majority of oncologists used the Internet on almost a daily basis, they felt that it had both positive and negative effects on their patients. Fifty-seven percent of those surveyed felt the Internet made their patients more hopeful, but in general they felt additional Internet information increased patients' level of confusion and anxiety. To advocate for patients, nurses and physicians must allow additional time to be spent talking with patients regarding the information they obtain from the Internet and educating them on how this information applies to their particular disease.

At the present time, legislation is being written to reimburse health professionals for patient education [31]. Because the amount of education for cGHVD patients is so extensive during the majority of visits to a medical facility, it is imperative for health care professionals to record the time required to educate patients and confirm their understanding of the information. All care providers, including physicians and nurses, should be reimbursed for this important education time.

As stated earlier, cGVHD patients often have returned home and are only seen at a transplant center every few months or annually. Dealing with a chronic illness can lead to isolation and fear because patients and caregivers do not have the transplant community to fall back on when needing assessment, treatment, education, and psychosocial support. Web-based health information systems and patient portals are an effective method of communicating with patients and may lessen the isolation and fear for this population. Medical centers may

Table 35.2: Advocacy Organizations

HSCT and GVHD Advocacy Organizations

This list includes selected advocacy organizations that contain cGVHD-related information for patients and caregivers. They offer print materials, audio-visual media, patient education programs, professional education programs, webcasts, and telephone support programs

Association of Cancer Online Resource (www.acor.org)

BMT InfoNet (www.bmtinfonet.org)

BMT-Support (www.BMTSupport.org)

Leukemia and Lymphoma Society (www.leukemia-lymphoma.org)

Lymphomation (www.lymphomation.org)

National Bone Marrow Transplant Link (www.nbmtlink.org)

National Children's Cancer Society (www.children-cancer.com)

National Marrow Donor Program (www.marrow.org)

Young Adult and Adolescent Issues

This list provides resources for young adults and adolescents surviving cancer and living with the effects of cancer therapy. They do not address cGVHD specifically, but offer resources for young adults.

I'm Too Young For This (www.imtooyoungforthis.org)

Candlelighters (www.candlelighters.org)

Lance Armstrong Foundation (www.livestrong.org)

Planet Cancer (www.planetcancer.org)

The Sam Fund (www.thesamfund.org)

Ulman Cancer Fund for Young Adults (www.ulmanfund.org)

Professional Organizations

This list includes professional organizations that represent oncology/hematology professionals. These organizations have patient education materials, professional education materials, and conferences along with health policy and advocacy arms.

American Society for Blood and Marrow Transplant (www.asbmt.org)

American Society of Clinical Oncology (www.cancer.net)

American Society of Hematology (www.hematology.org)

Center for International Blood and Marrow Transplant Research (www.cibmtr.org)

Cure Search Children's Oncology Group (www.childrensoncologygroup.org/disc/LE/default/htm)

Oncology Nursing Society (www.ons.org)

Research Support Organizations

These organizations provide research funding and support for clinical trials related to HSCT and cGVHD.

Center for International Blood & Marrow Transplant Research (www.cibmtr.org)

Leukemia and Lymphoma Society (www.leukemia-lymphoma.org)

Oncology Nursing Foundation (www.onf.org)

National Cancer Institute (www.cancer.gov)

National Marrow Donor Program (www.marrow.org)

Patient and Research Advocacy

These organizations advocate for patients, families, and survivors. They also advocate for clinical trials and continued support for research grants and support.

American Society of Clinical Oncology (www.cancer.net)

Aplastic Anemia and MDS International Foundation, Inc. (www.aamds.org)

BMT InfoNet (www.bmtinfonet.org)

Lymphoma Research Foundation (www.lymphoma.org)

Cancer Care for Young Adults (www.cancercare.org/get_help/special_progs/young_adult.php)

Lance Armstrong Foundation (www.livestrong.org)

Leukemia and Lymphoma Society (www.leukemia-lymphoma.org)

National Bone Marrow Transplant Link (www.nbmtlink.org)

National Cancer Institute (www.cancer.gov)

National Marrow Donor Program (www.marrow.org)

Oncology Nursing Society (www.ons.org)

---

use patient portals to conduct e-mail communication with patients, review medications and provide web-based educational information [32] These portals may also allow patients access to support programs offered by the transplant center and facilitated by an experienced transplant professional. Virtual communities can now be established to provide such a service to post-transplant patients. Bringing patients together via electronic media may increase ones awareness of what others are facing and help to bring a mix of people together to advocate for one cause.

Table 35.3: Criteria for Evaluating Medical and Health-Related Online Resources

---

1. Authoritative
   - Authors are listed
   - Credentials for authors, educational background and contact information, are listed

2. Complementarity
   - Information should support, not replace, the doctor–patient relationship

3. Privacy and security
   - What information is collected about users and why?
   - How is privacy and confidentiality of personal information of site visitors respected

4. Information sources
   - References for information
   - Links to additional information sources
   - Date when the page was last modified clearly displayed
   - Citations for journal articles or sources of evidence

5. Sponsor
   - Site has information regarding the organization and its purpose
   - Web addresses ending in "gov" are government-sponsored sites
   - Web addresses ending in "edu" are educational institutions
   - Web addresses ending in "org" are often used by noncommercial or voluntary organizations
   - Web addresses ending in "com" denote commercial organizations

6. Funding source(s)
   - Identify funding sources

7. Advertising policy
   - Distinguish advertising from editorial content

Sources: www.hon.ch/HONcode/Conduct.html; http://understandingrisk.cancer.gov/media/internet/cfm; Anderson, A. and Klemm, P. 2008.

Advocacy organizations use public meetings to educate patients, caregivers, and healthcare professionals. These organizations may partner with a medical center, professional organization, industry sponsor, or another nonprofit organization to offer a public meeting for a particular target audience. Patients and members of their support networks have the opportunity to talk with health professionals, become educated on new treatment options, and/or clinical trials while having questions answered. They also can meet others who understand what it means to live with a chronic illness and share methods of coping [33].

PEER SUPPORT

Many patients with cancer or another chronic illness benefit from peer support. These groups use a variety of formats (peer support, psychoeducational, and informational), but the underlying purpose is to offer emotional and social support to patients and their caregivers while serving as a form of advocacy. Gottlieb and Wachala [34] performed a review of professionally facilitated cancer support groups and found that participants reported high satisfaction and felt less alone, better understood their disease, and were more hopeful following their group experience. Peer support programs have been found to improve satisfaction with medical care, personal relationships, and social support [35]. While this substantiates the importance of support groups, many cGVHD patients do

not feel that general cancer support groups meet their needs. Hence, the importance of offering support networks specifically for HSCT survivors living with cGVHD.

Face-to-face support groups are offered at some academic centers and in communities with transplant advocacy organizations. Participants report feeling happier and more relaxed, receiving practical and emotional support, and experiencing a sense of comfort and comradery [33]. Disadvantages of face-to-face groups are that they are only available for those who have access to the group; participation may be limited for those living distances away, and/or with limited financial support or transportation.

Technology allows patients to access web-based support groups. Patients participate in these groups from the comfort of their own home without worrying about transportation, risking infection by going out in public, or using extra energy when fatigue is a problem. Internet groups offer greater flexibility, allowing patients to access them at any time of day or night when they are feeling in need of support [36]. Computer-mediated support has been found to be an effective means to reach populations that are dispersed and have restrictions on their time [37].

Meier et al. [38] reported a desire for information, rather than emotional support, as the primary reason patients participate in online support groups. After sampling 10 different online cancer groups for 5 months, the most common expressions of support were offers of technical information and explicit advice about how to communicate with health care providers. This qualitative study found that patients can and do find what they seek, while also finding opportunities to play rewarding roles as support givers. Three well-established Internet support groups are available to patients with cGVHD. Two are electronic mailing lists (list-servs), where patients may send and respond to e-mails from a large group of participants. The third is an online chat room that meets at a specified time each week.

BMT-Talk is a list-serv hosted by the Association of Cancer Online Resources (www.acor.org) [39] More than 1,400 people currently subscribe to the list, including newly diagnosed patients, long-term survivors and their caregivers. cGVHD is a frequent thread of discussion on this list-serv. Survivors share experiences about various treatments, exchange information about experiences with physicians who treat the disease, and provide emotional support to one another.

A second list-serv called GVHD is also hosted on www.acor.org. This electronic mailing list focuses specifically on GHVD and its treatment. Three hundred and sixty people subscribed to the list. Participants have had experience with a wide range of treatment options and are generally very well informed. BMT-Support.org [40] is an online chat room that addresses a range of HSCT issues including cGVHD, both from the patient and caregiver perspective.

Concerns regarding the accuracy of online information and ideas exchanged are valid. However, since patients are instructed to review with their physicians the therapies discussed online before initiating the treatment, the information obtained from online support forums serve largely as a catalyst for discussion, not as a replacement for physician recommended treatment.

Telephone support groups offer many of the benefits of web-based groups along with increased flexibility. Participants need only have access to a phone, without concerns of online access. Since cGVHD may affect patient's eyes and their ability to read along with peripheral neuropathy affecting their ability to type, telephone support groups may be a good option for many cGVHD patients. Hoey et al. (2008) performed a systematic review of peer support programs for people with cancer and found that telephone support group participants reported feeling less isolated, receiving empathy, empowerment, and increased assertiveness when communicating with health professionals. Disadvantages of the telephone groups included a lack of follow-up support and not being able to see other members. The National Bone Marrow Transplant Link (www.nbmtlink.org) has partnered with transplant providers at the National Institutes of Health to create a series of ongoing telephone education and support groups convened exclusively for cGVHD patients using a psychoeducational support format. Group participants cite the ability to discuss their concerns with others who truly understand the disease and symptoms, gaining new knowledge, talking with experts regarding cGVHD, and the convenience of being able to take part in the group from anywhere as benefits of the telephone group [41]. Telephone support groups can also be effective for caregivers who may be experiencing more stress than the patient and

have more responsibilities that may limit their ability to take part in a face-to-face group [42].

While some patients prefer the convenience and anonymity of the Internet and telephone support groups, others find the personal interaction with survivors at local educational/support sessions more rewarding. Many BMT-related advocacy organizations, such as the National Marrow Donor Program, BMT InfoNet, the National Bone Marrow Transplant Link, The Leukemia & Lymphoma Society, and Lymphoma Research Foundation host various educational forums throughout the United States. Workshops on cGVHD enable survivors and caregivers to better understand their diagnosis and treatment options. Patients with cGVHD and their families can interact with their peers in person, discuss their unique concerns, and learn from medical professionals. These programs also enable patients to identify cGVHD medical experts in their geographic area or at nationally recognized research facilities with whom they can consult, should the need arise. These organizations also provide webinars that may include presentations on cGVHD and are usually archived for later review by those unable to attend.

Providing information about the benefits of advocacy organizations and empowering patients and caregivers to seek out methods of meeting their psychosocial needs is a critical role of transplant professionals. Advocacy groups have a number of valuable tools available to assist patients. These include print information about cGVHD, referrals to physicians/programs that specialize in cGVHD, peer support networks, telephone support groups, webcasts, teleconferences, patient education meetings. Online list-servs and a weekly online BMT-Support chat group are also available.

Disseminating the information and support available to these patients and their families is of critical importance. Patients cannot avail themselves of these educational and support resources unless they are aware of them. Transplant centers that provide the patient and transplant professionals with information about available resources will empower patients and their caregivers to better cope with the medical and psychological stress of cGVHD and to take a constructive, active role in managing their disease and treatment.

PUBLIC POLICY

"The world of advocacy is one of diversity, unity and collaboration." [10] The concerns facing cGVHD patients and transplant survivors are complex. Advocacy and health policy are important parts of most professional organizations and patient advocacy groups. Groups with an interest in cancer must work together to resolve these complex issues. Professional organizations are in a perfect position to utilize the leadership, knowledge, expertise, and their membership to help move public policy legislation for cancer patients forward. The cGVHD population is small; however, their policy efforts can be leveraged by collaboration with other groups working on issues that affect the cGVHD patient as well, such as prescription drug benefits and reimbursement for patient education. The Oncology

Nursing Society (ONS) has allocated organizational resources in the form of budgeted staff positions, educational programs for members, use of volunteer time and skills, and production and dissemination of position statements to move public policy on issues related to cancer patients and survivors [43].

Professional organizations form key partnerships with others such as American Society of Clinical Oncology, the Association of Community Cancer Centers, the Intercultural Cancer Council, Oncology Nursing Society and the American Nurses Association [43]. These key partnerships are critical when attempting to meet define and meet advocacy goals on the national, state, and local level.

Standardized grading and treatments for cGVHD continue to be developed. The cGVHD consensus working group is an example of the benefits of bringing together the intellectual properties of transplant experts to move the field of cGVHD patient care forward [44]. Funding and support for clinical trials will allow the transplant community to answer many questions surrounding cGVHD that remain unanswered. Fewer than 50 clinical trials are currently active or recruiting cGVHD patients [45]. Advocacy groups and professional organizations can make the general public aware of the importance of clinical trials and encourage increased congressional funding for cancer research. The Oncology Nursing Foundation offers investigators funding for a variety of research trials that help professionals understand quality of life and long-term survivor issues.

As we move into the future, patients, advocacy organizations, and professional organizations need to work to develop and maintain national networks of well-informed and easily accessible advocates to carry the message. They need to negotiate funding from a variety of sources and nurture collaborative relationships in which assets, political capital, and intellectual properties are shared for the greater good [43].

cGVHD patients and their support systems encounter physical, emotional, and social obstacles. As health care professionals, we are responsible for not only educating patients and offering support groups but also for demonstrating to patients and their support networks the importance of advocating for public and research advocacy. To truly make a difference for cGVHD patients, health professionals, patients, advocacy organizations, and professional organizations must come together to raise their voice for one cause.

REFERENCES

1. Worel N, Biener D, Kalhsm P, et al. Long-term outcome and quality of life of patients who are alive and in complete remission more than two years after allogeneic stem cell transplantation. *Bone Marrow Transplant.* 2002;30:619–626.
2. Ness K, Bhatia S, Baker S, et al. Performance limitations and participation restrictions among childhood cancer survivors treated with hematopoietic stem cell transplantation. *Arch Pediatr Transplant Med.* 2005;159:706–713.
3. Williams LA. Whatever it takes: informal caregiving dynamics in blood and marrow transplantation. *Oncol Nurs Forum.* 2007;34:370–387.
4. *Blood & Marrow Transplant Information Network,* www. bmtinfonet.org. Accessed June 8, 2008.
5. *Blood & Marrow Transplant Newsletter,* www.bmtinfonet.org/newsletters/index.html. Accessed June 8, 2008.
6. Andrykowski MA, Bishop MM, Hahn EA, et al. Long-term health related quality of life, growth, and spiritual well-being after hematopoietic stem-cell transplantation. *J Clin Oncol.* 2005;23:599–608.
7. Bishop, MM, Beaumont, JL, Hahn, EA, et al. Late effects of cancer and hematopoietic stem-cell transplantation on spouses or partners compared with survivors and survivor-matched controls. *J Clin Oncol.* 2007;25;1403–1411.
8. Committee on Psychosocial Services to Canter Patients/Families in a Community Setting, Institute of Medicine. ISBN:0–309–11104–8. pp. 1–16.
9. The Advocacy Continuum: Self-advocacy and Policy Advocacy. Silver Spring, MD: National Coalition for Cancer Survivorship. Accessed March 15, 2008, at http://www.canceradvocacy.org/get-involved/educate/policy/intro.html.
10. Davenport-Ennis N, Cover M, Ades T, Stoval E. An analysis of advocacy: A collaborative essay. *Semin Oncol Nurs.* 2002;18:290–296.
11. Mayer D, Dow K. *The cancer of politics.* 1993;20(9):1305.
12. Falvo, D. Patient compliance: a brief overview. In: Falvo D, ed. Effective patient education: A guide to increased compliance. Sudbury, MA, Jones and Barlett Publishing, 2004.
13. Anderson A, Klemm P. The internet: friend or foe when providing patient education? *Clin J Oncol Nurs.* 2008;12(1):55–63.
14. Redman, B. Status of patient education. In: Redman B, ed. Advances in patient education. New York, NY, Springer Publishing, 2004.
15. National Marrow Donor Program. (2008). Long-term survival guidelines. Available at www.marrow.org/physicians. Accessed June 6, 2008.
16. BMT InfoNet (2008). Available at www.bmtinfonet.org. Accessed June 8, 2008.
17. National Bone Marrow Transplant Link (2008). Available at www.nbmtlink.org. Accessed June, 8, 2008.
18. Leukemia and Lymphoma Society (2008). Disease information, blood and marrow stem cell transplantation. Available at www.leukemia-lymphoma.org. Accessed June 8, 2008.
19. American Society for Blood and Marrow Transplantation. Chronic GVHD Consensus Project. Available at http://www.asbmt.org/policystat/policy.htm. Accessed June, 2008.
20. Basch E, Thaler H, Shi W, et al. Use of information resources by patients with cancer and their companions. *Cancer.* 2004;100(1):2476–2483.
21. Harrisinteractive.com Harris poll shows number of "cyberchondiacs–adults who have ever gone online for health information–increases to an estimated 160 million nationwide. Available at www.harrisinteractive.com/harris_poll/index.asp?PID=792. Accessed June 7, 2008.
22. Eysenbach G. The impact of the Internet on cancer outcomes. *CA Cancer J Clin,* 2003;53(6):256–371.
23. Haung G, Penson D. Internet health resources and the cancer patient. *Cancer Invest.,* 2008;26:202–207.
24. Rains, S. Perceptions of traditional information sources and use of the world wide web to seek health information: findings from the health information national trends survey. *J Health Commun.* 2007;12:667–680.

25. Rutten L, Squiers L, Hesse B. Cancer-related information seeking: hints from the 2003 health information national trends survey (HINTS), *J Health Commun.*, 2006;11:147–156.

26. Baker L, Wagner T, Singer S. Use of the internet and e-mail for health care information: Results from a national survey. *JAMA*, 2003;289:2400–2406.

27. Hesse B, Nelson D, Kreps G, et al. Trust and sources of health information. The impact of the internet and its implications for health care providers: findings from the first health information national trends survey. *Arch Intern Med*, (2005);165: 2618–2624.

28. Health on the Net Foundation. HON Code of Conduct (HONcode) for medical and health web sites. Available at http://www.hon.ch/HONcode/Conduct.html, Accessed June 7, 2008.

29. National Cancer Institute. Is Information on the Web Reliable? Available at http://understandingrisk.cancer.gov/medica/internet.cfm. Accessed June 7, 2008

30. Helft P, Hlubocky F, Daugherty C. American oncologists' views of internet use by cancer patients: a mail survey of American Society of Clinical Oncology members, *J Clin Oncol.*, 2003;21(5):942–947.

31. Oncology Nursing Society. Legislative Action Corner. www.ons.org/lac/pdf/HR5585/DC-01538525.pdf Accessed: June 27, 2008.

32. Rodriquez E, Salvaggio R, O'Sullivan M, et al Using a patient portal for electronic communication with oncology patients: implications for nurses, *Oncol Nurs Forum*, 2008;35(3):533 (Abstract).

33. Castro K, Sampl K, Grasmeder S, et al. Supporting community education: a collaborative effort between volunteer organizations to develop a hematopoietic stem cell transplant patient and caregiver educational symposium, 2007; *Oncol Nurs Forum*, 34(2):544 (Abstract)

34. Gottlieb BH, Wachala ED. Cancer support groups: a critical review of empirical studies, *Psychooncology*, 2007;16:379–400.

35. Hoey L, Ieropoli S, White V, Jefford M. Systematic review of peer-support programs for people with cancer, *Patient Educ Couns*, 2008;70:315–317.

36. Im E, Chee W, Lim H, et al. Patients' Attitudes Toward Internet Cancer Support Groups, *Oncol Nurs Forum*, (2007);34(3): 705–712.

37. Bragadòttir H. Computer-mediated support group intervention for parents, *J Nurs Sch.*, (2008);40(1):32–38.

38. Meier A, Frydman G, Forlenza M, Rimer B. How Cancer Survivors Provide Support on Cancer-Related Internet Mailing Lists. *J Med Internet Res.* 2007;9(2):e12

39. Association of Cancer Online Resources (www.acor.org)

40. BMT-Support.org. www.bmtsupport.org Accessed: June 18, 2008.

41. Castro K, Mitchell S, Heath T, Jacobs M. A chronic graft-versus-host disease (cGVHD) telephone support group: partnering with an advocacy organization to address an underserved population of cancer survivors. *Oncol Nurs Forum*, 2008;35(3):514 (Abstract).

42. Bank A, Arguelles S, Rubert M, et al The value of telephone support groups among ethnically diverse caregivers of persons with dementia, *Gerontologist*, 2006;46(1):134–138.

43. Rieger P, Moore P. Professional organizations and their role in advocacy. *Semin Oncol Nurs.* 2002;18(4):276–289.

44. Martin PJ, Weisdorf D, Przepiorka D, et al. National Institutes of Health consensus development project on criteria for clinical trials in chronic graft-versus-host disease: VI. design of clinical trials working group. *Biol Blood Marrow Transplant.*, 2006;12(5):491–505.

45. National Institutes of Health Clinical Trials.gov. Chronic graft-versus-host disease studies. Available at http://clinicaltrials.gov/ct2/results?term=chronic+graft+versus+host+disease. Accessed June 4, 2008.

36

FUTURE DIRECTIONS

Stephanie J. Lee

Dr. Ernie Beutler wrote an amusing "what if" chapter about the future of hematopoietic cell transplantation (HCT) for the Thomas textbook. I'd like to recapitulate his tone and approach here in the final chapter of the Chronic GVHD book edited by Pavletic and Vogelsang.

What if in the future, chronic graft versus host disease (GVHD) as we know it was a historical footnote in the remarkable developmental history of HCT? Starting from myeloablative procedures using bone marrow from human leukocyte antigen (HLA)-identical siblings, the majority of transplants in the future would use minimal chemotherapy or targeted immunosuppressive agents to achieve donor engraftment from a variety of sources. The donor selection process will focus on testing the malignant and healthy tissues of the patient and the immune cells of the donor to precisely identify the risks for recurrent malignancy, acute and chronic GVHD, and treatment-related complications. Each patient's risk profile would be determined prospectively and the most appropriate donor selected to optimize the chance for disease-free, cGVHD free survival.

After transplantation, patients would receive prophylaxis and preemptive treatment for GVHD based on biomarker studies suggesting impending risk, an approach currently practiced in 2008 for *Cytomegalovirus* and *Epstein Barr* virus reactivation. However, future interventions for GVHD are largely intended to protect end organs so that other treatments have time to delete the offending cells, block the causative cytokines, or remove the recipient signals inciting the immune response. End organ dysfunction, disability, and death attributable to GVHD are largely prevented. After several prominent papers note the statistically significant decrease in GVHD in recent years, the HCT community celebrates and renames the syndrome GVHR for "graft-versus-host reaction" to distinguish the new experience from the bad memories of the past.

Lacking sufficient patients, several clinical trials of secondary therapy, conceived and finally funded during a time of National Institutes of Health (NIH) reexpansion, are shuttered and resources directed to studies of relapse prevention, which remains a problem and is in fact exacerbated by faster progress

in treating GVHR than understanding the graft-versus-malignancy effects.

The NIH consensus criteria have been revisited and modified several times based on empirical data collected by many investigators energized by the original 2005 NIH conference. Much discussion occurs at these conferences about whether to hone definitions further, improving the criteria even more, or to leave well enough alone so that people don't get confused by ever changing criteria. Eventually, the practitioners triumph over the methodologists and the Consensus Criteria are renamed simply "the chronic GVHD criteria" to reflect their exhaustive validation in multiple populations. The Food and Drug Administration (FDA) adopts the criteria formally as acceptable guidance for registration trials, and just in time. Many targeted therapies are being used off-label but companies are clamoring for FDA approval since new health care regulations provide full coverage only for FDA-approved treatments.

The Pavletic and Vogelsang textbook is in its fifth edition. Although the third edition had peaked as a 2,000 page, two volume set, the fifth edition has shrunk to a small manual, largely focused on historical background, review of pathophysiology and outlines of best practices. Historical slides show patients with severe joint contractures, oral ulcers, sclerotic skin changes and wasting, and are popular background slides in "history of medicine" talks to illustrate old scourges successfully treated with modern medicine. Chronic GVHD joins the ranks of rickets, leprosy, Ebola, and AIDS.

Medical residents and fellows simply order "GVHD biomarker panels" whenever a transplant patient appears in the emergency room, much to the annoyance of older physicians who think they should examine the patient first. Teaching physicians have not gone extinct, and quiz students about elements of basic cGVHD pathophysiology and how to recognize full blown GVHR if they were to see it, which they almost never do. Trainees furtively consult their portable electronic medical resources when they can't quite recall the details of the textbook diagram outlining the biologic interactions that results in GVHR. Recertification Boards in Hematology and Oncology ask "A patient who has been lost to follow-up after an allogeneic HCT returns complaining of a skin rash and mouth ulcers.

You suspect GVHR. You prescribe…." and the *incorrect* answer is "Prednisone at a dose of 1 mg/kg/day."

I'm sure new problems will arise in HCT because its history thus far is rife with thinking that we have solved one problem only to create fertile ground for another. But it is hard to imagine a more challenging problem than cGVHD, or one whose solution would improve the lives of so many patients otherwise cured of their malignancies.

INDEX

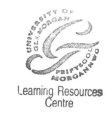

Learning Resources
Centre